FUNDAMENTALS OF
PHARMACOGNOSY
AND PHYTOTHERAPY

Commissioning Editor: Pauline Graham
Development Editor: Fiona Conn
Project Manager: Sruthi Viswam
Design Direction: Charles Gray
Illustration Manager: Merlyn Harvey

FUNDAMENTALS OF PHARMACOGNOSY AND PHYTOTHERAPY

SECOND EDITION

Michael Heinrich Dr rer nat habil MA(WSU) Dipl. Biol. FLS
*Professor and Head, Centre for Pharmacognosy and Phytotherapy, UCL School of Pharmacy,
University of London, London, UK*

Joanne Barnes BPharm PhD MRPharmS FLS
Associate Professor in Herbal Medicines, School of Pharmacy, University of Auckland, Auckland, New Zealand

Simon Gibbons BSc PhD CChem CSci FRSC FLS
*Professor of Phytochemistry, Department of Pharmaceutical and Biological Chemistry,
UCL School of Pharmacy, University of London, London, UK*

Elizabeth M. Williamson BSc(Pharm) PhD MRPharmS FLS
Professor of Pharmacy, School of Pharmacy, University of Reading, UK

Foreword

A. Douglas Kinghorn BPharm MSc PhD DSc FRPharmS FAAAS FAAPS FLS FSP
*Professor and Jack L. Beal Chair of Natural Products Chemistry and Pharmacognosy, College of Pharmacy,
The Ohio State University, Columbus, Ohio, USA*

Epilogue

J. David Phillipson DSc PhD MSc BSc(Pharm) FRPharmS FLS
*Emeritus Professor of Pharmacognosy, Centre for Pharmacognosy and Phytotherapy, School of Pharmacy,
University of London, London, UK*

Illustrations by
Debbie Maizels and Simon Gibbons

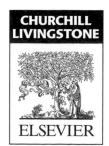

CHURCHILL LIVINGSTONE

ELSEVIER

EDINBURGH LONDON NEW YORK OXFORD PHILADELPHIA ST LOUIS SYDNEY TORONTO 2012

First edition 2004
Second edition 2012

ISBN 978-0-7020-3388-9

British Library Cataloguing in Publication Data
A catalogue record for this book is available from the British Library

Library of Congress Cataloging in Publication Data
A catalog record for this book is available from the Library of Congress

Notices

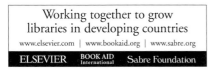

Working together to grow
libraries in developing countries

www.elsevier.com | www.bookaid.org | www.sabre.org

ELSEVIER   BOOK AID International   Sabre Foundation

your source for books, journals and multimedia in the health sciences

www.elsevierhealth.com

The Publisher's policy is to use paper manufactured from sustainable forests

Printed in China

Contents

Foreword

Worldwide, drugs derived from organisms continue to be important for the treatment and prevention of many diseases. Pharmacognosy, which is defined in this book as 'the science of biogenic or nature-derived pharmaceuticals and poisons', has been an established basic pharmaceutical science that has been taught in institutions of pharmacy education for about two centuries. This subject area has changed considerably since its initiation, having metamorphosed from a largely descriptive botanical and mycological field in the late 19th and early 20th centuries, to having more of a chemical and biological focus within the last 50 years or so. Today, pharmacognosy embraces the scientific study of compounds from plants, animals and microbes, of both terrestrial and marine origin, and has evolved relatively recently to also include phytotherapy and nutraceuticals. The teaching of pharmacognosy has become even more relevant than previously over the last decade, as a result of the increasing use of herbal remedies (phytomedicines) by the public in Europe, North America and Australasia. When entering a pharmacy today it becomes apparent that considerable shelf space is devoted to a selection of 'herbs', to a degree which would have been quite unimaginable even 20 years ago. If the United States is taken as an example, community pharmacists nowadays have to deal with a rather bewildering array of botanical 'dietary supplements', many of which were introduced soon after the passage of the Dietary Supplement Health and Education Act of 1994. In a major National Health Interview Survey, commissioned by the Centers for Disease Control and Prevention (CDC), it was found that in 2007 about 20% of the US adult population consumed 'nonvitamin, nonmineral natural products', amounting to the sum of $14.8 billion. Therefore, societal interest in pharmacognosy is likely to increase in the future as the biochemical role of phytomedicines, nutraceuticals and natural drugs in general becomes more clearly defined.

This second edition of this volume, *Fundamentals of Pharmacognosy and Phytotherapy*, by Michael Heinrich, Joanne Barnes, Simon Gibbons and Elizabeth Williamson, aims to provide a contemporary and in-depth perspective of natural product drugs used in the practice of pharmacy. The book is organized into two major parts, entitled 'Fundamentals of pharmacognosy' (Part A) and 'Important natural products and phytomedicines used in pharmacy and medicine' (Part B). Part A is divided into five sections, dealing, in turn, with: the history and importance of pharmacognosy and phytotherapy in pharmacy and medicine; relevant principles of botany and ethnobotany; the chemistry of secondary metabolites of organisms pertinent to drug therapy; the characterization and standardization of phytomedicines and nutraceuticals; and the use of medicinal plants in Oriental and South Asian systems of traditional medicine, as well as in Western complementary and alternative medicine. Part B provides coverage of the use of phytomedicines in various therapeutic categories, affecting, respectively: the gastrointestinal and biliary systems; the cardiovascular system; the respiratory system; the central nervous system; infectious diseases; the endocrine system; the reproductive and urinary tracts; the musculoskeletal system; the skin; the eyes; the ear, nose and pharynx; and miscellaneous supportive therapies.

This comprehensive pharmacognosy textbook integrates effectively the traditional elements of pharmacognosy and phytotherapy. The four talented co-authors have been successful in this endeavour in large part because they have contributed their collective technical expertise in several diverse areas, including ethnobotany and ethnopharmacology, classical botanical pharmacognosy, natural product chemistry, phytochemistry, phytotherapy and clinical pharmacy.

This book may be confidently recommended for purchase by undergraduate and professional doctoral students in pharmacy, as well as beginning graduate students in programmes in the pharmaceutical sciences. It will also be of great interest for use in continuing education courses by pharmacists, dentists, nurses and physicians. In addition, all those with a scientific interest in herbalism and complementary and alternative medicine will also find the content of value. The book will also serve as a reliable source of information on natural product drugs for the informed lay reader. It is predicted that *Fundamentals of Pharmacognosy and Phytotherapy* will soon become a classic in its field. This volume will be especially warmly welcomed by educators of future pharmacists and of other healthcare professionals.

Professor A. Douglas Kinghorn,
Columbus, Ohio

Preface

In the last few decades pharmacognosy as an academic discipline, and its application in health care, has changed almost beyond recognition. With the revival of interest in natural drugs, phytotherapy and herbal remedies, new courses are springing up to educate students of pharmacy, medicine, medical herbalism, nursing and related professions. Knowledge about plant-derived products is essential in all areas of health care, not only because these forms of treatment are a popular and widely used healthcare choice (often as over-the-counter products), but also because of the importance of them in many medical traditions. Here, we aim to provide a modern, therapy-oriented perspective, as well as an overview which any reader or educated layperson will find interesting and useful. This book is not a guide to treatment, but a textbook presenting the scientific principles and the evidence, where applicable, underpinning the use of herbal- and other plant-derived medicines.

The content arose in part from the new lecture courses developed by the authors, and is intended to cover all fundamental aspects of pharmacognosy (the study of drugs of natural origin) as well as adding topics on the therapeutic use of such drugs, which is phytotherapy. There is no other book which covers the subject of medicinal plants as an important element of contemporary health care in quite this way and which reflects the current public interest in natural health care. We have combined sections on the scientific study of plant drugs – phytochemistry, ethnopharmacy and botany – with accounts of alternative medicine systems such as medical herbalism, traditional Chinese and Ayurvedic medicine, aromatherapy and others, and a comprehensive section on plant drugs arranged into therapeutic categories. Our purpose is to equip the student with the knowledge to evaluate these therapies, use them when looking to develop drugs and herbal products, and when advising the patient who wishes to try them.

Natural product-derived drugs also include those produced by biotechnology and from animal and microbial sources, but we considered that, as vast and important subjects in their own right, no comprehensive coverage was possible in this text.

Chemical structures are included whenever necessary and appropriate, and we hope to encourage students to appreciate the relevance of the information they impart. In this new edition, we have increased the references and further reading material in each section, so the reader can delve further into the subject, and consult the original work from which our information was taken.

We thank all those who have contributed advice, suggestions and support, including our colleagues, and not forgetting our families of course.

Michael Heinrich, Lismore (Australia) and London (UK)
Joanne Barnes, Auckland (New Zealand)
Simon Gibbons, London (UK)
Elizabeth M. Williamson, Reading (UK)

PART A

Fundamentals of pharmacognosy

Why are plants and their extracts still important in pharmacy and medicine? Historically, plants have yielded some of our most important drugs, but, with the great advances in medicinal chemistry of the last century, synthetic drugs have superseded them as the main focus of research. However, the development of drugs using natural products as 'lead' molecules continues, and many plant-derived pure compounds (or **natural products**) are used in modern, conventional medicine; other compounds are potentially useful to humans or are of toxicological relevance.

There has also been a huge rise in the use of phytopharmaceuticals and herbal medicines in recent years, especially in North America, Europe and Australasia. Traditional medicine, which uses many plant remedies, remains an important (and in some cases, the only) form of treatment in many developing countries, but it is now used increasingly worldwide. People in many countries now want to cure minor health problems with something 'natural' and ageing populations have an increasing demand for medicines and foods ('nutraceuticals') to help combat the symptoms and problems of ageing. This public demand is an enormous challenge for all health professionals, many of whom have little specialist knowledge of natural medicines. This book is divided into two parts. The first part addresses the concepts that help in the understanding of the pharmacognostical basis of such medical products, including the pharmaceutical, pharmacological, toxicological and phytochemical aspects. The second part is devoted to important plant-derived medicines, which are arranged in therapeutic categories.

Part A deals with the *basic scientific principles* underlying the use of medicinal plants, and the extracts and pure compounds (sometimes referred to as 'natural products') derived from them. This part is selective, and highlights those aspects most relevant to everyday practice. In the first chapter, a general introduction to the scientific field of pharmacognosy, and one of its main applications, phytotherapy, is given. Chapter 2 provides an overview of the historical development of plants in pharmacy and medicine, showing how the modern use of medicinal plants has evolved. In Chapters 3–5, the botanical basis of the discipline is summarized, covering classification and the use of plants by people with little or no access to modern medicine – known as ethnobotany and ethnopharmacy. Chapters 6–8 deal mainly with phytochemistry. Here, the types of compounds that may be present are discussed, together with their isolation and identification, using chromatographic and spectroscopic techniques. In Chapter 9 a very short overview of the process is given, from agricultural production or collection from the wild, to the processing of the pharmaceutical product or health food supplement. Phytomedicines have particular attributes not encountered using synthetic drugs or single compounds, in that the botanical drug or an extract derived from it may be combined with other herbal drugs or extracts. This may involve synergistic and other interactions; this is discussed in Chapters 10 and 11. Some ancient written traditions, such as Chinese and Ayurvedic medicine, have been passed on for centuries, and their practical use and philosophical basis is presented in Chapter 12. Chapter 13 looks at complementary and alternative therapies which are currently popular in Europe, Australasia and North America. These are non-science-based approaches to healing, to which pharmacists and members of the medical professions are now being more frequently exposed. More detailed information on these topics can be found in the further reading sections of each chapter. Due to lack of space, there is no section on biotechnology (e.g. fermentation and tissue culture), which is a more specialized area and of less relevance to practising pharmacists and medical doctors.

Section 1

Phytotherapy and pharmacognosy

SECTION CONTENTS

Chapter 1

Importance of plants in modern pharmacy and medicine

AIMS AND DEFINITIONS

This introductory textbook aims to provide a scientific basis for the use of plants in pharmacy (pharmacognosy) and also to describe the main characteristics of herbal medicines (herbal medicinal products, herbal remedies, phytomedicines) and their clinical uses [herbal medicine (UK), phytotherapy (Continental Europe)]. There is also an overview of some of the historical aspects of medicinal plant use in different societies (ethnobotany, ethnopharmacology) and of the role of plants in a variety of popular 'non-scientific' medical systems (traditional medicine).

Pharmacognosy (derived from Greek *pharmakon*, 'remedy', and *gignosco*, 'knowledge') is the science of biogenic or nature-derived pharmaceuticals and poisons. It deals with all medicinal plants, including those yielding complex mixtures, which are used in the form of crude herbs (comminuted herbal substance) or extracts (phytotherapy), pure compounds such as morphine, and foods having additional health benefits only in the context of having preventive effects (nutraceuticals).

TYPES OF DRUGS DERIVED FROM PLANTS

HERBAL DRUGS DERIVED FROM SPECIFIC PARTS OF A MEDICINAL PLANT

Botanical drugs which form the basis for herbal remedies or phytomedicines include, for example:

- the herb of St John's wort (*Hypericum perforatum*), used in the treatment of mild to moderate depression

- the leaves of *Ginkgo biloba*, used for cognitive deficiencies (often in the elderly), including impairment of memory and affective symptoms such as anxiety
- the flower heads of chamomile (*Chamomilla recutita*), used for mild gastrointestinal complaints and as an anti-inflammatory agent
- the leaves and pods of senna (*Cassia* spp.), used for constipation.

From the perspective of pharmacognosy and rational phytotherapy, such products lie alongside, and in some cases are, conventional pharmaceutical medicines. Herbal medicines are often considered to be part of complementary and alternative medicine (CAM), and the use of herbal medicinal products (HMPs) and of CAM has increased across the developed world.

NATURAL PRODUCTS OR COMPOUNDS ISOLATED FROM NATURE

These are pure chemical entities, often used in the form of licensed medicines. They are sometimes produced synthetically and referred to as 'nature identical' (if that is the case), but were originally discovered from plant drugs. Examples include:

- morphine, from opium poppy (*Papaver somniferum*), used as an analgesic
- digoxin and other digitalis glycosides, from foxglove (*Digitalis* spp.), used to treat heart failure
- taxol, from the Pacific yew (*Taxus brevifolia*), used as an anticancer treatment

- quinine, from *Cinchona* bark (*Cinchona* spp.), used in the treatment of malaria
- galanthamine from *Galanthus* and *Leucojum* species, used in the management of cognitive disorders.

NUTRACEUTICALS OR 'FUNCTIONAL FOODS'

Many foods are known to have beneficial effects on health. Examples include:

- garlic, ginger, turmeric and many other herbs and spices
- anthocyanin- or flavonoid-containing plants such as bilberries, cocoa and red wine
- carotenoid-containing plants such as tomatoes, carrots and many other vegetables.

USE OF HERBAL MEDICINES

The use of these remedies is extensive, increasing and complex. In several surveys 20–33% of the UK population claimed to regularly use CAM alone or in addition to orthodox or conventional medicine and treatments. In the UK, usage is particularly frequent amongst those who are over-the-counter medicines-users. There is not, on the whole, a wide understanding of what herbal medicines are (or are not) (IPSOS-MORI 2008). Healthcare professionals and students also commonly use such products. Forty-three percent of students at a University School of Pharmacy reported using at least one type of CAM during the last 12 months (Freymann et al 2006).

In the United States, approximately 38% of adults and approximately 12% of children are using some form of CAM (NIH/NCCAM). Kennedy et al (2008) showed that in the preceding 12 months about 38 million adults in the US (18.9% of the population) used herbal medicines or supplements, but that only one-third revealed this use to their physician. Data for other regions are even more limited, but the usage of herbal medicines is widespread in countries like India, Indonesia, Australia and China, to name just a few.

In addition, market research data reveal high levels of expenditure on herbal medicines, although it is difficult to obtain precise figures for sales of such products since some are classed as food supplements and are sold through numerous outlets. For similar reasons, it is usually not possible to compare properly the estimates for expenditure

on herbal medicines using different studies and in different countries. For 2009, it is estimated that the total value of the global market in herbal medicines was around $83 billion. In 2009 in the USA alone consumers spent an estimated total of $5 billion on herbal dietary supplements. In the UK in 2007, the market for herbal medicines was estimated to be almost £700 million, which, compared with many other European countries, is rather low. The European market for herbal supplements and herbal medicines is currently worth about $7.4 billion. Germany is the largest European market, with a 27% share, followed by France (24%), Italy (12%) and the UK (9%). The Indian healthcare market is valued at $7.3 billion, 60% of which is controlled by pharmaceutical drug manufacturers, while 30% is controlled by Ayurvedic medicine manufacturers; the Chinese market comes in at around $8 billion.

In most continental European countries, such phytomedicines are licensed medicinal products and are used under medical supervision. However, the widespread use of herbal medicines by the general public raises several important issues. Some of these relate to how individuals, whether consumers or healthcare professionals, perceive and use these preparations; other concerns relate to the quality, safety and efficacy of the herbal medicines themselves.

As part of the primary healthcare team, pharmacists, as well as nurses and general practitioners, need to be competent in advising consumers on the safe, effective and appropriate use of all medicines, including herbal medicines. Healthcare professionals also need to be aware of the products and healthcare choices that patients are making, often without their knowledge.

There are many reasons for the increased use of herbal medicines. These may range from the appeal of products from 'nature' and the perception that such products are 'safe' (or at least 'safer' than conventional medicines, which are often derogatorily referred to as 'drugs'), to more complex reasons related to the philosophical views and religious beliefs of individuals.

In developed countries, most purchases of HMPs are made on a self-selection basis from pharmacies and health-food stores, as well as from supermarkets, by mail order and via the Internet. **Normally, with the exception of pharmacists, there is no requirement for a trained healthcare professional to be available on the premises to provide**

information and advice. In any case, most HMPs can be sold or supplied without the involvement of a healthcare professional and several studies have confirmed that many individuals do not seek professional advice before purchasing or using such products, even when purchased from a pharmacy (Barnes et al 1998, Gulian et al 2002). Rather, consumers of HMPs tend to rely on their own (usually limited) knowledge, or are guided by advice from friends and relatives or the popular media. Consumers who do seek professional advice (e.g. from their pharmacist or general practitioner) may find that he or she is not able to answer their question(s) fully. In some cases this may be because the information simply is not available, but it is also recognized that, at present, many healthcare professionals are not adequately informed about herbal medicines, particularly with regard to their quality, safety and efficacy. This book attempts to redress that omission.

HMPs are used for general health maintenance, as well as for treating diseases, including serious conditions such as cancer, HIV/AIDS, multiple sclerosis, asthma, rheumatoid arthritis and osteoarthritis. Older patients, pregnant and breastfeeding women, and children also take HMPs, and this raises concerns because, as with conventional medicines, precautions need to be taken. For example, few medicines (whether conventional or herbal) have been established as safe for use during pregnancy and it is generally accepted that no medicine should be taken during pregnancy unless the benefit to the mother or fetus outweighs any possible risk to the fetus. Similarly, HMPs should be used with caution in children and the elderly, who, as with conventional medicines, differ from adults in their response to, and metabolism and clearance of drugs. The use of herbal medicines by patients who are already taking prescribed medicines is of particular concern as there is the potential for drug–herb interactions to occur. For example, important pharmacokinetic and pharmacodynamic interactions between St John's wort (*Hypericum perforatum*) and certain conventional medicines have been documented (Williamson et al 2009) and mechanisms for such interactions have been identified. Generally, information on interactions between HMPs and conventional medicines is limited, although potential drug–herb interactions can sometimes be identified based on the known phytochemistry and pharmacological properties of the herbs involved.

These issues illustrate once more the need for healthcare professionals, and especially pharmacists,

to be knowledgeable about HMPs, and professional bodies are increasingly mindful of their responsibilities regarding herbal medicines and have taken steps to address the issue. It is now recognized by the UK Committee on Safety of Medicines and the Medicines and Healthcare Products Regulatory Agency that pharmacists have an important role to play in pharmacovigilance with regard to HMPs; this involves reporting suspected adverse reactions and disseminating information to patients and the public about safety concerns. Calls for healthcare professionals to be competent with regard to herbal medicines and other 'complementary' therapies are now coming from outside the professions.

In summary, the use of herbal products continues to be a popular healthcare choice among patients and the general public. Most pharmacies sell herbal medicines and it is likely that pharmacists will be asked for advice on such products or that they will have to consider other implications of herbal product use, such as interactions with conventional medicines. This book provides the scientific background to the use of plants as medicines.

SOME FUNDAMENTAL ASPECTS OF THE REGULATION OF HERBAL MEDICINES

The regulation of herbal medicines is complex, varies greatly and is constantly changing. These diverse regulatory frameworks form an essential basis for the activities of all healthcare professionals and for research on such products. For example, in the UK, until recently *Ginkgo biloba* was considered a food and now is, as in other European countries, regulated as a traditional herbal medical product; it is a herbal medical product in Germany and a food supplement in the USA. In the UK Echinacea may be a traditional herbal medical product or a food supplement or a registered medicine. It is classed as a dietary supplement in the USA and a medicine in Germany. Therefore here a brief and selective overview of the regulation of herbal medicines in key English-speaking countries is given, excluding the regulation of the professions involved in their production, prescription and dispensing.

UNITED KINGDOM

In essence, today's regulatory framework in the UK, is very similar to the ones in other countries of the European Union. Historically, in the UK, many of the concerns regarding herbal medicinal products have arisen from the lack of regulation of such products. Consequently, such products lacked evidence for acceptable standards for quality, safety and efficacy. A range of safety problems occurred as a result of the use of unlicensed herbal preparations of inadequate pharmaceutical quality.

The basis for the current regulatory regime for the licensing of medicines in the UK is set out by the 1968 Medicines Act and other regulations which have arisen from the implementation of relevant European Commission legislation, namely Directive 65/65/EEC, now revised as Directive 2001/83/EC. Under this legislation, manufacturers of products, including herbal remedies, which are classed as medicinal products must hold a marketing authorization (MA, or product licence, PL) for that product unless it satisfies the criteria for exemption from the requirement for a MA. In essence, medicinal products are defined as those that are medicinal by presentation *or* (not *and*) by function. Manufacturers of products comprising new chemical entities, including isolated constituents from plant or other natural sources, are required to submit applications for MAs for those products, based on the full dossier of chemical, pharmaceutical, pharmacological, toxicological and clinical data.

Herbal products are available on the UK market as:

- licensed herbal medicines
- traditional herbal medical products registered under the European 'Traditional Herbal Medicinal Product Directive' (THMPD)
- herbal medicines exempt from licensing
- unlicensed herbal products, sold as food or dietary supplements
- prescription-only medicines (POM); these potentially hazardous plants may only be dispensed by order of a prescription by a registered doctor
- pharmacy-only medicines (P); certain others may only be supplied by a registered pharmacist, or may be subject to dose (but not duration of treatment) and route of administration restrictions.

Licensed herbal medicines

Most licensed herbal products in the UK were initially granted a product licence of right (PLR) because they were already on the market when the licensing system was introduced in the 1970s. When PLRs were reviewed, manufacturers of herbal products

intended for use in minor self-limiting conditions were permitted to rely on bibliographic evidence to support efficacy and safety, rather than being required to carry out new controlled clinical trials. So, many licensed herbal medicinal products have not necessarily undergone stringent testing. The 'well-established use' directive (99/83/EC) was intended to allow greater flexibility on the use of bibliographic data to demonstrate safety and efficacy, and it was hoped that this legislation would provide a regulatory framework for the many unlicensed herbal products on the market. Unfortunately, interpretations of the provisions of the directive vary between EU member states and this directive is not widely accepted in the UK.

Traditional herbal medical products

The THMPD 2004/24/EC (see http://www.mhra.gov.uk) is a regulatory process established to provide a mechanism whereby manufacturers of good-quality herbal medicines can register their products as medicinal products and make (restricted) medicinal claims on the packaging and the patient information leaflet (PIL). Examples of the types of information that may be displayed are given here:

- Evidence that a corresponding herbal product (i.e. one derived from the same botanical drug and prepared in a similar way) has been used traditionally for at least 30 years (15 years' non-EU and 15 years in the EU, or more than 30 years in the EU).
- Bibliographic data on safety with an expert report.
- A quality dossier specifying how the company complies with the quality guidance requirements of the regulators.
- Details on the patient information leaflet (PIL), packaging, naming and labelling.

Products registered under this Directive can only be used for minor, self-limiting conditions. Overall, it provides an assurance that the patient is receiving not only a good-quality product, but also more reliable advice on its use.

Unlicensed herbal medicines

HMPs still exempt from licensing are those 'compounded and supplied by herbalists on their own recommendation' [specified under Section 12(1) of the Medicines Act 1968] and those consisting solely of dried, crushed or comminuted (fragmented) plants. They must not contain any non-herbal 'active' ingredients and are sold under their botanical name and with no written recommendations for use [specified under Section 12(2) of the Medicines Act]. The exemptions were initially intended to give herbalists the flexibility to prepare remedies for their patients, although, at present, there is no statutory regulation of herbalists in the UK (this is under review).

Traditional medicines used by ethnic groups include Traditional Chinese Medicines (TCM) and Ayurvedic medicines. These products are subject to the same legislation as are 'Western' herbal medicines. Some toxic species, like *Aristolochia* sp., are banned. There still remain problems associated with some imported medicines: in addition to containing non-herbal ingredients such as animal parts and/or minerals, some manufactured ('patent') 'herbal' products have been found to contain conventional drugs which may have POM status in the UK (e.g. dexamethasone and glibenclamide) or which are banned. Non-herbal active ingredients of any type (chemically synthesized, animal products) cannot legally be included in herbal remedies, and inclusion of drugs with POM status represents an additional infringement of European and US legislation. Some ingredients, such as certain species of plants, are also restricted under the Convention on International Trade in Endangered Species of Wild Fauna and Flora (CITES).

AUSTRALIA

In Australia, Western herbal medicine is one of the most popular forms of CAM and a range of ethnic medicines, especially TCM, are increasingly becoming popular. All medicines, including herbal and other complementary medicines, are covered by the Therapeutic Goods Act (1989) and regulated by a federal agency, the Therapeutic Goods Administration (TGA, http://www.tga.gov.au/). A statutory expert committee, the Advisory Committee on Complementary Medicines (formerly the Complementary Medicines Evaluation Committee) provides the TGA with advice on the regulation of complementary medicines. The Australian regulatory guidelines for complementary medicines (http://www.tga.gov. au/docs/html/argcm.htm) provide information to help producers and distributors of complementary medicines to meet their obligations under therapeutic goods legislation.

Australia adopts a two-tiered, risk-based approach to the regulation of all medicines. Low-risk medicines, including most herbal and complementary medicines, are included in the Australian Register of Therapeutic Goods (ARTG) as listed medicines and identified by a unique AUST L number of the label. Medicines deemed to be of higher risk are entered on the register as registered medicines and identified by an AUST R number. While registered medicines undergo full pre-market safety and efficacy evaluation, listed medicines are not evaluated for efficacy, but product sponsors must hold evidence to support the claims they make about the product. Random and targeted post-market audits of this evidence are carried out by the regulator. Indications and claims for listed medicines are limited to health maintenance, health enhancement or non-serious, self-limiting conditions and may be supported by evidence from traditional use or scientific evidence. Both listed and registered medicines must be made to pharmaceutical GMP standards, and herbal ingredients must conform to the relevant BP (AH thu EurPhar) monograph, if one exists.

Medicines extemporaneously compounded for a specific patient following consultation are exempt from inclusion on the ARTG; this allows herbalists and other practitioners to compound individualized formulae for their patients.

CANADA

In Canada herbal medicines are classified as 'natural health products' which require a product licence before they can be marketed. The relevant agency is 'Health Canada'. Since 2004 this is regulated in the The Natural Health Products Regulations. The system is intended to find an equilibrium between openness towards various health paradigms (e.g. Traditional Chinese Medicine, Ayurveda, Western traditional herbalism, etc.) and scientific rigor. Hence, specific health claims are allowed on the basis of a variable evidence base that becomes more stringent with the severity of the condition treated with a product. A manufacturer has to submit detailed information on the product to Health Canada, including: medicinal ingredients, source, potency, non-medicinal ingredients and recommended use(s). Once a product has been assessed and granted market authorization by Health Canada, the product label will bear an eight digit product licence number preceded by the distinct letters NPN (Natural Product Number), or, in the case of a homeopathic medicine, by the letters DIN-HM (Homeopathic Medicine Number).

This number on the label will inform consumers that the product license application has been reviewed and approved by Health Canada to meet the standards in terms of safety, efficacy and quality. GMPs (Good Manufacturing Practices) must be guaranteed in the products production in order to ensure the product's quality and thus its safety. In addition the system requires that all Canadian producers and importers of natural health products are licensed.

Similar to the UK, an Adverse Reaction Reporting System for natural health products is in place and is used to warn the public (http://www.hc-sc.gc.ca/dhp-mps/prodnatur/about-apropos/index-eng.php).

INDIA

India has an ancient heritage of traditional medicine (see Chapter 12) with a well-recorded and widely practised knowledge of herbal medicine. The Department of Ayurveda, Yoga & Naturopathy, Unani, Siddha and Homoeopathy (AYUSH) within the Ministry of Health & Family Welfare focuses on its regulation and on the improvement of standards in the areas of quality control and standardization of drugs, the availability of raw material, research and development, education/training of professionals, and a wider outreach with regard to these traditional medical systems.

The **Traditional Herbal Medicines Act, 2006** regulates the sale of the traditional herbal medicines which are marketed without any licence and control on the basis of being from ancient texts. According to the Act every retailer or seller of traditional herbal medicines needs to have a licence to sell traditional herbal medicines from the Authority. Every manufacturer of traditional herbal medicine needs to work under the principles of GMP and has to list the ingredients of each medicine on the packing of the medicine along with their accurate quantity. Side effects and warning of contraindications need to be stated on the package. Pharmacopoeia Committees have been established to develop quality standards for the main groups of therapeutically relevant drugs of Ayurveda, Unani, Siddha and homoeopathy (Mukherjee et al 2007).

The Indian Government also established an independent body – the 'National Medicinal Plants Board' under the Ministry of Health and Family Welfare. It is responsible for co-ordinating all matters relating to the development of medicinal plants, including policies and strategies for conservation, proper harvesting, cost-effective cultivation and marketing of raw material in order to protect, sustain and develop this sector.

Uniquely, the Indian government has established programmes for the documentation of traditional Indian knowledge, which is already available in public domain. The political goal is to safeguard the sovereignty of this traditional knowledge and to protect it from being misused in patenting on non-patentable inventions. The **Traditional Knowledge Digital Library (TKDL)** is an original proprietary database, which is fully protected under national and international laws of Intellectual Property Rights and is maintained and developed by the government. TKDL also allows automatic conversion of information from Sanskrit into various languages. The information includes names of plants, Ayurvedic description of diseases under their modern names and therapeutic formulations (Mukherjee et al 2007).

UNITED STATES OF AMERICA (USA)

In the USA, herbal medicines are generally regulated as 'dietary supplements'. The US Food and Drug Administration (FDA, www.fda.gov/Food/DietarySupplements/) is in charge of these comparatively loose regulations (http://nccam.nih.gov/health/supplements/wiseuse.htm). Some key characteristics stand out:

- Prior to marketing, dietary supplements do not have to be assessed for safety and effectiveness. Limited therapeutic claims may be made, e.g. that a dietary supplement addresses a nutrient deficiency, supports health, or is linked to a particular body function (e.g. immunity). However, this requires supportive prior research. Such a claim must be followed by the words 'This statement has not been evaluated by the U.S. Food and Drug Administration (FDA). This product is not intended to diagnose, treat, cure, or prevent any disease.'
- Since 2008 'Good manufacturing practices' (GMPs) is expected in order to ensure that dietary supplements are processed consistently and meet quality standards.
- Once a dietary supplement is on the market, the FDA monitors the claims made and the product's safety. If inappropriate claims are made the manufacturer receives a warning letter or is required to remove the product from the marketplace. If a product is found to be unsafe, the FDA takes similar action against the manufacturer and/or distributor.

References

Barnes, J., Mills, S.Y., Abbot, N.C., et al., 1998. Different standards for reporting ADRs to herbal remedies and conventional OTC medicines: face-to-face interviews with 515 users of herbal remedies. Br. J. Clin. Pharmacol. 45, 496–500.

Freymann, H., Rennie, T., Bates, I., Nebel, S., Heinrich, M., 2006. Knowledge and use of herbal medical products and other CAM among British undergraduate pharmacy students. Pharm. World Sci. 27, 13–18.

Gulian, C., Barnes, J., Francis, S.A., et al., 2002. Types and preferred sources of information concerning herbal medicinal products: face-to-face interviews with users of herbal medicinal products. International Journal of Pharmaceutical Practice 10 (Suppl.), R33.

IPSOS – Mori, 2008. Public perceptions of herbal medicines general public qualitative & quantitative research. IPSOS-Mori, London, UK.

Kennedy, J., Wang, C.C., Wu, C.H., 2008. Patient disclosure about herb and supplement use among adults in the US. Evid. Based Complement. Alternat. Med. 5, 451–456.

Williamson, E.M., Driver, S., Baxter, K. (Eds.), 2009. Stockley's herbal medicines. Interactions Pharmaceutical Press, London.

Further reading

Barnes, J., Phillipson, J.D., Anderson, L.A., 2009. Herbal medicines. A guide for healthcare professionals, third ed. Pharmaceutical Press, London.

Bruneton, J., 1995. Pharmacognosy, phytochemistry, medicinal plants. Springer-Verlag, Berlin.

Cavaliere, C., Rea, P., Lynch, M.E., Blumenthal, M., 2010. Herbal supplement sales rise in all channels in 2009. HerbalGram 86, 82–85.

Evans, W.C., 2009. Trease and Evans's pharmacognosy, sixteenth ed. WB Saunders, London.

Hänsel, R., Sticher, O. (Eds.), 2010. Pharmakognosie – phytopharmazie. Springer, Berlin.

McEwen, J., 2004. What does TGA approval of medicines mean? Australian Prescriber 27, 156–158.

Mills, S., Bone, K., 2000. Phytotherapy. Principles and practice. Churchill Livingstone, London.

Mukherjee, P.K., Venkatesh, M., Kumar, V., 2007. An overview on the development in regulation and control of medicinal and aromatic plants in the Indian system of medicine. Boletín Latinoamericano y del Caribe de Plantas Medicinales y Aromáticas (BLACPMA) 6, 129–136.

Robbers, J.E., Speedie, M.K., Tyler, V.E., 1996. Pharmacognosy and pharmacobiotechnology. Williams & Wilkins, Baltimore.

Ross, I., 1999. Medicinal plants of the world, vol. I. Humana Press, Totawa, NJ.

Ross, I., 2000. Medicinal plants of the world, vol. II. Humana Press, Totawa, NJ.

Schulz, V., Haensel, R., Tyler, V., 1998. Rational phytotherapy. Springer-Verlag, Berlin.

Thomas, K.J., Nicholl, J.P., Coleman, P., 2001. Use and expenditure on complementary medicine in England: a population based survey. Complement Ther. Med. 9, 2–11.

Williamson, E., 2003. Potter's herbal cyclopedia. CW Daniels, Saffron Walden.

Chapter 2

Pharmacognosy and its history: people, plants and natural products

The history of pharmacy was for centuries identical to that of pharmacognosy, or the study of **materia medica,** which were obtained from natural sources – mostly plants, but also minerals, animals and fungi. While European traditions are particularly well known and have had a strong influence on modern pharmacognosy in the West, almost all societies have well-established customs, some of which have hardly been studied at all. The study of these traditions not only provides insight into how the field has developed, but it is also a fascinating example of our ability to develop a diversity of cultural practices. The use of medicinal plants in Europe has been influenced by early European scholars, the concepts of lay people and, more recently, by an influx of people and products from non-European traditions. This historical overview only covers Europe and the most well-known traditions of Asia: **Traditional Chinese Medicine** (TCM), **Ayurveda** and **Jamu**. TCM and Ayurveda will be discussed further in a separate chapter, because they are still used widely today.

SOURCES OF INFORMATION

The sources available for understanding the history of medicinal (as well as nutritional and toxic) plant use are archaeological records and written documents. The desire to summarize information for future generations and to present the writings of the classical (mostly early Greek) scholars to a wider audience was the major stimulus for writing about medicinal plants. The traditions of Japan, India and China were also documented in many early manuscripts and books (Mazar 1998, Waller 1998). No written records are available for other regions

of the world either because they were never produced (e.g. Australia, many parts of Africa and South America, and some regions of Asia) or because documents were lost or destroyed by (especially European) invaders (e.g. in Meso-America). Therefore, for many parts of the world the first written records are reports by early travellers who were sent by their respective feudal governments to explore the wealth of the New World. These people included missionaries, explorers, salesmen, researchers and, later, colonial officers. The information was important to European societies for reasons of potential dangers, such as poisoned arrows posing a threat to explorers and settlers, as well as the prospect of finding new medicines.

EARLY ARABIC AND EUROPEAN RECORDS

Humans have always used plants in a multitude of ways in a tradition spanning human evolution. The selection of medicinal plants is a conscious process which has led to an enormous number of medicinal plants being used by the numerous cultures of the world.

An early European example is medicinal mushrooms, which were found with the Austrian/ Italian 'iceman' of the Alps of Ötztal (3300 BCE). Two walnut-sized objects were identified as the birch polypore (*Piptoporus betulinus*), a bracket fungus common in alpine and other cooler environments. This species contains toxic natural products, and one of its active constituents (agaric acid) is a very strong and effective purgative, which leads to strong and short-lasting diarrhoea. It also has antibiotic effects against mycobacteria and toxic effects on diverse organisms (Capasso 1998). Since the iceman also harboured eggs of the whipworm (*Trichuris trichiuria*) in his gut, he may well have suffered from gastrointestinal cramps and anaemia. The finding of *Piptoporus betulinus* points to the possible treatment of gastrointestinal problems using these mushrooms. Also, scarred cuts on the skin of the iceman might indicate the use of medicinal plants, since the burning of herbs over an incision on the skin was a frequent practice in many ancient European cultures (Capasso 1998).

THE DOCUMENTS OF SHANIDAR IV

The earliest documented record, which presumably relates to medicinal (or ritual) plants, dates from 60,000 BCE in the grave of a Neanderthal man from Shanidar IV, an archaeological site in Iraq. Pollen of several species of plants was discovered (Leroi-Gourhan 1975, Solecki 1975, Lietava 1992):

Centaurea solstitialis L. (knapweed, Asteraceae)
Ephedra altissima (ephedra, Ephedraceae)
Achillea sp. (yarrow, Asteraceae)
Althea sp. (mallow, Malvaceae)
Muscari sp. (grape hyacinth, Liliaceae/Hyacinthaceae)
Senecio sp. (groundsel, Asteraceae).

These species were possibly laid on the ground and formed a carpet on which the dead were laid. These plants could have been of major cultural importance to the people of Shanidar IV. Whether they were used as medicine cannot be determined, but it seems likely. Today, these species are important medicinal plants used for a range of indications. However, others have criticized these reports, because:

- detailed archaeobotanical descriptions of the pollen were never published
- normally, pollen does not survive well in the Near East
- there is good evidence that ants often hoard pollen in a similar context (Sommer 1999).

Thus, although this may be a finding with no direct bearing on the culture of Shanidar, these species (or closely related ones from the same genus) are still important today in the phytotherapy of Iraq and are also known from other cultural traditions. These species may well be typical for the Neanderthal people, and may also be part of a tradition for which Shanidar IV represents the first available record.

CLASSICAL ARABIC, GREEK AND ROMAN RECORDS

The oldest written information in the European–Arabic traditions comes from the Sumerians and Akkadians of Mesopotamia, thus originating from the same area as the archaeological records of Shanidar IV. Similar documents have survived millennia in Egypt. The Egyptians documented their knowledge (including medical and pharmaceutical) on papyrus, which is paper made from *Cyperus aquaticus*, an aquatic sedge (also called papyrus) found throughout southern Europe and northern Africa. The most important of these writings is the Ebers Papyrus, which originates from around 1500 BC. This document was reputedly found in a tomb, and bought in 1873 by Georg Ebers, who deposited it at the University of Leipzig and 2 years later published a facsimile edition. The Ebers Papyrus is a medical handbook covering all sorts of illnesses and includes empirical as well as symbolic forms of treatment. The diagnostic precision documented in this text is impressive. Other papyri focus on recipes for pharmaceutical preparations (e.g. the so-called Berlin Papyrus).

Greek medicine has been the focus of historical pharmaceutical research for many decades. The Greek scholar Pedanius Dioscorides (Fig. 2.1) from Anarzabos (1 BC) is considered to be the 'father of [Western] medicine'. His works were a doctrine governing pharmaceutical and medical practice for more than 1500 years, and which heavily influenced European pharmacy. He was an excellent pharmacognosist and described more than 600 medicinal plants. Other Greek and Roman scholars were also influential in developing related fields of health care and the natural sciences. Hippocrates, a Greek medical doctor (ca. 460–375 BC)

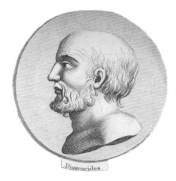

Fig. 2.1 Pedanius Dioscorides. *Reproduced with permission from The Wellcome Library, London.*

came from the island of Kos, and heavily influenced European medical traditions. He was the first of a series of (otherwise largely unknown) authors who produced the so-called *Corpus Hippocraticum* (a collection of works on medical practice). The Graeco-Roman medical doctor Claudius Galen (Galenus) (130–201 AD) summarized the complex body of Graeco-Roman pharmacy and medicine, and his name survives in the pharmaceutical term 'galenical'. Pliny the Elder (23 or 24–79 AD, killed in Pompeii at the eruption of Vesuvius) was the first to produce a 'cosmography' (a detailed account) of natural history, which included cosmology, mineralogy, botany, zoology and medicinal products derived from plants and animals.

CLASSICAL CHINESE RECORDS

Written documents about medicinal plants are essential elements of many cultures of Asia. In China, India, Japan and Indonesia, writings pointing to a long tradition of plant use survive. In China, the field developed as an element of Taoist thought: followers tried to assure a long life (or immortality) through meditation, special diets, medicinal plants, exercise and specific sexual practices. The most important work in this tradition is the *Shen nong ben caojing* (the 'Drug treatise of the divine countryman') which is now only available as part of later compilations (Waller 1998; see also Chapter 12, p. 177 et seq). This 2200-year-old work includes 365 drugs, most of botanical origin. For each, the following information is provided:

- Geographical origin
- Optimum period for collection
- Therapeutic properties
- Forms of preparation and dose.

These scholarly ideas were passed on from master to student, and modified and adapted over centuries of use. Unfortunately, in none of the cases do we have a surviving written record. Table 2.1 summarizes some of the Chinese works that include important chapters on drugs.

In the 16th century the first systematic treatise on (herbal) drugs using a scientific method was produced. The *Ben Cao Gang Mu* ('Drugs', by Li Shizhen, 1518–1593) contains information about 1892 drugs (in 52 chapters) and more than 11,000 recipes are given in an appendix. The drugs are classified into 16 categories (e.g. herbs, cereals, vegetables, fruits). For each drug the following information is provided (Waller 1998):

- Definition of the drug
- Selected commentaries
- Classification according to the four characteristics of temperatures and the five types of taste
- Uses (detailed information on uses according to the criteria of Chinese medicine)
- Corrections of previous mistakes
- Methods of preparing the drug
- New features
- Examples of recipes.

The recognition of the need to further develop the usage of a plant, to correct earlier mistakes and to include new information is particularly noteworthy. However, the numerous medicopharmaceutical traditions of the Chinese minorities were not included in these works and we, therefore, have no historical records of their pharmacopoeias.

OTHER ASIAN TRADITIONAL MEDICINE

Overall, the written records on other Asian medicine are less comprehensive than for Chinese medicine. The oldest form of traditional Asian medicine is Ayurveda, which is basically Hindu in origin and which is a sort of art-science-philosophy of life. In this respect it resembles Traditional Chinese Medicine, and like TCM has influenced the development of more practical, less esoteric forms of medicine,

Table 2.1	Chinese works that include important sections on drugs (after Waller 1998)	
YEAR	**AUTHOR IF KNOWN**	**TITLE**
200 BC	Shen Nong	*Shen nong ben cao jing* (the drug treatise of the divine countryman)
2nd century		*Shang han za bing lun* (about the various illnesses caused by cold damage)
6th century	Tao Hongjing	*Shen nong ben cao jing fi zhu* (collected commentaries on *Shen nong ben cao jing*)
10th to 12th centuries		*Ben cao tu jing*
16th century	Li Shizhen	*Ben cao gang mu* (information about medicinal drugs: a monographic treatment)
1746		*Jing shi zheng lei bei ji ben cao*

which are used for routine or minor illnesses in the home. Related types of medicine include Jamu, the traditional system of Indonesia, which will be described briefly below. All these forms of traditional medicine use herbs and minerals and have many features in common. Naturally, many plants are common to all systems and to various official drugs that were formerly (or still) included in the British Pharmacopoeia (BP), European Pharmacopoeia (Eur. Ph.) and US Pharmacopoeia (USP).

Ayurveda

Ayurveda is arguably one of the most ancient of all recorded medicinal traditions. It is considered to be the origin of systemized medicine, because ancient Hindu writings on medicine contain no references to foreign medicine whereas Greek and Middle Eastern texts do refer to ideas and drugs of Indian origin. Dioscorides (who influenced Hippocrates) is thought to have taken many of his ideas from India, so it looks as though the first comprehensive medical knowledge originated there. The term 'Ayurveda' comes from *ayur* meaning 'life' and *veda* meaning 'knowledge' and is a later addition to Hindu sacred writing from 1200 BC called the *Artharva-veda*. The first school to teach Ayurvedic medicine was at the University of Banaras in 500 BC and the great Samhita (or encyclopaedia of medicine) was written. Seven hundred years later another great encyclopaedia was written and these two together form the basis of Ayurveda. The living and the non-living environment, including humans, is composed of the elements earth (*prithvi*), water (*jala*), fire (*tejac*), air (*vaju*) and space (*akasa*). For an understanding of these traditions, the concept of impurity and cleansing is also essential. Illness is the consequence of imbalance between the various elements and it is the goal of treatment to restore this balance (see Chapter 12 for details).

Jamu

Indonesian traditional medicine, Jamu, is thought to have originated in the ancient palaces of Surakarta and Yogyakarta in central Java, from ancient Javanese cultural practices and also as a result of the influence of Chinese, Indian and Arabian medicine. Carvings at the temple of Borobudur dating back to 800–900 AD depict the use of *kalpataruh* leaves ('the tree that never dies') to make medicines. The Javanese influence spread to Bali as links were established, and in 1343 an army of the Majapahit

kingdom of eastern Java was sent to subjugate the Balinese. Success was short-lived and the Balinese retaliated, regaining their independence. After Islam was adopted in Java and the Majapahit Empire destroyed, many Javanese fled, mainly to Bali, taking with them their books, culture and customs, including medicine. In this way, Javanese traditions survived in Bali more or less intact, and the island remained relatively isolated until the conquest by the Dutch in 1908. Other islands in the archipelago use Jamu with regional variations.

There are a few surviving records, but often those that do exist are closely guarded by healers or their families. They are considered to be sacred and, for example those in the palace at Yogyakarta, are closed to outsiders. In Bali, medical knowledge was inscribed on *lontar* leaves (a type of palm) and in Java on paper. Consequently, they are often in poor condition and difficult to read. Two of the most important manuscripts – *Serat kawruh bab jampi-jampi* ('A treatise on all manner of cures') and *Serat Centhini* ('Book of Centhini') – are in the Surakarta Palace library. The former contains a total of 1734 formulae made from natural materials and indications as to their use. The *Serat Centhini* is an 18th century work of 12 volumes and, although it contains much information and advice of a general nature and numerous folk tales, it is still an excellent account of medical treatment in ancient Java.

The status of Jamu started to improve ca. 1940 with the Second Congress of Indonesian Physicians, at which it was decided that an in-depth study of traditional medicine was needed. A further impetus was the Japanese occupation of 1942–1944, when the Dai Nippon government set up the Indonesian Traditional Medicines Committee; another boost occurred during Indonesia's War of Independence when orthodox medicine was in short supply. President Sukarno decreed that the nation should be self-supporting, so many people turned to the traditional remedies used by their ancestors (see Beers 2001).

Jamu contains many elements of TCM, such as treating 'hot' illnesses with 'cold' remedies, and of Ayurveda, in which religious aspects and the use of massage are very important. Remedies from Indonesia such as clove (*Syzygium aromaticum*), nutmeg (*Myristica fragrans*), Java tea [*Orthosiphon stamineus* (=*O. aristatus*) and *Orthosiphon* spp], jambul (*Eugenia jambolana*) and galangal (*Alpinia galanga*) are still used around the world as medicines or culinary spices.

Kampo

Kampo, or traditional Japanese medicine, is sometimes referred to as low-dose TCM. Until 1875 (when the medical examination for Japanese doctors became restricted to Western medicine), the Chinese system was the main form of medical practice in Japan, having arrived via Korea and been absorbed into native medicine. Exchange of scholars with China meant that religious and medical practices were virtually identical; for example, the medical system established in Japan in 701 was an exact copy of that of the T'ang dynasty in China. In the Nara period (710–783), when Buddhism became even more popular, medicine became extremely complex and included facets of Ayurveda as well as of Arabian medicine. Native medicine remained in the background and, after concerns that it would be subsumed into Chinese medicine, the compendium of Japanese medicine, *Daidoruijoho*, was compiled in 808 on the orders of the Emperor Heizei. In 894, official cultural exchange with China was halted, and native medicine was temporarily reinstated. Knowledge gained from China, however, continued to be assimilated, and in 984 the court physician Yasuyori Tamba compiled the *Ishinho*, which consisted of 30 scrolls detailing the medical knowledge of the Sui and T'ang dynasties. Although based entirely on Chinese medicine, it is still invaluable as a record of medicine as practised in Japan at that time.

In 1184 the framework began to change when a reformed system was introduced by Yorimoto Minamoto in which native medicine was included, and by 1574 Dosan Manase had set down all the elements of medical thought which became a form of independent Japanese medicine during the Edo period. This resulted in Kampo, and it remained the main form of medicine until the introduction of Western medicine in 1771, by Genpaku Sugita. Although Sugita did not reject Kampo, and advocated its use in his textbook book *Keieiyawa*, it fell into decline because of a lack of evidence and an increasingly scholastic rather than empirical approach to treatment. Towards the end of the 19th century, despite important events such as the isolation of ephedrine (Fig. 2.2) by Nagayoshi Nagai, Kampo was still largely ignored by the Japanese medical establishment. However, by 1940, a university course on Kampo had been instituted, and now most schools of medicine in Japan offer courses on traditional medicine integrated with

(–)-Ephedrine

Fig. 2.2

Western medicine. In 1983, it was estimated that about 40% of Japanese clinicians were writing Kampo herbal prescriptions and today's research in Japan and Korea continues to confirm the validity of many of its remedies (Takemi et al 1985).

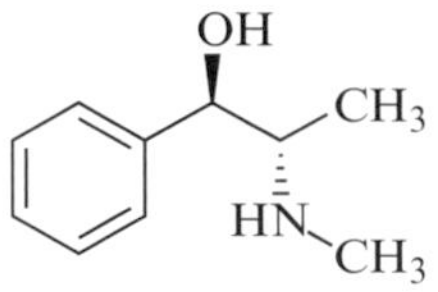

THE EUROPEAN MIDDLE AGES AND ARABIA

After the conquest of the southern part of the Roman Empire by Arab troops, Greek medical texts were translated into Arabic and adapted to the needs of the Arabs. Many of the Greek texts survived only in Arab transcripts. Ibn Sina, or Avicenna from Afshana (980–1037), wrote a monumental treatise *Qânûn fi'l tibb* ('Canon of medicine'; ca. 1020), which was heavily influenced by Galen and which in turn influenced the scholastic traditions especially of southern Europe. This five-volume book remained the most influential work in the field of medicine and pharmacy for more than 500 years, together with direct interpretations of Dioscorides' work. While many Arab scholars worked in eastern Arabia, Arab-dominated parts of Spain became a second centre for classical Arab medicine. An important early example is the *Umdat at-tabîb* ('The medical references') by an unknown botanist from Seville. Thanks to the tolerant policies of the Arab administration, many of the most influential representatives of Arab scholarly traditions were Jews, including Maimoides (1135–1204) and Averroes (1126–1198). In Christian parts of Europe, the texts of the classical Greeks and Romans were copied from the Arabian records and annotated, often by monks. The Italian monastery of Monte Cassino is one of the earliest examples of such a tradition; others developed around the monasteries of Chartres (France) and St Gall (Switzerland).

A common element of all monasteries was a medicinal plant garden, which was used both for growing herbs to treat patients and for teaching about medicinal plants to the younger generation. The species included in these gardens were common to most monasteries and many of the species are still important medicinal plants today. Of particular interest is the *Capitulare de villis* of Charles the Great (Charlemagne, 747–814), who ordered that medicinal (and other plants) should be grown in the King's gardens and in monasteries, and specifically listed 24 species. Walahfri(e)d Strabo (808 or 809–849), Abbot of the monastery of Reichenau (Lake Constance), deserves mention because of his *Liber de cultura hortum* ('Book on the growing of plants'), the first 'textbook' on (medical) botany, and the *Hortulus*, a Latin poem about the medical plants grown in the district. The *Hortulus* is not only famous as a piece of poetry, but also because of its vivid and excellent descriptions of the appearance and virtues of medicinal plants. Table 2.2 lists the plants reported in the *Capitulare de villis* and in some other sources of the 10th and 11th centuries. Today, many

Table 2.2	Species of plants listed in the *Capitulare de villis*		
BOTANICAL NAME	**FAMILY**	**ENGLISH NAME**	**GEOGRAPHICAL ORIGIN**
Achillea millefolium[a,b]	Asteraceae	Milfoil	Northern hemisphere
Agrimonia eupatoria[a,b]	Rosaceae	Agrimony	Europe, south-eastern Asia
Allium ascalonicum	Alliaceae	Shallot	Western Asia
Allium cepa	Alliaceae	Onion	Western Persia
Allium porrum (?)	Alliaceae	Leek	Western Mediterranean
Allium sativum	Alliaceae	Garlic	South-eastern Asia
Allium schoenoprasum	Alliaceae	Chives	Southern Europe
Althea officinalis	Malvaceae	Marsh mallow	Eastern Mediterranean
Anethum graveolens	Apiaceae	Dill	Western Asia, southern Europe
Anthriscus cerefolium[a]	Poaceae	Chervil	Western Asia, south-eastern Europe
Apium graveolens[a]	Apiaceae	Celery	Western Asia, southern Europe
Artemisia abrotanum[a]	Asteraceae	Southernwood, old man	Eastern Europe, western Asia
Artemisia absinthium[a,b]	Asteraceae	Wormwood	Europe, Asia
Beta vulgaris	Chenopodiaceae	Beetroot	Mediterranean and Atlantic Coast
Betonica officinalis (Stachys officinalis)[a,b]	Lamiaceae	Betonica	Western Europe, Mediterranean
Brassica oleracea	Brassicaceae	Kale, borecole	Mediterranean and Atlantic Coast
Brassica oleracea var. gongyloides	Brassicaceae	Kohlrabi	Mediterranean and Atlantic Coast
Castanea sativa	Fagaceae	Sweet chestnut	Southern Europe, Africa, south-eastern Asia
Chrysathemum balsamita[a]	Asteraceae	Balsamite, costmary	South-eastern Europe
Chrysanthemum vulgare	Asteraceae	Tansy	Europe, Caucasus
Cichorium intybus	Asteraceae	Chicory	Europe, Asia
Coriandrum sativum	Apiaceae	Coriander	Orient
Corylus avellana	Betulaceae	Hazel	Europe, Asia
Cucumis melo[a]	Cucurbitaceae	Melon	Africa, southern Asia
Cucumis sativus	Cucurbitaceae	Cucumber	Western India
Cuminum cyminum	Apiaceae	Cumin	Turkey, eastern Europe
Cydonia oblonga	Rosaceae	Quince	Western Asia
Ficus carica	Moraceae	Fig	Western Mediterranean
Foeniculum vulgare[a]	Apiacae	Fennel	Mediterranean
Iris germanica[a]	Iridaceae	Iris	South-eastern Europe
Juglans regia	Juglandaceae	European walnut	Western Asia, eastern Europe
Juniperus sabina	Juniperaceae	Juniper	Alps, southern Europe
Lactuca sativa	Asteraceae	Lettuce	Western Asia, southern Europe
Lagenaria siceraria[a]	Cucurbitaceae	Calabash, bottle gourd	Africa, Asia (America)
Laurus nobilis	Lauraceae	(Bay) laurel	South-eastern Europe, south-western Asia
Lepidium sativum	Brassicaceae	Pepperwort	Orient
Levisticum officinale[a]	Apiaceae	Lovage	Persia/Iran
Lilium candidum[a]	Liliaceae	Lily	Western Asia
Malus communis	Rosaceae	Apple	Europe, western Asia
Malva neglecta	Malvaceae	Mallow	Europe, Asia
Marrubium vulgare[a,b]	Lamiaceae	Horehound	Mediterranean

Continued

Table 2.2	Species of plants listed in the *Capitulare de villis*—cont'd		
BOTANICAL NAME	**FAMILY**	**ENGLISH NAME**	**GEOGRAPHICAL ORIGIN**
Mentha crispa	Lamiaceae	True spearmint	Mediterranean
Mentha pulegium[a]	Lamiaceae	Pennyroyal	Mediterranean
Mentha spp.[a]	Lamiaceae	Mint	Southern Europe, Mediterranean
Mespilus germanica	Rosaceae	Medlar	South-eastern Europe, western Asia
Morus nigra	Moraceae	Mulberries	Western Asia
Nepeta cataria[a]	Lamiaceae	Catnip	Eastern Mediterranean
Nigella sativa	Ranunculaceae	Nigella, black cumin	Western Asia, southern Europe
Papaver somniferum[a]	Papaveraceae	Opium poppy	Mediterranean
Pastinaca sativa	Apiaceae	Parsnip	Europe, Caucasus
Petroselinum crispum	Apiaceae	Parsley	South-eastern Europe, western Asia
Prunus avium/P. cerasus	Rosaceae	Wild cherry, mazzard	Europe, Asia, Persia
Prunus domestica	Rosaceae	Plum	Western Asia
Prunus amygdalus (= P. dulcis)	Rosaceae	(Sweet) almond	Western Asia
Prunus persica	Rosaceae	Peach	China
Pyrus communis	Rosaceae	Pear	Central and southern Europe, south-western Asia
Raphanus sativus[a]	Brassicaceae	Radish	Western Asia
Rosa gallica[a]	Rosaceae	French rose	Southern Europe
Rosmarinus officinalis	Lamiaceae	Rosemary	Mediterranean
Ruta graveolens[a]	Rutaceae	Rue	South-eastern Europe
Salvia officinalis[a]	Lamiaceae	Sage	South-eastern Europe, Mediterranean
Salvia sclarea[a]	Lamiaceae	Clary (sage)	Mediterranean
Satureja hortensis	Lamiaceae	Summer savoury	Western Mediterranean
Sorbus domestica	Rosaceae	Service tree	Central and southern Europe, south-western Asia
Trigonella foenum-graecum[a]	Fabaceae	Fenugreek	Mesopotamia
Vigna sinensis	Fabaceae	Cow pea, cow bean	Central Africa

[a]Species listed by Walahfried Strabo in his *Hortulus* (information based on Vogellehner [1987]).
[b]Not in the *Capitulare de villis* but in other sources from the period.

of these plants are still important medicinally or in other ways. Many are vegetables, fruits or other foods. The list shows not only the long tradition of medicinal plant use in Europe, but also the importance of these resources to the state and religious powers during the Middle Ages. Although these were not necessarily of interest as scholarly writings, they were at least a practical resource.

A plan (which was not executed) for a medicinal herb garden for the Cloister of St Galls (Switzerland), dating from the year 820, has been preserved and gives an account of the species that were to be grown in a cloister garden. In general, pharmacy and medicine were of minor importance in the European scholastic traditions, as shown for example by the fact that in the Monastery of St Gall there were only six books on medicine, but 1000 on theology. Scholastic traditions, influenced by Greek–Arab medicine and philosophy, were practised in numerous European cloisters. In Arab-dominated Sicily, the first medical centre of medieval Europe was developed in Salerno (12th century). Until 1130, before the Council of Clermont, the monks combined medical and theological work, but after this date only lay members of the monastery were permitted to practise medicine. Simultaneously, the first universities (Paris 1110, Bologna 1113, Oxford 1167, Montpellier 1181, Prague 1348) were founded which provided training in medicine.

The climax of medieval medico-botanical literature was reached in the 11th century with *De viribus herbarum* ('On the virtues of herbs') and *Macer floridus*, a Latin poem from around 1070 AD, presumed to be by Odo of Meune (Magdunensis), the Abbot of Beauprai. In this educational poem, 65 medicinal plants and spices are presented. Other frequently cited sources are the descriptions of the medical virtues of plants by the Benedictine nun, early mysticist and abbess Hildegard of Bingen (1098–1179). In her works *Physica* and *Causae et curae* she included many remedies that were popularly used during the 12th century. Her writings also focus on prophetic and mystical topics. The works of both scholars are only available as later copies in other texts, which unfortunately give a rather distorted idea of the originals, as they are heavily re-interpreted.

PRINTED REPORTS IN THE EUROPEAN TRADITION (16TH CENTURY)

For over 1500 years the classical and most influential book in Europe had been Dioscorides' *De materia medica*. Until the Europeans' (re-)invention of printing in the mid-15th century (by Gutenberg), texts were hand-written codices, which were used almost exclusively by the clergy and scholars in monasteries. A wider distribution of the information on medicinal plants in Europe began with the early herbals, which rapidly became very popular and which made the information about medicinal plants available in the languages of lay people. These were still strongly influenced by Graeco-Roman concepts, but influences from many other sources came in during the 16th century (see Table 2.3).

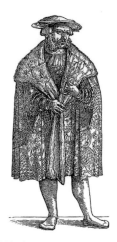

Fig. 2.3 Leonhard Fuchs. *Reproduced with permission from The University Library, Tübingen.*

Table 2.3	Examples of early European herbals from the 15th and 16th centuries (based on Leibrock-Plehn 1992 and Arber 1938)		

YEAR	AUTHOR	TITLE	LANGUAGE
1478	Dioscorides	De materia medica	Latin
1481	Anon.	The Latin Herbarius	Latin
1485	Anon.	The German Herbarius (*Gart der Gesundheit*)	German
1525	Anon.	Herball (*Rycharde Banckes' Herball*)	English
1526 (ca.)	Anon.	*Le grand herbier en francoys*	French
1530	Otto Brunfels	*Herbarium vivae eicones ad naturae imitationem*	Latin
1530–1574	Nicolás Monardes	*Historia medicinal de las cosas que se traen de nuestras Indias Occidentales que sirven en medicina*	Spanish
1532	Otto Brunfels	*Contrafayt Kreüterbuch*	German
1533	Eucharius Rösslin/Adam Lonitzer	*Kreüterbuch von allen Erdtgewächs*	German
1534	Various	*Ogrod zdrowia* ('The garden of health')	Polish
1541	Conradus Gesnerus	*Historia plantarum et vires ex Dioscorides*	Latin
1542	Leonhard Fuchs (Fig. 2.3)	*De historia stirpium commentarii insignes*	Latin
1543	Leonhard Fuchs	*New Kreüterbch*	German
1546	Hieronymus Bock	*Kreüterbuch*	German
1546	Dioskorides	*Kreüter Buch* (translated by J Dantzen von Ast)	German
1548	William Turner	*Libellus de re herbaria novus, in quo herbarium*	Latin
1554	Remibertus Dodonaeus	*Cruÿterboeck*	Flemish
1554	Pietro A Mattioli	*Commentarii, in libros sex pedacii Dioscoridis Anazarbi*	Latin/Italian
1560 (ca.)	(Pseudo) Albertus Magnus	*Ein neuer Albert Magnus*	German
1563	Garcia ab Horto (Orto/d'Orta)	*Orto/coloquios dos simples, e drogas he cousas medicinais da India* (Portuguese d'Orta; first published in Goa, India)	Portuguese
1576	Carolus Clusius	*Rariorum aliquot stirpium per hispanias observatum historia*	Latin
1588	Jakob Theodor (Tabernae montanus)	*Neuw Kreüterbuch*	German
1596	Casparus Bauhinus	*Phytopinax*	Latin
1596	John Gerard	*General historie of plantes* (or The 'Herball')	English
1597	Antoine Constantin	*Brief traicté de la pharmacie provinciale...*	French

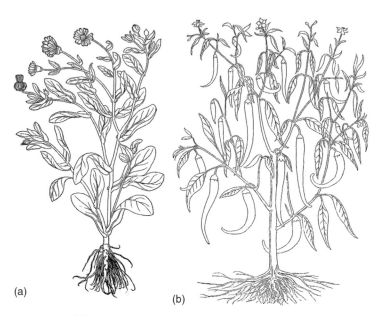

(a)

(b)

Fig. 2.4 Examples of early woodcuts: (a) marigold or Ringelblume (*Calendula officinalis*), one of the most important medicinal plants in historical and modern phytotherapy; (b) capsicum (chilli pepper; *Capsicum frutescens*). *Reproduced with permission from The University Library, Tübingen.*

Herbals were rapidly becoming available in various European languages and, in fact, many later authors copied, translated and re-interpreted the earlier books. This was especially so for the woodcuts used for illustration (see Fig. 2.4); these were often used in several editions or were copied. The herbals changed the role of European pharmacy and medicine and influenced contemporary orally transmitted popular medicine. Previously there had been two lines of practice: the herbal traditions of the monasteries and the popular tradition, which remains practically unknown. Books in European languages made scholastic information much more widely available and it seems that the literate population was eager to learn about these medicopharmaceutical practices. These new books became the driving force of European 'phytotherapy', which developed rapidly over the next centuries.

The trade in botanical drugs increased during this period. From the East Indies came nutmeg (*Myristica fragrans*, Myristicaceae), already used by the Greeks as an aromatic and for treating gastrointestinal problems. Rhubarb (*Rheum palmatum* and *Rh. officinale*, Polygonaceae) arrived in Europe from India in the 10th century and was employed as a strong purgative. Another important change at this time was the discovery of healing plants with new properties, during the exploration and conquest of

the 'New Worlds' – the Americas, as well as some regions of Asia and Africa. For example, 'guayacán' (*Guaiacum sanctum*, Zygophyllaceae), from Meso-America, was used against syphilis, despite its lack of any relevant pharmacological effects.

Nicolás Monardes was particularly important in the dissemination of knowledge about medicinal plants from the New World. His principal work, *Historia medicinal de las cosas que se traen de nuestras Indias Occidentales que sirven en medicina* ('Medical history of all those things which are brought from our Western India and may be used as medicines') was published in 1574. Some parts had appeared as early as ca. 1530. Another influential scholar during this period was Theophrastus Bombastus of Hohenheim, better known as Paracelsus (1493–1541). His importance lies less in the written record he left but more in his medical and pharmaceutical inventions and concepts. He rejected the established medical system and, after a fierce fight with the medical faculty of Basel in 1528, fled to Salzburg. According to some sources, he had publicly burned the 'Canon of medicine' by Avicenna. He introduced minerals into medical practice and called for the extraction of the active principle from animals, plants or minerals, a goal that was not achieved until the beginning of the 19th century (see below). He regarded the human body as a 'microcosm', with its substances and powers needing to be brought into harmony with the 'macrocosm' or universe. According to Paracelsus, healing was due to 'the power of life, which is only supported by the medical doctor and the medicine'. Although some of his ideas anticipated later ones, at the time they were largely rejected. The first pharmacopoeias were issued by autonomous cities, and became legally binding documents on the composition, preparation and storage of pharmaceuticals.

THE FIRST PHARMACOPOEIAS

- *Ricettario Fiorentino* (Florence, Italy), 1498.
- *Pharmacopoeia of Nuremberg* (Frankonia, Germany) or *Pharmacorum omnium*, 1546.
- *Pharmacopoeia Londiniensis* (UK), 1618, one of the most influential early pharmaceutical treatises.

These pharmacopoeias were mainly intended to bring some order to the many forms of preparation available at the time and the varying composition of medicines, and to reduce the problems arising out of their variability.

Another development was the establishment of independent guilds specializing in the sale of medicinal plants, even though apothecaries had practised this for centuries. In 1617, the Worshipful Society of Apothecaries was founded in London, and in 1673 it formed its own garden of medicinal plants, known today as the Chelsea Physic Garden (Minter 2000). One of the most well-known English apothecaries (and astrologers) of the 17th century is Nicholas Culpeper (1616–1654), best known for his 'English physician' – more commonly called 'Culpeper's herbal'. This is the only herbal that rivals in popularity John Gerard's *General historie of plantes*, but his arrogant dismissal of orthodox practitioners made him very unpopular with many physicians. Culpeper describes plants that grow in Britain and which can be used to cure a person or to 'preserve one's body in health'. He is also known for his translation *A physicall directory* (from Latin into English) of the London Pharmacopoeia of 1618 published in 1649 (Arber 1938).

MEDICAL HERBALISM

The use of medicinal plants was always an important part of the medical systems of the world, and Europe was no exception. Little is known about

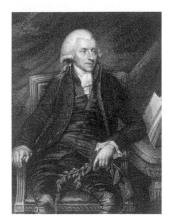

Fig. 2.5 William Withering. *Reproduced with permission from The Wellcome Library, London.*

popular traditions in medieval and early modern Europe and our knowledge starts with the availability of written (printed) records on medicinal plant use by common people. As pointed out by Griggs (1981, p. 88), a woman in the 17th century was a 'superwoman' capable of administering 'any wholesome receipts or medicines for the good of the family's health'. A typical example of such a remedy is foxglove (*Digitalis purpurea*), reportedly used by an English housewife to treat dropsy, and then more systematically by the physician William Withering (1741–1799; Fig. 2.5). Withering transformed the orally transmitted knowledge of British herbalism into a form of medicine that could be used by medical doctors. Prior to that, herbalism was more of a clinical practice interested in the patient's welfare, and less of a systematic study of the virtues and chemical properties of medicinal plants.

EUROPEAN PHARMACOGNOSY AND NATURAL PRODUCT CHEMISTRY IN THE 18TH AND 19TH CENTURIES

In the 17th and 18th centuries, knowledge about plant-derived drugs expanded, but all attempts to 'distillate' the active ingredients from plants were unsuccessful. The main outcome during this period was detailed observations on the clinical usefulness of medicinal products, which had been recorded in previous centuries or imported from non-European countries. The next main shift in emphasis came in the early 19th century when it became clear that the pharmaceutical properties of plants are due to specific molecules that can be isolated and characterized. This led to the development of a field of

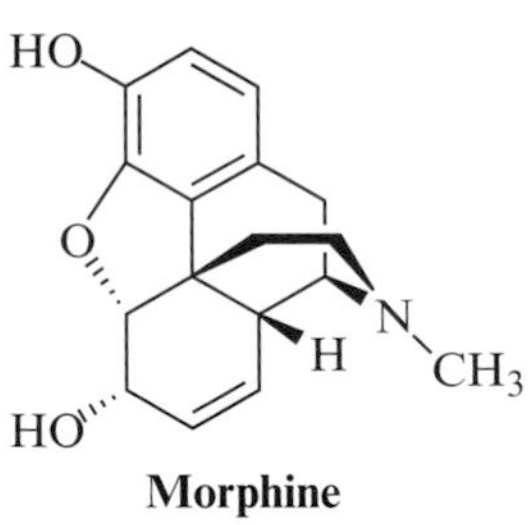

Morphine

Fig. 2.6

Quinine

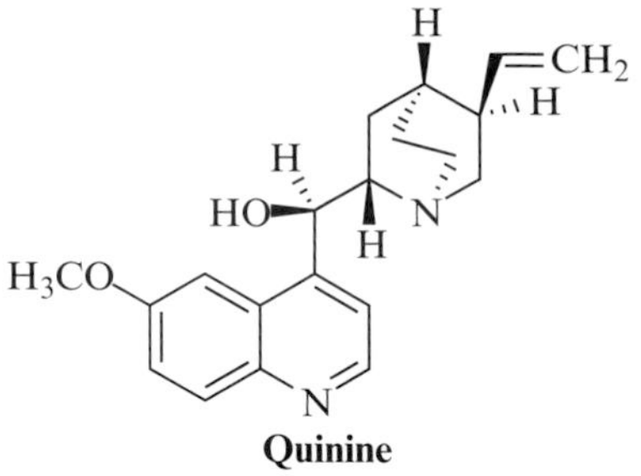

Fig. 2.8

research now called **natural product chemistry** or, specifically for plants, **phytochemistry**. Pure chemical entities were isolated and their structures elucidated. Some were then developed into medicines or chemically modified for medicinal use. Examples of such early pure drugs include:

● **morphine** (Fig. 2.6) from opium poppy (*Papaver somniferum*, Papaveraceae), which was first identified by FW Sertürner of Germany (Fig. 2.7) in 1804 and chemically characterized in 1817 as an alkaloid. The full structure was established in 1923, by JM Gulland and R Robinson, in Manchester

● **quinine** (Fig. 2.8), from cinchona bark (*Cinchona succirubra* and others), was first isolated by Pierre Joseph Pelletier and Joseph Bienaime Caventou

of France in 1820; the structure was elucidated in the 1880s by various laboratories. Pelletier and Caventou were also instrumental in isolating many of the alkaloids mentioned below

● **salicin**, from willow bark (*Salix* spp., Salicaceae), was first isolated by Johannes Buchner in Germany. It was derivatized first (in 1838) by Rafaele Pirea (France) to yield salicylic acid, and later (1899) by the Bayer company, to yield acetylsalicylic acid, or **aspirin** – a compound that was previously known but which had not been exploited pharmaceutically (Fig. 2.9).

EXAMPLES OF PURE COMPOUNDS ISOLATED DURING THE EARLY 19TH CENTURY

Atropine (1833), from belladonna (*Atropa belladonna*, Solanaceae), was used at the time for asthma.

Caffeine (1821), from the coffee shrub (*Coffea arabica* and *C. canephora*, Rubiaceae); its structure was elucidated in 1882.

Coniine, a highly poisonous natural product, was first isolated in 1826 from hemlock (*Conium maculatum*, Apiaceae). Its properties had been known for years (Socrates used hemlock to commit suicide) and it was the first alkaloid to have its structure elucidated (1870). Some years later it was synthesized (1889).

Emetine (1817), from ipecacuanha (*Cephaelis ipecacuanha*, Rubiaceae), was fully characterized as late as 1948 and used as an emetic as well as in cough medications.

Strychnine (1817), from *Strychnos* spp. (Loganiaceae), was used as a tonic and stimulant (Sneader 1996).

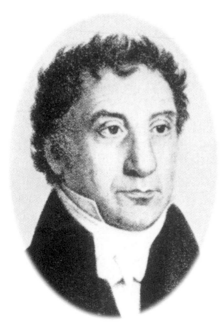

Fig. 2.7 FW Sertürner. *Reproduced with permission from The Wood Library-Museum of Anesthesiology, Park Ridge, IL, London.*

Also, early in the 19th century, the term 'pharmacognosy' was coined by the Austrian professor Johann Adam Schmidt (1759–1809) and was included in his

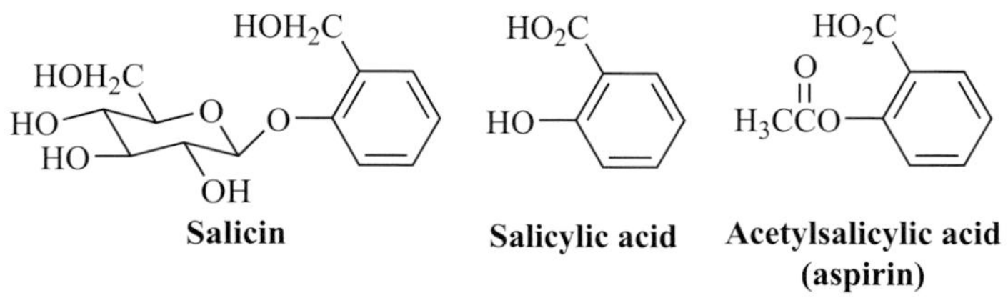

Salicin   **Salicylic acid**   **Acetylsalicylic acid (aspirin)**

Fig. 2.9

posthumously published book *Lehrbuch der Materia Medica* (1811). This period thus saw the development of a well-defined scientific field of inquiry, which developed rapidly during the century.

One of the main achievements of 19th century science in the field of medicinal plants was the development of methods to study the pharmacological effects of compounds and extracts. The French physiologist Claude Bernard (1813–1878), who conducted detailed studies on the pharmacological effects of plant extracts, must be considered one of the first scientists in this tradition. He was particularly interested in curare – a drug and arrow poison used by the American Indians of the Amazon, and the focus of research of many explorers. The ethnobotanical story of curare is described further in Chapter 5.

Bernard noted that, if curare was administered into living tissue directly, via an arrow or a poisoned instrument, it resulted in death more quickly, and that death occurred more rapidly if dissolved curare was used rather than the dried toxin (Bernard 1966: 95–96). He was also able to demonstrate that the main cause of death was by muscular paralysis, and that animals showed no signs of nervousness or pain. Further investigations showed that, if the blood flow in the hind leg of a frog was interrupted using a ligature (without affecting the innervation) and the curare was introduced via an injury of that limb, the limb retained mobility and the animal did not die [Bernard 1966:95–96, 115 (orig. 1864)]. One of the facts noted by all those who reported on curare is the lack of toxicity of the poison in the gastrointestinal tract, and, indeed, the Indians used curare both as a poison and as a remedy for the stomach.

Bernard went on to say:

In our physiological studies we were able to identify the effect of the American arrow poison curare as one on the nervous motoric element and subsequently to determine a mechanism which results in death, which is an inert ability of this poisoned substance, but do we have to stop

here and have we reached the border which our current [19th century] science allows us to reach? I do not think so. One has to separate the active principle of curare from the foreign substances, with which it is mixed, and one also has to study which physical and chemical changes the toxic substance imprints onto the organic element [i.e. the body] in order to paralyse its activity.

[Bernard 1966:121 (orig. 1864), translation MH]

Later, the botanical source of curare was identified as *Chondrodendron tomentosum* Ruiz et Pavon, and the agent largely responsible for the pharmacological activity first isolated. It was found to be an alkaloid, and named D-tubocurarine because of its source, 'tube curare', so-called because of the bamboo tubes used as storage containers. In 1947 the structure of this complex alkaloid, a bisbenzylisoquinoline, was finally established (Fig. 2.10). The story of this poison is one of the most fascinating examples of transforming a drug used in an indigenous culture into a medication and research tool, and, although D-tubocurarine is now used less frequently for muscular relaxation during surgery, it has been used as a template for the development of newer and better drugs.

The 19th century thus saw the integration of ethnobotanical, pharmacological and phytochemical studies, a process that had taken many decades

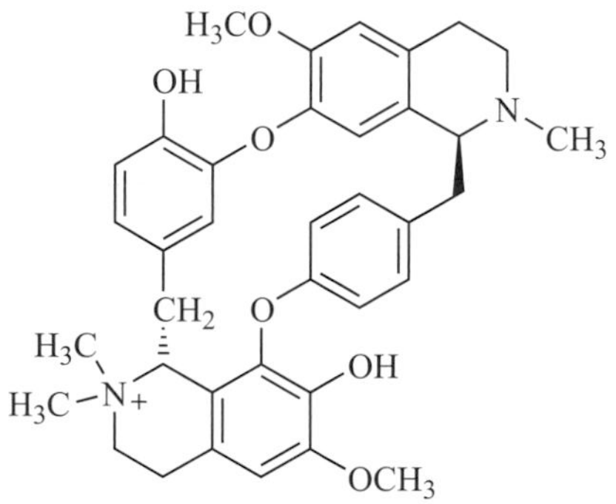

Tubocurarine

Fig. 2.10

but which allowed the development of a new approach to the study and the pharmaceutical use of plants. Ultimately, herbal remedies became transformed into chemically defined drugs.

THE 20TH CENTURY

One of the most important events that influenced the use of medicinal plants in the Western world in the last century was the serendipitous discovery of the antibacterial properties of fungal metabolites such as benzylpenicillin, by Florey and Fleming in 1928 at St Mary's Hospital (London). These natural products changed forever the perception and use of plant-derived metabolites as medicines by both scientists and the lay public. Another important development came with the advent of synthetic chemistry in the field of pharmacy. Many of these studies involved compounds that were synthesized because of their potential as colouring material (Sneader 1996). The first successful use of a synthetic compound as a chemotherapeutic agent was achieved by Paul Ehrlich in Germany (1854–1915); he successfully used methylene blue in the treatment of mild forms of malaria in 1891. Unfortunately, this finding could not be extended to the more severe forms of malaria common in the tropics. Many further studies on the therapeutic properties of dyes and of other synthetic compounds followed.

The latter part of the 20th century saw a rapid expansion in knowledge of secondary natural products, their biosynthesis, and their biological and pharmacological effects. A large number of natural products or their derivatives were introduced as medicines, including many anti-cancer agents (paclitaxol, the vinca alkaloids; see Chapter 6, pp. 103), the anti-malarial agent artemisinin and the anti-dementia medication galanthamine, to name just a few (Cragg et al 2005, Heinrich 2010, Heinrich & Teoh 2004). Numerous examples of drugs which are natural products, their deriviates or a pharmacophore based on a natural product have been introduced. There is now a better understanding of the genetic basis of the reactions that give rise to such compounds, as well as the biochemical (and in many cases genetic) basis of many important illnesses. This has opened up new opportunities and avenues for drug development.

References

Arber, A., 1938. Herbals. Their origin and evolution. A chapter in the history of botany 1470–1670. Cambridge University Press, Cambridge.

Bernard, C., 1966. Physiologische Untersuchungen über einige amerikanische Gifte. Das Curare. In: Bernard, C., Mani, N. (Eds.), Ausgewählte physiologische Schriften, Huber Verlag, Bern, pp. 84–133. (orig. French 1864).

Bernard, C. 1966. Physiologische Untersuchungen über einigeamerikanische Gifte. Das Curare. Bernard, C. und N. Mani (Übs.) Ausgewählte physiologische Schriften. Huber Verlag. Bern. (frz. orig. 1864) S. 84-133.

Beers, S.-J., 2001. Jamu. The ancient art of Indonesian herbal healing. Periplus Editions (HK) Ltd, Singapore Burger A, Wachter H 1998 Hunnius pharmazeutisches Wörterbuch, 8 Aufl. Walter de Gruyter, Berlin.

Capasso, L., 1998. 5300 years ago, the ice man used natural laxatives and antibiotics. Lancet 352, 1894.

Cragg, G.M., Newman, D.J., 2005. Plants as a source of anti-cancer agents. J. Ethnopharmacol 100, 72–79.

Griggs, B., 1981. Green pharmacy. A history of herbal medicine. Norman & Hobhouse, London.

Heinrich, M., 2010. Ethnopharmacology and drug development. In: Mander, L., Lui, H.W. (Eds.), Comprehensive natural products II Chemistry and biology, vol. 3. Elsevier, Oxford, pp. 351–381.

Heinrich, M., Teoh, H.L., 2004. Galanthamine from snowdrop – the development of a modern drug against Alzheimer's disease from local Caucasian knowledge. J. Ethnopharmacol. 92, 147–162.

Leibrock-Plehn, L., 1992. Hexenkräuter oder Arznei: die Abtreibungsmittel im 16 und 17 Jahrhundert. Heidelberger Schriften zur Pharmazie- und Naturwissenschaftsgeschichte, Bd 6. Wissenschaftliche Verlagsgesellschaft, Stuttgart.

Leroi-Gourhan, A., 1975. The flowers found with Shanidar IV, a Neanderthal burial in Iraq. Science 190, 562–564.

Lietava, J., 1992. Medicinal plants in a Middle Paleolithic grave Shanidar IV. J. Ethnopharmacol. 35, 263–266.

Mazar, G., 1998. Ayurvedische Phytotherapie in Indien. Z. Physiother. 19, 269–274.

Minter, S., 2000. The Apothecaries' Garden. Sutton Publications, Stroud.

Solecki, R.S., 1975. Shanidar IV, a Neanderthal flower burial in Northern Iraq. Science 190, 880–881.

Sneader, W., 1996. Drug prototypes and their exploitation. Wiley, Chichester.

Sommer, J.D., 1999. The Shanidar IV 'flower burial': a re-evaluation of Neanderthal burial ritual. Cambridge Archaeological Journal 9 (1), 127–137.

Takemi, T., Hasegawa, M., Kumagai, A., Otsuka, Y., 1985. Herbal medicine: Kampo, past and present. Tsumura Juntendo Inc., Tokyo.

Vogellehner, D., 1987. Jardines et verges en Europe occidentale (VIII–XVIII siècles). Flaran 9, 11–40.

Waller, F., 1998. Phytotherapie der traditionellen chinesischen Medizin. Z. Physiother. 19, 77–89.

Further reading

Adams, M., Caroline Berset, C., Kessler, M., Hamburger, M., 2009. Medicinal herbs for the treatment of rheumatic disorders—A survey of European herbals from the 16th and 17th century. J. Ethnopharmacol. 121, 343–359.

von Humboldt, A. (Beck H, Hrsg.), 1997. Die Forschungsreise in den Tropen Amerikas [Studienausgabe Bd 2, Teilband 3]. Wissenschaftliche Buchgesellschaft, Darmstadt.

Section 2

Basic plant biology

SECTION CONTENTS

Chapter 3

General principles of botany: morphology and systematics

The chapters in this section provide a short introduction to the bioscientific basis for all aspects of the use of plants in pharmacy required for understanding herbal medicines and pure natural products.

The following case study shows that knowledge about medicinal plants is not only relevant, because pharmacy uses many pure natural products derived from plants, but also that pharmacists can and should advise patients about common medicinal plants.

A (HYPOTHETICAL) CASE STUDY BASED ON G HATFIELD'S RESEARCH ABOUT THE USAGE OF MEDICINAL PLANTS IN NORFOLK

While you are working as a locum pharmacist, a patient informs you that his general practitioner is worried about unexplained low levels of potassium (hypokalaemia). Among other things, the patient is complaining of chronic constipation and requests several pharmaceuticals. He also reports that he uses a 'herbal tea', which he prepares from the plant he calls 'pick-a-cheese' and grows in his back garden. This tea helps him to overcome the problem of constipation.

How do you react? Is the patient using a little known, but unproblematic, herbal product? Further inquiry about the case gives you the following information:

- 'Pick-a-cheese' may be a widely distributed garden plant and weed known also as 'common mallow' which has the botanical name of *Malva sylvestris* or it may be some other botanical species known under the same common name.

- Upon your request the patient brings you a branch of the plant and with the help of the scientific (botanical) literature you make a positive identification of this plant as *Malva sylvestris*. The identification is based on the features of the plant (leaves, fruit, flowers) that you are able to observe.

- In checking the active constituents (especially polysaccharides) you come to the conclusion that the plant is unlikely to contribute to the symptoms as they were reported by the patient. The plant is widely used as a local food item (also, for example, in Mediterranean France) and as a household remedy. Toxic natural products seem to be absent. Therefore, the search for a cause of the hypokalaemia continues. . .

[For further information on Norfolk country remedies readers are referred to Hatfield G 1994 Country remedies. The Boydell Press, Woodbridge.]

PLANTS AND DRUGS

Pharmacognosy is the study of medical products derived from our living environment; especially those derived from plants and fungi. From the botanical point of view, the first concern is how to define a pharmaceutical (or medical) plant-derived drug.

In the context of pharmacy a botanical drug is a product that is either:

- derived from a plant and transformed into a drug by drying certain plant parts, or sometimes the whole plant, or

- obtained from a plant, but no longer retains the structure of the plant or its organs and contains a complex mixture of biogenic compounds (e.g. fatty and essential oils, gums, resins, balms).

The term 'drug' is linguistically related to 'dry' and is presumably derived from the Middle Low German *droge* ('dry').

Isolated pure natural products such as the numerous pharmaceuticals used in pharmacy are thus not 'botanical drugs', but rather chemically defined drugs derived from nature. Botanical drugs are generally derived from specific plant organs of a plant species. The following plant organs are the most important, with the Latin name that is used, for example in international trade, in parentheses:

- Aerial parts or herb (herba).
- Leaf (folia).
- Flower (flos).
- Fruit (fructus).
- Bark (cortex).
- Root (radix).
- Rhizome (rhizoma).
- Bulb (bulbus).

The large majority of botanical drugs in current use are derived from leaves or aerial parts.

Botanically speaking, a plant-derived drug should be defined not only in terms of the species from which it is obtained but also the plant part that is used to produce the dried product. Thus, a drug is considered to be adulterated if the wrong plant parts are included (e.g. aerial parts instead of leaves).

In the following sections of this chapter a brief overview of botanical taxonomy is given; then the higher plants are discussed on the basis of their main organs, function, morphology and anatomy. Since most of the pharmaceutical products derived from plants are from the higher plants (or Magnoliopsida), little reference is made here to other plants such as lichens, mosses, algae, or to mushrooms or micro-organisms.

Microscopic characteristics play an important role in identifying a botanical drug. Although microscopy is now only rarely used in everyday pharmaceutical practice, there are a large number of features that allow the identification of botanical material. Since classical textbooks provide an extensive description of such features, microscopic identification is only occasionally discussed in this introductory work.

These days, drug identification is achieved using a combination of methods, including thin-layer chromatography, high-performance liquid chromatography and microscopic methods. In large (phyto-)pharmaceutical companies, near-infrared spectroscopy has become an essential tool.

TAXONOMY

The **species** is the principal unit within the study of **systematics**. Biological diversity is subdivided into >500,000 discontinuous units (the botanical species) and >2 million zoological species. The species is thus the basic unit for studying relationships among living organisms. Systematicists study the relationships between species.

Taxonomy is the science of naming organisms and their correct integration into the existing system of nomenclature. Each of these names is called a **taxon** (pl. taxa), which thus stands for any named taxonomic unit. In order to make this diversity easier to understand, it is structured into a series of highly hierarchical categories, which ideally should represent the natural relationship between all the taxa.

EXAMPLE OF BOTANICAL CLASSIFICATION

The opium poppy, *Papaver somniferum* L.

Binomial: this is the genus and species names, plus the authority. Thus, in this example, *Papaver somniferum* is the binomial (the basic unit of taxonomy and systematics). It is followed by a short acronym (in this case 'L.'), which indicates the botanist who provided the first scientific description of the species and who assigned the botanical name [in this example, 'L.' stands for Carl von Linnaeus (or Linné), a Swedish botanist (1707–1778) who developed the binomial nomenclature].*

Species: *somniferum*, here meaning 'sleep-producing'.

Genus: *Papaver* (a group of species, in this case poppies, which are closely related).

Family: Papaveraceae (a group of genera sharing certain traits, named after one of the genera).

Order: Papaverales.

Class: Magnoliatae.

Subphylum: Magnoliphytina (seed-bearing plants with covered seeds).

Division (=Phylum): Spermatophyta (seed-bearing plants).

Kingdom: Plantae (the plants), one of three kingdoms, the others being the animals and fungi.

*In some cases, there is first a name in parentheses, followed by a second name not in parentheses. For example, in the case of the common aloe, *Aloe vera* (L.) Burm. f., the name in parentheses indicates the author (Linnaeus) who first described the species but assigned it to a different genus. The second name in this case, Burm. f., stands for the 18th century botanist Nicolaas Laurens Burman; f. stands for *filius* (son), since he is the son of another well-known botanist who provided numerous first descriptions of botanical species.

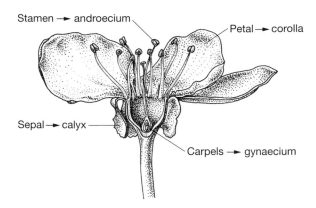

Fig. 3.1 Schematic line drawing of a flower.

A species is generally characterized as having morphologically similar members and being able to inbreed. Since Carl Linnaeus, the names of species are given in binomial form: the first part of the name indicates the wider taxonomic group, the **genus**; the second part of the name is the **species**. In order to better understand biological diversity, the species are arranged into clusters of varying degree of similarity, forming a hierarchy.

The basic classification of the plant kingdom into divisions circumscribes the main groups of plants, including the following:

- Algae, including the green algae (Chlorophyta) and the red algae (Rhodophyta)
- Mosses (Bryophyta)
- Ferns (Pteridophyta)
- Seed-bearing plants (Spermatophyta).

As mentioned above, only a few algae, mosses and ferns have yielded pharmaceutically important and will therefore only be discussed very cursorily.

THE IMPORTANCE OF TAXONOMY

The exact naming (taxonomy) and an understanding of the species' relationship to other species is an essential basis for pharmacognostical work. Only such endeavour allows the correct identification of a botanical drug, and consequently is the basis for further pharmacological, phytochemical, analytical or clinical studies.

MORPHOLOGY AND ANATOMY OF HIGHER PLANTS (SPERMATOPHYTA)

FLOWER

The flower (Fig. 3.1) is the essential reproductive organ of a plant. It is frequently very showy in order to attract pollinators, but in other instances the flowers are minute and difficult to distinguish from the neighbouring organs or from other flowers.

For an inexperienced observer, two characteristics of a flower are particularly noteworthy: the size and the colour. Although these are often good characteristics of a species, others aspects are more important from a botanical point of view.

Such characteristics include the form of the various parts of a flower, whether these parts are fused (joined) or separate (free), how many of each of these structures normally exist per flower, whether or not all flowers on a plant (or in a group of plants of the same species) are similar. Morphologically speaking, many parts of the flower are modified leaves, which during the development of higher plants have taken on specific functions for reproduction:

- The **calyx**, with individual sepals, generally serves as an outer protective cover during the budding stage of the flower. It is often greenish in colour, can be either fused or separate, and may sometimes drop off at the beginning of the flowering phase (e.g. *Chelidonium majus* L., greater celandine).
- The **corolla**, with individual petals, serves as an important element to attract the pollinator in animal-pollinated flowers. It is either fused or separate and may be very reduced, for example in plants pollinated with the help of the wind. Most commonly, the number of petals is regarded as a key feature and can vary from a well-defined number (e.g. four, five or six) to a large number that is no longer counted (written as ∞). The colour of the petals is not a good characteristic generally, since it may vary within a genus or even within a species. All of these features – i.e. the number and form of the petals, whether they

are fused or not and their size – are important information for identifying a plant.

- The **androecium**, with its individual **stamens** (also known as 'stamina') which produce the pollen, forms a ring around the innermost part of the flower. In some species, the anther is restricted to only some of the flowers on a plant (whereas the others only have a gynaecium). In other species, androecium-bearing flowers are restricted to some plants, whereas the others bear flowers with only a gynaecium. Again, their number is important for identifying a plant.
- **Gynaecium** (pl. gynaecia; also called gynoecium) with individual carpels. This develops into the fruit (i.e. the seed covered by the pericarp) and includes the ovules (the part of the fruit bearing the reproductive organs which develop into the seeds).
- The **stigma** and **style** – together with the gynaecium – form the **pistil**. Their size and form are important differences between species.

Another essential aspect of the flower's morphology is the position of the gynaecium with respect to the position of the corolla on the pistil: i.e. epigynous (the corolla and other elements of the flower are attached to or near the summit of the ovary), or hypogynous (the corolla and other elements of the flower are attached at or below the bottom of the ovary).

Inflorescences

The way in which flowers are arranged to form an inflorescence is another useful feature for recognizing (medicinal) plants, but this is beyond the scope of this introduction (see Heywood 1993).

Drugs

Although the flowers are of great botanical importance, they are only a minor source of drugs used in phytotherapy or pharmacy. A very important example is:

- chamomile, *Matricaria recutita* L. (Matricariase flos)

Other examples include:

- calendula, *Calendula officinalis* L. (Calendulae flos)
- arnica, *Arnica montana* L. (Arnicae flos)
- hops, *Humulus lupulus* L. (Humuli flos).

FRUIT AND SEED

The development of seeds occurred relatively late in the evolution of plants. The lower plants, such as algae, mosses and ferns, do not produce seeds. Gymnosperms such as the maiden hair tree (*Ginkgo biloba*) (see below) were the first group of organisms to produce seeds, from which the angiosperms or fruit-bearing plants evolved. The gymnosperms are characterized by seeds that are not covered by a secondary outer protective layer, but only by the testa – the seed's outer layer.

In the angiosperms, the ovule and, later, the seed are covered with a specialized organ (the carpels) which in turn develops into the pericarp (Fig. 3.2). This, the outer layer of the fruit, can either be hard as in nuts, all soft as in berries (dates, tomatoes), or hard and soft as in a drupe (cherry, olives). Drugs from the fruit thus have to be derived from an angiosperm species.

The morphology of a fruit provides important information as to the identity of a plant species or medicinal drug. Another distinction of fruits is based on the number of carpels and gynaecia per fruit, which may be:

- simple (developed from a single carpel)
- aggregate (several carpels of one gynaecium are united in one fruit, as in raspberries and strawberries)
- multiple (gynaecia of more than one flower form the fruit).

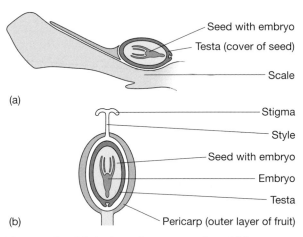

(a)

(b)

Fig. 3.2 Simplified schematic representation of (a) a gymnosperm seed sitting on a scale (as in a fir tree) and (b) an angiosperm fruit, covered by both the testa and the pericarp.

Drugs

Fruits and seeds have yielded important phytotherapeutic products, including:

Fruit
- Caraway, *Carum carvi* L. (Carvi fructus)
- Fennel, *Foeniculum vulgare* Miller (Foeniculi fructus)
- Saw palmetto, *Serenoa repens* (Bartram) Small (Sabal fructus)
- Schizandra/schisandra, *Schisandra chinensis* Baillon (Schisandrae fructus).

Seed
- (White) mustard, *Sinapis alba* L. (Sinapi semen)
- Horse chestnut seeds, *Aesculus hippocastanum* L. (Hippocastani semen)
- Ispaghula, *Plantago ovata* Forsskaol and *Plantago* spp. (Plantago ovatae semen), and psyllium, *Plantago afra* L. (=*P psyllium*, Psylli semen).

LEAVES

The leaves arise out of the stem; their key function is the assimilation of glucose and its derivative, starch, from water and carbon dioxide (photosynthesis) using energy provided by sunlight.

PHOTOSYNTHESIS

The net photosynthetic reaction is:

$$6CO_2 + 6H_2O \xrightarrow{hv} C_6H_{12}O_6 \text{ (glucose)} + 6O_2$$

This process is key, not only to the survival of all plants, but also in providing the energy and, ultimately, the basic building blocks for the secondary metabolites, which are used as pharmaceuticals.

The function of the leaves, as collectors of the sun's energy and its assimilation, results in their typical general anatomy with a petiole (stem) and a lamina (blade). In many cases, the petiole is reduced and may be missing completely. Plants have adapted to a multitude of environments and this adaptation is reflected in anatomical and morphological features of the leaf. For example, adaptation to dry conditions gives rise to leaves that conserve moisture, which may be fleshy or possess a thick cuticle. These are termed xerophytic leaves, and include oleander (*Nerium oleander* L.).

The lower surface of the leaf is generally covered with stomata, pores which are surrounded by specialized cells and which are responsible for the gaseous exchange between the plant and its environment (uptake of CO_2 and emission of water vapour and O_2).

The nodes (or 'knots') are the parts of the stem where the leaves and lateral buds join; the intermediate area is called the internodium. A key characteristic of a species is the way in which the leaves are arranged on the stem. For example, they may be (Fig. 3.3):

- **alternate**: the leaves form an alternate or helical pattern around the stem, also called spiral
- **distichous**: there is a single leaf at each node, and the leaves of two neighbouring nodes are disposed in opposite positions
- **opposite**: the leaves occur in pairs, with each leaf opposing the other at the nodes
- **decussate**: this is a special case of opposite, where each successive pair of leaves is at a right angle to the previous pair (typical for the mint family)
- **whorled**: three or more leaves are found at one node.

Another important characteristic is the form of the leaves. Typically, the main distinction is between simple or compound. Simple leaves have blades that are not divided into distinct morphologically separate leaflets, but form a single blade, which may be deeply lobed. In compound leaves, there are two or more leaflets, which often have their

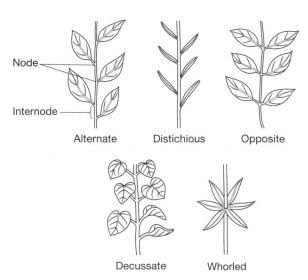

Fig. 3.3 Types of arrangements of leaves.

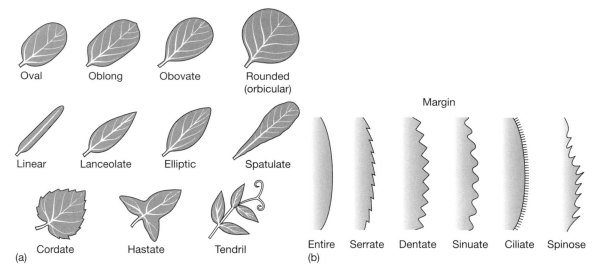

Fig. 3.4 (a) Characteristic shapes of leaves. (b) Characteristic margins of leaves.

own small petioles (called petiolules). The form and size of leaves are essential characteristics (Fig. 3.4a). For example, leaves may be described as oval, oblong, rounded, linear, lanceolate, ovate, obovate, spatulate or cordate. The margin of the leaf is another characteristic feature. It can be entire (smooth), serrate (sawtoothed), dentate (toothed), sinuate (wavy) or ciliate (hairy) (Fig. 3.4b). Also, the base and the apex often have a very characteristic form.

Microscopic characteristics of leaves include the form and number of stomata, the inner structure of the leaves, specialized secretory tissues including trichomes (glandular hairs), covering trichomes or bristles, and the presence of calcium oxalate structures which give a characteristic refractive pattern under polarized light.

The powdered leaves of several members of the nightshade family (Solanaceae), which yield some botanical drugs that are important for the industrial extraction of the alkaloid atropine, cannot be distinguished using normal chemical methods since they all contain similar alkaloids. On the other hand, they can easily be distinguished microscopically by the presence of different forms of crystals formed by the different species and deposited in the cells (see Fig. 3.5).

Drugs

Numerous drugs contain leaf material as the main component. Some widely used ones include the following:

- (Common) balm, *Melissa officinalis* L. (Melissae folium)
- Deadly nightshade, *Atropa belladonna* L. (Belladonnae folium) (and other solanaceous species).

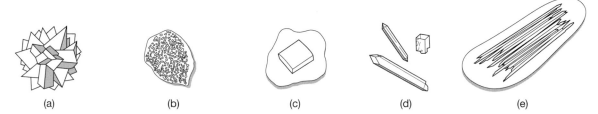

Fig. 3.5 Calcium oxalate crystals, main forms: (a) rosette (e.g. *Datura stramonium*, Solanaceae); (b) sand (e.g. *Atropa belladonna*, Solanaceae); (c) monoclinic prism (e.g. *Hyosyamus niger*, Solanaceae); (d) needles (e.g. *Iris germanica*, Iridaceae); (e) raphides (e.g. *Urginea maritima*, Hyacinthaceae).

(Deadly nightshade is not used, Belladonna and related Solanaceous plants are rarely used in Phytotherapy but rather for the extraction of alkaloids, of which they have a high content.)

- Ginkgo, *Ginkgo biloba* L. (Ginkgo folium)
- Green tea, *Camellia sinensis* (L.) Kuntze (Theae folium)
- Peppermint, *Mentha × piperita* L. (Menthae folium)
- (Red) bearberry, *Arctostaphylos uva-ursi* (L.) Sprengel (Uvae ursi folium).

SHOOTS (=STEM, LEAVES AND REPRODUCTIVE ORGANS)

An essential differentiation needs to be made between herbaceous ('herbs') and woody plants (trees and shrubs). In both cases, the function of the stem is to provide the physical strength required for positioning the leaves/flowers and fruit in the most adaptive way. The stem is a cylindrical organ which, together with the root, forms the main axis of a plant. Herbaceous species are generally short-lived and often grow rapidly and the distinction between the outside and the inner stem can only be made by detailed examination. Woody species, on the other hand, show a clear distinction between the bark and the (inner) wood.

In the stem, the transport of water and inorganic nutrients (upward transport) is achieved in the **xylem**, which only occurs in the inner parts of the stem and forms an essential part of the wood. The **phloem**, on the other hand, is the plant part responsible for the transport of assimilates (sugars and polysaccharides), which generally occurs from the leaves downwards. Between the wood and the bark is the cambium, the tissue that gives rise to new cells which then differentiate and form the outer (bark) and inner (wood) parts of a secondary stem. The fine structure of a bark or wood is an important diagnostic criterion for identifying a drug. The bark as an outer protective layer frequently accumulates biologically active substances; for example, several of the pharmaceutically important barks accumulate tannins.

Drugs: stem

Stem material is often part of those drugs that are derived from all above-ground parts (herb or herba). No stem-derived drug is currently of major importance. Some underground organs used as drugs (rhizome of tormentil) or food (potato) are in fact modified stems that have taken on specific new functions (storage, spreading of the plant) (see below).

Drugs: bark

- Frangula, *Rhamnus frangula* L. (syn. *Frangula alnus*) (Frangulae cortex)
- Red cinchona, *Cinchona succirubra* Weddell, *C. calisaya* Weddell (the main cultivated species in southern Asia) and *Cinchona* spp. (Cinchonae cortex)
- Oak, *Quercus petrea* (Mattuschka) Lieblein and *Qu. robur* L. (Quercus cortex)
- Willow, *Salix alba* L. and *Salix* spp. (Salicis cortex).

Drugs: aerial parts (=stem, leaves plus flowers/fruit)

- Ephedra, *Ephedra sinica* Stapf (Ephedra herba)
- Hawthorn, *Crataegus monogyna* Jacquin and *C. laevigata* (Poiret) DC. (syn. *C. oxycantha*) (Crataegi herba or Crataegi folium cum flore)
- Passion flower, *Passiflora incarnata* L. (Passiflora herba)
- Wormwood, *Artemisia absinthium* L. (Absinthii herba); in Africa and Asia, sweet or annual wormwood (*Artemisia annua* L.) is used in the treatment of malaria.

The substitution of leaves with aerial parts of the same species is a common problem with cheap phytopharmaceuticals used as 'health food supplements'. These adulterated drugs often contain fewer and/or other active constituents and this issue points to the need to define not only the species, but also the plant part to be used pharmaceutically.

ROOT

Three functions of a typical root are of particular importance to a plant:

- It provides an anchor in the ground or any other substrate and thus allows the development of the plant's above-ground organs (anchorage).
- It is the main organ for the uptake of water and inorganic nutrients (absorption and conduction).

- It often serves to store surplus energy, generally in the form of polysaccharides such as starch and inulin (storage).

The root is generally composed of an outer layer (the bark of the root including the hypodermis) and an inner cylinder, containing the xylem and the phloem. The two organs of the root are separated by the endodermis, an inner protective layer. Water and inorganic nutrients are transported upwards in the xylem; assimilates are transported in the phloem.

Very young plants have a primary root, which during development soon becomes thicker and adds layers of secondary tissue. It is the secondary roots – often roots or rootstocks with a special storage function – that are used in pharmacy.

ROOTSTOCK AND SPECIALIZED UNDERGROUND ORGANS

Some underground organs can be distinguished on botanical grounds from the root. Although they may have some functions similar to roots, botanically they are derived from other parts of the plants; they are therefore a separate group of plant organs and yield another group of botanical drugs. They include rhizomes and tubers (generally, both are morphologically a stem) and underground bulbs (morphologically derived from parts of the leaves).

Rhizome and root (radix) drugs

Underground organs of only a few species have yielded pharmaceutically important drugs. Examples include the following:

- Devil's claw, *Harpagohytum procumbens* DC. ex Meissner (Harpagophyti radix, thickened roots)
- Korean ginseng, *Panax ginseng* C. A. Meyer (Ginseng radix)
- Tormentill, *Potentilla erecta* (L.) Raeuschel (syn. *P. tormentilla*, Potentillae radix)
- Echinacea, *Echinacea angustifolia* DC., *E. pallida* Nuttall and *E. purpurea* (L.) Moench (Echinacea radix)
- Siberian ginseng, *Eleutherococcus senticosus* Maximimowicz (Eleutherococci radix)
- Kava-kava, *Piper methysticum* Forster f. (kava-kava rhizoma)
- Chinese foxglove root, *Rehmannia glutinosa* Libosch (Rehmannia radix)
- Rhubarb, *Rheum palmatum* L. and *Rh. officinale* Baillon, as well as their hybrids (Rhei radix, thickened roots)
- Sarsaparilla, *Smilax regelii* Killip & Morton and *Smilax* spp. (Sarsaparillae radix).

DIVERSE AND UNSPECIFIED BOTANICAL DRUGS

Some drugs are derived from the whole plant or from specialized organs (e.g. the bulbs in the case of garlic, *Allium sativum* L.). The exudates of *Aloe vera* (L.) Burman f. (syn. *Aloe barbadensis*) leaves are used as a strong purgative.

Reference

(For further references see Chapter 4)
Heywood, V.H., 1993. Flowering plants of the world. Batsford, London

Chapter 4

Families yielding important phytopharmaceuticals

Systematics has always been an important tool in pharmacognostical practice and research. Related families often contain similar types of compounds and, therefore, may have similar beneficial or toxic effects. Consequently, an understanding of the systematic position of a medicinal plant species allows some deductions to be made about the (biologically active) secondary natural products from the species. For example, many members of the mint family are known to contain essential oil.

In this chapter, the pharmaceutically most important families are highlighted, especially those that have yielded many, or very important, botanical drugs. Since a species may yield several botanical drugs (e.g. from the flowers and the leaves), these are not included in this chapter, but can be found in Part B. Here, 20 families (out of a total of more than 200 recognized families) have been selected as being particularly important or interesting and are presented in alphabetical order within the groupings angiosperms and gymnosperms. The families are not classified further; more detailed information on the systematic position of these families can be found in relevant botanical textbooks (see further reading).

ANGIOSPERMS (MAGNOLIPHYTA)

These are the plants we commonly know as 'fruit-bearing plants' – i.e. the seed is covered by closed carpels. The fruit are sometimes very large and yield many of the economically important botanical products used because of their nutritional properties.

An important characteristic of these plants is double fertilization, in which cells other than the egg unite during the fertilization to give a triploid endosperm. This then develops into the fruit, which may also include other parts of the flowers. The flowers are typically fertilized by animals (i.e. zoogamous; mostly insects, but also birds, bats and spiders). Many species of this huge group have secondarily lost this trait and are fertilized with the help of the wind (e.g. oak, birch). At least 240,000 species of angiosperms are known, making it the largest group of plants. Many estimates, however, are much higher.

The taxon was originally split into two large groups – the Dicotyledoneae and the Monocotyledoneae – distinguished, *inter alia*, by the different number of cotyledons (primary leaves), but modern systematic classifications reject this division into only two groups.

ALLIACEAE ('MONOCOTYLEDONEAE')

Allium is the only important genus of this family, which includes not only important food plants such as the common onion (*Allium cepa* L.), leek (*A. porrum* L.) and chives (*A. schoenoprasum* L.), but also the medicinal plant garlic (*A. sativum* L.). The genus is often included in the Liliaceae (i.e. the broadly defined lily family).

Important medicinal plants from the family

- *Allium sativum* L. (garlic, see p. 225, Chapter 15).

Morphological characteristics of the family

These perennial herbs have underground storage organs (onions), which are used for hibernation. Typically, the flowers are composed of a perianth of two whorls of three with the sepals and petals having identical shape (i.e. the calyx and corolla are indistinguishable), six stamens and three superior, fused gynaecia. This is, in fact, the typical composition of the flowers of many related families that were previously united with the Liliaceae. The leaves are simple, annual, spirally arranged, parallel-veined and often of a round shape. The fruit is a capsule.

Distribution

The 700 species of family are found in northern temperate to Mediterranean regions.

Chemical characteristics of the family

The genus *Allium* is particularly well known for very simple sulphur-containing compounds, especially alliin and allicin (Fig. 4.1), which are thought to be involved in the reported pharmacological activities of the plant as a bactericidal antibiotic, in the treatment of arterial hypertension and in the prevention of arteriosclerosis and stroke.

APIACEAE (ALSO CALLED UMBELLIFERAE)

Important medicinal plants in the family
(see p. 215-216, Chapter 14)

- *Carum carvi* L. (caraway), a carminative and also important as a spice
- *Coriandrum sativum* L. (coriander), a carminative and also important as a spice
- *Foeniculum vulgare* Miller (fennel), a mild carminative
- *Levisticum officinale* Koch (lovage), a carminative and antidyspeptic
- *Pimpinella anisum* L. (anise-fruit, wrongly called 'seed'), an expectorant, spasmolytic and carminative.

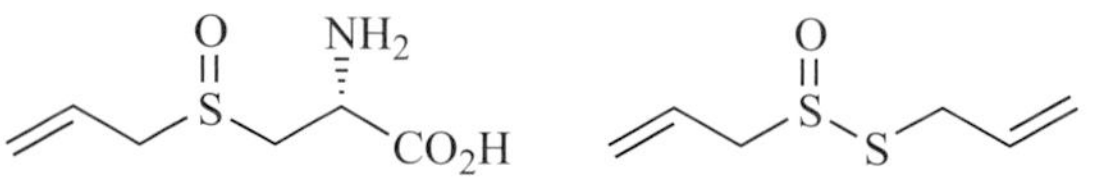

Morphological characteristics of the family

This family of nearly exclusively herbaceous species is characterized by hermaphrodite flowers in a double umbel (Fig. 4.2); note that the closely related Araliaceae have a simple umbel. Typical for the family are the furrowed stems and hollow internodes, leaves with a sheathing base and generally a much divided lamina. The flowers are relatively inconspicuous, with two pistils, an inferior gynaecium with two carpels, a small calyx and generally a white to greenish corolla, with free petals and sepals.

Distribution

Members of this family, which has about 3000 species, are mostly native to temperate regions of the northern hemisphere.

Chemical characteristics of the family

Unlike the Araliaceae, members of this family are often rich in essential oil, which is one of the main reasons for the pharmaceutical importance of many of the apiaceous drugs (see above). Also common are 17-carbon skeleton polyacetylenes, which are sometimes poisonous, and (furano-)coumarins, which are responsible for phototoxic effects (e.g. in *Heracleum mantegazzianum* Sommier and Levier, hogweed). Some species accumulate alkaloids (e.g. the toxic coniine from hemlock, *Conium maculatum* L.).

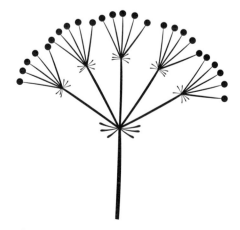

Alliin

Allicin

Fig. 4.1

Fig. 4.2 Double umbel.

ARALIACEAE

Important medicinal plants from the family

- *Hedera helix* L. [(common) ivy], used as a cough remedy
- *Panax ginseng* C. A. Meyer (ginseng), used as an adaptogene (a very ill-defined category) and to combat mental and physical stress [and sometimes replaced by *Eleutherococcus (Acanthopanax) senticosus* (Rupr. and Maxim) Maxim from the same family].

Morphological characteristics of the family

This family consists mostly of woody species, characterized by hermaphrodite flowers in a simple umbel (see the closely related Apiaceae with a double umbel). The leaf lobes are hand-shaped, and the flowers relatively inconspicuous with two pistils, an inferior gynaecium, a small calyx and generally a white to greenish corolla, with free petals and sepals.

Distribution

This family of >700 species is widely dispersed in tropical and subtropical Asia and in the Americas. *Hedera helix* is the only species native to Europe.

Chemical characteristics of the family

Of particular importance from a pharmacognostical perspective are the saponins, triterpenoids and some acetylenic compounds. The triterpenoids (ginsengosides) are implicated in the pharmacological effects of *Panax ginseng*, while saponins (hederasaponins) are of relevance for the secretolytic effect of *Hedera helix*.

ASPHODELACEAE ('MONOCOTYLEDONEAE')

This family is often included in the Liliaceae (lily family).

Important medicinal plants from the family

- *Aloe vera* (L.) Burman f. (syn. *Aloe barbadensis*, Barbardos aloe) and A. *ferox* Miller (Cape aloe), both strong purgatives (see p206 and 208). Aloe leaves contain a gel which is also applied topically for skin conditions; for botanical description. (see p. 286, Chapter 22).

Morphological characteristics of the family

Members of this family are generally perennials, and, in the case of *Aloe*, usually woody, with a basal rosette and the typical radial hermaphrodite flower structure of the Liliales. The petals and sepals are identical in form and colour, and composed of 3+3 free or fused, 3+3 free stamens and three fused superior carpels.

Distribution

This family, with about 600 species, is widely distributed in South Africa (a characteristic element of the Cape flora); some species occur naturally in the Mediterranean (*Asphodelus*).

Chemical characteristics of the family

Typical for the genus *Aloe* are anthranoids and anthraglycosides (aloe-emodin), which are responsible for the species' laxative effects, as well as polysaccharides accumulating in the leaves. Contrary to other related families, the Asphodelaceae do not accumulate steroidal saponins.

ASTERACEAE – THE 'DAISY' FAMILY (ALSO KNOWN AS COMPOSITAE)

This large family has kept botanists busy for many centuries and still no universally accepted classification exists. All members of the family have a complex inflorescence (the capitula), which gave rise to the older name of the family: Compositae (=inflorescence composed of many flowers). In other features, the family is rather diverse, especially with respect to its chemistry.

Important medicinal plants from the family

- *Arnica montana* L. (arnica), used topically, especially for bruises
- *Artemisia absinthum* L. (wormwood or absinthium), used as a bitter tonic and choleretic
- *Calendula officinalis* L. (marigold), used topically, especially for some skin afflictions
- *Cnicus benedictus* L. (cnicus), used as a cholagogue (a bitter aromatic stimulant)
- *Cynara scolymus* L. (artichoke), used in the treatment of liver and gallbladder complaints and several other conditions

- *Echinacea angustifolia* DC., *E. pallida* Nuttall and *E. purpurea* (L.) Moench (Cone flower), now commonly used as an immunostimulant
- *Matricaria recutita* L. (chamomille/camomille; several botanical synonyms are also commonly used, including *Chamomilla recutita* and *Matricaria chamomilla*) (see Chapter 14, p. 208).
- *Tussilago farfara* L. (coltsfoot), a now little used expectorant and demulcent.

Morphological characteristics of the family (Fig. 4.3)

The family is largely composed of herbaceous and shrubby species, but some very conspicuous trees are also known. The most important morphological trait is the complex flower head, a flower-like structure, which may in fact be composed of a few or many flowers (**capitulum** or **pseudanthium**). In some sections of the family (e.g. the subfamily

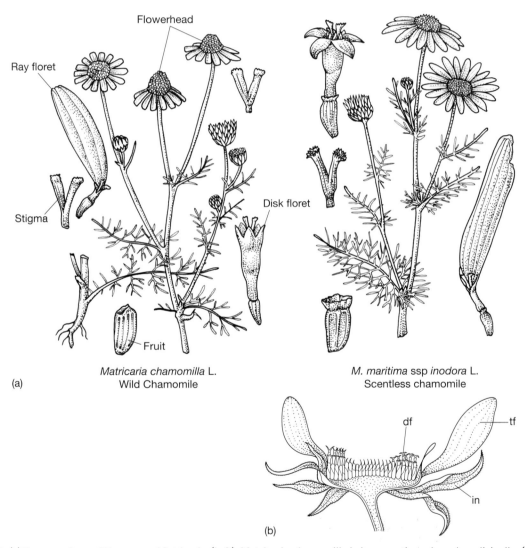

(a)

Flowerhead

Ray floret

Stigma

Fruit

Disk floret

Matricaria chamomilla L.
Wild Chamomile

M. maritima ssp *inodora* L.
Scentless chamomile

(b)

df   tf

in

Fig. 4.3 (a) Two members of the genus *Matricaria*. (Left) *Matricaria chamomilla* L. is aromatic and used medicinally. (Right) *Matricaria maritima* L. subsp. *inodora* Schultz [= *Tripleurospermum perforatum* (Mérat) Wagenitz], also known as *Matricaria inodora*, is not aromatic and is not used medicinally. The illustration shows typical morphological differences in these two species, such as the form of the flower heads and the fruit, but it also shows how similar the two species are in many other characteristics. From Fitch (1924). (b) Schematic of typical flower heads (a capitulum) of the Asteraceae (compositae). df, disk flowers; tf, tubular flowers; in, involucre, from Brimble (1942).

Lactucoideae, which includes lettuce and dande-lion), only ligulate (tongue- shaped) or disk (ray) florets are present in the dense heads. In the other major segment (subfamily Asteroideae), both ligu-late and radiate/discoid flowers are present on the same flower head, the former generally forming an outer, showy ring with the inner often containing large amounts of pollen. The flowers are epigynous, bisexual or sometimes female, sterile or functionally male. The (outer) calyx has five fused sepals and in many instances later develops into a pappus (feath-erlike in dandelions, in other instances more bristly), which is used as a means for dispersing the fruit; it is lacking in many other taxa. The fused petals (generally five) form a tubus or a ligula. The two gynaecia are epigynous and develop into tiny, nut-like fruits (achene or cypsela). The leaves are generally spirally arranged, simple, dissect or more or less compound.

Distribution

More than 21,000 species are known from practi-cally all parts of the world, with the exception of Antarctica, and the family has found niches in a large variety of ecosystems. The family is particu-larly well-represented in Central America and southern North America (Mexico).

Chemical characteristics of the family

A typical chemical trait of this family is the presence of polyfructanes (especially inulin) as storage carbo-hydrates (instead of polysaccharides) in perennial taxa. Inulin-containing drugs are used for preparing malted coffee (e.g. from the rootstocks of *Cichorium intybus*, chicory). In many taxa, some segments of the family accumulate sesquiterpene lactones (typi-cally with 15-carbon atoms such as parthenolide; Fig. 4.4), which are important natural products responsible for the pharmacological effects of many botanical drugs such as *Chrysanthemum parthenium* (feverfew) and *Arnica montana* (arnica). Polyacetylenic compounds (polyenes), and essential oil, are also widely distributed. Some taxa accumu-late pyrrolizidine alkaloids, which, for example, are present in *Tussilago farfara* (coltsfoot) in very small amounts. Many of these alkaloids are known for their hepatotoxic effects. Other taxa accumulate unusual diterpenoids; the diterpene glycoside stevioside (Fig. 4.4), for example, is of interest because of its intensely sweet taste.

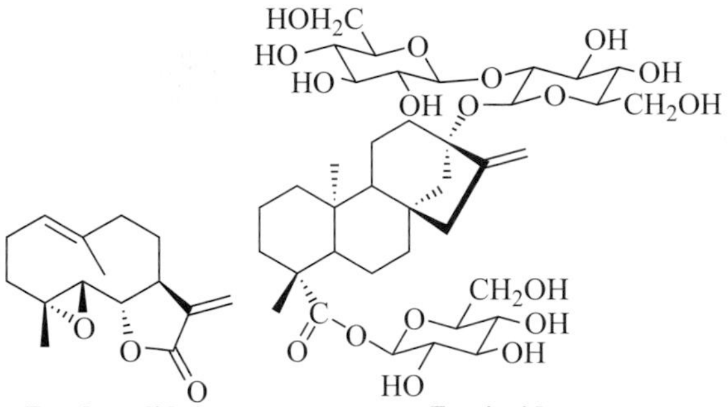

Parthenolide   Stevioside

Fig. 4.4

CAESALPINIACEAE

This family was formerly part of the Leguminosae (or Fabaceae) and is closely related to two other families: the Fabaceae (see below) and the Mimosaceae (not dis-cussed). Many contain nitrogen-fixing bacteria in root nodules. This symbiotic relationship is beneficial to both partners (for the plant, increased availability of physiologically usable nitrogen; for the bacterium, protection and optimal conditions for growth).

Important medicinal plants from the family

● *Cassia senna* L. and *C. angustifolia* Vahl (Senna), used as a cathartic.

Morphological characteristics of the family
(Fig. 4.5)

Nearly all of the taxa are shrubs and trees. Typically the leaves are pinnate. The free or fused calyx is composed of five sepals, the corolla of five generally free petals, the androecium of ten stamens, with many taxa showing a reduction in the number of stamens (five) or the development of staminodes instead of stamens. The flowers are zygomorphic and have a very characteristic shape, if seen from above, resembling a shallow cup.

Distribution

The 2000 species of this family are mostly native to tropical and subtropical regions, with some species common in the Mediterranean region. The family includes the ornamental *Cercis siliquastrum* L. (the Judas tree), native to the western Mediterranean, which according to (very doubtful) legend was the tree on which Judas Iscariot hanged himself.

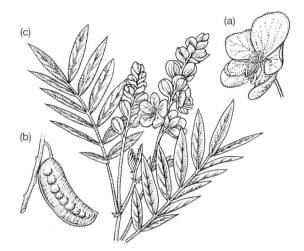

Fig. 4.5 *Cassia angustifolia*, a typical Caesalpiniaceae: (a) typical zygomorphic flower (yellow in its natural state); (b) fruit (one of the botanical drugs obtained from the species); (c) flowering branch showing the leaves composed of leaflets, and the inflorescence. *Modified after Frohne & Jensen (1998).*

Chemical characteristics of the family

From a pharmaceutical perspective the presence of anthranoides with strong laxative effects is of particular interest. Other taxa accumulate alkaloids, such as the diterpene alkaloids of the toxic *Erythrophleum*.

FABACEAE

This family is also classified together with the Mimosaceae and the Caesalpiniaceae as the Leguminosae (or Fabaceae, s.l.; see note under Caesalpiniaceae). One of its most well-known characteristics is that many of its taxa are able to bind atmospheric nitrogen.

Important medicinal plants from the family

- *Cytisus scoparius* (L.) Link (common or Scotch broom), which yields sparteine (formerly used in cardiac arrhythmias, as an oxytoxic, and in hypotonia to raise blood pressure)
- *Glycyrrhiza glabra* L. (liquorice), used as an expectorant and for many other purposes
- *Melilotus officinalis* L. (melilot or sweet clover); the anticoagulant drug warfarin was developed from dicoumarol, first isolated from spoiled hay of sweet clover

- *Physostigma venenosum* Balfour (Calabar bean), a traditional West African arrow poison, which contains the cholinesterase inhibitor physostigmine, used as a myotic in glaucoma, in postoperative paralysis of the intestine and to counteract atropine poisoning.

Morphological characteristics of the family

This family is characterized by a large number of derived traits. Most of the taxa of this family are herbaceous, sometimes shrubby and only very rarely trees. Typically, the leaves are pinnate and sometimes the terminal one is modified to form a tendril, used for climbing. Bipinnate leaves are not found in this family. The five sepals are at least basally united. The corolla is formed of five petals and has a very characteristic butterfly-like shape (papilionaceous), with the two lower petals fused and forming a keel-shaped structure, the two lateral ones protruding on both sides of the flower and the largest petal protruding above the flower, being particularly showy. The androecium of ten stamens generally forms a characteristic tubular structure with at least nine out of ten of the stamens forming a sheath. Normally, the fruit are pods, containing beans (technically called legumes) with two sutures, which open during the drying of the fruit (Fig. 4.6).

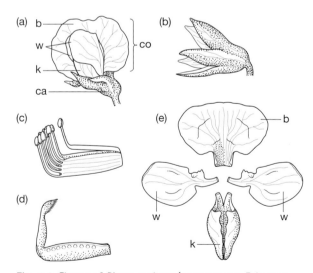

Fig. 4.6 Flower of *Pisum sativum* (common pea, Fabaceae, sensu stricto): (a) entire flower showing the various elements of the corolla (co; b, banner; w, wing (two); k, keel; ca calyx); (b) calyx; (c) stamens (nine fused and one free); (d) gynaecium; (e) the four petals of the corolla. *Modified after Frohne & Jensen (1998).*

Distribution

This is a cosmopolitan family with about 11,000 species, and is one of the most important families. It includes many plants used as food: for example, numerous species of beans (*Phaseolus* and *Vigna* spp., *Vicia faba* L.), peas (*Pisum sativum* L.), soy [*Glycine max* (L.) Merrill], fodder plants (*Lupinus* spp.) and medicines (see above).

Chemical characteristics of the family

This large family is characterized by an impressive phytochemical diversity. Polyphenols (especially flavonoids and tannins) are common, but from a pharmaceutical perspective various types of alkaloids are probably the most interesting and pharmaceutically relevant groups of compounds. In the genera *Genista* and *Cytisus* (both commonly called broom) as well as *Laburnum*, quinolizidine alkaloids, including cytisine and sparteine (Fig. 4.7), are common. The hepatotoxic pyrrolizidine alkaloids are found in this family (e.g. in members of the genus *Crotolaria*).

Other important groups of natural products are the isoflavonoids, known for their oestrogenic activity, and the coumarins used as anticoagulants (see *Melilotus officinalis* above). *Glycyrrhiza glabra* L. (licorice) is used because of its high content of the triterpenoid glycyrrhic acid, which, if joined to a sugar, is called glycyrrhizin (a saponin) and is used in confectionery as well as in the treatment of gastric ulcers (controversial). Last but not least, the lectins must be mentioned. These large (MW 40,000–150,000), sugar-binding proteins agglutinate red blood cells and they are a common element of the seeds of many species. Some are toxic to mammals, for example phasin from the common bean (*Phaseolus* spp.), which is the cause of the toxicity of uncooked beans.

HYPERICACEAE

This small family was formerly part of the Guttiferae and is of pharmaceutical importance because of St John's wort, which in the last decade of the 20th century became one of the most important medicinal plants in Western medicine.

Important medicinal plants from the family

- *Hypericum perforatum* L. (St John's wort) has clinically well-established effects in mild forms of depression. It has also been employed topically for inflammatory conditions of the skin.

Morphological characteristics of the family

The leaves are opposite, often dotted with glands. A characteristic feature of this family is a secondary increase in the number of stamens (polyandrous flowers). The fruit are usually capsules, but berries may occur in some species.

Distribution

This family, with about 900 species, has its main area of distribution in the tropics and in temperate regions.

Chemical characteristics of the family

The former name Guttiferae is an important indicator of a characteristic chemical feature: the presence of resins, balsam and other glands containing excretory products. For example, the hypericin glands, with a characteristic red colour, are present especially in the flowers and contain naphthodianthrones, including hypericin (Fig. 4.8) and pseudohypericin, which are characteristic for some sections of the genus. Typical for the family in general are also xanthones (found nearly exclusively in this family and in the Gentianaceae). The genus is known to accumulate flavonoids and their glycosides (rutoside, hyperoside), as well as hyperforin (Fig. 4.8) and its derivatives, which are derived from the terpenoid pathway.

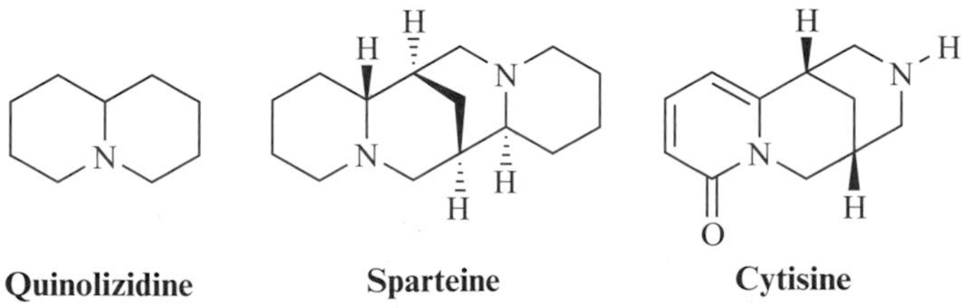

Quinolizidine   **Sparteine**   **Cytisine**

Fig. 4.7

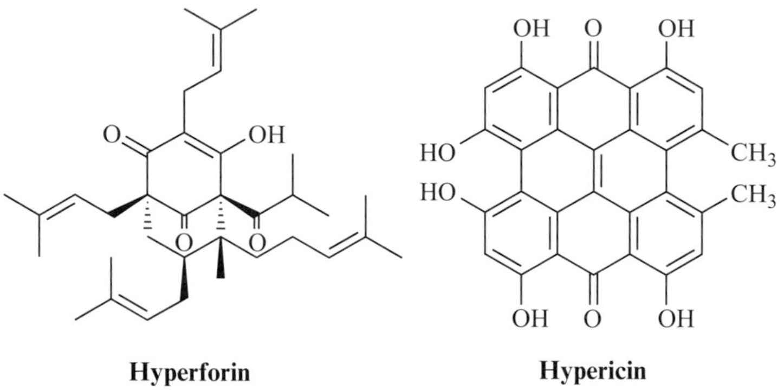

Hyperforin   **Hypericin**

Fig. 4.8

LAMIACEAE

The Lamiaceae is a family yielding a high number of medicinal taxa, especially due to their high content of essential oil.

Important medicinal plants from the family

- *Lavandula angustifolia* Miller (lavender), a mild carminative and spasmolytic
- *Melissa officinalis* L. (balm), a mild sedative, carminative and spasmolytic
- *Mentha arvensis* L. var. *piperascens* Malinvand (Japanese mint), yields a commonly used essential oil (e.g. for respiratory problems)
- *Mentha × piperita* L. (peppermint), a commonly used carminative and spasmolytic and a hybrid between *M. spicata* L. and *M. aquatica* L. (see Chapter 14, p. 214-215)
- *Mentha spicata* L. (spearmint), commonly used in toothpaste and chewing gum, with mild carminative effects
- *Rosmarinus officinalis* L. (rosemary), a carminative and spasmolytic
- *Salvia officinalis* L. (sage), used as a topical antiseptic (gargling) and orally as a carminative and spasmolytic
- *Thymus vulgaris* L. (thyme), a carminative and spasmolytic.

Morphological characteristics of the family
(Fig. 4.9)

Most of the taxa in this family are herbs or small shrubs with the young stems often being four-angled. All have opposite simple or rarely pinnate

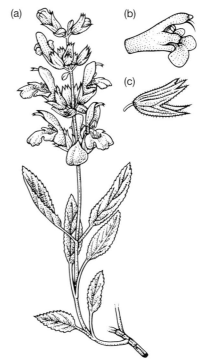

Fig. 4.9 *Salvia officinalis* (sage, Lamiaceae): (a) flowering branch showing typical leaves and the inflorescence; (b) corolla; (c) calyx. *After Frohne & Jensen (1998).*

leaves. The zygomorphic flowers, with very characteristic short-stalked epidermal glands, are very typical. They are bisexual, with five fused sepals, five generally zygomorphic petals, four or two stamens and two very characteristic fused gynaecia each divided into two partial units developing into a nut with a secondary division into nutlets.

Distribution

This important family with 5600 species is cosmopolitan and has a centre of distribution spanning from the Mediterranean to Central Asia.

Chemical characteristics of the family

Essential oil in the epidermal glands is very common. Some segments of the family are known to accumulate monoterpenoid glycosides (iridoids). Many species also accumulate rosmarinic acid and other derivatives of caffeic acid. Rosmarinic acid (Fig. 4.10) is of some pharmaceutical importance because of its non-specific complement activation and inhibition of the biosynthesis of leukotrienes (leading to an anti-inflammatory effect), as well as its antiviral activity.

PALMACEAE (ARECACEAE, PALMAE, 'MONOCOTYLEDONEAE')

The palms are particularly important because they include many species widely used as food, but in recent years at least one has become medically important.

Important medicinal plants from the family

- *Serenoa repens* (Bartram) Small (saw palmetto, sabal), for difficulty in micturition in benign prostate hyperplasia in the early stages.

Morphological characteristics of the family

These are generally unbranched, mostly erect, trees with primary thickening of the stem and a crown of large, often branched, leaves. The flowers are generally unisexual and radial, consisting of two whorls with three perianth leaves and six stamens. The three-lobed carpels may be free or united and develop into a berry, drupe or nut.

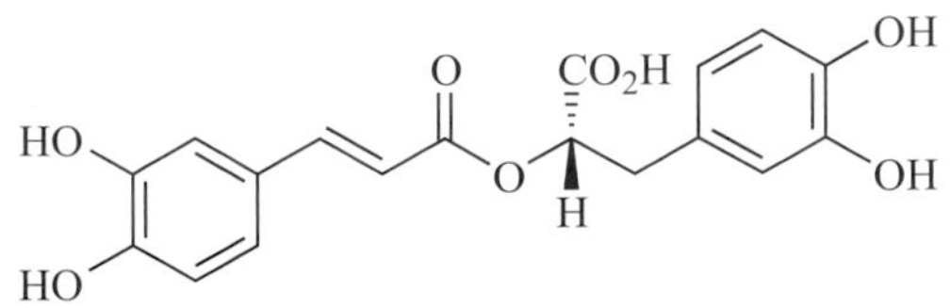

Rosmarinic acid

Fig. 4.10

Distribution

The family, with about 2700 exclusively evergreen woody species, is widely distributed in the tropics and subtropics.

Chemical characteristics of the family

The accumulation of polyphenols, some relatively simple alkaloids (especially pyridine derivatives) and steroidal saponins, as well as fatty acids [coconut (*Cocos nucifera* L.) and oil palm (*Elaeis guineensis* Jacq.)] is typical. The pharmaceutical use of *Serenoa repens*, on the other hand, seems to be due to the presence of relatively large amounts of the ubiquitous triterpenoid β-sitosterol.

PAPAVERACEAE

This rather small family has yielded a multitude of pharmaceutically or toxicologically important genera (e.g. *Chelidonium, Eschholzia, Glaucium, Papaver*) and natural products from two of its representatives are particularly widely used.

Important medicinal plants from the family

- *Chelidonium majus* L. (greater celandine), which yields the alkaloid chelidonine, sometimes employed as a cholagogue
- *Papaver somniferum* L. [(opium) poppy], which yields a multitude of pharmacologically active alkaloids and is a well-known and dangerous narcotic.

Morphological characteristics of the family
(Fig. 4.11)

This family of (generally) herbs or sub-shrubs typically has spirally arranged leaves which are entire or lobed or dissected. The generally large flowers are bisexual, have an inferior gynaecium, a reduced number of sepals (two to occasionally four), often four petals and numerous stamens. The fruit is a capsule (e.g. *Papaver somniferum*, which is lanced to obtain opium), with valves or pores for seed dispersal.

Distribution

This small family with about 200 species is mostly confined to the northern temperate regions of the world.

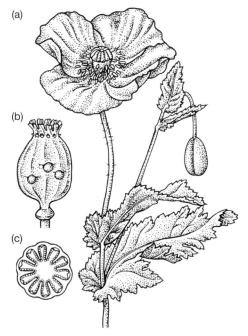

Fig. 4.11 *Papaver somniferum* (Papaveraceae). Botanical line drawings showing: (a) a flowering shoot; (b) the fruit (a capsule), with the latex shown at the lanced parts; (c) a cross-section of the fruit. *After Frohne & Jensen (1998).*

Chemical characteristics of the family

The laticifers (or latex vessels) are rich in isoquinoline alkaloids, including morphine (Fig. 4.12), papaverine, codeine, thebaine and noscapine. Some of these alkaloids are typical benzylisoquinoline alkaloids (papaverine, noscapine); others are chemically modified and have two additional ring systems (morphinane-type skeleton).

PIPERACEAE

Important medicinal plants from the family

- *Piper methysticum* Forster f. (kava-kava), traditionally used as a mild stimulant in Oceania

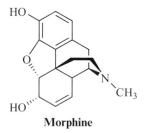

Morphine

Fig. 4.12

and now used for conditions of nervous anxiety; recent reports of liver toxicity has resulted in withdrawal in many countries
- *Piper nigrum* L. (black and white pepper), occasionally used in rubefacient preparations and as a spice.

Morphological characteristics of the family (Fig. 4.13)

This family of shrubs and herbs or small trees generally has simple, spirally arranged, leaves. The flowers are drastically reduced and sit in dense fleshy spikes.

Distribution

The family, with about 2000 species, is restricted to the tropics. The most important genera are *Piper* (including black pepper and kava-kava) and *Peperomia*. Some species are epiphytic (grow on other plants).

Chemical characteristics of the family

Pungent acidic amides, such as piperine, are known from several members of this family, and sometimes essential oil is present. The α-pyrone derivatives (e.g. kavain) from *Piper methysticum* are another group of commonly found compounds known from species of *Piper*.

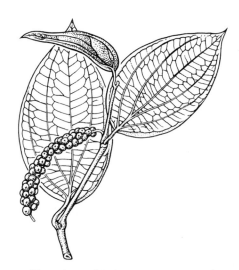

Fig. 4.13 *Piper nigram* (black pepper, Piperaceae). Line drawing of a fruiting shoot showing the typical leaves and the fruiting inflorescence. *After Frohne & Jensen (1998).*

POACEAE ('MONOCOTYLEDONEAE')

The 'grass' family is not very important with respect to their bioactive contents, but many pharmaceuticals contain starches derived from corn, rice or wheat as excipients.

Important medicinal plants from the family

- *Zea mays* L. (maize, corn) and other cereals, a common staple food; starches are also used in antidiarrhoeal preparations.

Morphological characteristics of the family

Most are herbs, often with rhizomes, and sometimes perennial. The leaves are distichous (with a single leaf at each node and the leaves of two neighbouring nodes disposed in opposite position), elongate with parallel main veins and often with a characteristic sheath at the base. A typical feature of the family is the wind-pollinated flowers, which form spike-like inflorescences (panicles).

Distribution

This cosmopolitan family has about 9000 species. Many of the economically important food staples are from this family and are grown all over the world.

Chemical characteristics of the family

Members of this family often accumulate silicates and some members have fruits rich in polysaccharides (starch) and proteinaceous tissue, mostly in the endosperm.

RHAMNACEAE

Important medicinal plants from the family

- *Rhamnus purshiana* DC. (American cascara) and *Rhamnus frangula* L. (syn. *Frangula alnus*, European alder, buckthorn), both used as strong purgatives.

Morphological characteristics of the family

This family mostly consists of trees with simple leaves, which are arranged spirally or opposite.

The flowers are small and unisexual with an epigynous gynaecium and four or five small petals. The fruit is a drupe (fleshy exo- and mesocarp with a hard endocarp).

Distribution

A relatively small cosmopolitan, mainly tropical and subtropical, family, with about 900 species.

Chemical characteristics of the family

The family is best known pharmaceutically because some taxa accumulate anthraquinones. Also alkaloids of the benzylisoquinoline type and the cyclopeptide type are known from many taxa.

RUBIACEAE

The family yields one of the most important stimulants, coffee (*Coffea arabica* L. and *C. canephora* Pierre ex Froehner) and one of the first and most important medicinal plants brought over from the 'New World', cinchona bark (see below).

Important medicinal plants from the family

- *Cinchona succirubra* Weddell, *C. calisaya* Weddell and *Cinchona* spp. (cinchona, Peruvian bark), used as a bitter tonic, febrifuge and against malaria.

Morphological characteristics of the family

This family consists mostly of trees or shrubs, with some lianas (climbing plants) and herbs. It has simple, entire and generally decussate leaves, which are nearly always opposed and which usually have connate stipules (sometimes as large as the leaves themselves, e.g. *Gallium*). The usually bisexual and epigynous, insect-pollinated flowers have four to five petals and four to five sepals, and five (or four) stamens and two gynaecia. The type of fruit varies (berry, drupe capsule).

Distribution

This is a large cosmopolitan family with more than 10,000 species, particularly prominent in the tropical and warmer regions of the world.

Chemical characteristics of the family

The family is known for a large diversity of classes of natural products, including iridoids (a group of monoterpenoids), alkaloids (including indole alkaloids such as quinine from *Cinchona* spp.), methylxanthines such as caffeine, theobromine and theophylline, and anthranoids in some taxa (e.g. the now obsolete medicinal plant *Rubia tinctorum*, which was withdrawn because of its genotoxic effect).

RUTACEAE

The family includes some of the most important fruitbearing plants known: the genus *Citrus* with orange, lemon, lime, mandarin, grapefruit, etc.

Important medicinal plants from the family

- *Pilocarpus jaborandi* Holmes and *Pilocarpus* spp. (pilocarpus), for the isolation of pilocarpine, which is used in ophthalmology
- *Ruta graveolens* L. (rue), formerly widely used as an emmenagogue and spasmolytic, shows strong phototoxic side effects
- Many species (especially of the genus *Citrus*) are aromatic and used as foods as well as in pharmacy and perfumery.

Morphological characteristics of the family

Most members of this family are trees or shrubs with spirally arranged, three pinnate or foliate (rarely simple) leaves. The bisexual flowers generally have five sepals and petals, 5+5 stamens and four or five hypogynous gynaecia.

Distribution

There are approximately 1700 species of this family distributed all over the world, but the tropics are particularly rich in them.

Chemical characteristics of the family

Essential oil is common in many taxa (*Citrus*, *Ruta*) and can be found in lysigenous secretory cavities in the parenchyma and pericarp. Alkaloids are also frequently found, especially benzyltetrahydroisoquinoline, acridone and imidazole types (pilocarpine; Fig. 4.14). The acridone

Pilocarpine

Fig. 4.14

alkaloids have so far only been reported from the Rutaceae. Other groups of natural products typically encountered are furano- and pyranocoumarins (e.g. bergapten from *Citrus aurantium* subsp. *bergamia*, used to flavour Earl Grey tea), as well as simple coumarins.

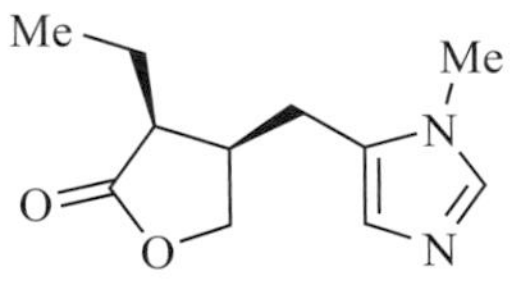

SOLANACEAE

This family includes one of the most important staples *Solanum tuberosum* (potato) and many medicinal and toxic plants known for their highly active natural products.

Important medicinal plants from the family

- *Atropa belladonna* L. (deadly nightshade, atropa), *Datura stramonium* L. (stramonium) and *Hyoscyamus niger* L. (henbane), which yield alkaloids with spasmolytic and anticholinergic properties; atropine is used in ophthalmology.

Morphological characteristics of the family
(Fig. 4.15)

The usually simple, lobed or pinnate/three-foliate leaves of these shrubs, herbs or trees are generally arranged spirally. The taxa have bisexual, radial flowers with five fused sepals, mostly five fused petals, five stamens and two gynaecia, which generally develop into a berry or a capsule.

Distribution

This family of about 2600 species is particularly well represented in South and Central America, but is widely distributed in most parts of the world.

Chemical characteristics of the family

Typical for the family are alkaloids, especially of the tropane, nicotine and steroidal type (Fig. 4.16). Many taxa are characterized by oxalic acid, which

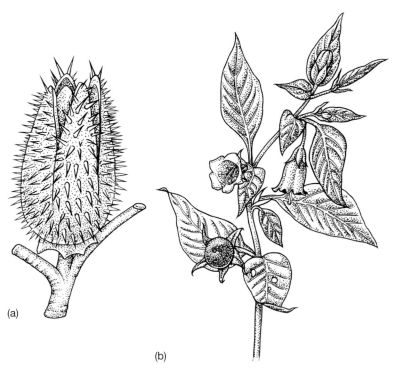

(a)

(b)

Fig. 4.15 (a) *Datura stramonium* (datura, Solanaceae), showing capsule enclosing the highly toxic seeds. (b) *Atropa belladonna* (deadly nightshade, atropa, Solanaceae), showing a flowering and fruiting branch with the violet-brown (outside) and dirty yellow (inside) flowers and the shiny black berries (highly toxic). *After Frohne & Jensen (1998).*

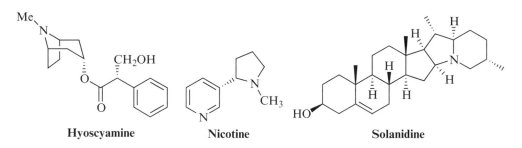

| **Hyoscyamine** | **Nicotine** | **Solanidine** |

Fig. 4.16

often forms typical structures (e.g. sand-like in *Atropa belladonna*, irregular crystals in *Datura stramonium*).

ZINGIBERACEAE ('MONOCOTYLEDONEAE')

In terms of pharmaceutical usage, this family is the most important of the former class Monocotyledoneae, which includes the Liliaceae, Palmaceae and Poaceae. Many members of this family are native to the Indo-Malayan region and are thus particularly important in Asian medical systems.

Important medicinal plants from the family

- *Curcuma zanthorrhiza* Roxburgh (Temu lawak, Javanese turmeric)
- *Curcuma longa* L. (syn. *C. domestica*, turmeric), a commonly used spice and popular remedy used, for example, for inflammatory and liver diseases, and in most Asian medical systems for a large variety of illnesses
- *Elettaria cardamomum* (L.) Maton (cardamom), which is mostly used as a spice but also as a medicine

- *Zingiber officinale* Roscoe (ginger), used for a large variety of illnesses, including travel sickness, respiratory and gastrointestinal disorders.

Morphological characteristics of the family

Generally, the species of this family are aromatic herbs with very prominent thickened rhizomes. The latter are often rich in essential oil, stored in typical secretory cells. The leaves are arranged spirally or are distichous with a sheath around the stem (similar to the grasses). However, these sheaths are arranged in such a way that they form a stem-like structure, which supports the real, rather weak, stem. The zygomorphic and bisexual flowers are often very large and prominent and are pollinated by large, often nocturnal, insects, birds or bats.

Distribution

The family is distributed throughout the tropics, but many species are native to Asia (Indo-Malayan region).

Chemical characteristics of the family

This family is one of the few families of the former Monocotyledons which is rich in essential oil with terpenes such as borneol, camphor and cineole (all oxygen-containing monoterpenes), camphene, pinene (monoterpenes) and zingiberene (a sesquiterpene), as well as phenylpropanoids (cinnamic acid derivatives) (Fig. 4.17). Typically, these compounds accumulate in oil cells, an important microscopical characteristic of the rhizomes of the Zingiberaceae.

GYMNOSPERMS

This much smaller group of seed-bearing plants differs from the angiosperms in not having the seeds enclosed in carpels (the seeds are naked) and in not having double fertilization. The gymnosperms are generally fertilized with the help of the wind and are often characterized as having needles instead of broad leaves (the most important exception being *Ginkgo biloba*, the Chinese maidenhair tree). Only about 750 species are known, but some species are extremely important in the production of timber [European fir (*Abies* spp.), spruce (*Picea* spp.), Douglas fir (*Pseudotsuga menziesii* (Mirbel) Franco), all Pinaceae] and some yield medically important essential oil. The most important medicinal plant is *Ginkgo biloba*.

GINKGOACEAE

This is one of the most ancient families of the seed-bearing plants and had been widely distributed during the Mesozoic (180 million years ago). Only one species survives today.

Important medicinal plants from the family

- *Ginkgo biloba* L. (Chinese maidenhair tree), used for its memory-improving properties.

Morphological characteristics of the family
(Fig. 4.18)

The characteristic fan-shaped leaves, which often have an indention at the apex, are well known. The tree does not bear fruit but has a pseudo-fruit, with the outer part of the seed (testa) developing into a fleshy cover, which has a strong unpleasant smell of butyric acid and a hard inner part. Fertilization is not by pollen but by means of microspermatozoids, a characteristic of less well-advanced plants. Another typical aspect is the separation of the deposition of the microspermatozoids on the gametophytes and fertilization (the unification of macro- and microspermatozoid). Thus the seeds found on the ground during the autumn are not yet fertilized, but will be during the winter.

Distribution

Ginkgo biloba is native to a small region in south-eastern Asia and is now widely planted in many temperate regions of the world.

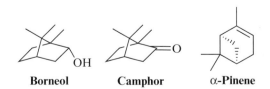

Borneol   **Camphor**   α-**Pinene**

Fig. 4.17

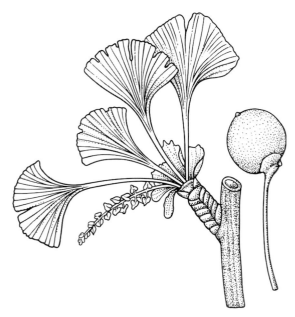

Fig. 4.18 *Ginkgo biloba* (Chinese maidenhair tree, Ginkgoaceae) showing the typical fan-shaped young leaves and a seed (sometimes wrongly called fruit). *After Frohne & Jensen (1998).*

Chemical characteristics of the family

The most important and a unique group of natural products are the ginkgolides (Fig. 4.19), which are unusual two-ringed diterpenoids with three lactone functions. Biflavonoids and glycosylated flavonoids are other groups of typical natural products.

Pinaceae

Important medicinal plants from the family

- *Abies* spp. (fir)
- *Picea* spp. (spruce).

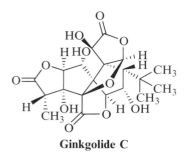

Ginkgolide C

Fig. 4.19

Morphological characteristics of the family
(Fig. 4.20)

The trees of this family (conifers) are evergreen and usually have opposed or whorled branches. Typically, the leaves of this family are needle-shaped and linear ('pine needles'). The pollen- and gynoecium-producing flowers are separate, but on one plant (monoecious). The pollen-producing cones are small and herbaceous. They produce large amounts of pollen, which is transported by the wind. The female cones are usually woody with spirally arranged scales, each usually with two ovules on the upper surface, and subtended by a more or less united bract. There are usually two winged, wind-distributed seeds per scale.

Distribution

This small family (about 200 species) is widely distributed in the north temperate regions of the world [including regions with long annual periods of extreme frost such as high mountains (Alps), the

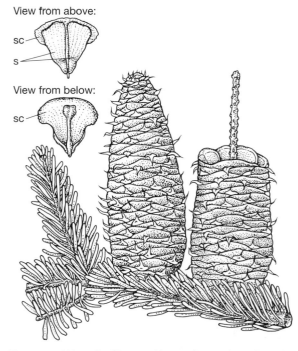

View from above:

sc

s

View from below:

sc

Fig. 4.20 *Abies alba* (fir tree, Pinaceae), showing a branch with cones, and a single scale viewed from above and below. s, seed; sc, scale. *After Frohne & Jensen (1998).*

northernmost parts of Western Europe and the Asian tundra] and extends into the warmer regions of the northern hemisphere. Many members of this family are accordingly very frost- and drought-resistant, and form large tree- or shrub-dominated zones of vegetation.

Chemical characteristics of the family

The best known pharmaceutical products from this family are essential oils and balsams, which are typically found in the schizogenic excretion ducts of the leaves as well as in the excretion pores of the wood and bark. Both are rich in monoterpenoids such as α-pinene and borneol. Mixtures of oil and resin from these species are called **turpentine**, while the resinous part is called **colophony** and is particularly rich in terpenoids (including diterpenoids such

Pinoresinol   **Abietic acid**

Fig. 4.21

as abietic acid). Other widely reported groups of compounds from members of this family are flavonoids, condensed tannins and lignans (e.g. pinoresinol) (Fig. 4.21).

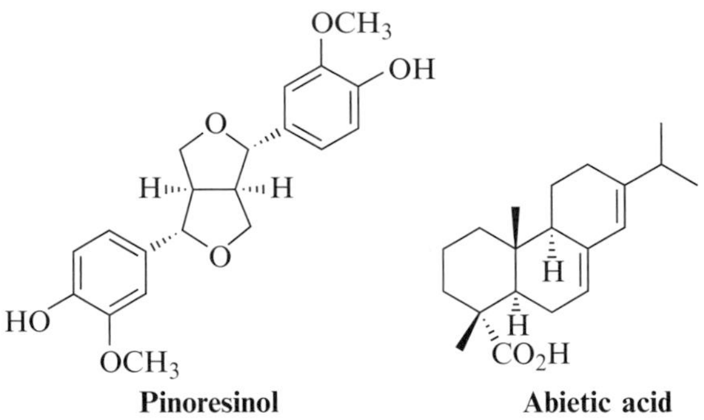

References

Brimble, L.F.J., 1942. Intermediate botany. Macmillan, London.

Fitch, W.H., 1924. Illustrations of the British flora. Reeve, London.

Frohne, D., Jensen, U., 1998. Systematik des Pflanzenreichs, 5 Aufl. Wissenschaftliche Verlagsgesellschaft, Stuttgart.

Further reading

Evans, W.C., 2000. Trease and Evans' pharmacognosy, fifteenth ed. WB Saunders, London.

Heywood, V.H., 1993. Flowering plants of the world. Batsford, London.

Judd, W.S., Campbell, C.S., Kellogg, E.A., et al., 2002. Plant systematics.

A phylogenetic approach, second ed. Sinauer, Sunderland, MA.

Mabberly, D.J., 1990. The plant book. Cambridge University Press, Cambridge.

Raven, P.H., Evert, R.F., Eichhorn, S.E., 1999. Biology of plants, sixth ed. WH Freeman, New York.

Robbers, J.E., Speedie, M.K., Tyler, V.E., 1996. Pharmacognosy and pharmacobiotechnology. Williams & Williams, Baltimore.

Sitte, P., Ziegler, H., Ehrendorfer, F., Bresinsky, A., 1997. Lehrbuch der Botanik ('Strasburger'), 34 Aufl. Gustav Fischer Verlag, Stuttgart.

Chapter 5

Ethnobotany and ethnopharmacy

Many drugs that are commonly used today (e.g. aspirin, ephedrine, ergometrine, tubocurarine, digoxin, reserpine, atropine) came into use through the study of indigenous (including European) remedies – that is, through the bioscientific investigation of plants used by people throughout the world. Table 5.1 lists just a few of the many examples of drugs derived from plants. As can be seen, most plant-derived pharmaceuticals and phytomedicines currently in use were (and often still are) used by native people around the world. Accordingly, our information is derived from local knowledge as it was and is practised throughout the world, although European and Mediterranean traditions have had a particular impact on these developments. The historical development of this knowledge is discussed in Chapter 2. This chapter is devoted to traditions as old as, or older than the written records but which have been passed on orally from one generation to the next. Some of this information, however, may have not been documented in codices or studied scientifically until very recently.

Ethnobotany and ethnopharmacology are interdisciplinary fields of research that look specifically at the empirical knowledge of indigenous peoples concerning medicinal substances and their potential health benefits, and (as with all drugs) the potential toxicological risks associated with such remedies. Empirical knowledge was sometimes recorded in herbals and other texts on materia medica (examples are given in Chapter 12). Written traditions are obviously better documented and easier to access, but both written and oral forms of indigenous phytotherapy are important factors influencing the use of medicinal plants in the Western world. Each year new plants become popular with some sections of the population (and often are as

quickly forgotten again). Only a few are sufficiently well-studied scientifically and can be recommended on the basis of bioscientific and/or clinical evidence.

ETHNOBOTANY

Shortly before the start of the 20th century (1896), the American botanist William Harshberger coined the term 'ethnobotany' – the study of plant use by humans.

> **Ethnobotany** studies the relationship between humans and plants in all its complexity, and is generally based on a detailed observation and study of the use a society makes of plants, including all the beliefs and cultural practices associated with this use.

It is usual for ethnobotanists to live with indigenous people, to share the everyday life of their community and, of course, to respect the underlying cultures. Ethnobotanists have a responsibility both to the scientific community and to the indigenous cultures. According to the above definition, ethnobotany focuses not only on medicinal plants, but also on other natural products derived from nature, such as:

- food
- plants used in rituals
- colouring agents
- fibre plants
- poisons
- fertilizers

Table 5.1 Botanical drugs used in indigenous medicine and of importance in the development of modern drugs

BOTANICAL NAME	ENGLISH NAME	INDIGENOUS USE	ORIGIN (REGIONAL AND ETHNIC)	USES IN BIOMEDICINE	RELEVANT BIOLOGICALLY ACTIVE COMPOUNDS
Adhatoda vasica Nees (syn. *Justicia adhatoda* L., Acanthaceae)	–	Antispasmodic, antiseptic, anti-asthmatic, fish poison, insecticide	India, Sri Lanka	Antispasmodic, oxytocic, cough suppressant	Vasicin (model for expectorants bromhexin and ambroxol)
Aesculus hippocastanum L. (Hippocastanaceae)[a]	Horse chestnut	Anti-inflammatory	South-eastern Europe	Chronic inflammatory conditions, circulatory problems	Aescin (a saponin mixture)
Ammi visnaga (L.) Lam. (Apiaceae)	Visnaga	Inflammatory and infectious conditions of the mouth, diuretic, 'palpitations of the aorta'	Northern Africa	Increase of cardiac activity	Khellin, and development of cromoglycate
Ananas comosus (L.) Merr. (Bromeliaceae)	Pineapple	Anthelmintic, expectorant, abortifacient	South America (today pantropical)	Anti-inflammatory	Bromelain
Atropa belladonna L. (Solanaceae)	Deadly nightshade	Pain relief, asthma, inflammatory conditions	Europe, Middle East	Parkinsonism, anti-emetic	(–)-Hyoscyamine
Camptotheca acuminata Decne (Nyssaceae)	–	?	South and South-eastern Asia	Cancer chemotherapy (inhibitor of topoisomerase 1)	Camptothecin (under development)
Cassia senna L. and other *Cassia* spp. (Caesalpiniaceae)	Senna	Laxative	North-eastern Africa, Middle East	Laxative	Sennoside anthraquinones
Catharanthus roseus (L.) G. Don. f. (Apocynaceae)	Madagascar periwinkle	Diabetes mellitus	Madagascar (today a pantropical garden plant)	Cancer chemotherapy	Vincristine, vinblastine
Cephaelis ipecacuanha (Brot.) Tussac (Rubiaceae)	Ipecacuanha	Amoebiasis, expectorant, emetic	Tropical regions of South America	Expectorant, emetic, amoebiasis	Emetine
Chondrodendron tomentosum Ruiz & Pavon (Menispermaceae)	–	Arrow poison	Brazil, Peru	Muscular relaxation (during operations)	D-Tubocurarine (Fig. 5.1) (and derivatives)
Cinchona succirubra Pav. [= C. pubescens Vahl and spp. (Rubiaceae)]	Jesuits' bark	No indigenous uses were recorded during the 16th and 17th centuries	Northern South America	Malaria, cardiac arrhythmia	Quinine
Colchicum autumnale L. (Colchicaceae)	Meadow saffron	Poison	Europe	Gout	Colchicine
Combretum caffrum Kuntze (Combrataceae)	–	?	South Africa	Cancer chemotherapy	Combretastatin A-4
Cryptolepis sanguinolenta (Lindl.) Schltr. (Asclepiadaceae)	–	Various symptoms, which may possibly be associated with diabetes	West Africa (e.g. Ghana)	Diabetes	Cryptolepine
Curcuma xanthorrhiza Roxb. and spp. (Zingiberaceae)	Turmeric (curcuma)	Cholagogue, stomachic, carminative	India (?), today widely distributed in the tropics	Hepatic disorders	Curcumin, essential oil
Datura metel L./D. innoxia Mill. (Solanaceae)	Thorn-apple	Hallucinogen	Africa and Asia, Middle America	Travel sickness, preoperative medication	Scopolamine (hyoscine)

Digitalis spp. (Scrophulariaceae)	Foxglove	Dropsy	Europe	Cardiac arrhythmia, atrial fibrillation	Digitalis glycosides
Drimia maritima (L.) Stearn (syn. Urginea maritima (L.) Baker (Hyacinthaceae)	Sea onion	Dropsy, emetic, diuretic	Mediterranean	Coronary insufficiency	C_{24}-steroidal cardiac glycosides
Echinacea angustifolia DC. and E. purpurea (L.) Moench (Asteraceae)[a]	Echinacea	Pain relief, anti-inflammatory, wounds	North America	Immunostimulant	Combined effect of several groups of compound
Ephedra sinica Stapf (Ephedraceae)	Ephedra	Chronic cough	China	Cough suppressant	Forskolin
Filipendula ulmaria (L.) Maxim (Rosaceae)	Meadowsweet	Various uses including as diuretic, kidney problems	Europe, northern Asia	Pain	Acetylsalicylic acid
Galanthus nivalis L. (Amaryllidaceae)	Snowdrop	According to Fuchs (1543), not used pharmaceutically (?)	Warmer regions of Europe	Dementia, including Alzheimer's disease	Galanthamine
Ginkgo biloba L. (Ginkgoaceae)[a]	Ginkgo	Asthma, anthelmintic (fruit)	Eastern China, today widely cultivated	Dementia, cerebral deficiencies, cerebral circulatory problems	Ginkgolides
Harpagophytum procumbens DC. ex Meissner (Pedaliaceae)[a]	Devil's claw	Fever, unspecified illnesses of the blood, pain relief (especially after parturition), inflammatory conditions, as digestive	Southern Africa	Pain, especially rheumatism	Harpagoside (?), caffeic acid derivatives
Hyoscyamus niger L. (Solanaceae)	Henbane	Pain relief (topical as ointment and plaster), fever, respiratory illnesses	Europe	Anticholinergic	Hyoscyamine
Hypericum perforatum L. (Hypericaceae)[a]	St John's wort	Very diverse uses including wounds, rheumatism, gout, menstrual problems	Europe	Mild forms of depression, topical for inflammatory conditions (oil)	Hyperforin, flavonoids, hypericin
Papaver somniferum L. (Solanaceae)	(Opium) poppy	Pain relief, tranquilizer, hallucinogen	Western Mediterranean	Pain (P), cough (C), antispasmodic (S)	Morphine (P), Codeine (C), Papaverine (S)
Physostigma venenosum Balfour (Fabaceae sensu stricto)	Calabar bean	Poison ('ordeal' and arrow poison)	Tropical West Africa (Sierra Leone–Zaire)	Glaucoma	Physostigmine
Pilocarpus jaborandi Holmes (Rutaceae)	Jaborandi	Poison	Africa	Parasympathomimetic, glaucoma	Pilocarpine
Piper methysticum Forst. f. (Piperaceae)[a]	Kava-kava	Ritual stimulant and tonic	Polynesia	Anxiolytic, mild stimulant	Kava pyrones and others
Podophyllum peltatum L. (Berberidaceae)	May apple	Especially as laxative, also for skin infections	North-eastern North America	Cancer chemotherapy, warts	Podophyllotoxin (and other lignans)
Prunus africana (Hook. f.) Kalkman (Rosaceae)[a]	African plum	Laxative (veterinary) and diverse other uses	Tropical Africa	Prostate hyperplasia	Especially sitosterol
Psoralea corylifolia L. (Fabaceae sensu stricto)	–	Stomachic, various skin infections	Asia	Psoriasis	Psoralen

Continued

Table 5.1 Botanical drugs used in indigenous medicine and of importance in the development of modern drugs—cont'd

BOTANICAL NAME	ENGLISH NAME	INDIGENOUS USE	ORIGIN (REGIONAL AND ETHNIC)	USES IN BIOMEDICINE	RELEVANT BIOLOGICALLY ACTIVE COMPOUNDS
Rauvolvia spp.	Snake root	Emetic, cholera	Widely distributed in the tropics	Cardiac arrhythmia (A), high blood pressure (B)	Ajmalin (A), reserpine (B)
Rhamnus purshiana DC. [syn. *Frangula purshiana* (DC.) Cooper] and other *Frangula* spp. (Rhamnaceae)[a]	Cascara sagrada	Widely used as a laxative	Western North America	Purgative	Anthraquinones
Salix spp. (Salicaceae)[a]	Willow	A variety of uses, especially for chronic and acute inflammatory conditions	Europe, Asia, North America	Various types of pain (lower back pain), chronic inflammatory conditions	Salicin and derivatives (model for aspirin)
Strophanthus gratus (Hook.) Bail. and *Strophanthus* spp. (Apocynaceae)	–	Arrow poison	Tropical Africa	Coronary insufficiency	Strophantin, ouabain
Syzygium aromaticum (L.) Merr. (Myrtaceae)[a]	Clove	Stomachic, digestive, antidiarrhoea, oil for toothache and rheumatism	Molucca Islands (formerly Spice Islands)	Toothache	Eugenol
Taxus brevifolia Nutt. (Taxaceae)	Californian yew	Very diverse uses including for 'cancer' (Tsimshian)	Western USA	Cancer chemotherapy (induction of tubulin aggregation)	Paclitaxel

[a]Examples of plants commonly used in Europear phytotherapy. In general, the others are not used as an extract, but as pure compounds, or served as a model for developing semi-synthetic drugs or as standardized (normalized) extractcts.

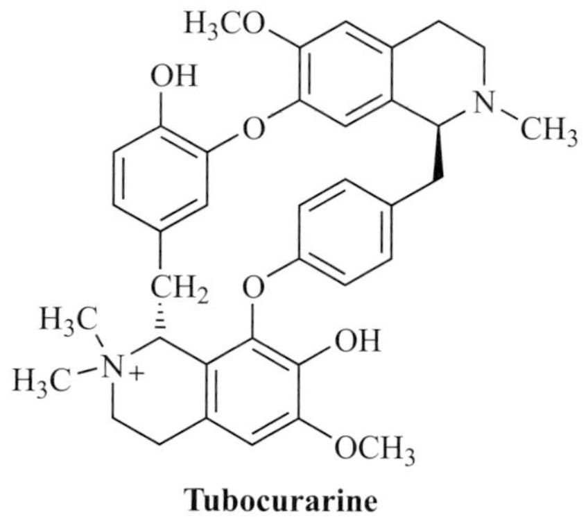

Tubocurarine

Fig. 5.1

- building materials for houses, household items, boats, etc.
- ornamentals
- oil plants.

This broad definition is still used today, but modern ethnobotanists face a multitude of other tasks and challenges (see below). Medicinal plants have always been one of the main research interests of ethnobotany and the study of these resources has also made significant contributions to the theoretical development of the field (Berlin 1992); however, the more anthropologically oriented fields of research are beyond the scope of this introductory chapter.

ETHNOPHARMACOLOGY

Ethnopharmacology as a specifically designated field of research has had a relatively short history. The term was first used in 1967 in the title of a book on hallucinogens (see Efron et al 1970). The field is nowadays much more broadly defined.

The observation, identification, description and experimental investigation of the ingredients, and of the effects of the ingredients, and the effects of such indigenous drugs, is a truly interdisciplinary field of research which is very important in the study of traditional medicine. **Ethnopharmacology** is here defined as 'the interdisciplinary scientific exploration of biologically active agents traditionally employed or observed by man' (Bruhn & Holmstedt 1981: 405–406).

This definition draws attention to the bioscientific study of indigenous drugs but does not explicitly address the issue of searching for new drugs. Medicinal plants are an important element of indigenous medical systems in many parts of the world, and these resources are usually regarded as part of the traditional knowledge of a culture. Europe has for many years profited from the exchange of ideas with other continents, and many of the natural products and phytomedicines used today are derived from plants used in indigenous cultures. Examples of 18th century explorers who described indigenous plant use in detail are Richard Spruce (British), Hipolito Ruiz (Spanish) and Alexander von Humboldt (German), who co-discovered curare.

THE STORY OF CURARE

An interesting example of an early ethnopharmacological approach is provided by the study of the botanical origin of the arrow poison curare, its physiological effects and the compound responsible for these effects. Curare was used by certain, wild, tribes in South America for poisoning their arrows and many early explorers documented this usage. The historical aspects of the scientific investigation of curare by Bernard (1966) are outlined in Chapter 2, but the detailed descriptions made by Alexander von Humboldt in 1800, of the process used to prepare poisoned arrows in Esmeralda on the Orinoco River, are equally interesting. von Humboldt had met a group of native people who were celebrating their return from an expedition to gather the raw material for making the poison and he described the 'chemical laboratory' used to prepare the poison (Humboldt 1997:88, from the original text published 1800):

> He [an old Indian] was the chemist of the community. With him we saw large boilers (Siedekessel) made out of clay, to be used for boiling the plant sap; plainer containers, which speed up the evaporation process because of their large surface; banana leaves, rolled to form a cone-shaped bag [and] used to filter the liquid which may contain varying amounts of fibres. This hut transformed into a laboratory was very tidy and clean.

The botanical source of curare was eventually identified as the climbing vine *Chondrodendron tomentosum* Ruiz and Pavón; other species of the Menispermaceae (*Curarea* spp. and *Abuta* spp.) and Loganiaceae (*Strychnos* spp.) are also used in the production of curares of varying types (Bisset

1991). von Humboldt then eloquently described one of the classical problems of ethnopharmacology:

> We are unable to make a botanical identification because this tree [which produces the raw material for the production of curare] only grows at quite some distance from Esmeralda and because [it] did not have flowers and fruit. I had mentioned this type of misfortune previously, that the most noteworthy plants cannot be examined by the traveller, while others whose chemical activities are not known [i.e. which are not used ethnobotanically] are found covered with thousands of flowers and fruit.

THE ROLE OF THE ETHNOBOTANIST

The role of the ethnobotanist in the search for new drugs was important until the second half of the 20th century, when other approaches became more 'fashionable'. More recently, the study of ethnobotany has again received considerable interest in the media and in some segments of the scientific community. Also the 'Western' use of such information has come under increasing scrutiny, and the national and indigenous rights of these resources have become acknowledged by most academic and industrial researchers. These developments result in a considerable challenge to (and increasing responsibilities for) ethnobotanists and ethnopharmacologists. Simultaneously, the need for basic scientific investigation of plants used in indigenous medical systems is becoming ever more relevant. The public availability of research results is as essential for further developing and 'upgrading' indigenous and traditional medicine as it is for any other medical or pharmaceutical system.

ETHNOPHARMACOLOGY AND THE CONVENTION ON BIOLOGICAL DIVERSITY (CONVENTION OF RIO)

None of the studies discussed so far took the benefits for the providers (the states and their people) into account. This has changed in recent years. Ethnopharmacological and related research using the biological resources of a country are today based on agreements and permits, which in turn are based on international and bilateral treaties. The most important of these is the Convention of Rio or the Convention on Biological Diversity (see http://www.biodiv.org/chm/conv.htm), which looks in particular at the rights and responsibilities associated with biodiversity on an international level:

> The objectives of this Convention, to be pursued in accordance with its relevant provisions, are the conservation of biological diversity, the sustainable use of its components and the fair and equitable sharing of the benefits arising out of the utilization of genetic resources, including by appropriate access to genetic resources and by appropriate transfer of relevant technologies, taking into account all rights over those resources and to technologies, and by appropriate funding.

The basic principles of access are regulated in article 5:

> States have, in accordance with the Charter of the United Nations and the principles of international law, the sovereign right to exploit their own resources pursuant to their own environmental policies, and the responsibility to ensure that activities within their jurisdiction or control do not cause damage to the environment of other States or of areas beyond the limits of national jurisdiction.

The rights of indigenous peoples and other keepers of local knowledge are addressed in article 8j:

> Subject to its national legislation, respect, preserve and maintain knowledge, innovations and practices of indigenous and local communities embodying traditional lifestyles relevant for the conservation and sustainable use of biological diversity and promote their wider application with the approval and involvement of the holders of such knowledge, innovations and practices and encourage the equitable sharing of the benefits arising from the utilization of such knowledge, innovations and practices.

This and subsequent treaties significantly changed the basic conditions for ethnopharmacological research. Countries that provide the resources for natural product research and drug development now have well-defined rights. This specifically includes the sharing of any benefits that may accrue from the collaboration. Access to resources is addressed in article 15, which is crucial for an understanding of this and any other activity which may yield economically important products:

> 15.1. Recognizing the sovereign rights of States over their natural resources, the authority to determine access to genetic resources rests with the national governments and is subject to national legislation. 15.5. Access to genetic resources shall be subject to prior informed consent of the

Contracting Party providing such resources, unless otherwise determined by that Party.

15.7. Each Contracting Party shall take legislative, administrative or policy measures. . .with the aim of sharing in a fair and equitable way the results of research and development and the benefits arising from the commercial and other utilization of genetic resources with the Contracting Party providing such resources. Such sharing shall be upon mutually agreed terms.

In the case of ethnopharmacological research, the needs and interests of the collaborating community become an essential part of the research, and in fact there is an inextricable link between cultural and biological diversity. This principle was first formulated at the 1st International Congress on Ethnobiology held in Belem (Brazil) in 1988. No generally agreed upon standards have so far been accepted, but the importance of obtaining the 'prior informed consent' of the informants has been stressed by numerous authors (e.g. Posey 2002).

BIOPROSPECTING AND ETHNOPHARMACOLOGY

Studies dealing with medicinal and other useful plants and their bioactive compounds have used many concepts and methodologies. These are interdisciplinary or multidisciplinary studies, combining such diverse fields as anthropology, pharmacology, pharmacognosy or pharmaceutical biology, natural product chemistry, toxicology, clinical research, plant physiology and others. In order to analyse their strengths and weaknesses, and especially the outcomes of research, two different but closely related approaches can be distinguished: **bioprospecting** and **ethnopharmacology** (see Table 5.2).

Bioprospecting focuses on the development of new drugs for the huge markets of the northern hemisphere. Potentially highly profitable pharmaceutical products are developed, based on the biological and chemical diversity of the various ecosystems of the earth; this requires an enormous financial input. The research starts with the collection of biogenic

Table 5.2 Ethnopharmacology and bioprospecting compared	
ETHNOPHARMACOLOGY	**BIOPROSPECTING**
Overall goals	
(Herbal) drug development, especially for local uses	Drug discovery for the international market
Complex plant extracts (phytotherapy)	Pure natural products as drugs
Social importance of medicinal and other useful plants	–
Cultural meaning of resources and understanding of indigenous concepts about plant use and of the selection criteria for medicinal plants	–
Main disciplines involved	
Anthropology	–
Biology (ecology)	Biology including (very prominently) ecology
Pharmacology/molecular biology	Pharmacology and molecular biology
Pharmacognosy and phytochemistry	Phytochemistry
Number of samples collected	
Very few (up to several hundred)	As many as possible, preferably several thousand
Selected characteristics	
Detailed information on a small segment of the local flora (and fauna)	Limited information about many taxa
Database on ethnopharmaceutical uses of plants	Database on many taxa (including ecology)
Development of autochthonous resources (especially local plant gardens, small-scale production of herbal preparations)	Inventory (expanded herbaria) economically sustainable alternative use to destructive exploitation (e.g. logging)
Pharmacological study	
Preferably using low-throughput screening assays which allow a detailed understanding of the local or indigenous uses	The assay is not selected on the basis of local usage, instead high-throughput screening systems are used
Key problem	
Safety and efficacy of herbal preparations	Local agendas (rights) and compensation to access

samples (plants, fungi, other micro-organisms and animals), progresses through analysis of the chemical, biological and pharmacological activities to the development of drug templates or new drugs. A key process in this search is high-throughput screening systems such as those that have been established by major international pharmaceutical companies. Huge libraries of compounds (and sometimes extracts) are screened for biological activity against specific targets. Active natural products are only one of the many sources of material for these batteries of tests but serve as a starting point for drug development. Currently, some companies envision screening 500,000 samples a week against a single target; thus it becomes essential to have an enormous number of chemically diverse samples available.

The other approach may best be termed ethnopharmacological. Ethnobotanical studies generally result in the documentation of a rather limited set of well-documented useful plants, mostly medicinal, but also those known to be toxic or used in nutrition. In ethnopharmacology, an important goal is the development of improved preparations for use by local people. Thus it is essential to obtain information on the bioactive compounds from these plants, their relative contribution to the effects of the extract (including, for example, synergistic or antagonistic effects), the toxicological profile of the extract and its constituents. By restricting ethnopharmacology to the bioscientific study of indigenous uses, attention is drawn to the need for improving indigenous phytomedical systems, especially in developing countries. This requires research strategies for studying indigenous medicinal plants and their uses.

The importance of conserving such nature-derived products in the health care of the original keepers of such knowledge must be the main goal of truly interdisciplinary research. Ethnopharmacology may contribute to the development of new pharmaceutical products for the markets of the northern hemisphere, but this is only one of several targets. Truly multidisciplinary research on medicinal plants requires the inclusion of other methodologies from such fields as medical or pharmaceutical anthropology or sociology. Not only do we need a detailed understanding, incorporating social scientific and bioscientific methods, but we also need to support all means available of making better use of these products. It has been pointed out that the two approaches – ethnopharmacology and biodiversity prospecting – are not mutually exclusive and the two concepts as they are outlined here are rarely realized in such extreme forms. Instead, any discussion should specifically draw attention to particular strengths and roles of both approaches. In bioprospecting programmes, which are directed specifically towards infectious diseases, the use of 'ethnobotanical' information is very useful and promising (Lewis 2000). However, this is not necessarily the case in cancer chemotherapy, for example, where highly toxic plants are not used in traditional medicine because the dose cannot be controlled sufficiently well to ensure safety.

EXAMPLES OF MODERN ETHNOPHARMACOLOGICAL STUDIES

A project focusing on the bioscientific study of indigenous uses of *Hyptis verticillata* (Lamiaceae) is a good example. This plant is prepared in different ways by the Lowland Mixe people of Oaxaca, Mexico, depending on the disease to be treated. For skin infections and inflammation, the plant is ground up with a little alcohol or the mashed leaves are applied directly to the affected part. However, for gastrointestinal problems, a tea is prepared using 'a handful' of fresh leaves (Heinrich 2001).

Phytochemical investigation using an inflammatory model as well as antibacterial activity led to the isolation of several lignans, rosmarinic acid and sideritoflavone (see Fig. 5.2). These compounds help to explain the rationale behind the indigenous uses. The lignans are known to have strong antibacterial activity, which was also corroborated in these studies, and both rosmarinic acid and sideritoflavone were shown to be active in anti-inflammatory models.

It was also possible to show that the lignans are only extracted to a very limited degree if the plant material is prepared as a tea, whereas relatively large amounts are extracted in a process mimicking the indigenous extraction with 'aguardiente' (40–70% ethanol). The more toxic lignans are thus present in much smaller quantities in the tea, reducing the health risk of this preparation.

The second example is drawn from ethnobotanical fieldwork in Eastern Guatemala with a Mayan-speaking people, the Chorti. The Chorti use the fruit of *Ocimum micranthum* Willd. (Lamiaceae) in the treatment of infectious and inflammatory eye diseases (Kufer et al, unpublished). The fruits are approximately 1 mm in diameter and hard, and several of these are applied directly into the eye. At first glance this seems an unlikely remedy for

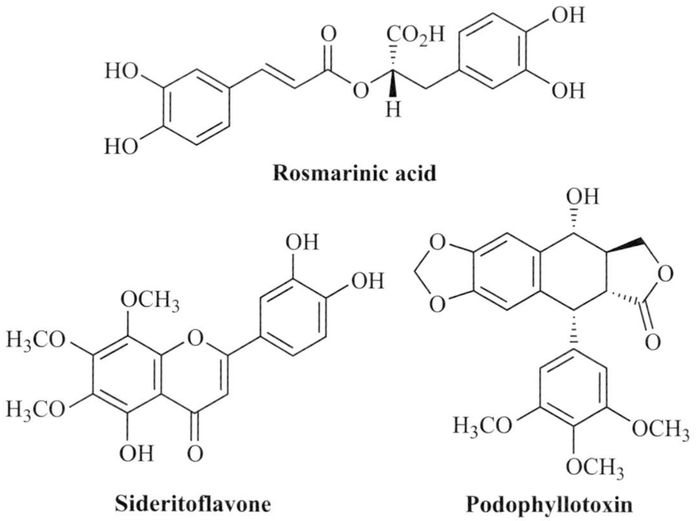

Fig. 5.2

eye problems, but the rationale behind it becomes evident when considering the morphological and chemical make-up. The fruits are covered with a mucilaginous layer containing complex polysaccharides which form a soft layer around the fruit if it is put into water (Heinrich 1992). This layer may well have a cleansing effect, and polysaccharides are known to be useful in the treatment of inflammatory conditions and bacterial or viral infections. Although there are no pharmacological data from experimental studies available to corroborate this use, information on the histochemical structure of the fruit makes it likely that the treatment has some scientific basis.

The above two examples demonstrate the relevance of ethnopharmacology in relation to the scientific study of indigenous medical products. However, ethnopharmacology, as the science bridging the gap between natural sciences and anthropology, should also look at symbolic and cognitive aspects. People may select plants because of their specific pharmacological properties, but also because of the symbolic power they may believe is in a plant. Understanding these aspects requires cognitive and symbolic analysis of field data. Another example from field studies with the Mixe in Mexico can be used. At the end of a course of medical treatment, the patient is sometimes given a petal of *Argemone mexicana* L. (known to the Mixe as San Pedro Agats, Papaveraceae). This plant is known to contain a large number of biologically active alkaloids, including protopine. However, the yellow petals are presumably used, not because they exert a

pharmacological effect (at this dose) but because they symbolize the bread of the Last Supper according to Christian mythology. Thus they are a powerful symbol for the end of the healing process (for other examples of symbolic and empirical forms of plant use see Heinrich 2010).

The role of ethnopharmacology can be extended beyond that defined previously. It looks not only at empirical aspects of indigenous and popular plant use, but also at the cognitive foundations of this use. Only if these issues are to be included will it truly be a interdisciplinary field of research (Bruhn & Holmstedt 1981:406). The key tasks of pharmaceutical researchers in this interdisciplinary process will be to:

- study the pharmacological effects of the most widely used species (for selection criteria for the ethnopharmacologically most important taxa, see Heinrich et al 1998)
- further develop local ethnopharmacopoeias
- characterize the relevant constituents
- formulate improved (but relatively simple) galenical preparations.

This will result in a truly ethnopharmaceutical approach to medicinal plants which encompasses all subdisciplines of pharmacy and medicine. The value of integrating ethnobotanical with phytochemical and pharmacological studies has been clearly demonstrated. While, for example, the likelihood of developing new therapeutic agents for use in biomedicine is relatively low (although it is certainly much higher than with many other approaches), such studies confirm the therapeutic value and contribute to our general scientific knowledge about medicinal plants (Heinrich 2010).

Some plants have many side effects or are highly toxic. In an example from the Highlands of Mexico, Bah et al (1994) showed that a species popularly used there contains hepatotoxic pyrrolizidine alkaloids, which pose potential health risks. Although this information is available to the scientific community, the general public may not be aware of these risks. Such data must be summarized appropriately and made available to local people in regions where the plants are used. It is now essential to develop partnerships with institutions capable of translating these findings into an effective strategy.

CONCLUSION

The examples given in this chapter are intended to show the breadth of the contribution of ethnobotany and ethnopharmacology, from the study of indigenous, orally transmitted medical systems to drug development, and to illustrate that the pharmaceutical sciences may profit in many ways by including such approaches. It is also important to further consolidate local knowledge. Ethnopharmacology in this context will provide patients with access to some evidence-based forms of their own 'traditional' medicine, in developing countries in Africa, South and Central America, Asia and South-East Asia.

> The term **'ethnopharmacy'** may well be the most appropriate to stress the breadth of such an approach, since it encompasses all the relevant disciplines: pharmacognosy, pharmacology, pharmaceutics (especially relating to Oalenicals), drug delivery, toxicology, bioavailability and metabolism studies, as well as pharmacy practice and policy development. This would allow the development of local resources into elements to be used in primary health care.

References

(NB: a relatively large selection of sources has been included because of the complexity of this multidisciplinary topic and the brevity of this introduction.)

Bah, M., Bye, R., Pereda-Miranda, R., 1994. Hepatotoxic pyrrolizidine alkaloids in the Mexican medicinal plant *Packera candidissima* (Asteraceae: Senecioneae). J. Ethnopharmacol. 43, 19–30.

Berlin, B., 1992. Ethnobiological classification. Principles of categorization of plants and animals in traditional societies. Princeton University Press, Princeton, NJ.

Bernard, C., 1966. Physiologische Untersuchungen über einige amerikanische Gifte. Das Curare. In: Bernard, C., Mani, N. (Eds.), Ausgewählte physiologische Schriften. Huber Verlag, Bern, [frz. orig. 1864]. pp. 84–133.

Bisset, N.G., 1991. One man's poison, another man's medicine. J. Ethnopharmacol. 32, 71–81.

Bruhn, J.G., Holmstedt, B., 1981. Ethnopharmacology: objectives, principles and perspectives. In: Beal, J.L., Reinhard, E. (Eds.), Natural products as medicinal agents. Hippokrates Verlag, Stuttgart, pp. 405–430.

Efron, D., Farber, S.M., Holmstedt, B., 1970. Ethnopharmacologic search for psychoactive drugs. Public Health Service Publications no. 1645. Government Printing Office, Washington, DC (reprint, orig. 1967).

Heinrich, M., 1992. Economic botany of American Labiatae. In: Harley, R.M., Reynolds, T. (Eds.), Advances in Labiatae Science. Royal Botanical Gardens, Kew, pp. 475–488.

Heinrich, M., 2001. Ethnobotanik und Ethnopharmakologie. Eine Einführung. Wissenschaftliche Verlagsgesellschaft, Stuttgart.

Heinrich, M., 2010. Ethnopharmacology and drug development. In: Mander, L., Lui, H.W. (Eds.), Comprehensive natural products II. Chemistry and biology, vol. 3. Elsevier, Oxford, pp. 351–381.

Heinrich, M., Ankli, A., Frei, B., et al., 1998. Medicinal plants in Mexico: healers' consensus and cultural importance. Soc. Sci. Med. 47, 1863–1875.

Lewis, W., 2000. Ethnopharmacology and the search for new therapeutics. In: Minnis, P.E., Elisens, W.J. (Eds.), Biodiversity and native America. University of Oklahoma Press, Norman, OK.

Posey, D.A., 2002. Kayapó ethnoecology and culture. In: Plenderleith, K. (Ed.), Studies in environmental anthropology, vol 6. Routledge, London.

Further reading

Brett, J., Heinrich, M., 1998. Culture perception and the environment. Journal of Applied Botany 72, 67–69.

Cotton, C.M., 1997. Ethnobotany. Wiley, Chichester.

Etkin, N.L., 1985. Ethnopharmacology: biobehavioral approaches in the anthropological study of indigenous medicines. Ann. Rev. Anthropol. 17, 23–42.

Etkin, N.L., Harris, D.R., Prendergast, H.D.V., et al., 1998. Plants for food and medicine. Royal Botanical Gardens, Kew.

Heinrich, M., 1994. Herbal and symbolic medicines of the Lowland Mixe (Oaxaca, Mexico): disease concepts, healers' roles, and plant use. Anthropos 89, 73–83.

Heinrich, M., Robles, M., West, J.E., et al., 1998. Ethnopharmacology of Mexican Asteraceae (Compositae). Annu. Rev. Pharmacol. Toxicol. 38, 539–565.

Moerman, D.E., 1998. Native American ethnobotany. Timber Press, Portland, OR.

Neuwinger, D., 2000. African traditional medicines. Medpharm, Stuttgart.

Okpako, D.T., 1989. Principles of pharmacology: a tropical approach. Cambridge University Press, Cambridge.

Okpako, D.T., 1999. Traditional African medicine: theory and pharmacology explored. Trends Pharmacol. Sci. 20, 482–485.

Schultes, R.E., 1962. The role of the ethnobotanist in the search for new medicinal plants. Lloydia 25, 257–266.

Schultes, R.E., 1983. Richard Spruce: an early ethnobotanist and explorer of the Northwest Amazon and Northern Andes. J. Ethnobiol. 3, 139–147.

Schultes, R.E., Nemry von Thenen de Jaramillo-Arango, M.J., 1998. The journals of Hipólito Ruiz: Spanish botanist in Peru and Chile 1777–1788. Timber Press, Portland, OR.

Schultes, R.E., Raffauf, R., 1990. The healing forest. Medicinal and toxic plants of the Northwest Amazonia. Dioscorides Press, Portland, OR.

Sofowara, A., 1979. African medicinal plants: proceedings of a conference. University of Ife Press, Nigeria.

Thomas, O.O., 1989. Perspectives on ethno-phytotherapy of Yoruba medicinal medicinal plants and preparations. Fitoterapia 60, 49–60.

von Humboldt, A., (Hrsg. H Beck), 1997. Die Forschungsreise in den Tropen Amerikas. Studienausgabe Bd 2, Teilband 3. Wissenschaftliche Buchgesellschaft, Darmstadt.

Section 3

Natural product chemistry

Chapter 6

Natural product chemistry

This chapter looks briefly at the chemistry of natural products. This is the study of chemicals produced by the many diverse organisms of nature, including plants, microbes (fungi and bacteria), marine organisms and more exotic sources such as frog skins and insects.

> Natural products are defined here as organic compounds in the molecular weight range 100–2000. In a broader sense, the term natural products can also be applied to bulk substances from nature, such as crude plant material, foodstuffs, resins and exudates from plants (e.g. myrrh and frankincense) or extracts of plant material (water or alcoholic extracts). The treatment of this subject will be confined to pure **single chemical entities** (i.e. chemicals with a well-defined structure and purity).

Historically, natural products have formed the basis of medicines and, even now, many of the compounds that are pharmaceutically and medicinally important are derived from natural sources. The reasons for this are complicated, but probably stem from the ability of nature to produce a fantastic array of **structurally complex** and **diverse** molecules. A number of theories have been proposed as to why these compounds are produced and although we can only theorize as to why these products occur in nature, it is highly likely that many of them are produced as part of a chemical defence system to protect the producing organism from attack. Examples of this defence include the synthesis of antimicrobial

compounds by plants that are infected by bacteria and fungi (compounds known as **phytoalexins**), or the synthesis of highly toxic natural products in the skins of Central American frogs to deter predation by other animals. Whatever the reasons for the presence of these compounds in nature, they are an invaluable and under-exploited resource that can be used to find new drug molecules.

NATURAL PRODUCTS IN DRUG DISCOVERY

A survey of any pharmacopoeia will show that natural products have a key role as biologically active agents; in fact, it has been estimated that 20–25% of all medicines are derived from such sources. In this definition, the medicinal agent may be a natural product isolated straight from the producing organism (e.g. the β-lactamase inhibitor **clavulanic acid** isolated from the bacterium *Streptomyces clavuligerus*), a natural product that has undergone a minor chemical modification (semisynthetic) (e.g. **aspirin**, derived from **salicylic acid**, which occurs as esters and glycosides in *Salix* spp.), or a compound that was totally synthesized based on a particular natural product possessing biological activity (e.g. **pethidine**, which was based on **morphine** from the opium poppy, *Papaver somniferum*). It is sometimes difficult to see how the fully synthetic compound was modelled on the natural product (Fig. 6.1).

Natural products are historically the core of medicines and they are still a major source of **drug leads**, which is a term used to describe compounds that may be developed into medicines. A particular example of a natural product that is currently one

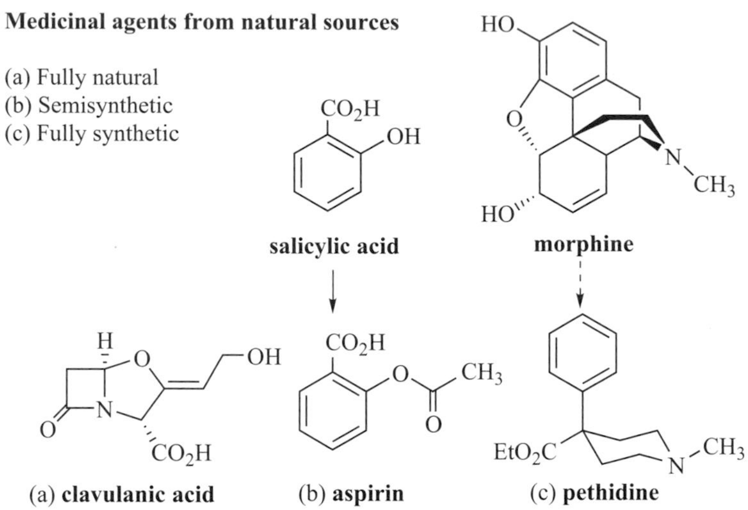

Medicinal agents from natural sources

(a) Fully natural
(b) Semisynthetic
(c) Fully synthetic

salicylic acid

morphine

(a) clavulanic acid   **(b) aspirin**   **(c) pethidine**

Fig. 6.1

of the best selling drugs is **paclitaxel**, marketed as **Taxol** (Fig. 6.2). This drug was developed by BristolMyers Squibb and marketed for the treatment of ovarian and mammary cancers, and became available for use in the USA in 1993. The compound was initially isolated from the bark of the Pacific yew tree, *Taxus brevifolia*, and demonstrates the best possible qualities of a natural product, being highly functional and chiral. Additionally, paclitaxel occurs in the bark with a wide range of structurally related compounds (taxanes diterpenes); this is a further important and valuable quality of natural products when they are considered as a source in

the search for biologically active drug leads. Paclitaxel has many functional groups and chiral centres (11) and these qualities give rise to its distinct shape and fascinating biological activity. It is important not to be overwhelmed at such a complex molecule, but to look at the functional groups that make up the total structure of the compound. Even a natural product that is as structurally complex as paclitaxel can be broken down into the simple chemical features of functional groups and chiral centres.

Interest in natural drugs has long captured the imagination of the general public who has the impression that natural products are safe and non-toxic, but, as we will see, some of the most potent poisons are derived from nature. This view of natural medicines is in part based on the romantic notion of **bioprospecting** for new **drug leads** from areas with an exceptionally high level of **biodiversity** and beauty, such as the Amazonian rain forest. Although public interest in natural drugs is high, investment in the discovery of natural drugs by industry has been highly fashionable and cyclical, due to the development of alternative ways of finding new drug leads (e.g. **combinatorial chemistry**). An additional perceived benefit of compounds derived from nature is that they are 'eco-friendly' and that they may be produced as a renewable resource by growing the plants or by fermenting the micro-organisms that produce them. This approach has both advantages and disadvantages over the synthetic production of biologically active agents, but synthetic chemistry cannot yet readily mimic the ability of organisms to

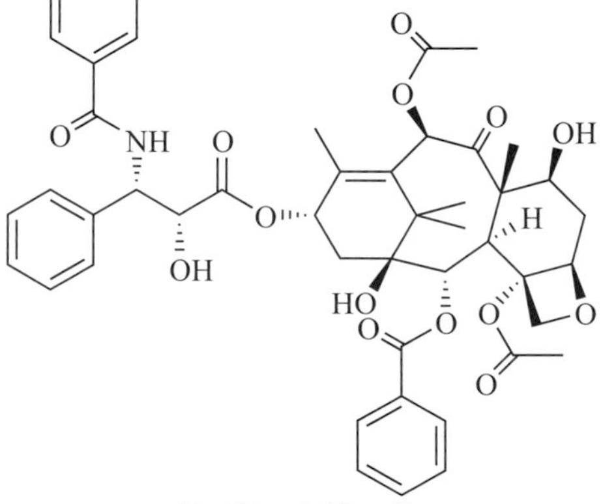

Paclitaxel (Taxol)

Fig. 6.2

produce such structurally complex and diverse natural product molecules.

There are a number of approaches that can be used to discover new drug leads from nature, and all of the following have been used by large and small pharmaceutical companies in an attempt to harness the biological potential of natural products.

In the **ethnobotanical** approach, knowledge of the use of a particular plant by an indigenous people is used to direct a search for a drug lead. In this case, observation of a particular usage of a plant, usually made by a highly trained observer (ethnobotanist), allows the collection of that plant and its subsequent testing for biological activity. Examples of such uses include arrow poisons made from trees by South American Indians as a way of hunting animals for food. One of these agents, curare (from the liana *Chondrodendron tomentosum*) acts as a muscle relaxant, which kills by paralysing the muscles required to breathe. The active component in curare is **tubocurarine**. This ethnobotanical observation of curare used as an arrow poison led to the development of a muscle relaxant used in surgery known as atracurium. The use of ethnobotanical information is greatly under-exploited and, as many of the more remote regions of the planet become more readily accessible, without trained personnel to interview and retrieve this information, it is highly likely that much valuable local medicinal knowledge will be lost.

In the **chemotaxonomic** approach, knowledge that a particular group of plants contains a certain class of natural product may be used to predict that taxonomically related plants may contain structurally similar compounds. This approach is highly useful when the chemistry and biological activity of a compound is well described and compounds with similar chemical structure are needed for further biological testing. A good example of this is the plant family Solanaceae, which is a rich source of alkaloids of the tropane type. The knowledge that deadly nightshade (*Atropa belladonna*)

produces hyoscyamine (a smooth muscle relaxant) would enable one to predict that the thorn apple (*Datura stramonium*) would contain structurally related compounds, and this is certainly the case, with hyoscine being the major constituent of this solanaceous plant (Fig. 6.3).

Using the **random** approach, plants are collected regardless of any existing previous knowledge of their chemistry or biological activity. This approach relies on the availability of plants that are abundant in a certain area (and may previously have been extensively studied). Plants that are rare or only exist in a specific habitat (e.g. alpine or parasitic plants) may be neglected and access to chemical diversity lost. This approach is purely serendipitous in that there is a chance that random plant selection will give access to extracts (and therefore compounds) with biological activity (**bioactivity**).

The **information-driven** approach utilizes a combination of ethnobotanical, chemotaxonomic and random approaches together with a database that contains all of the relevant information concerning a particular plant species. The database is used to prioritize which plants should be extracted and screened for bioactivity. This approach is favoured by large organizations (particularly pharmaceutical companies) interested in screening thousands (in some cases hundreds of thousands) of samples for bioactivity as it may reduce costs by a process known as **dereplication** – the process of avoiding the repeated discovery of common or known drugs. This is most important where millions of dollars are spent in the natural product drug lead discovery process.

An example of when a database would be of use in the information-driven approach is in the discovery of anti-tumour agents. Should bioactivity be demonstrated upon screening extracts from the English yew (*Taxus baccata*), then chemotaxonomic knowledge could be entered into the database indicating that this species is related to *Taxus brevifolia* and consequently may produce related chemical

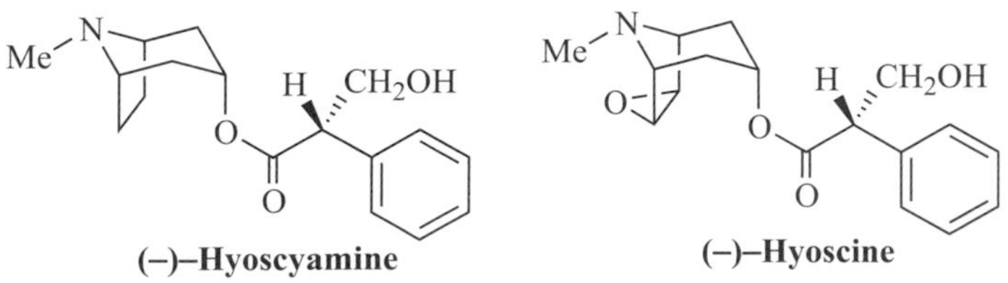

(–)–Hyoscyamine   (–)–Hyoscine

Fig. 6.3

constituents and should be prioritized accordingly. This is certainly the case as *Taxus brevifolia* produces the antitumour drug paclitaxel.

The discovery of drugs from nature is complex and is depicted schematically in Fig. 6.4. The **biomass** (plant, microbe, marine organism) is collected, dried and extracted into a suitable organic solvent to give an **extract**, which is then screened in a **bioassay** to assess its biological activity (bioactivity). Screening or assessment of biological activity is generally divided into two formats depending on the number of extracts to be assessed. In **low-throughput screening** (LTS), small numbers of extracts (a single extract up to hundreds of extracts) are dispensed into a format that is compatible with the bioassay (e.g. a microtitre plate, sample tubes). This approach is used widely in academic laboratories where only a relatively low number of extracts are assessed. In **high-throughput screening** (HTS), thousands of extracts are dispensed into a format (usually microtitre plates with many wells, e.g. 384 wells per plate) and screened in the bioassay. This approach is favoured by the pharmaceutical industry, which may have hundreds of thousands of samples (both natural and synthetic) for biological evaluation. This large-scale approach means that decisions can be made rapidly about the status of an extract, which has an impact on the cost of the discovery process.

Active extracts are **fractionated** using **bioassay-guided isolation**, in which **chromatographic techniques** are used to separate the extract into its individual components; the biological activity is checked at all stages until a pure active compound is obtained. The natural product isolated will be designated as a **lead compound** and will be assessed for biological activity in a bank of other assays. This process is known as **cross-screening** and will give information on how **selective** the compound is – i.e. is it active in all the assays or does it exhibit specificity for one particular assay? This is an important consideration as one of the criteria for the selection of a compound for further development is **specificity**. Whilst biological evaluation is on-going, **structure elucidation** will be necessary to determine the three-dimensional structure of the active molecule. This will enable a search to be done to establish whether the compound is novel, what chemical class it belongs to and whether that type of compound has previously been reported to possess biological activity in the bioassay of interest or other bioassays.

Once novelty and potent biological activity have been established, large amounts of the lead compound are isolated and the decision is made as to whether the compound can be synthesized *de novo* or whether **chemical modification** needs to be made to enhance the biological activity. The lead compound will undergo extensive *in vivo* **studies** to establish activity, toxicity and efficacy; these studies are sometimes known as **preclinical studies**. Only once all of these steps have been completed will a drug lead finally enter **clinical trials**, which is the most extensive evaluation stage of a drug candidate during which many drug leads fail through toxicity or lack of efficacy in humans. Successful completion of these trials usually results in a product licence, which means that the compound is now a **drug**.

Given the complexity of the process described above, it is not surprising that many natural product drug leads fail to make their way onto the market. Some estimates state that only 1 in 10,000 drug leads may actually make their way to the market.

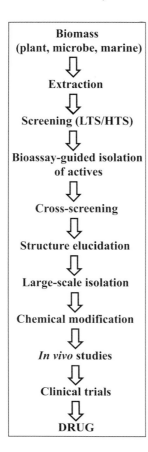

Fig. 6.4

The process is also very lengthy and it may take 12–15 years from the collection of the original biomass to the granting of a licence for a new natural product drug. Additionally, the process is very costly but the rewards are enormous. For example, although high costs could occur for the development of Taxol (US $300 million), these can be readily recovered, with initial sales in excess of US$1 billion per annum. In 2009 the best selling brand name drug was Lipitor (Atorvastatin), which made $13.3 billion; this highlights the potential value of the drug discovery process.

The expense, complexity and time of the natural drug lead process have militated against natural products in the past, but the fact remains that natural products are a tried and tested source and there are many examples of natural drugs. The most important strengths of natural products are their complex chemistry and structural diversity.

THE POLYKETIDES

Polyketide natural products form an immense group of therapeutically important compounds comprising many antibiotics (macrolides and tetracyclines), fatty acids and aromatic compounds (anthrone purgative glycosides and anthracyclic antitumour agents).

Polyketides are mainly acetate (C_2) derived metabolites and occur throughout all organisms (as fatty acids and glycerides), but it is the microbes, predominantly the filamentous bacteria of the genus *Streptomyces*, that produce structurally diverse types of polyketides, especially as antibiotic substances. The biosynthesis of these compounds begins (Fig. 6.5) with the condensation of one molecule of **malonyl-CoA** (CoA is short for coenzyme A) with one molecule of **acetyl-CoA** to form the simple polyketide acetoacetyl-CoA. In this reaction (Claisen reaction), one molecule of CO_2 and one molecule of HSCoA are generated. The reaction occurs because the carbon between both carbonyl groups of malonyl-CoA (the acidic carbon) is nucleophilic and can attack an electropositive (electron-deficient) centre (e.g. the carbon of a carbonyl group).

The curved arrows in Fig. 6.5 indicate the movement of a pair of electrons to form a bond. Further condensation reactions between another molecule of malonyl-CoA and the growing polyketide lead to chain elongation, in which every other carbon in the chain is a carbonyl group. These chains are known as **poly-β-keto esters** and are the reactive intermediates that form the polyketides. Using these esters, large chains such as fatty acids can be constructed and, in fact, reduction of the carbonyl groups and hydrolysis of the -SHCoA thioester leads to the fatty acid class of compounds. The expanding

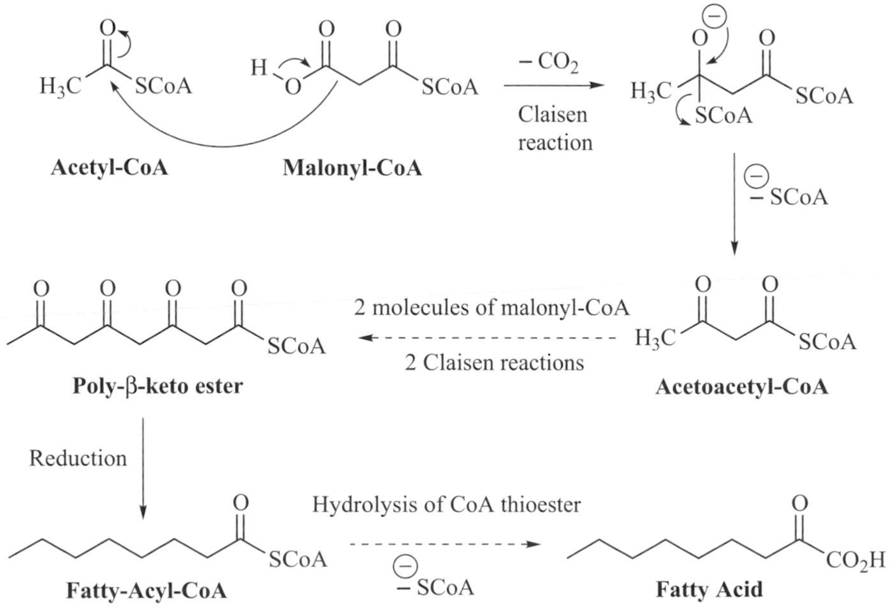

Fig. 6.5

polyketide chain may be attached as a thioester to either CoA or to a protein called an acyl-carrier protein. Multiple Claisen reactions with additional molecules of malonyl-CoA can generate long-chain fatty acids such as stearic acid and myristic acid.

The poly-β-keto ester can also cyclize to give aromatic natural products, and the way in which the poly-β-keto ester folds determines the type of natural product generated (Fig. 6.6). If the poly-β-keto ester folds as **A1**, then loss of a proton, followed by an intramolecular **Claisen reaction** of intermediate **A2** (by attack of the acidic carbon on the carbonyl), would result in the formation of a cyclic polyketide enolate **A3** which will rearrange to the keto compound with expulsion of the SCoA anion, resulting in the ketone **A4**. This ketone would readily undergo keto-enol tautomerism to the more favoured aromatic triphenol **A5** (**phloroacetophenone**).

Should the poly-β-keto ester fold as **B1**, then an aldol reaction on intermediate **B2** will occur by attack of the carbonyl by the acidic carbon, and, with the addition of a proton, an alcohol is formed, resulting in intermediate **B3**. This alcohol can then dehydrate to the conjugated alkene **B4**, which can also tautomerize and, via hydrolysis of the thioester-SCoA, the aromatic phenolic acid **orsellinic acid** (**B5**) is formed.

The reactive nature of poly-β-keto esters gives rise to many useful pharmaceuticals, and, because they are oxygen-rich starting precursors, the final natural products are generally rich in functional group chemistry. Ketone groups are often retained, but reduction to alcohols and the formation of ethers is common and many polyketides, particularly certain antibiotics and antitumour agents, also occur as glycosides.

FATTY ACIDS AND GLYCERIDES

This group of polyketides is widely distributed and present as part of the general biochemistry of all organisms, particularly as components of cell membranes. They are usually insoluble in water and soluble in organic solvents such as hexane, diethyl ether and chloroform. These natural products are sometimes referred to as fixed oils (liquid) or fats (solid), although these terms are imprecise as both fixed oils and fats contain mixtures of **glycerides** and free fatty acids and the state of the compound (i.e. liquid or solid) will depend on the temperature as well as the composition. Glycerides are fatty acid esters of **propane-1,2,3-triol (glycerol)**. They are sometimes referred to as saponifiable natural products, meaning that they can be converted into soaps by a strong base (NaOH). The term

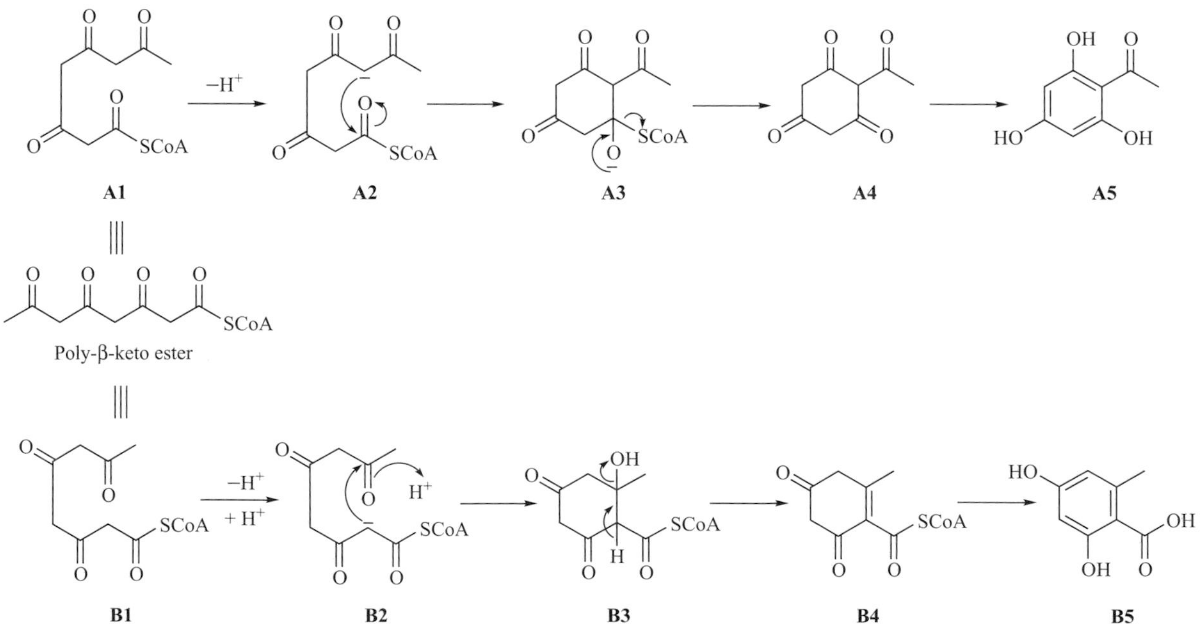

Fig. 6.6

saponifiable comes from the Latin word *sapo* meaning 'soap'. Saponification of fatty acids and glycerides with sodium hydroxide results in the formation of the sodium salts of the fatty acids (Fig. 6.7).

Glycerides can be very complicated mixtures as, unlike the example given in Fig. 6.7, the substituents on the glycerol alcohol may be different from each other, and it is not uncommon for lipophilic plant extracts to contain many types of glycerides.

Fatty acids are very important as formulation agents and vehicles in pharmacy and as components of cosmetics and soaps. Table 6.1 lists the common names, chemical formulae, sources and uses of the more common fatty acids.

The **saturated** fats are widespread in nature. The three most common (**myristic, palmitic** and **stearic acids**) differ in two methylene groups and contain no double bonds.

The **unsaturated** fatty acids contain a varying number of double bonds. This, together with the length of the carbon chain, is indicated after the name of the fatty acid. For example, **oleic acid** (18:1), which is widespread in plants and is a major component of olive oil from the olive tree *Olea europaea* (Oleaceae), has an 18-carbon chain and one double bond. **α-Linolenic acid** (18:3) is a constituent of linseed oil from *Linum usitatissimum* (Linaceae) and is used in liniments and as a highly valued additive in oil-based paints. The related acid, **γ-linolenic acid** (18:3), is found in evening primrose oil from *Oenothera biennis* (Onagraceae) and is widely used as a dietary supplement. This acid (like α-linolenic acid) is an essential fatty acid and is a precursor to the prostaglandins, which are involved in many biochemical pathways. Evening primrose oil has gained increasing popularity as an aid to alleviating symptoms associated with multiple sclerosis and premenstrual tension. **Ricinoleic acid** is the main purgative ingredient of castor oil from the seeds of *Ricinus communis* (Euphorbiaceae), which was used as a domestic purgative but is now used as a source of the oil for the manufacture of soap and as a cream base.

The **polyunsaturated** fatty acids contain three or more double bonds and are particularly beneficial in the diet as antioxidants. A number of health-food supplements are available as oils or capsules containing fish liver oils from **cod** and **halibut**, which are rich in polyunsaturated fats.

Natural oils that are high in fatty acids and glycerides are also used as components of oral formulations and vehicles for injections of pharmaceuticals. Some of the most common oils used in oral preparations include cocoa, olive, almond and coconut oils.

In man, the saturated fats are precursors for the biosynthesis of cholesterol, high serum levels of which are implicated in heart disease through the formation of atherosclerotic plaques in arteries. By reducing fat intake or by consuming foods that are high in unsaturated fats (particularly polyunsaturated fats), the risk of heart disease is reduced.

THE TETRACYCLINES

These polyketide-derived natural products are tetracyclic (i.e. have four linear six-membered rings, from which the group was named) and were discovered as part of a screening programme of extracts produced by filamentous bacteria (Actinomycetes), which are common components of soil. The most widely studied group of actinomycetes are species of the genus *Streptomyces*, which are very adept at producing many types of polyketide natural products of which the antibiotic **tetracycline** (Fig. 6.8) and the **anthracyclic** antitumour agents (see Chapter 8) are excellent examples.

The key features of this class of compound are shown in Fig. 6.8. Although tetracycline has numerous functional groups, including a tertiary amine,

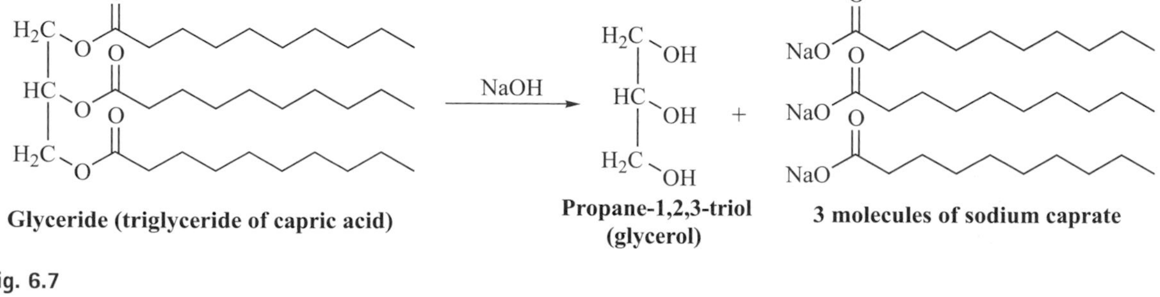

Glyceride (triglyceride of capric acid)   **Propane-1,2,3-triol (glycerol)**   **3 molecules of sodium caprate**

Fig. 6.7

Table 6.1 Common fatty acids

COMMON NAME	FORMULA	OIL AND SOURCE	OIL USE
Arachidic	$CH_3(CH_2)_{18}CO_2H$ (20:0)	Peanut oil, butter, *Arachis hypogaea* (Fabaceae)	Lubricant, food, emollient
Behenic	$CH_3(CH_2)_{20}CO_2H$ (22:0)	Carnauba wax, *Copernicia prunifera* (Arecaceae)	Polish for coated tablets
Butyric	$CH_3(CH_2)_2CO_2H$ (4:0)	Butter fat, cow, *Bovus taurus*	Food oil
Caproic	$CH_3(CH_2)_4CO_2H$ (6:0)	Coconut oil, *Cocos nucifera* (Arecaceae)	Manufacture of flavours
Caprylic	$CH_3(CH_2)_6CO_2H$ (8:0)	Coconut oil, *Cocos nucifera* (Arecaceae)	Dietary supplement, perfumes
Capric	$CH_3(CH_2)_8CO_2H$ (10:0)	*Cuphea viscosissima, C. lanceolata* (Lythraceae)	Artificial flavours, perfumes
Docosahexaenoic	$CH_3CH_2(CH=CHCH_2)_6CH_2CO_2H$ (22:6) all *cis*	Cod liver oil and halibut liver oil	Dietary supplement
Eicosapentaenoic	$CH_3CH_2(CH=CHCH_2)_5(CH_2)_2CO_2H$ (20:5) all *cis*	Cod liver oil and halibut liver oil	Dietary supplement
Erucic	$CH_3(CH_2)_7CH=CH(CH_2)_{11}CO_2H$ (22:1) *cis*	Rapeseed oil, *Brassica napus* var. *oleifera* (Brassicaceae)	Food
Lauric	$CH_3(CH_2)_{10}CO_2H$ (12:0)	Coconut and palm kernel oil, *Cocos nucifera, Elaeis guineensis* (Arecaceae)	Food, soaps, shampoos
Linoleic	$CH_3(CH_2)_4(CH=CHCH_2)_2(CH_2)_6 CO_2H$ (18:2) all *cis*	Vegetable oils, soybean, corn, *Glycine max* (Fabaceae)	Essential fatty acid
α-Linolenic	$CH_3CH_2CH=CHCH_2CH=CHCH_2CH=CH(CH_2)7CO_2H$	Linseed oil, *Linum usitatissimum* (Linaceae)	Liniments, paints, food
γ-Linolenic	$CH_3(CH_2)_4CH=CHCH_2CH=CHCH_2CH=CH(CH_2)_4CO_2H$	Evening primrose oil, *Oenothera biennis* (Onagraceae)	Dietary supplement
Myristic	$CH_3(CH_2)_{12}CO_2H$	Coconut and palm kernel oil, *Cocos nucifera, Elaeis guineensis*	Food, soaps, shampoos
Nervonic	$CH_3(CH_2)_7CH=CH(CH_2)_{13}CO_2H$ (24:1) all *cis*	Honesty oil, *Lunaria annua* (Brassicaceae)	Supplement for multiple sclerosis patients
Oleic	$CH_3(CH_2)_7CH=CH (CH_2)_7CO_2H$ (18:1) *cis*	Olive oil, *Olea europaea* (Oleaceae)	Food, emulsifying agent
Palmitic	$CH_3(CH_2)_{14}CO_2H$ (16:0)	Coconut and palm kernel oil, *Cocos nucifera, Elaeis guineensis*	Food, soaps, candles
Ricinoleic	$CH_3(CH_2)_5CH(OH)CH_2CH=CH(CH_2)_7CO_2H$ (18:1) *cis*	Castor oil, *Ricinus communis* (Euphorbiaceae)	Soap manufacture
Stearic	$CH_3(CH_2)_{16}CO_2H$ (18:0)	Olive oil, *Olea europaea* (Oleaceae)	Suppositories, tablet coatings

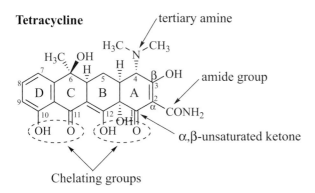

Fig. 6.8

hydroxyls, an amide, a phenolic hydroxy and keto groups, it is still possible to see that tetracycline is a member of the polyketide class of natural products by looking at the lower portion of the molecule. C_{10}, C_{11}, C_{12} and C_1 are oxygenated, indicating that the precursor of this compound was a poly-β-keto ester. C_{10} and C_{11} and C_{12} and C_1 form part of a chelating system that is essential for antibiotic activity and may readily chelate metal ions such as calcium, magnesium, iron or aluminium and become inactive. This is one of the reasons why oral formulations of the tetracycline antibiotics are never given with foodstuffs that are high in these ions (e.g. Ca^{2+} in milk) or with

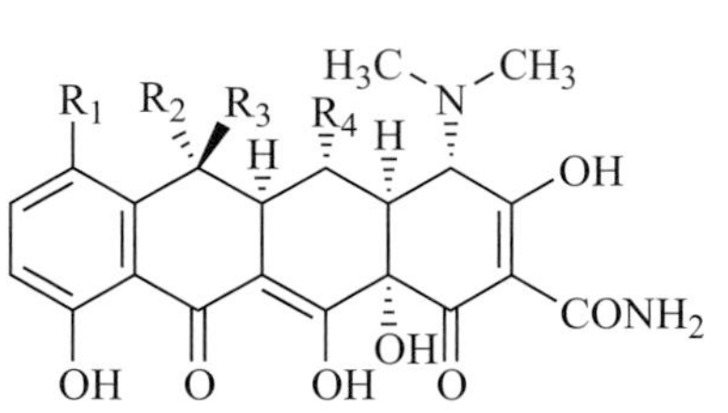

Tetracycline, R_1 = H, R_2 = CH$_3$, R_3 = OH, R_4 = H
Oxytetracycline, R_1 = H, R_2 = CH$_3$, R_3 = OH, R_4 = OH
Doxycycline, R_1 = H, R_2 = H, R_3 = CH$_3$, R_4 = OH
Minocycline, R_1 = N(CH$_3$)$_2$, R_2 = H, R_3 = H, R_4 = H

Fig. 6.9

antacids, which are high in cations such as Mg^{2+}. This group of antibiotics has been long known and they have a very broad spectrum of activity against Gram-positive and Gram-negative bacteria, spirochetes, mycoplasmae, rickettsiae and chlamydiae. **Tetracycline** comes from mutants of *Streptomyces aureofaciens*, and the related analogue **oxytetracycline** from *S. rimosus* (Fig. 6.9). These antibiotics are widely used as topical formulations for the treatment of acne, and as oral/injection preparations.

Minocycline and **doxycycline** are produced semisynthetically from natural tetracyclines. Minocycline has a very broad spectrum of activity and has been recommended for the treatment of respiratory and urinary tract infections and as a prophylaxis for meningitis caused by *Neisseria meningitides*. Doxycycline (Vibramycin) has use in treating chest infections caused by *Mycoplasma* and *Chlamydia* and has also been used prophylactically against malaria in regions where there is a high incidence of drug resistance.

GRISEOFULVIN

Another polyketide antibiotic is griseofulvin (Grisovin) from the fungus (mould) *Penicillium griseofulvum* (Fig. 6.10). This compound was originally

Griseofulvin

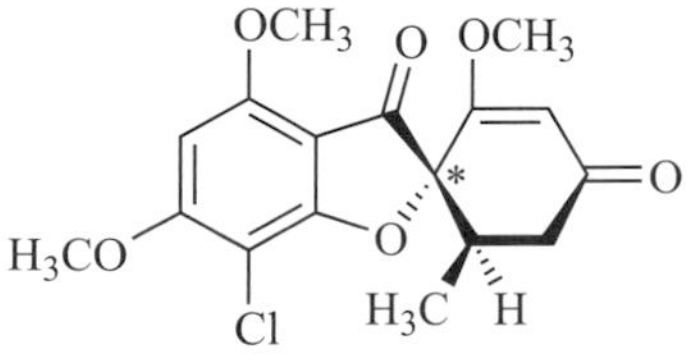

* denotes spiro carbon

Fig. 6.10

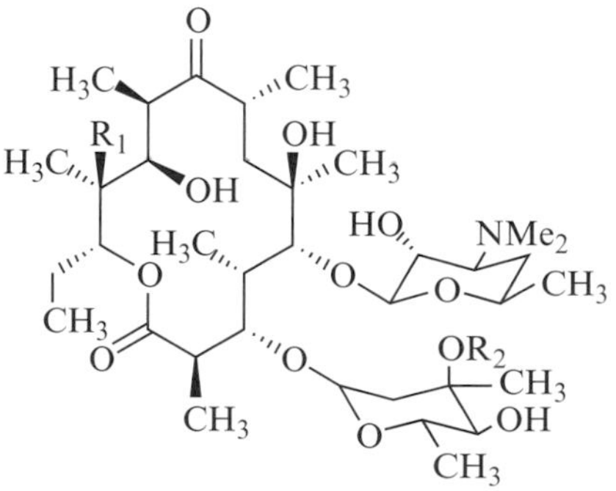

isolated by researchers at the London School of Hygiene and Tropical Medicine.

Griseofulvin is a **spiro** compound; that is, it has two rings that are **fused** at one carbon. Initially, the compound was used to treat fungal infections in animals and plants, but it is now recommended for the systemic treatment of fungal dermatophytic infections of the skin, hair, nails and feet caused by fungi belonging to the genera *Trichophyton, Epidermophyton* and *Microsporum*. Its main use is in veterinary practice for the treatment of ringworm in animals; it is marketed as Fulcin and Grisovin.

ERYTHROMYCIN A

Erythromycin A is a complex polyketide from *Saccharopolyspora erythrea* (Actinomycetes), which is a filamentous bacterium, originally classified in the genus *Streptomyces*. This compound is a member of the natural product class of **macrolide** antibiotics; these can contain 12 or more carbons in the main ring system. The term macrolide is derived from the fact that erythromycin is a large ring structure (**macro**) and is also a cyclic ester referred to as an **olide** (a lactone). As can be seen from Fig. 6.11, erythromycin A has the best features of natural products, being highly chiral (possessing many stereochemical centres) and having many different functional groups, including a sugar, an amino sugar, lactone, ketone and hydroxyl groups.

The therapeutic antibiotic is marketed as a mixture containing predominantly erythromycin A with small amounts of erythromycins B and C.

Erythromycin A, R_1 = OH, R_2 = CH$_3$
Erythromycin B, R_1 = H, R_2 = CH$_3$
Erythromycin C, R_1 =OH, R_2 =H

Fig. 6.11

Erythromycin is used to treat Legionnaire's disease and for patients with respiratory tract infections who are allergic to penicillin. A number of semisynthetic analogues (including **clarithromycin** and **azithromycin**) have been made and there has been interest in the genetic manipulation of *Saccharopolyspora erythrea* to produce 'un-natural' natural products. These compounds could potentially be analogues of the erythromycin class and might also have antibiotic activity.

THE STATINS

A further group of polyketide-derived natural products is the statins, so named for their ability to lower (bring into stasis) the production of cholesterol, high levels of which are a major contributing factor to the development of heart disease. The rationale behind the use of these compounds is as inhibitors of the enzyme hydroxymethylglutaryl-CoA (HMG-CoA) reductase, which catalyses the conversion of HMG-CoA (Fig. 6.12) to mevalonic acid, one of the key intermediates in the biosynthesis of cholesterol. HMG-CoA reductase became a target for the discovery of the natural product inhibitor **mevastatin**, which was initially isolated from cultures of the fungi *Penicillium citrinum* and *Penicillium brevicompactum* (Fig. 6.12).

Following this discovery, the methyl analogue **lovastatin** was isolated from *Monascus ruber* and *Aspergillus terreus* and is also an inhibitor of HMG-CoA reductase. **Simvastatin** (Zocor) is the dimethyl analogue of mevastatin and all three compounds are prodrugs, being activated by the hydrolysis (ring opening) of the lactone ring to β-hydroxy acids by liver enzymes. These acids are similar in structure to HMG-CoA and are inhibitors of the reductase enzyme. **Pravastatin** (Lipostat) is semisynthetically produced by microbial hydroxylation of mevastatin by *Streptomyces carbophilus*. Unlike the previous examples, the lactone ring has been opened to form the β-hydroxy acid which has then been converted into the sodium salt, increasing its hydrophilic water-soluble nature.

SHIKIMIC–ACID–DERIVED NATURAL PRODUCTS

Shikimic acid, sometimes referred to as shikimate, is a simple acid precursor for many natural products and aromatic amino acids, including phenylalanine, tyrosine, tryptophan, the simple aromatic acids that are common in nature (e.g. benzoic and gallic acids) and aromatic aldehydes such as vanillin and benzaldehyde that contribute to the pungent smell of many plants (Fig. 6.13).

A number of natural product groups can be constructed from the amino acid phenylalanine, in particular the **phenylpropenes, lignans, coumarins** and **flavonoids**, all of which possess a common substructure based on an aromatic 6-carbon ring (C_6 unit) with a 3-carbon chain (C_3 unit) attached to the aromatic ring (Fig. 6.14). Many reactions can occur to this 9-carbon unit, including oxidation, reduction, methylation, cyclization, glycosylation (addition of a sugar) and dimerization, all of which contribute to the value of natural products as a resource of biologically active compounds and enhance the qualities of structural complexity with the presence of chirality and functionality.

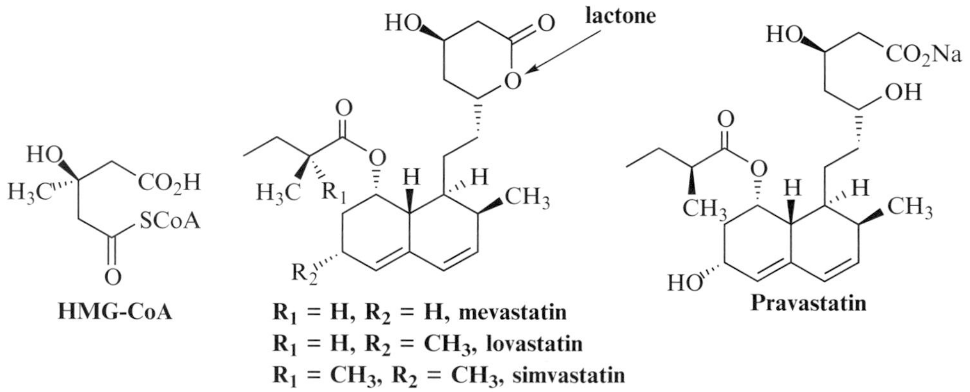

HMG-CoA

R$_1$ = H, R$_2$ = H, mevastatin
R$_1$ = H, R$_2$ = CH$_3$, lovastatin
R$_1$ = CH$_3$, R$_2$ = CH$_3$, simvastatin

Pravastatin

Fig. 6.12

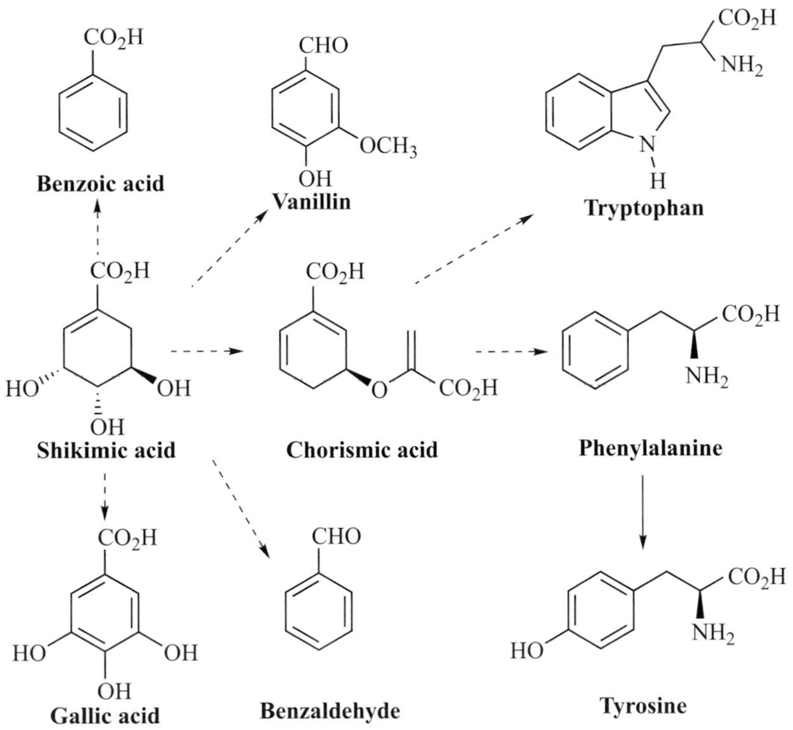

Fig. 6.13

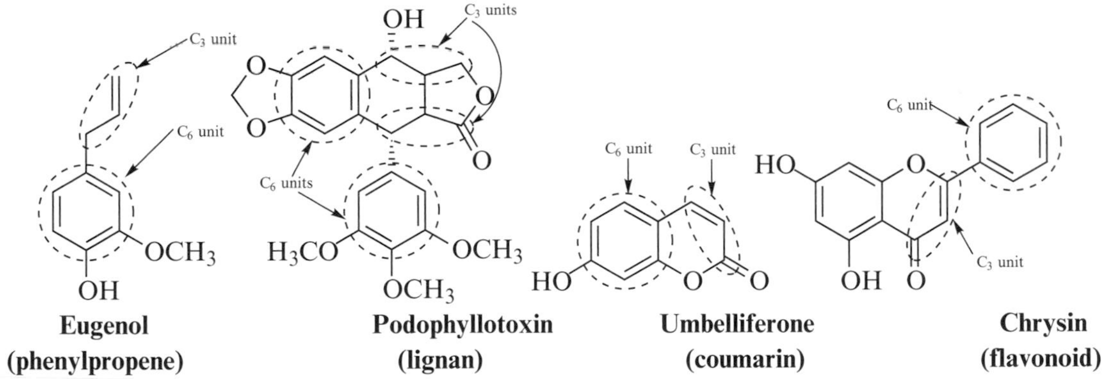

Fig. 6.14

PHENYLPROPENES

The phenylpropenes are the simplest of the shikimic-acid-derived natural products and consist purely of an aromatic ring with an unsaturated 3-carbon chain attached to the ring. They are biosynthesized by the oxidation of phenylalanine by the enzyme phenylalanine ammonia lyase, which through the loss of ammonia results in the formation of cinnamic acid. Cinnamic acid may then undergo a number of **elaboration reactions** to generate many of the phenylpropenes. For example, in Fig. 6.15, cinnamic acid is reduced to the corresponding aldehyde, **cinnamaldehyde**, which is the major component of cinnamon oil derived from the bark of *Cinnamomum zeylanicum* (Lauraceae) and used as a spice and flavouring. Cinnamon has a rich history, being used by the ancient Chinese as a treatment for fever and diarrhoea and by the Egyptians as a fragrant ingredient in embalming mixtures.

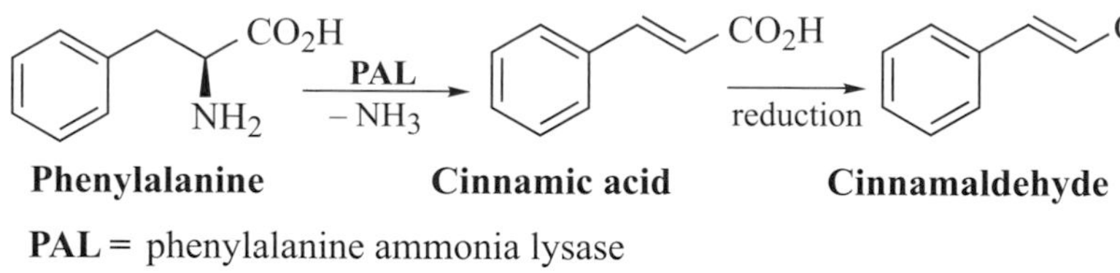

Phenylalanine → Cinnamic acid → Cinnamaldehyde

PAL = phenylalanine ammonia lysase

Fig. 6.15

Cinnamon leaf also contains **eugenol**, the major constituent of oil of cloves derived from *Syzygium aromaticum* (Myrtaceae). Clove oil was used as a dental anaesthetic and antiseptic, both properties of which are due to eugenol, and the oil is still widely used as a short-term relief for dental pain. These phenylpropenes may have many different functional groups (e.g. OCH_3, O-CH_2-O, OH) and the double bond may be in a different position in the C_3 chain (e.g. eugenol versus **anethole**) (Fig. 6.16). They are common components of spices, have highly aromatic pungent aromas and many are broadly antimicrobial, with activities against yeasts and bacteria. Some members of this class can also cause inflammation.

Myristicin is a component of nutmeg (*Myristica fragrans*, Myristicaceae) and is thought to be the hallucinogenic component when this spice is ingested in large quantities. This phenylpropene is very lipophilic due to the presence of methylenedioxy and methyl ether substituent groups and it has been proposed that *in vivo* the double bond of this compound is aminated (an amino group is added), resulting in the formation of an 'amphetamine-like' compound. It should be noted, however, that high doses can be fatal and the ingestion of large amounts of nutmeg should be avoided. **Safrole**, and particularly *trans*-**anethole**, are the major components of anise-flavoured essential oils from star anise (*Illicium verum*, Illiciaceae), aniseed (*Pimpinella anisum*, Apiaceae) and fennel (*Foeniculum vulgare* var. *vulgare*, Apiaceae). These oils are components of popular Mediterranean beverages such as anisette, ouzo and raki. When water is added to these drinks a cloudy white suspension results, which is attributable to a decrease in the solubility of these phenylpropenes as they are more soluble in ethanol than in water.

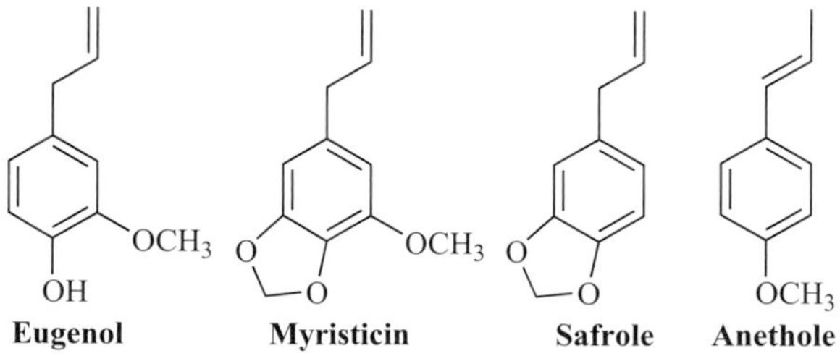

The phenylpropenes are generally produced by **steam distillation** of plant material (e.g. cloves) to produce an essential oil, which is normally a complex mixture of phenylpropenes and other volatile natural products such as **hemiterpenes, monoterpenes** and **sesquiterpenes** (see below). The steam distillation procedure involves boiling the plant material with water and trapping the vapour in a distillation apparatus. The condensed liquid is transferred to a separating funnel and, as the oils are immiscible with water and form a less dense layer, they can be readily removed.

LIGNANS

Lignans are low molecular weight polymers formed by the coupling of two phenylpropene units through their C_3 side-chains (Fig. 6.17) and between the aromatic ring and the C_3 chain. A common precursor of lignans is cinnamyl alcohol, which can readily form free radicals and enzymatically dimerize to form aryltetralin-type lignans of which the compounds **podophyllotoxin, 4′-demethylpodophyllotoxin** and **α-** and **β-peltatin** (from *Podophyllum peltatum* and *Podophyllum hexandrum*, Berberidaceae) are examples (Fig. 6.17).

This class of compound is common in the plant kingdom, especially in the heartwood and leaves and as major constituents of resinous exudates from roots and bark. The resin obtained from the roots of *P. peltatum* has long been used as a treatment for warts by North American Indians, and some preparations still exist which contain podophyllin, which is an ethanolic extraction of the resin rich in podophyllotoxin. This lignan is a dimer of two 9-carbon (C_6-C_3) units and is **polycyclic** (possessing more than one ring). This natural product has a five-membered lactone ring or cyclic ester and there

Eugenol   Myristicin   Safrole   Anethole

Fig. 6.16

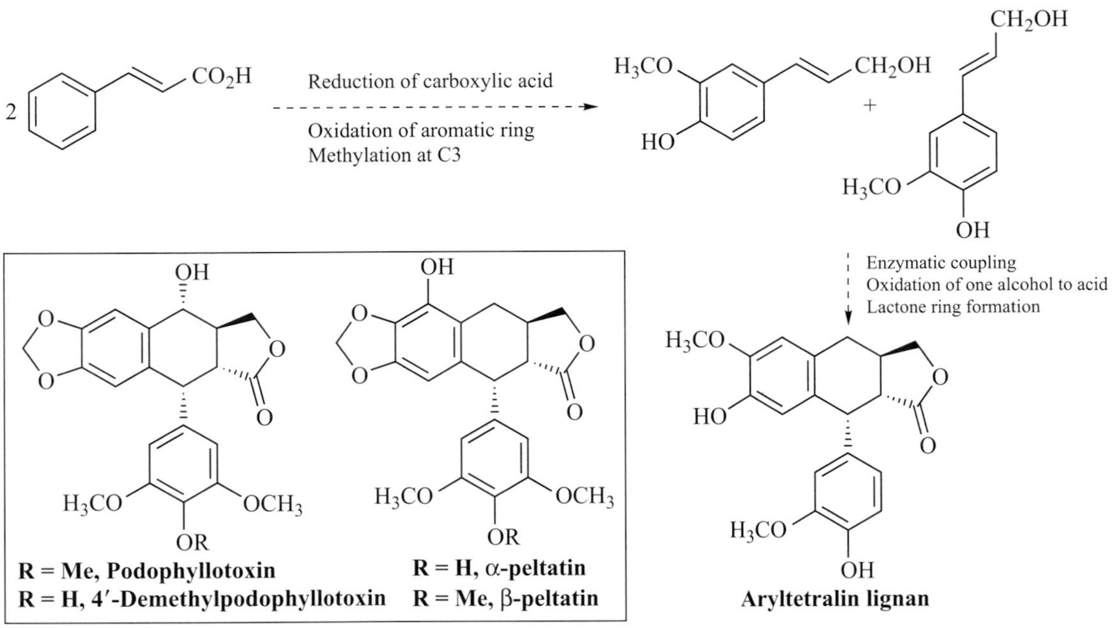

Fig. 6.17

are many examples of these types of lignans possessing this functional group.

Much work has been done on the podophyllotoxin (aryltetralin) class of lignans, the major active cytotoxic principle, podophyllotoxin, being isolated in the 1940s. This compound inhibits the enzyme tubulin polymerase which is needed for the synthesis of tubulin, a protein that is a vital component of cell division (mitosis). Podophyllotoxin is highly toxic and not used clinically for the treatment of cancers, but this class of compounds was an excellent template on which to base the semisynthetic analogues **etoposide** and **teniposide** (see Chapter 8).

COUMARINS

The coumarins are shikimate-derived metabolites formed when phenylalanine is deaminated and hydroxylated to *trans*-hydroxycinnamic acid (Fig. 6.18). The double bond of this acid is readily converted to the *cis* form by light-catalysed isomerization, resulting in the formation of a compound that has phenol and acidic groups in close proximity. These may then react **intramolecularly** to form a lactone and the basic coumarin nucleus, typified by the compound **coumarin** itself, which contributes to the smell of newly mown hay.

The majority of the coumarins are oxygenated at position C_7, resulting from *para* hydroxylation

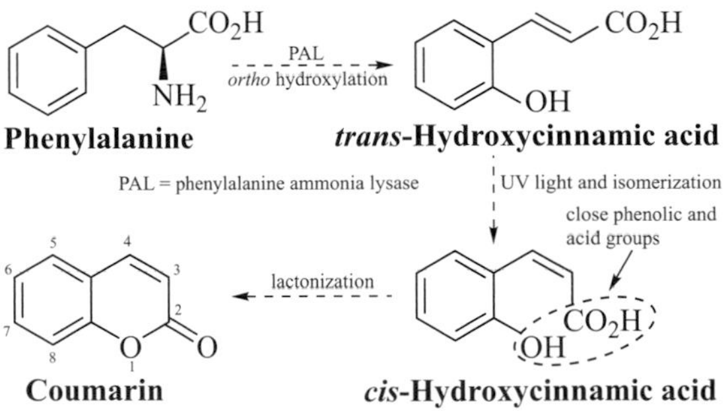

Fig. 6.18

of cinnamic acid to give coumaric acid prior to further *ortho* hydroxylation, isomerization and lactone formation.

Coumarins have a limited distribution in the plant kingdom and have been used to classify plants according to their presence (chemotaxonomy). They are commonly found in the plant families Apiaceae, Rutaceae, Asteraceae and Fabaceae and, as with all of the natural products mentioned so far, undergo many elaboration reactions, including hydroxylation and methylation and, particularly, the addition of terpenoid-derived groups (C_2, C_5 and C_{10} units) (Fig. 6.19).

Some coumarins are **phytoalexins** and are synthesized *de novo* by the plant following infection by a bacterium or fungus. These phytoalexins are

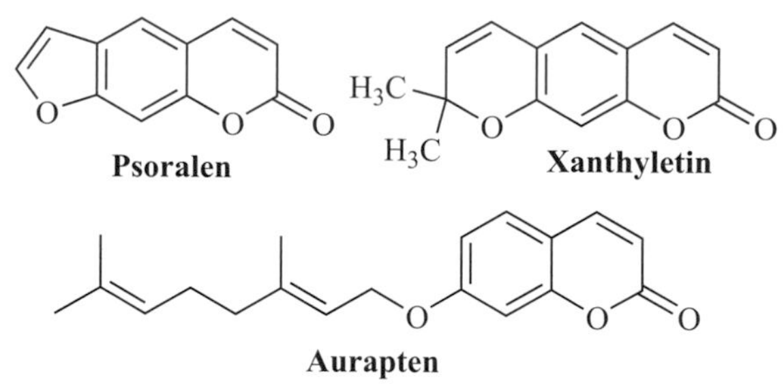

Fig. 6.19

broadly antimicrobial; for example, **scopoletin** is synthesized by the potato (*Solanum tuberosum*) following fungal infection. **Aesculetin** occurs in the horse chestnut (*Aesculus hippocastanum*) and phytotherapeutic preparations of the bark of this species are used to treat capillary fragility. *Hieracium pilosella* (Asteraceae), also known as mouse ear, contains **umbelliferone** and was used to treat brucellosis in veterinary medicine and the antibacterial activity of this plant drug may in part be due to the presence of this simple phenol (Fig. 6.20). **Khellin** is an **isocoumarin** (**chromone**) natural product from *Ammi visnaga* (Apiaceae) and has activity as a spasmolytic and vasodilator.

It has long been known that animals fed sweet clover (*Melilotus officinalis*, Fabaceae) die from haemorrhaging. The poisonous compound responsible for this adverse effect was identified as the bis-hydroxycoumarin (hydroxylated coumarin dimer) **dicoumarol** (Fig. 6.21).

Dicoumarol is used as an anticoagulant in the USA. It is used alone or in conjunction with heparin in the

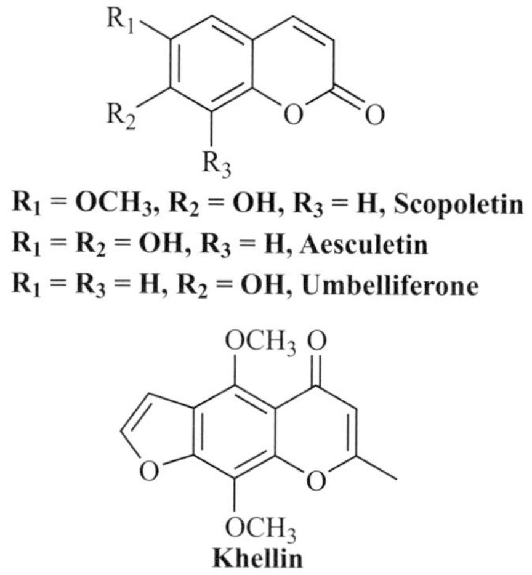

$R_1 = OCH_3$, $R_2 = OH$, $R_3 = H$, **Scopoletin**
$R_1 = R_2 = OH$, $R_3 = H$, **Aesculetin**
$R_1 = R_3 = H$, $R_2 = OH$, **Umbelliferone**

Khellin

Fig. 6.20

prophylaxis and treatment of blood clotting and to arrest gangrene after frostbite. A number of compounds have been synthesized based on the dicoumarol structure and include salts of **warfarin** and **nicoumalone**, which are widely used as anticoagulants. These agents interfere with vitamin K function in liver cells; this vitamin is necessary for the synthesis of 'normal' prothrombin. A deficiency of vitamin K leads to abnormal prothrombin synthesis and a reduction in activity of the blood-clotting mechanism. Warfarin has also been used as a rat poison.

Warfarin and nicoumalone are examples of fully synthetic agents that have been developed from a natural product template.

The **psoralens** are coumarins that possess a furan ring and are sometimes known as **furocoumarins** or **furanocoumarins** because of this ring. Examples are **psoralen, bergapten, xanthotoxin** and **isopimpinellin** (Fig. 6.22).

Because of the extended chromophore of these compounds, they readily absorb light and fluoresce blue/yellow under long-wave ultraviolet light (UV-A, 320–380 nm). These compounds may be produced by the plant as a protection mechanism against high doses of sunlight and some coumarins are formulated into sunscreens and cosmetics for this purpose. The psoralens are typical of the citrus (Rutaceae) and celery (Apiaceae) families. Some plants of these groups are known as 'blister bushes' as the psoralens they contain are known to cause phototoxicity. This can prove difficult for farmers who clear large amounts of giant hogweed (*Heracleum mantegazzianum*) and come into contact with sap from the plant, which is rich in psoralens and, in the presence of sunlight, can cause inflammation and, in severe cases, blistering of the skin. Other species that are known to be phototoxic include hogweed (*Heracleum sphondylium*), rue (*Ruta graveolens*) and some *Citrus* spp., particularly essential oils from bergamot (*Citrus aurantium* subsp. *bergamia*, Rutaceae) of which a major constituent is **bergapten**. A number of apiaceous herbs that have culinary significance, such as celery (*Apium graveolens*), parsley (*Petroselinum crispum*), parsnip (*Pastinaca sativa*) and angelica (*Angelica archangelica*), may even cause phototoxicity due to the presence of furanocoumarins.

The mechanism of this phototoxicity has yet to be fully elucidated, but it is known that the psoralens are carcinogenic and mutagenic due to the formation of adducts with pyrimidine bases of DNA, such as thymine, via cycloaddition (Fig. 6.23).

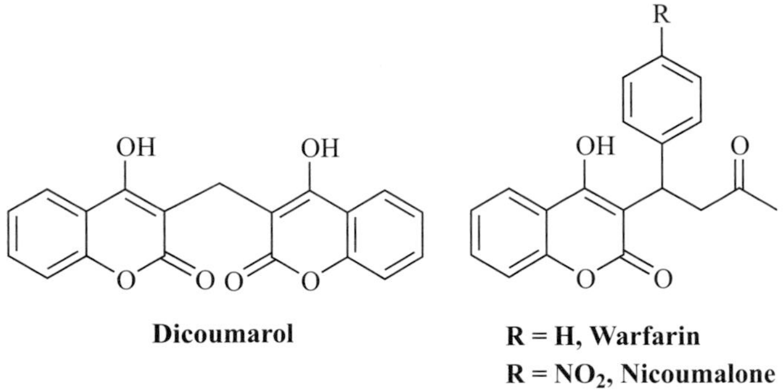
OH
OH
O
O O
O
Dicoumarol
R
OH
O
O
O
R = H, Warfarin
R = NO2, Nicoumalone

Fig. 6.21

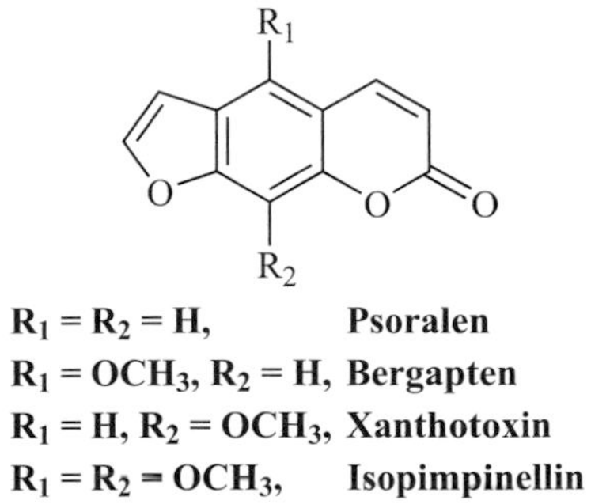
R1
O
O
O
R2
R1 = R2 = H, Psoralen
R1 = OCH3, R2 = H, Bergapten
R1 = H, R2 = OCH3, Xanthotoxin
R1 = R2 = OCH3, Isopimpinellin

Fig. 6.22

This reaction can occur with one (monoadduct) or two (diadduct) pyrimidine bases and may result in cross-linking of DNA.

Preparations using apiaceous and rutaceous plants containing psoralens have been used to promote skin pigmentation in the disease vitiligo, a disease that is common in the Middle East and results from patches of skin that are deficient in the pigment melanin. Pure **xanthotoxin** is used to treat severe vitiligo and psoriasis, and is given orally in combination with UV-A. This results in coloration and pigmentation of non-pigmented skin areas and an improvement in the psoriatic skin by reducing cell proliferation. The treatment is not without risks and requires careful regulation to prevent skin cancer or cataract formation. The therapy is referred to as PUVA (psoralen+UV-A) or photodynamic therapy in which a drug is activated by the application of UV light.

FLAVONOIDS

The flavonoids are derived from a C_6-C_3 (phenylpropane) unit which has as its source shikimic acid (via phenylalanine) and a further C_6 unit that is derived from the polyketide pathway. This polyketide fragment is generated by three molecules of malonyl-CoA, which combine with the C_6-C_3 unit (as a CoA thioester) to form a triketide starter unit (Fig. 6.24). Flavonoids are, therefore, of mixed biosynthesis, consisting of units derived from both shikimic acid and polyketide pathways.

The triketide starter unit undergoes cyclization by the enzyme chalcone synthase to generate the **chalcone** group of flavonoids. Cyclization can then

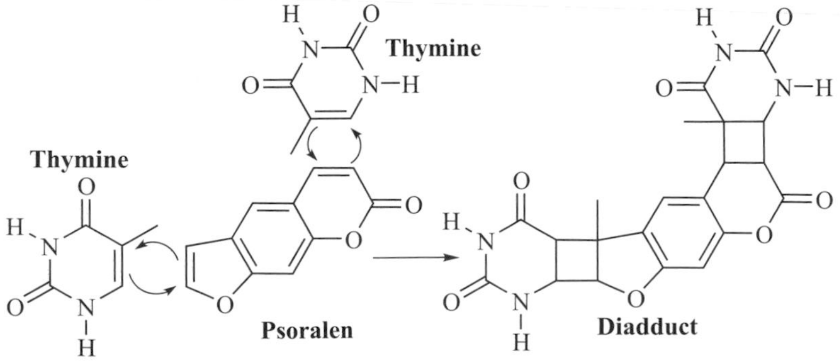
Thymine
Thymine
Psoralen
Diadduct

Fig. 6.23

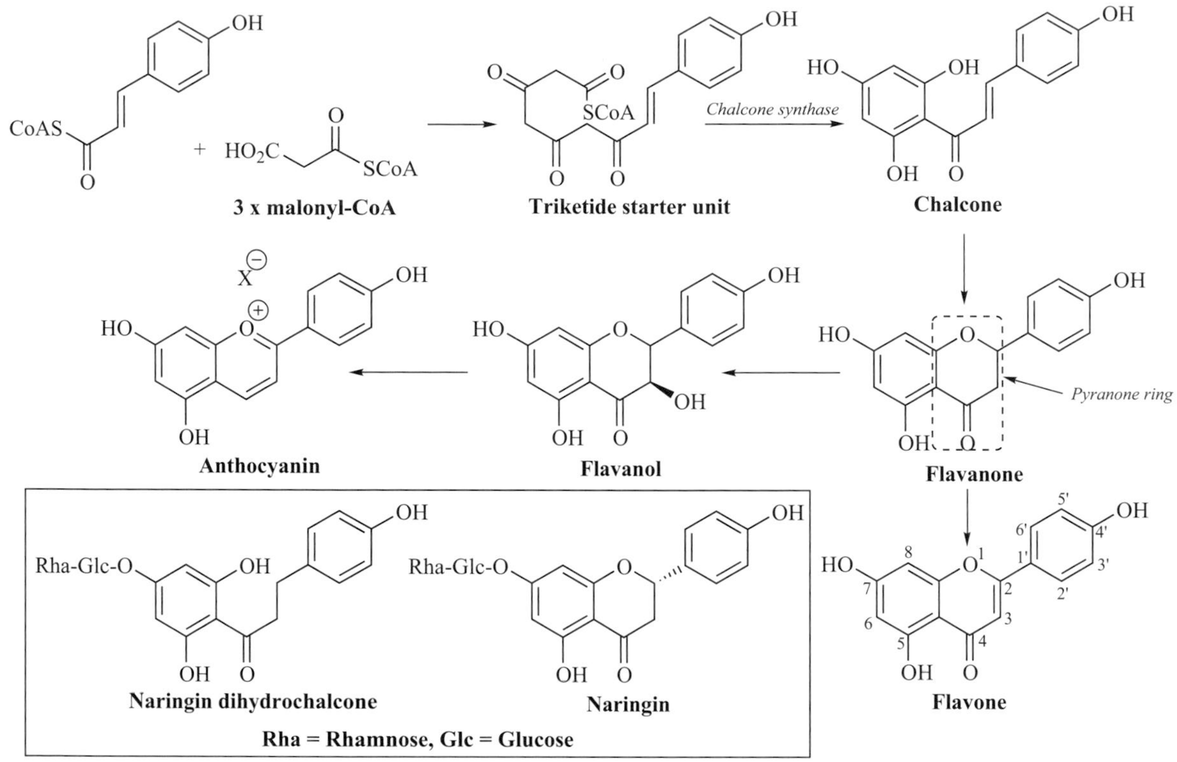

Fig. 6.24

occur to give a pyranone ring-containing **flavanone** nucleus, which can either have the C_2-C_3 bond oxidized (unsaturated) to give the **flavones** or be hydroxylated at position C_3 of the pyranone ring to give the **flavanol** group of flavonoids. The flavanols may then be further oxidized to yield the **anthocyanins**, which contribute to the brilliant blues of flowers and the dark colour of red wine. The flavonoids contribute to many of the other colours found in nature, particularly the yellow and orange of petals; even the colourless flavonoids absorb light in the UV spectrum (due to their extensive chromophores) and are visible to many insects. It is likely that these compounds have high ecological importance in nature as colour attractants to insects and birds as an aid to plant pollination. Certain flavonoids also markedly affect the taste of foods; for example, some are very bitter and astringent such as the flavanone glycoside **naringin** (Fig. 6.24), which occurs in the peel of grapefruit (*Citrus paradisi*). Interestingly, the closely related compound **naringin dihydrochalcone** (Fig. 6.24), which lacks the pyranone ring of naringin, is

exceptionally sweet, being some 1000 times sweeter than table sugar (sucrose).

It is likely that the flavonoids have important dietary significance because, being phenolic compounds, they are strongly antioxidant. Many disease states are known to be exacerbated by the presence of free radicals such as superoxide and hydroxyl, and flavonoids have the ability to scavenge and effectively 'mop up' these damaging oxidizing species. Foods rich in this group have, therefore, been proposed to be important in ameliorating diseases such as cancer and heart disease (which can be worsened by oxidation of low-density lipoprotein); **quercetin** (Fig. 6.25), a flavonoid present in many foodstuffs, is a strong antioxidant. Components of milk thistle (*Silybum marianum*), in particular **silybin** (Fig. 6.25), are antihepatotoxins; extracts of milk thistle are generally known as **silymarin** and are used to reduce the effects of poisoning by fungi of the genus *Amanita*, which produces the deadly peptide toxins the amanitins. The mechanism of action of these antihepatotoxins is not entirely clear, but it has been proposed that they

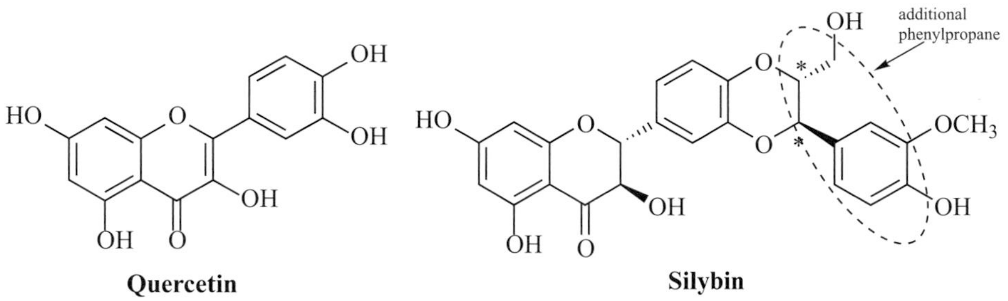

Quercetin   **Silybin**

Fig. 6.25

protect liver cells by reducing entry of the toxic peptides through the cell membrane and by acting as broad-spectrum antioxidants by scavenging the free radicals that can lead to hepatotoxicity. Silybin is a flavanol that has an additional phenylpropane unit joined to it as a di-ether and it exists in the extract as a mixture of enantiomers at one of the positions where this additional unit is joined (* in Fig. 6.25).

The **stilbenes**, sometimes referred to as **bisbenzyls** or **stilbenoids**, are related to the flavonoids and have the basic structure C_6-C_2-C_6 (Fig. 6.26) arising from the loss of one carbon (as CO_2) from the triketide starter unit. The simplest member of this class is **stilbene**. There is much interest in this class of compounds, especially in **resveratrol**, a component of red wine that has antioxidant, anti-cancer and anti-inflammatory activity. There is a low incidence of heart disease among the French population where large concentrations of fatty acids are sometimes present in the diet. It has been suggested that this low rate of heart disease is due to the consumption of red wine, which is rich in resveratrol and other flavonoids, and that the presence of these antioxidant compounds is cardioprotective. This phenomenon is known as 'the French paradox' and cardiologists advise patients who have a history of heart disease to consume a glass of red wine per day. Another group of stilbenoids of current interest are the **combretastatins**. For example, **combretastatin**

A_1, which is a cytotoxic drug lead, is a potent inhibitor of microtubule assembly and thought to have anti-tumour activity as a result of specifically targeting the vasculature of tumours. Combretastatin A_1 is derived from *Combretum caffrum* (Combretaceae) and there has been much work on the Combretaceae to look for other biologically active members of this class.

TANNINS

In addition to the flavonoids, another class of natural products that gives rise to the astringency and bitterness in plants and food are the **tannins**. This group comprises water-soluble polyphenolic compounds, which may have a high molecular weight. They are broadly divided into two groups: the **hydrolysable** tannins, which are formed by the esterification of sugars (e.g. glucose) with simple phenolic acids that are shikimate-derived (e.g. gallic acid), and the **non-hydrolysable** tannins, which are sometimes referred to as **condensed** tannins, that occur due to polymerization (condensation) reactions between flavonoids (Fig. 6.27).

As their name suggests, the hydrolysable tannins may be hydrolysed with base to simple acids and sugars. A key feature of tannins is their ability to bind to proteins, and they have been used to tan leather, clarify beer and as astringent preparations in pharmacy. They have a very wide distribution

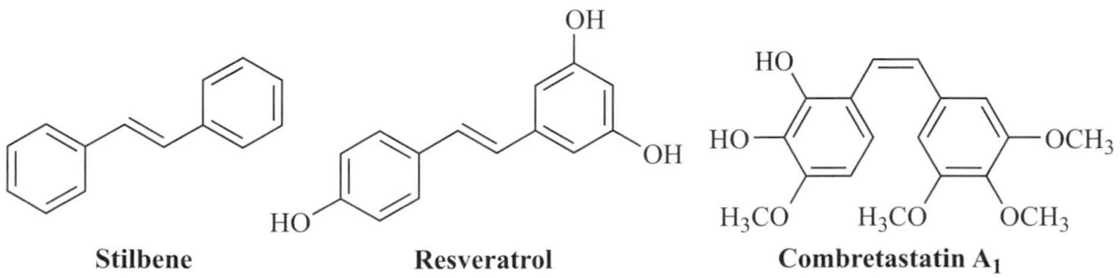

Stilbene   **Resveratrol**   **Combretastatin A₁**

Fig. 6.26

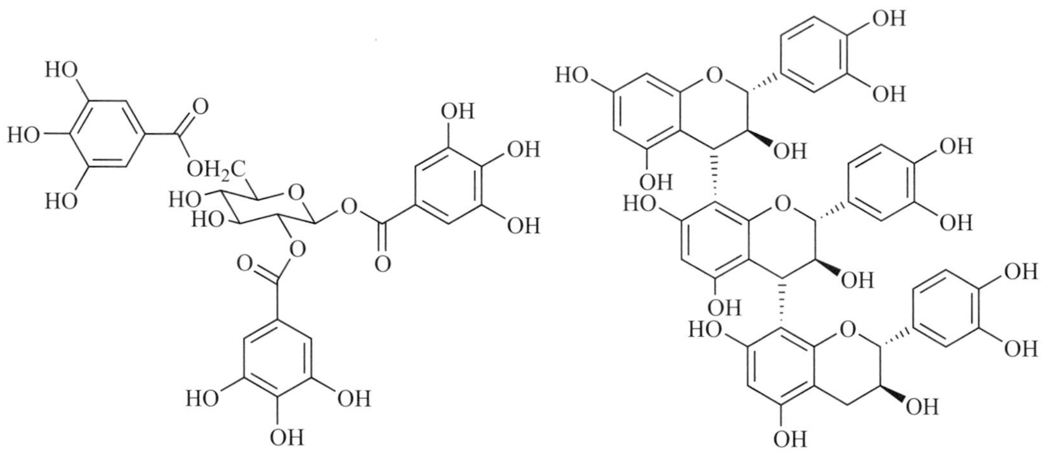

Hydrolysable tannin (trigalloyl glucose)   **Non-hydrolysable tannin (flavonoid trimer)**

Fig. 6.27

in the plant kingdom and may be produced by a plant as a feeding deterrent, as their binding to proteins may reduce the dietary value of the plant as a food.

Tannic acid is a mixture of gallic acid esters of glucose and is obtained from nutgall, which is an abnormal growth of the tree *Quercus infectoria* produced by insects. These growths (galls) are harvested and extracted with solvents (ether and water); the aqueous layer is collected and evaporated to yield tannic acid, which is further purified and used as a topical preparation for cold sores.

THE TERPENES

The terpenes are very widespread in nature and occur in most species, including man. They are sometimes referred to as **isoprenes** because a common recurring motif in their structure (the branched repeating C_5 unit, the **isopentane** skeleton) is similar to isoprene (Fig. 6.28). Terpenes (**hemiterpenes, monoterpenes and sesquiterpenes**) contribute to many of the aromas associated with plants and range in complexity from simple C_5 units (**hemiterpenes**) up to the **polyisoprenes**, which include latex, leaf waxes and rubber. Terpenes are derived from a number of extensive reactions between two C_5 units [**dimethylallyl pyrophosphate (DMAPP)** and **isopentenyl pyrophosphate (IPP)**] (Fig. 6.28); the products of these reactions will, therefore, have multiples of five carbons. DMAPP and IPP are biosynthesized from two sources (**mevalonic acid** or **deoxyxylulose phosphate**).

The terpenes are a perfect example of a natural product class that is highly structurally diverse, has many members that are chiral and have extensive functional group chemistry. The simplest are the hemiterpenes (C_5) produced by modification reactions to either DMAPP or IPP and include simple acids such as the structural isomers **tiglic acid** and **angelic acid** (Fig. 6.28), which form esters with many natural products. The monoterpenes (C_{10}), sesquiterpenes (C_{15}), **diterpenes** (C_{20}), **triterpenes** and **steroids** (C_{30}-derived) and the **tetraterpenes** (**carotenoids**, C_{40}) are all important medicinally and thus will be dealt with in more detail.

MONOTERPENES (C_{10})

Together with the phenylpropenes, the **monoterpenes** are major constituents of the volatile oils that are common in plants and which contribute to their

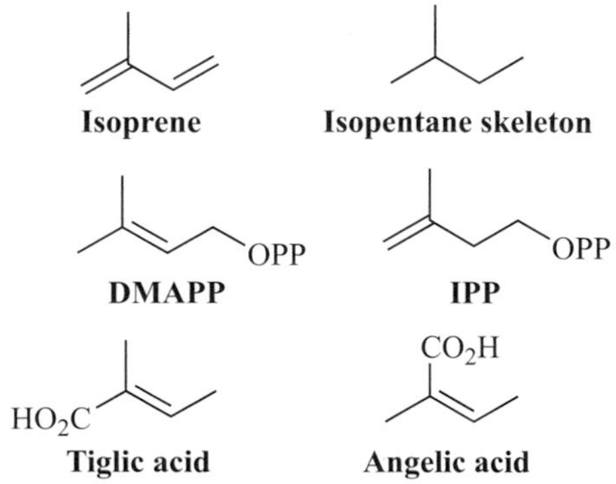

Isoprene   **Isopentane skeleton**

DMAPP   **IPP**

Tiglic acid   **Angelic acid**

Fig. 6.28

aroma. This group of compounds has highly characteristic odours and tastes and is used widely in the food and cosmetic industries in flavourings and perfumes. Monoterpenes are present in the leaf glands of plants and in the skin and peel of fruit (in particular *Citrus* spp.). The reasons for the presence of these compounds in the exterior organs of the plant are due to the many complex interactions that plants have with other organisms: some monoterpenes are insect attractants (to aid pollination), others have a broad spectrum of antimicrobial activity to inhibit growth and invasion by bacteria and fungi (e.g. **thymol**). Volatile oils in plants are highly complex and their analysis by gas chromatography (GC) can show the presence of hundreds of individual components, many of which are monoterpenoid. These oils are highly prized in the perfume industry; plants such as jasmine are cultivated and the monoterpene-rich oils harvested for the production of popular fragrances. Monoterpenes may be either aliphatic (**acyclic** or straight chain) or **cyclic** (saturated, partially unsaturated or fully aromatic) compounds. These natural products usually possess functional groups such as ethers, hydroxyls, acids, aldehydes, esters or ketone moieties, and are generally highly volatile and fat-soluble (lipophilic).

Biosynthetically, the monoterpenes are produced by the reaction between DMAPP and IPP in the presence of the enzyme **prenyltransferase** (Fig. 6.29).

The first step of this reaction is thought to be the ionization of DMAPP to a cation (through the loss of pyrophosphate), which is then attacked by the double bond of IPP to generate a further cationic intermediate. Loss of a proton from the carbon neighbouring the cation (resulting in double bond formation) occurs in a stereospecific fashion (the R proton is lost) and this generates **geranyl pyrophosphate** (a C_{10} unit).

Geranyl pyrophosphate can then undergo many reactions to generate the variety of monoterpenes observed, such as simple modification to give the acyclic monoterpene **β-citronellol**, which is a component of rose oil. Geranyl pyrophosphate can be cyclized to give cyclic monoterpenes, which may be fully saturated, partially unsaturated or fully aromatic products of which **menthol, piperitone** and **carvacrol** are examples, respectively (Fig. 6.30).

As with the polyketides, some key features of monoterpenes (and terpenes in general) are the presence of stereochemical centres (chiral centres) and wide-ranging functional group chemistry. The extensive structural diversity of this group is astounding considering that all of the monoterpenes are derived from just one C_{10} unit, geranyl pyrophosphate.

Linalool, a major constituent of coriander oil (*Coriandrum sativum*), is used as a flavouring and carminative. **Myrcene**, which is present in hop oil, is also used as a flavouring. Tea tree oil (from

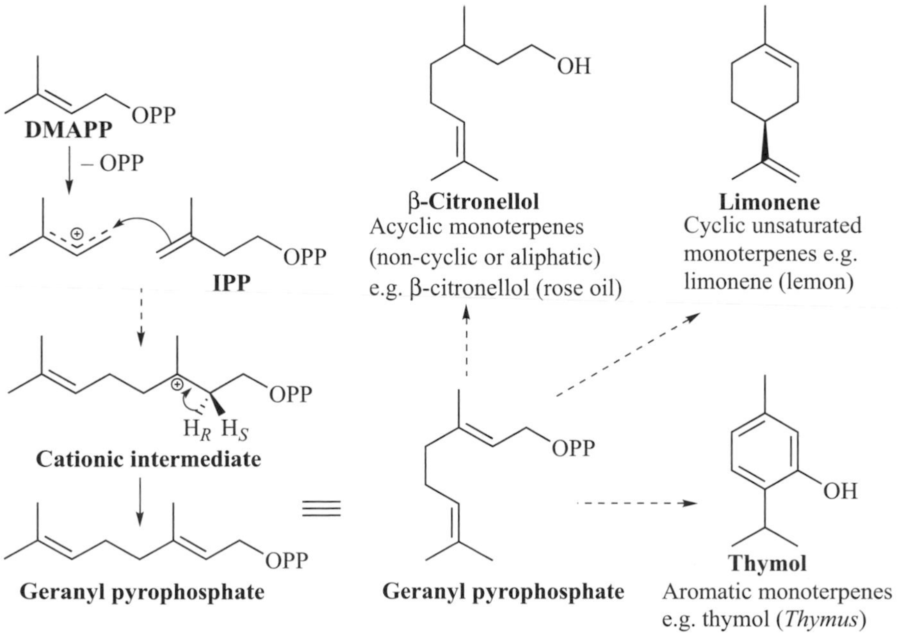

DMAPP

$-$ OPP

IPP

Cationic intermediate

H_R H_S

Geranyl pyrophosphate

β-Citronellol
Acyclic monoterpenes
(non-cyclic or aliphatic)
e.g. β-citronellol (rose oil)

Limonene
Cyclic unsaturated
monoterpenes e.g.
limonene (lemon)

Geranyl pyrophosphate

Thymol
Aromatic monoterpenes
e.g. thymol (*Thymus*)

Fig. 6.29

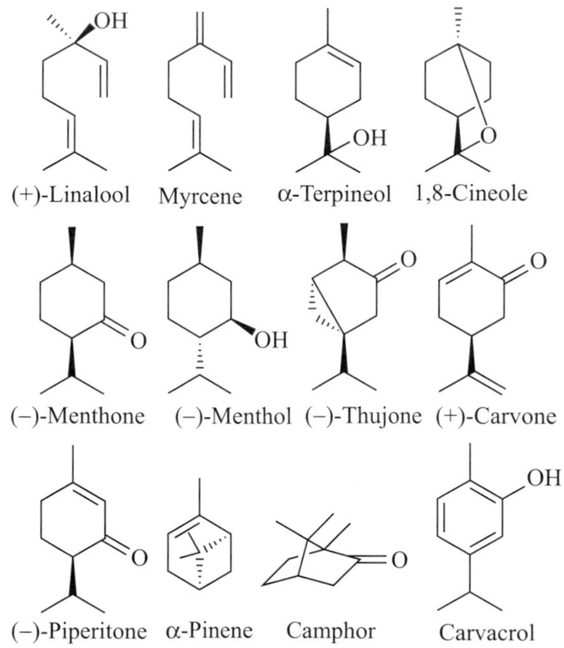

Fig. 6.30

Melaleuca alternifolia) has been used by the indigenous peoples of Australia as a treatment for skin infections; a main ingredient of this volatile oil is the tertiary hydroxylated monoterpene **α-terpineol**. **1,8-Cineole**, the structurally related ether, also has antibacterial properties and comes from species of *Eucalyptus* that are in the same plant family as *Melaleuca*, the Myrtaceae. **Menthol** and **menthone** are major constituents of oils of plants belonging to the genus *Mentha* (Lamiaceae); in particular, peppermint (*Mentha* × *piperita*) is used as a flavouring and carminative tea, and menthone is included in some pharmaceutical preparations as a nasal decongestant. **Thujone** has a cyclopropane ring as a functional group and is a constituent of *Artemisia absinthium*, an extract of which was used as an anthelmintic by the French army, hence the common name for this plant, wormwood. The liqueur absinthe was prepared by making an alcoholic extract of wormwood; this was highly popular amongst artists and literati in 19th century France. Unfortunately, high doses of this beverage induce hallucinations and the drink is addictive (not just the alcohol), and these effects led to the term 'absinthism' to describe the side effects associated with absinthe. Due to these problems, the production of absinthe was banned in 1915. **Carvone** is derived from dill (*Anethum graveolens*) and caraway

oils (*Carum carvi*), which have use as calming ingredients in gripe water preparations. **α-Pinene**, which has a cyclobutane ring system, is the major constituent of juniper oil (*Juniperus communis*), which is antiseptic and used in aromatherapy and as a flavouring. Oil from *Cinnamomum camphora* (Lauraceae) is produced by the steam distillation of the wood and is rich in **camphor**, which is antiseptic and used in soaps.

Although oils from plants such as caraway, coriander, dill, peppermint and eucalyptus are widely used as flavouring agents and perfumes for many preparations (including foods, cosmetics and pharmaceuticals), at present not a great deal is known about the biological activity of the monoterpene components present in these complex mixtures. Natural oils have a very specific aroma, which accounts for the preference to buy these complex natural mixtures rather than cheaper synthetic alternatives. They are produced by steam distillation (see Chapter 7) and, unless much is known about the stability of the oil components, care must be taken using this technique as some monoterpenes are **thermolabile** (i.e. they decompose on heating). The analysis of these complex mixtures is usually performed by GC or the combined technique of gas chromatography–mass spectrometry (GC-MS), which utilizes the separating power of GC with MS to yield the molecular ions of components of a mixture, and in some cases fragmentation information which can aid in determining the structure of these components.

The perfume industry has a great interest in monoterpene mixtures and uses preparative GC to separate and isolate individual components, which a highly qualified perfumer then smells to find compounds with a distinctive, novel or unusual aroma that can be blended with other volatiles to give a popular fragrance.

The **iridoids** are monoterpenes derived from the **iridane** skeleton, which is derived from geranyl pyrophosphate and, when oxidized, produces the iridoid skeleton (Fig. 6.31). These natural products are normally esterified and are common in the plant families Lamiaceae, Gentianaceae and Valerianaceae. The compounds are highly oxygenated and the esters are often derived from hemiterpenes; for example, valeric acid is esterified to form **valtrate** and **didrovaltrate**.

These compounds come from valerian (*Valeriana officinalis*, Valerianaceae), which was used as a sedative for the treatment of 'shell shock', a condition with which troops serving in the First World War

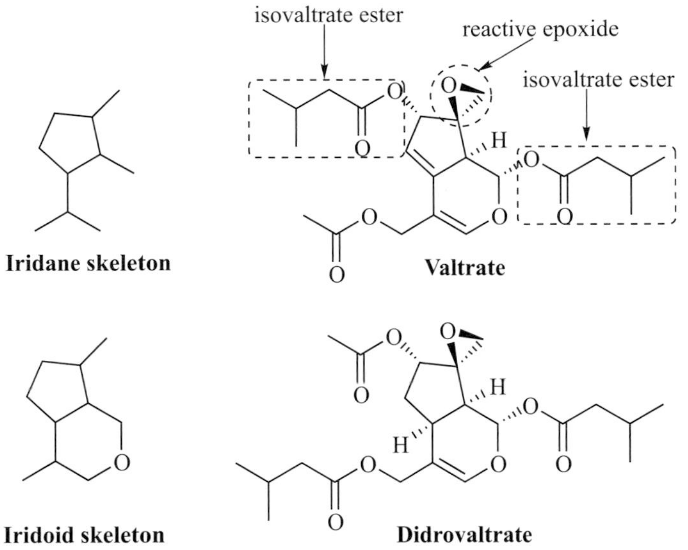

Fig. 6.31

were afflicted following extensive barrage by high explosive shells. This class of iridoids is often referred to as the **valepotriates**; they are highly functional, possessing isovalerate esters and an epoxide group that is possibly responsible for the *in vitro* cytotoxicity of valtrate and didrovaltrate. It is still not known exactly which class of compounds is responsible for the sedative activity, although the iridoids are widely regarded as the active components. However, it has been suggested that γ-aminobutyric acid (GABA), which is present in aqueous extracts of valerian, contributes to the sedative activity. Valerian also contains a number of small acids, such as isovaleric acid, that are structurally similar to GABA; these may, therefore, contribute to the sedative action of this herb extract. Valerian is commonly found in herbal remedies to improve sleep and is often used in conjunction with extracts from hops (*Humulus lupulus*) (e.g. in the preparation Valerina Night-Time).

SESQUITERPENES (C$_{15}$)

These natural products have properties similar to those of the monoterpenes, are constituents of many of the volatile oils and in some cases are broadly antimicrobial and anti-insecticidal, therefore contributing to the overall chemical defence of the producing organism. The starting unit for these compounds is **farnesyl pyrophosphate** (FPP), which is produced by the reaction of GPP (the

monoterpene precursor) with a molecule of IPP (Fig. 6.32). The reaction is analogous to that for the formation of the monoterpenes in which a cationic intermediate is formed that reacts with IPP with elimination of a hydrogen ion.

As with the monoterpenes, FPP can cyclize to form linear (acyclic) and cyclic sesquiterpenes. A key feature of these metabolites is their ability to undergo extensive elaboration chemistry, where they are highly functionalized, thus giving rise to the high structural diversity seen within this group of natural products. It is not always easy to

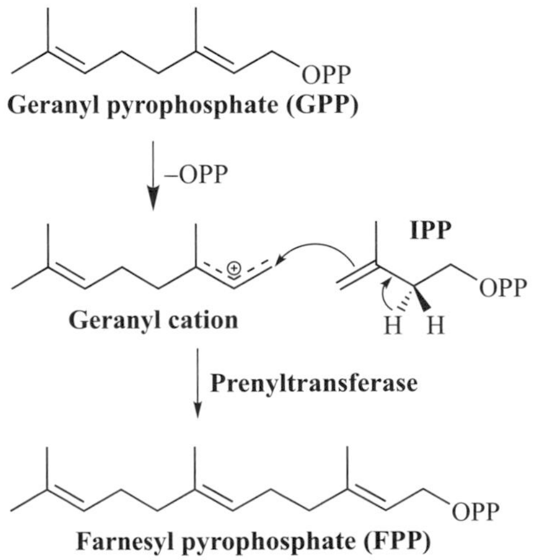

Fig. 6.32

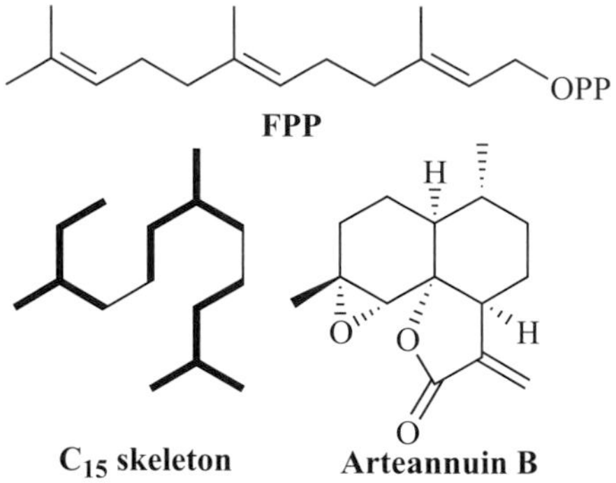

Fig. 6.33

see that these complex, functional, cyclic chiral compounds are derived from FPP due to these elaboration reactions. However, if the C_{15} **skeleton** of FPP is compared to **arteannuin B**, it can be seen how even complex structures are constructed (Fig. 6.33).

The most important sesquiterpene from the pharmaceutical perspective is the antimalarial product **artemisinin** (Fig. 6.34) from sweet wormwood (*Artemisia annua*, Asteraceae). This herb is widely distributed throughout Europe but also has a long history of use for the treatment of fevers and malaria in China where the drug is known as Qinghao. Artemisinin has a number of interesting features,

including an ether, a lactone (cyclic ester) and an unusual peroxide functional group.

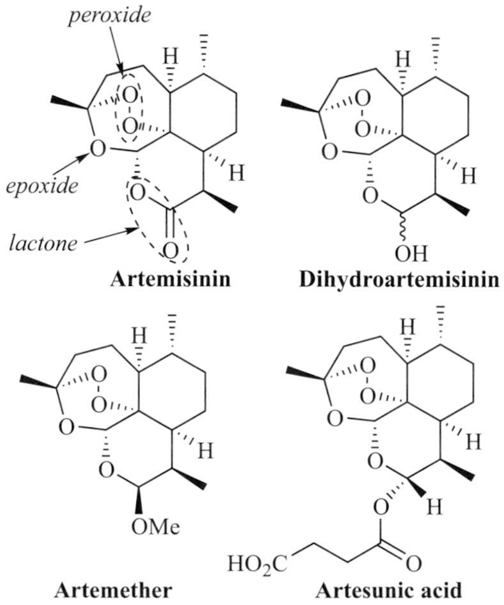

The peroxide is essential for the antimalarial activity and much work has been done to enhance the solubility of the compound whilst retaining the biological activity. **Artemether**, the methyl ether of **dihydroartemisinin** (which possesses an acetal functional group), is used for the treatment of chloroquine-resistant and multidrug-resistant *Plasmodium falciparum* under the trademark Paluther. **Artesunic acid** (a succinic acid derivative marketed as Artesunate) is more water-soluble than artemether and is hydrolysed *in vitro* to dihydroartemisinin. These compounds are very lipid-soluble, are rapidly absorbed into the central nervous system (CNS) and, therefore, may have potential in treating cerebral malaria. It has been proposed that these peroxides complex to the iron atom of haem (which is produced by the degradation of haemoglobin) resulting in the formation of oxy radicals. These radicals may then re-arrange to generate carbon-centred radicals, which can attack biomolecules such as DNA and proteins leading to parasite death.

Interestingly, another Chinese medicinal plant used for treating malaria, *Artabotrys uncinatus* (Annonaceae), also contains a series of sesquiterpene peroxides (typically, **yingzhaosu A**; Fig. 6.35), which are responsible for the antimalarial activity.

In China, studies have been conducted into cottonseed oil (*Gossypium hirsutum*), which has been shown to have contraceptive effects and restrict fertility in men and women when incorporated into the diet. In men, the oil has been shown to alter sperm maturation, motility and inhibit enzymes necessary for fertilization. In women, inhibition of implantation has been observed. The active component is the **bis-sesquiterpene (sesquiterpene dimer) (−)-gossypol**, which exists in the plant with the (+)-isomer. These compounds are optically active due to restricted rotation around the bond that joins the two naphthalene ring systems. Studies show that the antifertility effect is reversible after stopping administration, provided that the treatment has not been prolonged.

DITERPENES

There are few examples of C_{20} diterpenes as drugs, but a former best-selling antitumour agent, paclitaxel, is based on this class of natural products. These compounds are complex in structure and, until the use of multidimensional nuclear magnetic

Fig. 6.34

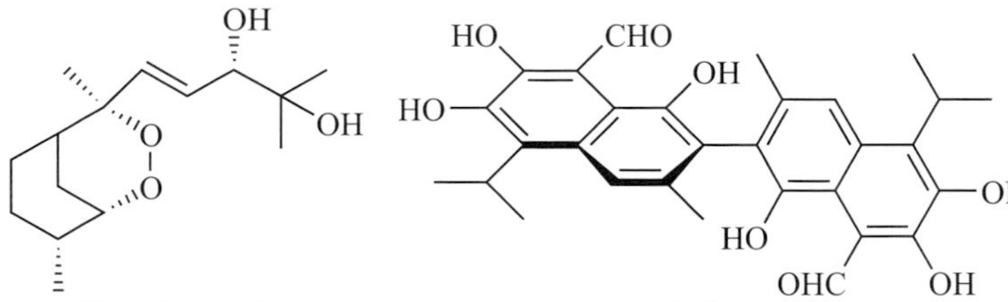

Yingzhaosu A   **(−)-Gossypol**

Fig. 6.35

resonance (NMR) spectroscopy, the structure elucidation of these compounds (along with other higher
terpenes, e.g. triterpenes) was not routine. NMR has
made the structure determination of these compounds readily achievable, even if only 1–2 mg of
natural product is available, and it is likely that
more examples of this class will become drug candi-
dates in the future. Historically, plants producing
diterpenes that contain a nitrogen atom (the so-called
diterpene alkaloids), such as *Aconitum* sp. and
Delphinium sp., have been used for a number of
illnesses, including decongestants; however, these
compounds (e.g. **aconitine**) are highly toxic and preparations containing these plants are no longer used.
    Members of the diterpene class are formed by the
reaction of farnesyl pyrophosphate (FPP), a C_{15} unit,

with isopentenyl pyrophosphate (IPP), the C_5 unit
that is the common building block for all of the
terpenes. The first step of this reaction is the formation of a **farnesyl allylic cation** (analogous to the other
examples of terpenes seen) which then reacts with
IPP with stereospecific loss of a proton, resulting
in the formation of **geranyl geranyl pyrophosphate**
(GGPP). Depending on how GGPP folds and
cyclizes, a very large number of products may result
(Fig. 6.36).
    Loss of a proton from an allylic methyl (* in
Fig. 6.36) and migration of bonds to form a bicyclic
structure results in the formation of **labdadienyl
pyrophosphate** (LDPP), which is a member of the
labdane class of diterpenes of which **sclareol** from
the clary sage (*Salvia sclarea*, Lamiaceae) is widely

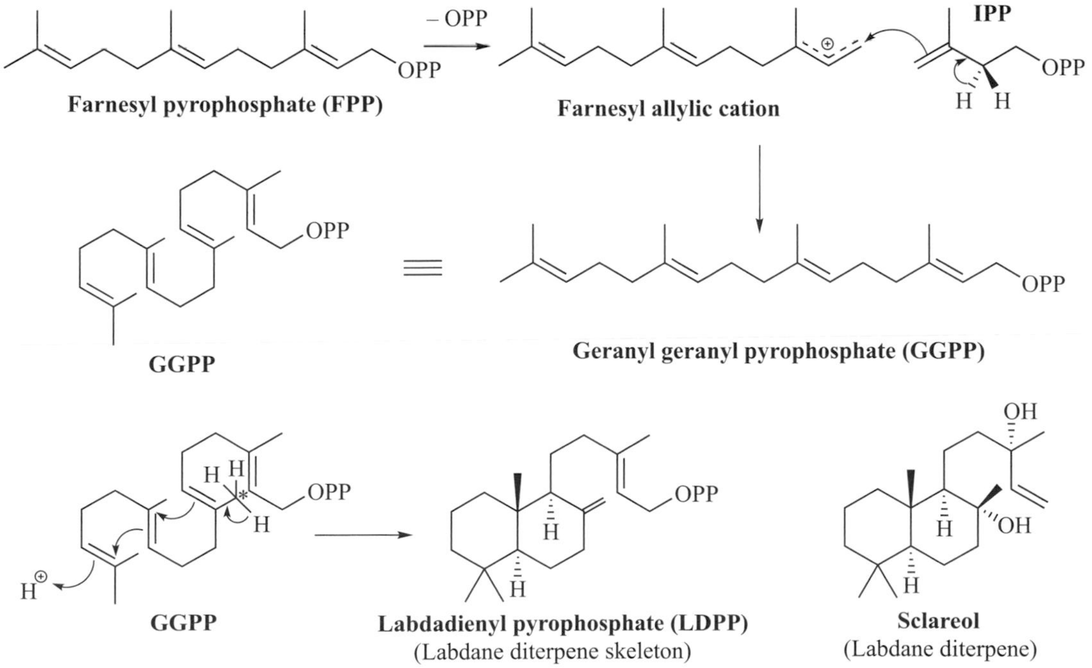

Farnesyl pyrophosphate (FPP)   Farnesyl allylic cation

GGPP   Geranyl geranyl pyrophosphate (GGPP)

GGPP   **Labdadienyl pyrophosphate (LDPP)**   **Sclareol**
              (Labdane diterpene skeleton)   (Labdane diterpene)

Fig. 6.36

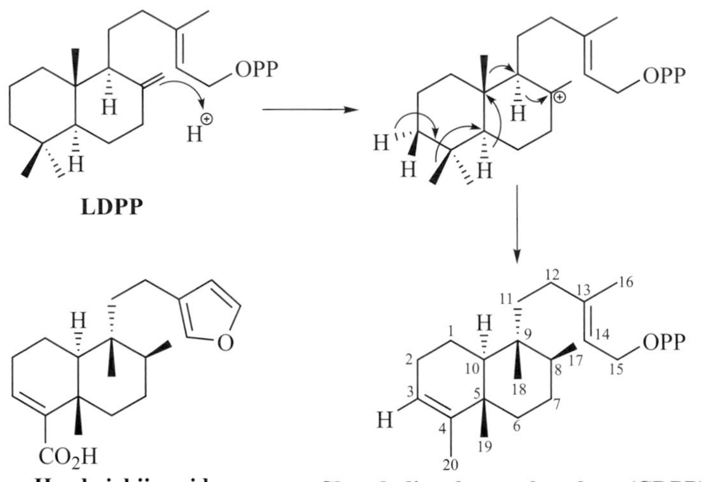

Fig. 6.37

used in the perfumery industry. Sclareol is generated by hydrolysis of LDPP. If the *exo*methylene of LDPP reacts with a proton to form a cationic intermediate, this may undergo a series of **Wagner–Meerwein** hydride and methyl shifts (Fig. 6.37).

These reactions are sometimes referred to as **1,2-shifts** (indicating a movement of a group from a position to a neighbouring carbon) or **NIH shifts** (after the National Institutes of Health, where this reaction was studied). The hydride on C_9 migrates to C_8, the methyl on C_{10} migrates to C_9, the hydride on C_5 migrates to C_{10}, the β-methyl on C_4 migrates to C_5 and, finally, a proton is lost at C_3 resulting in the formation of a C_3-C_4 double bond. This series of migrations yields **clerodadienyl pyrophosphate** (CDPP; a **clerodane** diterpene) with many members of this class; for example, **hardwickiic acid** which possesses a furan ring (produced by oxidation and cyclization of the six-carbon side-chain at C_9) and a carboxylic acid (produced by oxidation of C_{20}). An important facet of these Wagner–Meerwein shifts is the inversion of stereochemistry at the chiral centres where migration has occurred. For example, in LDPP, the methyl at C_{10} is β (coming up out of the plane of the page), whereas the corresponding group in CDPP is an α hydrogen (going down into the plane of the page).

GGPP can cyclize to give an extraordinarily wide range of diterpene groups, some of which are shown in Fig. 6.38.

It is important to understand that, once a simple skeleton has been produced, a wide array of further

elaboration reactions can occur, resulting in the highly complicated natural products of this class (e.g. paclitaxel; Fig. 6.39). This antitumour diterpene was discovered in 1971 by Monroe Wall and Mansukh Wani at the Research Triangle Institute as part of a programme funded by the National Cancer Institute. This compound is dealt with in further detail in Chapter 8. It was not until the 1980s that further work on the mode of action of this compound prompted its development and release onto the US market in 1993 under the trade name Taxol for the treatment of ovarian cancers.

Paclitaxel is present in the bark of the Pacific yew (*Taxus brevifolia*, Taxaceae), a slow growing tree from the forests of north-west Canada and the USA that takes 100 years before it can be exploited for processing. The wood of *T. brevifolia* is not suitable for timber production and was in danger of replacement by faster growing conifers, but this practice has been stopped. The yield of paclitaxel is also low (0.01–0.02%) as it takes three 100-year-old trees to produce 1 g of the drug. Thus, with a course of treatment being 2 g, it was quickly realized that the supply of paclitaxel had to come from another source. *Taxus brevifolia* produces a wide range of taxane diterpenes, and related compounds are also found in the common English yew, *Taxus baccata*. Paclitaxel belongs to a small class of taxanes that possess a four-membered ether (also called an oxirane) and a complex nitrogen-containing ester side-chain; both of these functional groups are essential for antitumour activity. The solution to

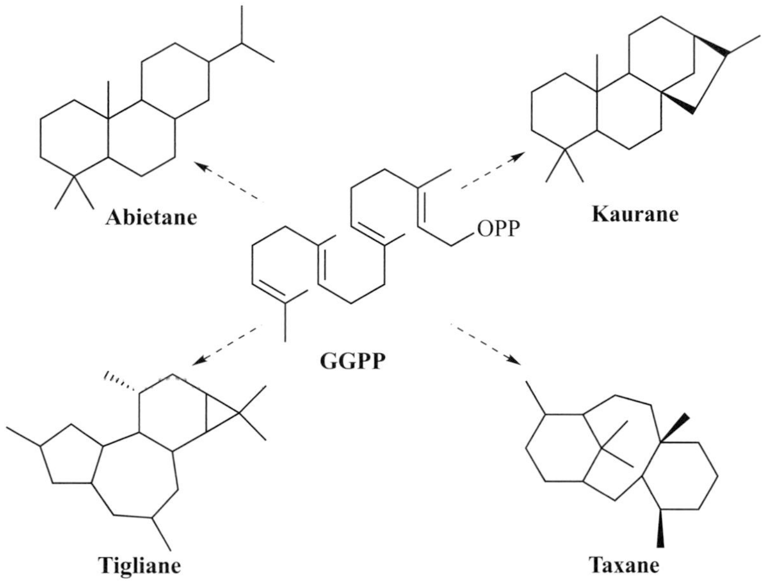

Fig. 6.38

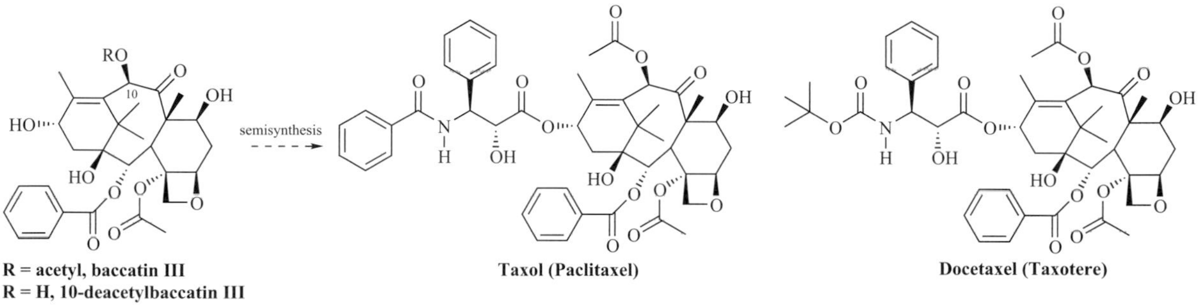

R = acetyl, baccatin III
R = H, 10-deacetylbaccatin III

Taxol (Paclitaxel)

Docetaxel (Taxotere)

Fig. 6.39

the problem of low concentration of the drug came from the knowledge that related compounds, such as **baccatin III** and **10-deacetylbaccatin III** (Fig. 6.39), were present in greater concentrations than paclitaxel and could be converted to paclitaxel by simple reactions.

Most importantly, 10-deacetylbaccatin III is also present in the needles (leaves) of the faster growing English yew (*T. baccata*) at a higher concentration (0.1%) and, unlike the bark, the needles can be harvested without destroying the tree. This is an example of a **renewable resource**, which is an important concept in natural product chemistry, for, if a biologically active compound is developed into a drug, then large-scale production is always necessary. This is not problematic if a compound from a plant can be synthesized (semi- or fully synthesized) or

produced by cell culture. Another route to this compound is to extract a mixture of taxanes and use enzymes that specifically cleave ester groups from the taxane nucleus, resulting in a higher concentration of 10-deacetylbaccatin.

It has also been shown that *Taxomyces andreanae*, a fungus that lives in close association with the yew tree, produces small concentrations of paclitaxel in fermentation culture. It is possible that the fungus has inherited the gene from the tree (or vice versa), which allows the organism to produce paclitaxel. Another fungus that has been isolated from the Himalayan yew tree (*Taxus wallachiana*) is *Pestalotiopsis microspora*, which produces higher concentrations of paclitaxel than *T. andreanae*. Taxol is now produced by large scale plant cell culture fermentation.

Docetaxel (Taxotere) (Fig. 6.39), a related semi-synthetically produced taxane diterpene, is also used clinically for the treatment of ovarian cancers and has a modified side-chain to that of paclitaxel.

TRITERPENES

The triterpenes are C_{30}-derived terpenoids with an exceptionally wide distribution, including man, plants, fungi, bacteria, soft corals and amphibia. The triterpenes include some very important molecules, such as the **steroids** (e.g. **testosterone**), which are degraded triterpenes with many important functions in mammals, notably as sex hormones. Other types include the **sterols** (e.g. **β-sitosterol**), which are common tetracyclic steroidal alcohols with ubiquitous distribution in plants, the **pentacyclic triterpenes** such as **glycyrrhetic acid** found in liquorice and the **limonoids** (e.g. **limonin**), which are highly oxidized bitter principles present in the *Citrus* plant family (Rutaceae) (Fig. 6.40).

Triterpenes are also components of **resins** and resinous exudates from plants (e.g. frankincense and myrrh); myrrh is derived from the Arabic word for bitter, a characteristic which many triterpenes display. These resins are common from trees belonging to the plant family Burseraceae (which includes the myrrh-producing *Commiphora* sp.) and are produced following damage to the tree as a physical barrier to attack by fungi and bacteria. Additionally, many of the terpenoid components of these resins have high antimicrobial activity, either killing potentially invasive microbes, slowing their growth until the tree has repaired the damage or providing a physical barrier toward further invasion.

Their biosynthesis starts with the reaction between two molecules of farnesyl pyrophosphate (FPP) to form the true precursor of all triterpenes, **squalene** (Fig. 6.41). Squalene is then enzymatically epoxidized to **squalene epoxide** which, when folded in a particular conformation such as the 'chair-boat-chair-boat' conformation, can cyclize to give **sterol intermediate 1** which is the precursor of the steroids and sterols (Fig. 6.42). This intermediate can undergo a series of Wagner–Meerwein shifts to give **lanosterol**, a common component of plants and of wool fat.

Oxidation and loss of methyls at positions C_4 and C_{14}, introduction of a C_5-C_6 double bond (oxidation) and loss of two double bonds (one at C_8-C_9 and one in the side-chain) would result in the formation of **cholesterol**. Cholesterol is the main animal sterol, a component of cell membranes and gallstones, and control of the levels of this sterol is important in the management of heart disease. The basic steroid nucleus and numbering of the ring system depicting the A, B, C and D rings is given for cholesterol (Fig. 6.43).

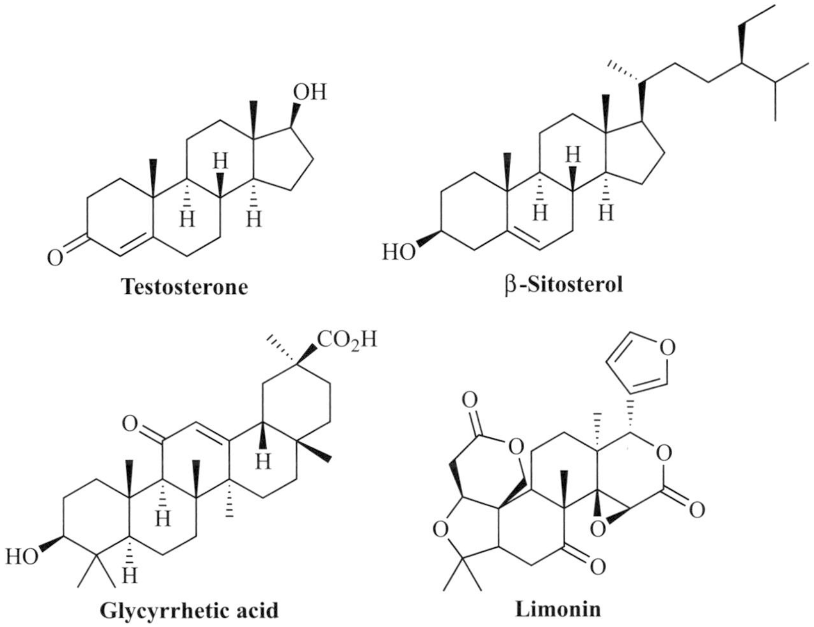

Testosterone

β-Sitosterol

Glycyrrhetic acid

Limonin

Fig. 6.40

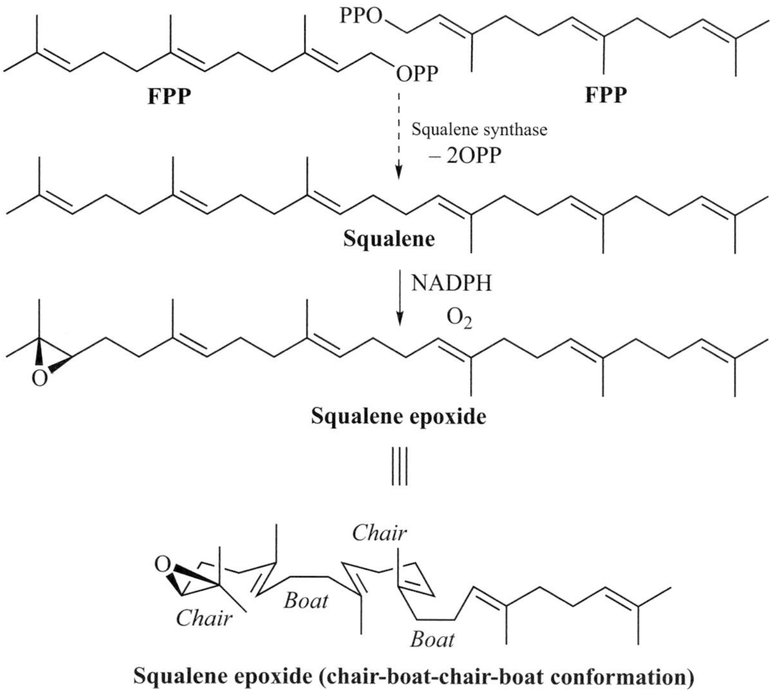

Squalene epoxide (chair-boat-chair-boat conformation)

Fig. 6.41

Other common sterols include the **phytosterols** (plant sterols) **β-sitosterol** and **stigmasterol** (which differs from β-sitosterol only by the presence of a double bond at position C_{22}-C_{23}), which are widespread in plants, and **ergosterol**, which is ubiquitous in fungi as a cell wall component (Fig. 6.43).

There is a great need for steroids in the pharmaceutical industry and this is met by using the plant sterol **diosgenin** from the wild yam (*Dioscorea* sp.). Diosgenin also occurs naturally as a glycoside (a sugar is attached at the hydroxyl position) and without the sugar the compound is referred to as a **genin**. Unlike the other plant sterols mentioned, the side-chain that is normally present at position C_{17} has been formed into two ring structures. Diosgenin can be converted into **progesterone** via a chemical process known as the Marker degradation, which gives access to many important steroids such as **testosterone** (a male sex hormone) and **oestradiol** (a female sex hormone) which has had the A ring aromatized, resulting in the loss of a methyl group from C_{10} (Fig. 6.44).

Another semi-synthetic compound that lacks this methyl is the oral contraceptive **norethisterone**, which has an unusual acetylene group at position

C_{17}. One of the most widely used steroids in pharmaceutical preparations is the anti-inflammatory drug **hydrocortisone** (cortisol). This compound has an hydroxyl group at C_{11} which is introduced into the molecule in a stereospecific manner in fermentation culture using fungi of the genus *Rhizopus*.

If squalene is folded in a different conformation (chair-chair-chair-boat), then cyclization mediated by a cyclase enzyme results in the formation of a different intermediate, **sterol intermediate II**, which is the precursor of the pentacyclic triterpenes (Fig. 6.45).

Migration of the C_{16}-C_{17} bond to satisfy the positive charge results in the formation of **sterol intermediate III**. This may undergo several rearrangements to give different triterpene skeletons. Pathway 1 involves formation of a bond between C_{18} and C_X, resulting in a positive charge on C_Y (through removal of one pair of electrons from the double bond to form the C_{18}-C_X bond). This may be satisfied by a series of Wagner–Meerwein methyl and hydride shifts with loss of a proton from C_{12} resulting in a C_{12} double bond. This pathway gives us the **ursane**-type triterpenes of which **α-amyrin** is an example, possessing a double bond in position C_{12} (referred to as a $\Delta 12$ ursene) (Fig. 6.45).

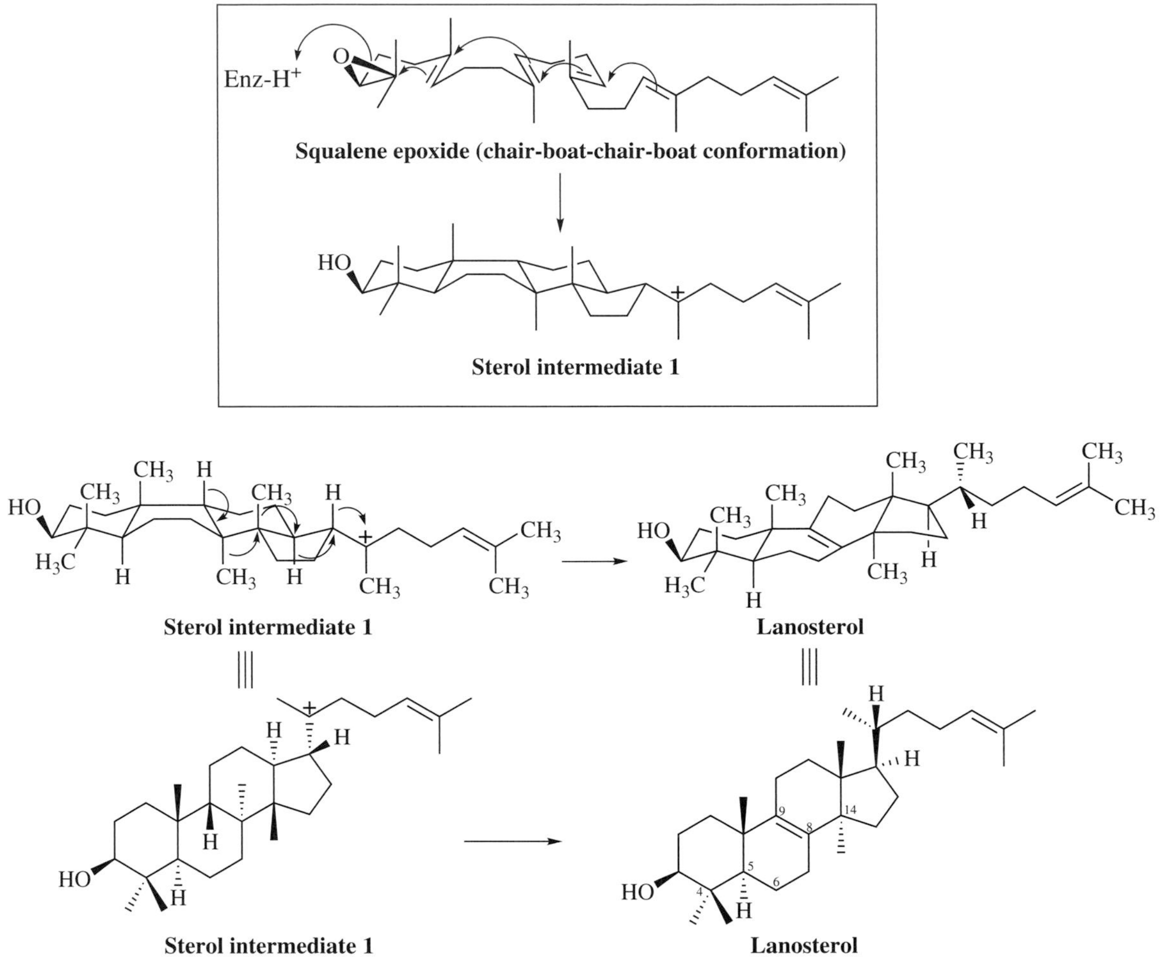

Fig. 6.42

Pathway 2 occurs through the formation of a C_{18}-C_Y bond, which leaves a positive charge on C_X which is stabilized by the two methyls attached to it. This intermediate may then lose a hydrogen ion from one of these methyls to forming a neutral double bond and the **lupane** skeleton (pathway a), or the bond between C_Y and C_Z may migrate to C_X, giving a carbocation at C_Y. Wagner–Meerwein migrations and loss of a hydrogen ion from C_{12} forming a double bond gives the **oleanane** triterpene skeleton, of which **β-amyrin** is typical, again possessing a double bond at C_{12}. This compound may be referred to as a Δ12 oleanene.

Pentacyclic triterpenes are common in plants and herbal remedies such as horse chestnut (*Aesculus hippocastanum*) and liquorice (*Glycyrrhiza glabra*). Examples such as **protoaescigenin, baringtogenol**

(both from horse chestnut) and **glycyrrhetic acid** (liquorice) (Fig. 6.46) have a high degree of functionality and chirality, and usually occur in the plant material in the form of glycosides.

Horse chestnut is used as an anti-inflammatory and antibruising remedy and liquorice has a long history of use as an anti-inflammatory (anti-ulcer) agent. **Carbenoxolone sodium** is a semi-synthetic derivative of glycyrrhetic acid that is widely prescribed for the treatment of gastric ulcers.

TETRATERPENES (C_{40})

The final class of terpenoids that will be dealt with are the **tetraterpenes**, which are C_{40} natural products derived from the reaction of two molecules of geranyl geranyl pyrophosphate (C_{20}). Members of this class are

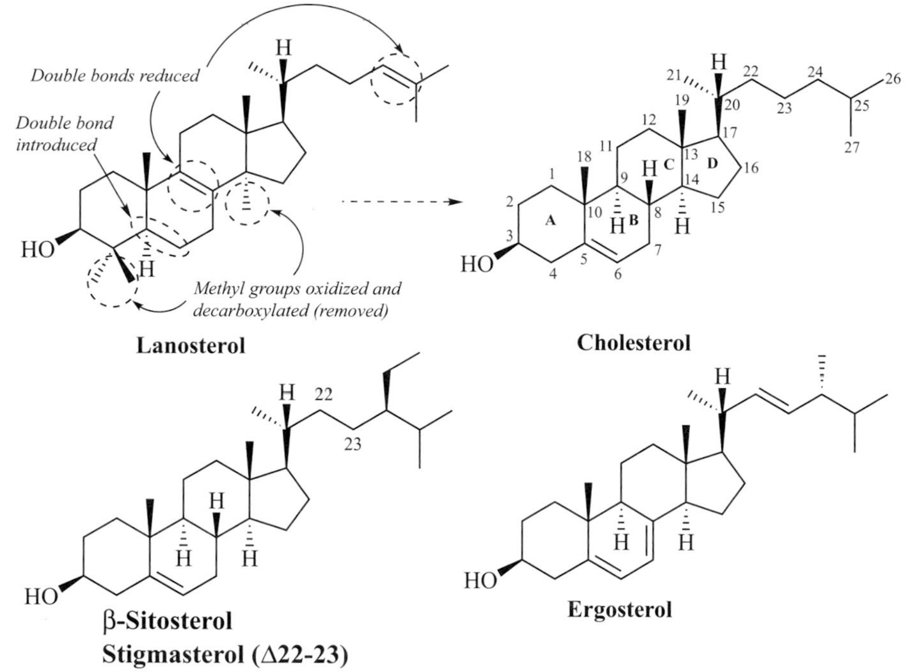

Fig. 6.43

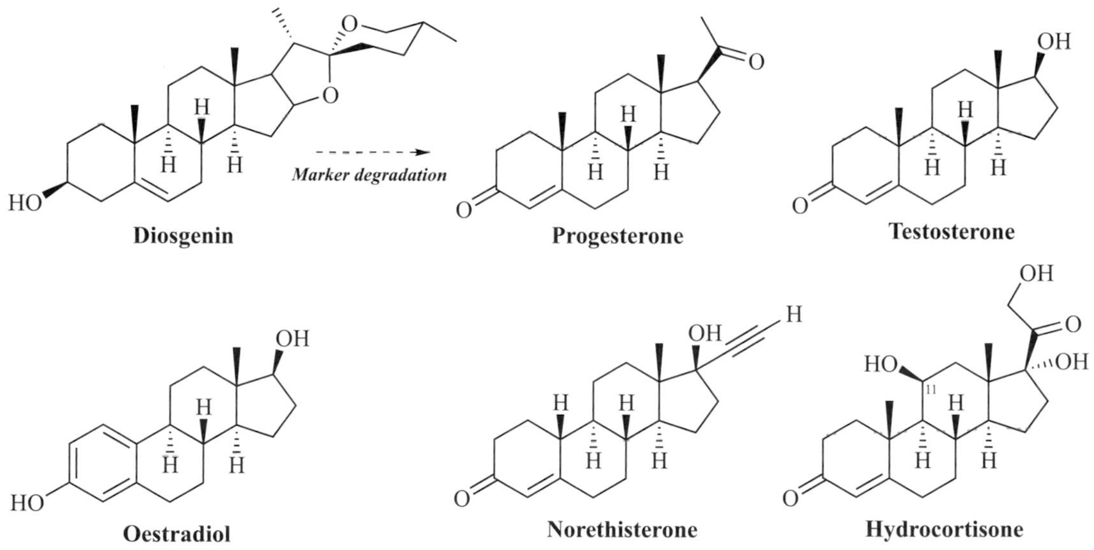

Fig. 6.44

sometimes referred to as **carotenes** or **carotenoids** because of their occurrence in the carrot (*Daucus carota*). As with the flavonoids, the tetraterpenes are highly pigmented natural products and are responsible for the very bright colours of certain plants, in particular the orange of carrots due to **β-carotene**, and the brilliant red colour of tomatoes (*Lycopersicon esculentum*) and peppers (*Capsicum anuum*), which is due to **lycopene** and **capsanthin**, respectively (Fig. 6.47). These compounds are highly conjugated

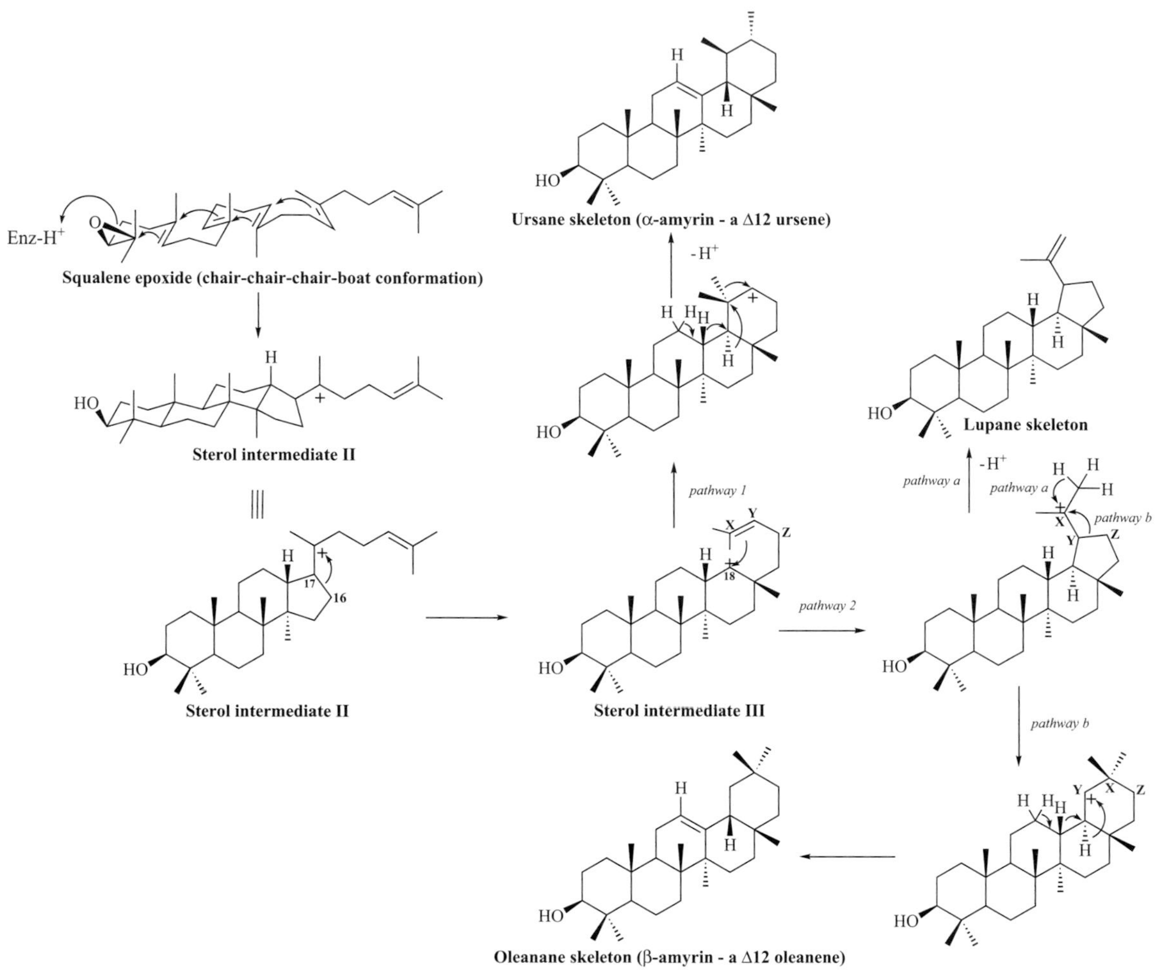

Fig. 6.45

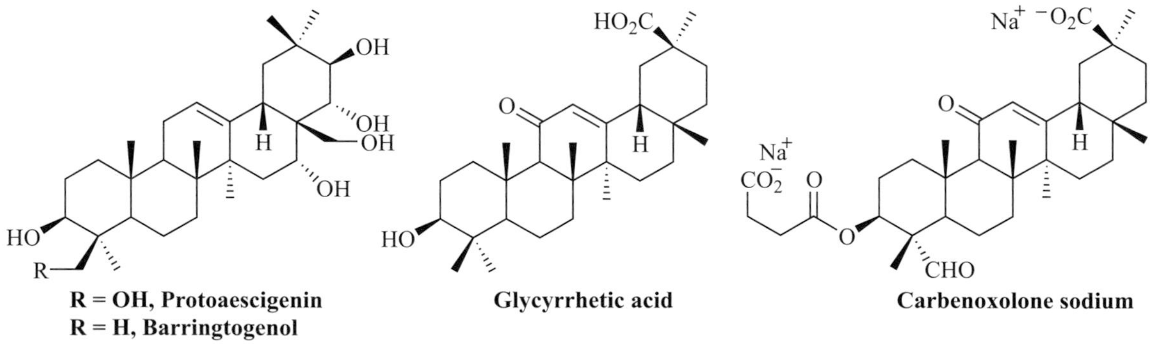

R = OH, Protoaescigenin
R = H, Barringtogenol

Glycyrrhetic acid

Carbenoxolone sodium

Fig. 6.46

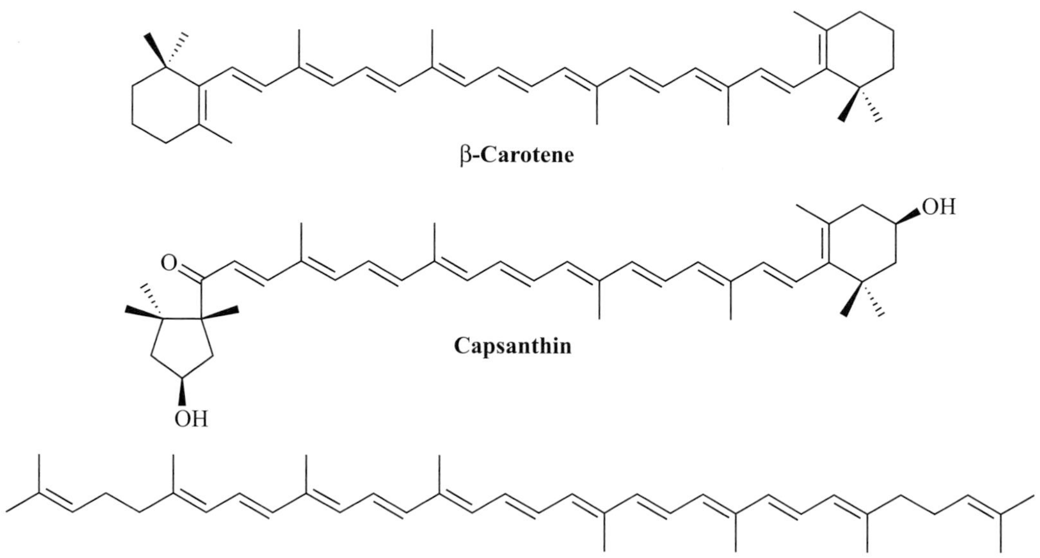

β-Carotene

Capsanthin

Lycopene

Fig. 6.47

and strongly UV light absorbing, and are involved in photosynthesis as light accessory pigments. They are widely distributed in plants and may also act as a protection factor against UV light damage. Because of their high colouration they are employed as colouring agents in foods, pharmaceuticals and cosmetics.

The tetraterpenes are strong antioxidants, being preferentially oxidized over biological molecules such as nucleic acids and proteins. It is thought that many disease states such as certain cancers and heart disease are exacerbated by species that cause oxidation; therefore, the presence of these compounds may retard the development of such diseases. The presence of lycopene in the diet has been shown to reduce the incidence of prostate cancer in men and it is likely that the tetraterpenes have high dietary significance and are important in cancer chemoprevention.

The tetraterpenes are precursors of **vitamin A$_1$** (**retinol**), a deficiency of which results in a reduction in sight efficiency through changes to the cornea and conjunctiva. Vitamin A$_1$ occurs naturally in fish liver oils, carrots, green and yellow vegetables, and dairy products. It is biosynthesized by the oxidative cleavage of β-carotene to **retinal**, which is then reduced to **retinol** (**vitamin A$_1$**) (Fig. 6.48).

Vitamin A preparations are also used to treat nappy rash, skin irritations and minor burns; vitamin A acid (retinoic acid) and vitamin A palmitate are used as treatments for acne.

THE GLYCOSIDES

The glycosides are discussed in a separate section here as they enhance the structural diversity of other natural product classes. The term glycoside is a generic term for a natural product that is chemically bound to a sugar. Thus the glycoside is composed of parts: the **sugar** and the **aglycone**. The aglycone may be a terpene, a flavonoid, a coumarin or practically any other natural product. If the aglycone is a triterpene, it is sometimes referred to as a **genin** (e.g. protoaescigenin; Fig. 6.46). Glycosides are very common in nature and provide extra chemical diversity and structural complexity in natural products.

There are two basic classes of glycosides: the **C-glycosides**, in which the sugar is attached to the aglycone through a carbon–carbon bond, and the **O-glycosides** in which the sugar is connected to the aglycone through an oxygen–carbon bond (Fig. 6.49).

Glycosides are usually more polar than the aglycone, and glycoside formation generally increases water solubility. This may allow the producing organism to transport and store the glycoside more effectively.

CYANIDE GLYCOSIDES

Some glycosides are undoubtedly used by plants as a chemical defence and this is certainly so with the cyanide glycosides. These compounds, in the presence of

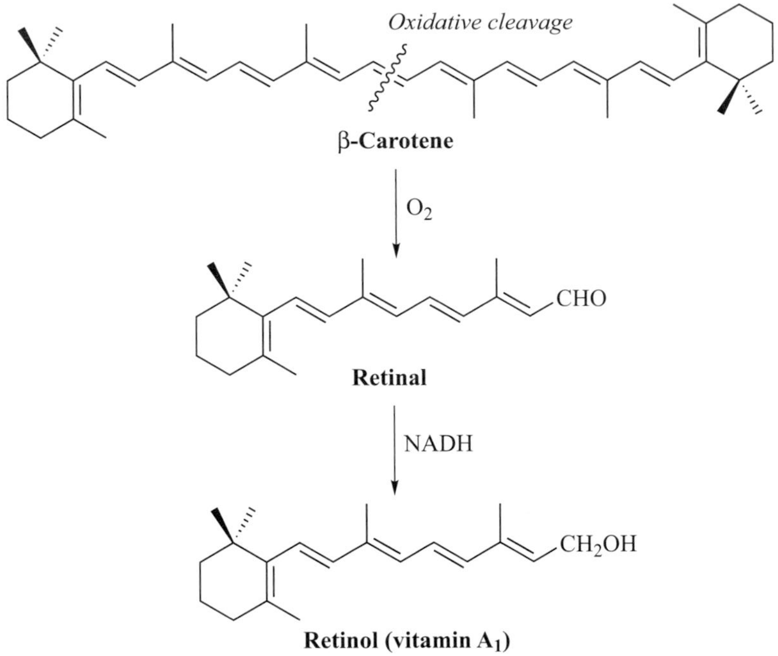

Fig. 6.48

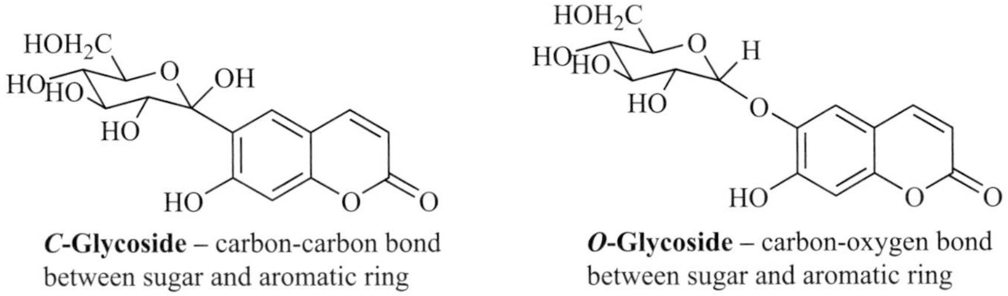

C-Glycoside – carbon-carbon bond
between sugar and aromatic ring

O-Glycoside – carbon-oxygen bond
between sugar and aromatic ring

Fig. 6.49

enzymes such as **β-glucosidase**, lose their sugar portion to form a **cyanohydrin** which, in the presence of water, can undergo hydrolysis to give **benzaldehyde** and the highly toxic **hydrogen cyanide** (HCN) (Fig. 6.50).

Cyanide glycosides such as **amygdalin** (Fig. 6.50) are present in many species of the genus *Prunus*, which includes commercially important fruit such as peaches, cherries, plums and apricots. Fortunately, the enzymes that convert these compounds to the cyanohydrins are localized in different parts of the plant or are absent. In the case of sweet almonds (*Prunus amygdalus* var. *dulcis*), the enzymes are present but there are no cyanide glycosides present.

Cassava (*Manihot esculenta*) is consumed widely in Africa as a food-stuff and both the enzymes and cyanide glycosides are present, although extensive boiling of the cassava before eating results in

the removal of the toxic HCN. Some cassavas are eaten raw, but it is highly likely that these are chemical races of the plant that lack either the glycosides or the enzymes, so raw cassava should certainly be avoided if there is doubt about the presence of these compounds.

GLUCOSINOLATES

The plant family Brassicaceae includes cabbages, sprouts and the mustards and produces a group of glycosides known as **glucosinolates**. These are sulphur- and nitrogen-containing glycosides previously referred to as nitrogen mustards. A common example of this group is **sinalbin** from white mustard (*Sinapis alba*), which in the presence of the enzyme **myrosinase** is converted into

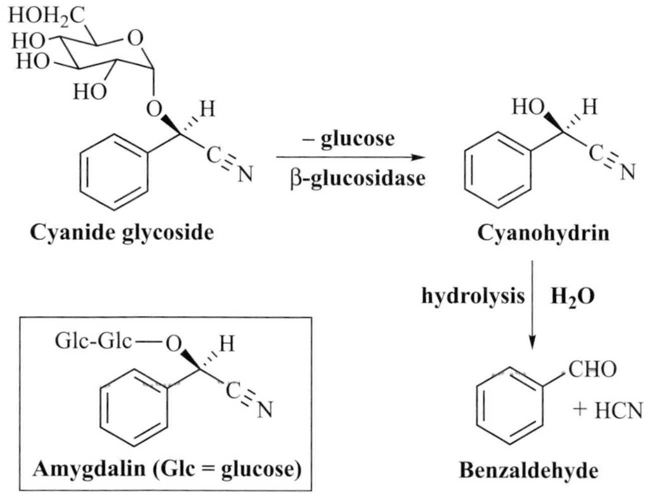

Fig. 6.50

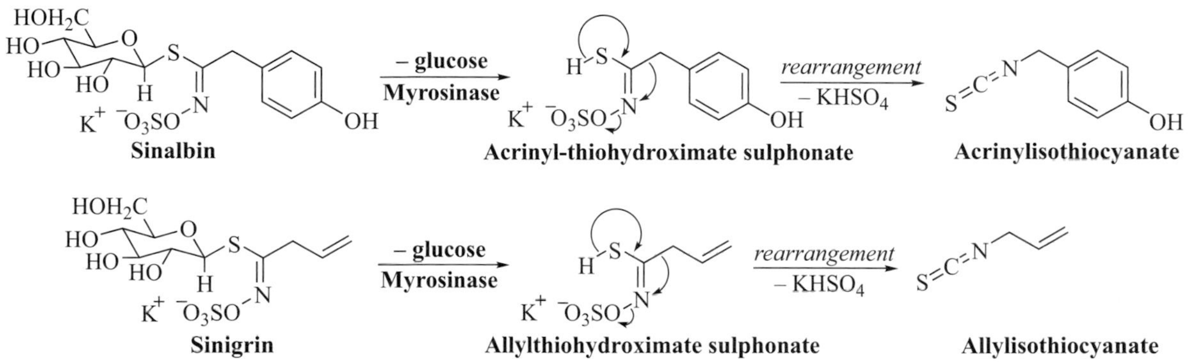

Fig. 6.51

a **thiohydroximate**, which rearranges with the loss of a hydrogen sulphate salt to the **isothiocyanate**, **acrinylisothiocyanate** (Fig. 6.51).

These isothiocyanates are exceptionally pungent and impart a strong aroma to mustards, which can be described as hot or even acrid to the taste. In black mustard (*Brassica nigra*), the simple glucosinolate **sinigrin** is converted in the same fashion to **allylisothiocyanate** (Fig. 6.51), which is an oil and far more volatile than acrinylisothiocyanate. The oils derived from mustards are rich in these isothiocyanates and are mildly irritant; they are used medicinally as externally applied treatments for muscular pain.

CARDIAC GLYCOSIDES

Many plants contain **cardioactive** or **cardiac glycosides**, which have a profound effect on heart rhythm. They are commonly found in the genera *Convallaria*,

Nerium, *Helleborus* and *Digitalis*. The aglycone portion is steroidal in nature and is sometimes referred to as a **cardenolide**, being **card**ioactive and possessing an alkene and an **olide** (a cyclic ester) (Fig. 6.52).

Being 'steroid-like', the aglycone (genin) portion is derived from the triterpenes and these compounds may have a wide variety of sugars attached to the steroid portion. The most widely studied plant that contains these compounds is the foxglove (*Digitalis purpurea*) of the plant family Scrophulariaceae, which was used as long ago as the 18th century for the treatment of heart disease described as 'dropsy'. The basis of this use was well founded as this plant contains the medicinal agents **digoxin** and **digitoxin** (Fig. 6.52). Digoxin is the most widely used cardiac glycoside in congestive heart failure and is now produced by isolation from the related species *Digitalis lanata*. Related cardiac glycosides, which because they are very fast-acting compounds are used in emergencies

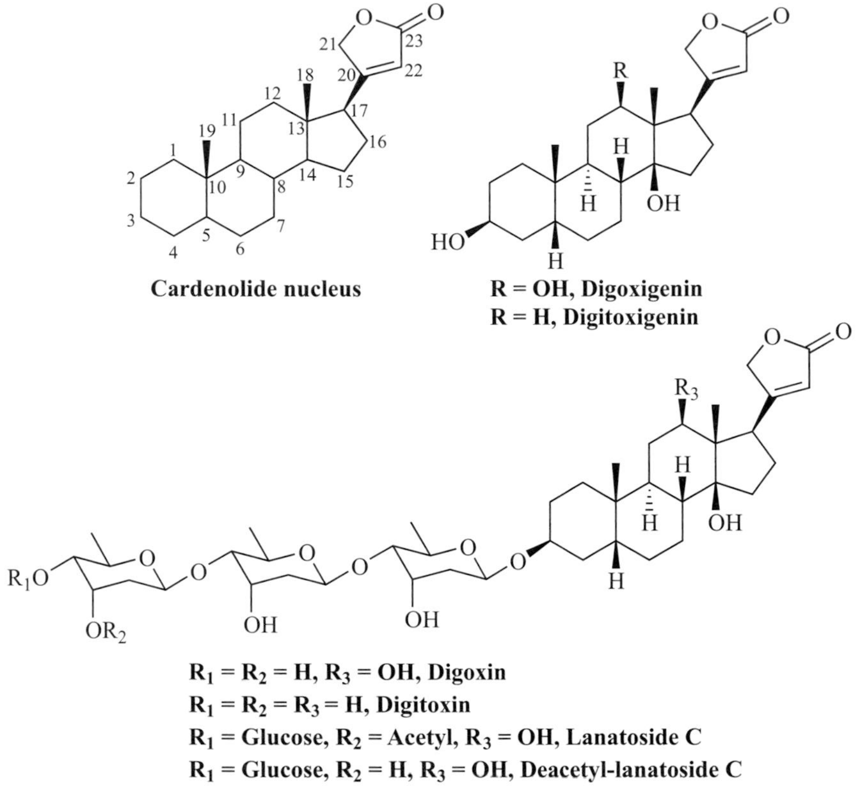

Cardenolide nucleus

R = OH, Digoxigenin
R = H, Digitoxigenin

$R_1 = R_2 = H$, $R_3 = OH$, **Digoxin**
$R_1 = R_2 = R_3 = H$, **Digitoxin**
$R_1 = Glucose$, $R_2 = Acetyl$, $R_3 = OH$, **Lanatoside C**
$R_1 = Glucose$, $R_2 = H$, $R_3 = OH$, **Deacetyl-lanatoside C**

Fig. 6.52

via the intravenous route, are **lanatoside C** and **deacetyl-lanatoside C**.

Triterpene glycosides have widespread distribution in plants and are sometimes referred to as **saponins** as they have soap-like properties and readily form foams. Medicinally important examples include **glycyrrhizic acid** from liquorice (*Glycyrrhiza glabra*) (Fig. 6.53), which is used as a treatment for stomach ulcers and the salts of which are intensely sweet. The sugars in Fig. 6.53 are of the **glucuronic acid** type and are shown as their Fisher projections.

Triterpene glycosides are steroid-like in structure and overuse can lead to similar symptoms associated with steroid overuse such as hypertension and thrombosis.

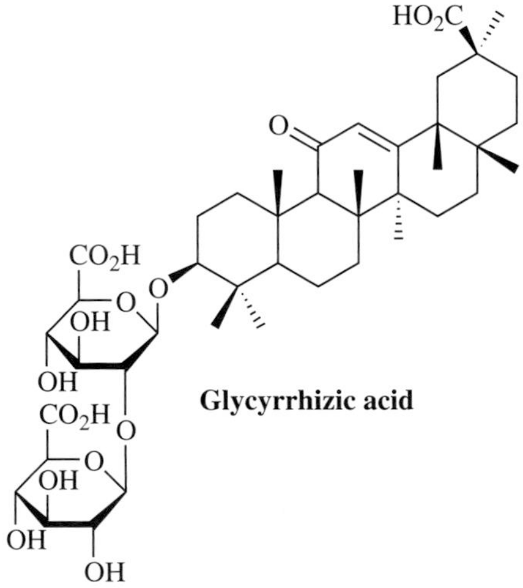

Glycyrrhizic acid

Fig. 6.53

ANTHRAQUINONE GLYCOSIDES

A number of plants that contain **anthraquinone** or **anthrone glycosides** (Fig. 6.54) have long been known for their laxative properties. They include **cascara** (*Rhamnus purshiana*), **aloe** (*Aloe vera*) and **senna**; the latter is divided into two species (*Cassia*

angustifolia, known as **Tinnevelly senna**, and *Cassia senna*, known as **Alexandrian senna**). Aloe is used as a laxative as well as a treatment for minor burns. It contains a mixture of anthraquinone glycosides of which **barbaloin** is the major component and is a

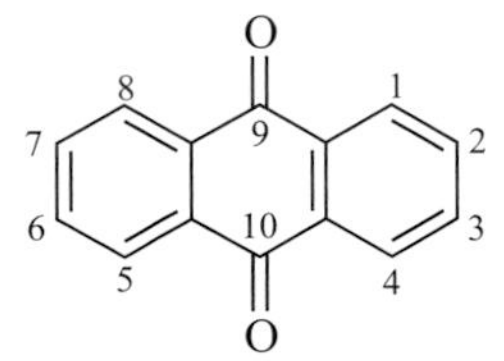

Anthraquinone nucleus

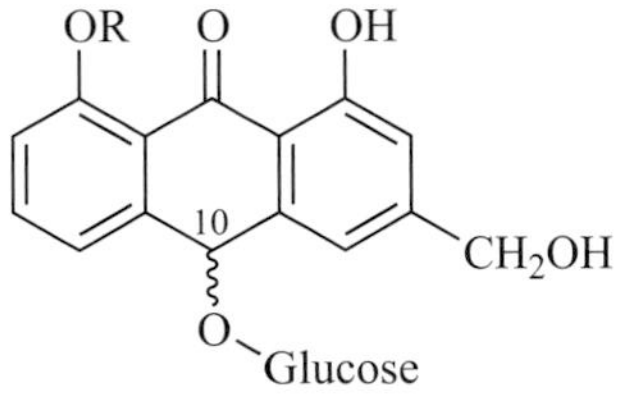

R = H, Barbaloin
R = Glucose, Cascaroside

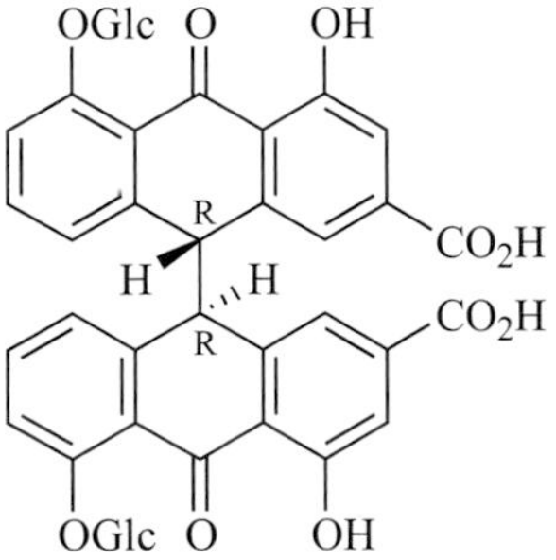

Sennoside A

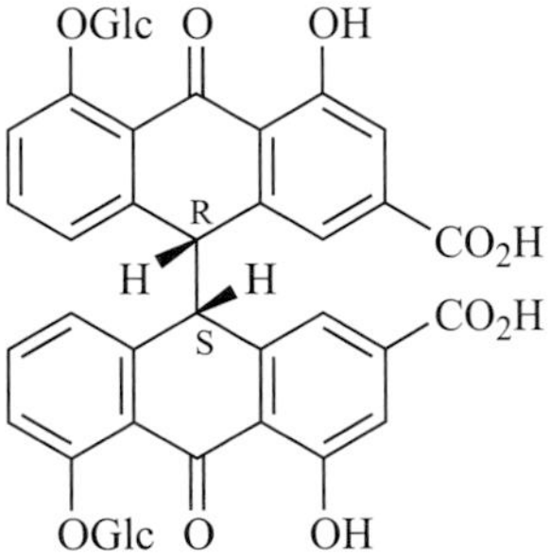

Sennoside B

Fig. 6.54

mixture of 10R and 10S isomers; the purified components are referred to as **aloin A** and **B**. The gel or mucilage from aloe is rich in polysaccharides and these anthraquinone glycosides, and is incorporated into creams and ointments to treat abrasions, burns and skin irritation.

Cascara was in use in the late 19th century as a laxative by the preparation of the bark of the tree. The main active principle is the diglucoside **cascaroside**, which, in common with barbaloin, exists as a mixture of epimers at position C10 as **cascaroside A** (10S) and **B** (10R).

There is little difference in the chemistry of the two senna species. The active constituents are **sennosides A** and **B** (Fig. 6.54). These natural products are **dianthrones** (dimers) of the **anthrone** skeleton. The fresh leaves of senna contain glycosides with additional sugar groups present and these are naturally hydrolysed to sennosides A and B. *In vivo*, the sennosides are then hydrolysed to the dianthrones (lacking the glucose sugars). Senna is widely prescribed for constipation; an example of a marketed product is Senokot.

THE ALKALOIDS

No other group of natural products has contributed more to medicines and pharmaceutical preparations than the alkaloids. As a group, they display an exceptionally wide array of biological activities and have an equally wide distribution, being present in plants, fungi, bacteria, amphibia, insects, marine animals and man. Plants and fungi rich in these natural products were used by early man to relieve pain, as recreational stimulants or, in religious ceremonies, to enter a psychological state to achieve 'communication' between his ancestors or God. The German pharmacist Karl Friedrich Wilhelm Meissner first coined the term 'alkaloid' in 1818, to describe substances that had alkaline (hence alkaloid) properties. Many alkaloids are, indeed, alkaline in nature (Fig. 6.55) as they possess either a **primary, secondary** or **tertiary amine** functional group and the alkaline (basic) properties of these groups may be exploited to aid their extraction and purification (see Chapter 7). However, some alkaloids exist as quaternary amine salts in which a lone pair of electrons from the nitrogen atom is used to form a bond with another group (e.g. methyl) and, therefore, a positive charge resides on the nitrogen making this group essentially neutral (neither basic nor acidic). Care must, therefore, be taken with the alkali or base definition of alkaloids as some are neutral, especially the amides (Fig. 6.55), and some alkaloids possess phenolic groups which actually contribute to the acidity of the molecule.

Alkaloids may also naturally exist as salts, which are the product of a reaction of a base (alkaloid) and

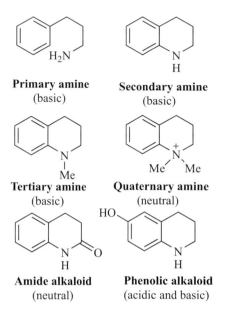

Primary amine
(basic)

Secondary amine
(basic)

Tertiary amine
(basic)

Quaternary amine
(neutral)

Amide alkaloid
(neutral)

Phenolic alkaloid
(acidic and basic)

Fig. 6.55

an acid (e.g. sulphuric acid to give the sulphate, or hydrochloric acid to give the hydrochloride). A further definition of this group is that they are heterocyclic natural products containing nitrogen, but in our definition we will include compounds that contain nitrogen in an aliphatic chain (e.g. the **phenyl-alkylamines**; see below). Biosynthetically, the alkaloids are produced from several different amino acids thereby giving rise to a diverse group of fundamental structures (Fig. 6.56). A biosynthetic treatment of this class is outside the scope of this

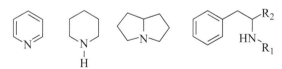

Pyridine Piperidine Pyrrolizidine Phenylalkylamine

Quinoline   Isoquinoline   Indole

Tropane   Xanthine   Imidazole

Fig. 6.56

chapter; consequently this group of natural products will be dealt with by alkaloid class.

PYRIDINE, PIPERIDINE AND PYRROLIZIDINE ALKALOIDS

The most widely studied member of the pyridine class is **nicotine**, the stimulant alkaloidal component of tobacco (*Nicotiana tabacum*, Solanaceae) (Fig. 6.57), which is responsible for the addictive nature of cigarettes and other tobacco preparations. Nicotine is used as a model for addiction to other drugs such as **heroin**. The compound has a pyrrole ring attached to the pyridine ring. Pharmaceutically, nicotine is formulated into chewing gum as an aid to cessation of smoking in products such as Nicorette.

The European plant hemlock (*Conium maculatum*, Apiaceae) produces the highly poisonous piperidine alkaloid **coniine**, which has an alkyl (C_3) side-chain at the 2-position of the piperidine ring. This plant is famous as it was used to execute the Greek philosopher Socrates who was found guilty of treason and forced to drink a preparation of hemlock. Occasional poisoning with this plant occurs when children use the hollow stems as 'pea shooters' and ingest small quantities of the poison.

In the Indian subcontinent, large quantities of betel nuts (*Areca catechu*, Arecaceae) are consumed by farm workers for their stimulant properties to alleviate fatigue. The nuts are red (due to the presence of tannins), which causes staining of the teeth. These nuts are addictive, the active stimulant component being the piperidine alkaloid **arecoline**. Like nicotine, arecoline binds to the nicotinic receptors and has a stimulant effect on the CNS.

Lobeline is found in the leaves and tops of *Lobelia inflata* (Campanulaceae), which is also known as wild tobacco or pukeweed. It has similar effects to those of nicotine and arecoline and has been used as a smoking deterrent. Much work has been done to find alkaloids with activity against HIV of which **castanospermine** from *Castanospermum australe* (Fabaceae) is exceptional. This compound is an inhibitor of α-glucosidase, an enzyme involved in glycoprotein processing, which is important in the formation of viral coating, abnormalities of which stop infection of white blood cells. Castanospermine is a **polyhydroxylated alkaloid** (PHA) and is in fact a sugar analogue (compare with glucose in Fig. 6.57), which explains its activity against the glucosidase enzymes involved in the formation of glycoproteins. The compound is sometimes classified as an indolizidine alkaloid,

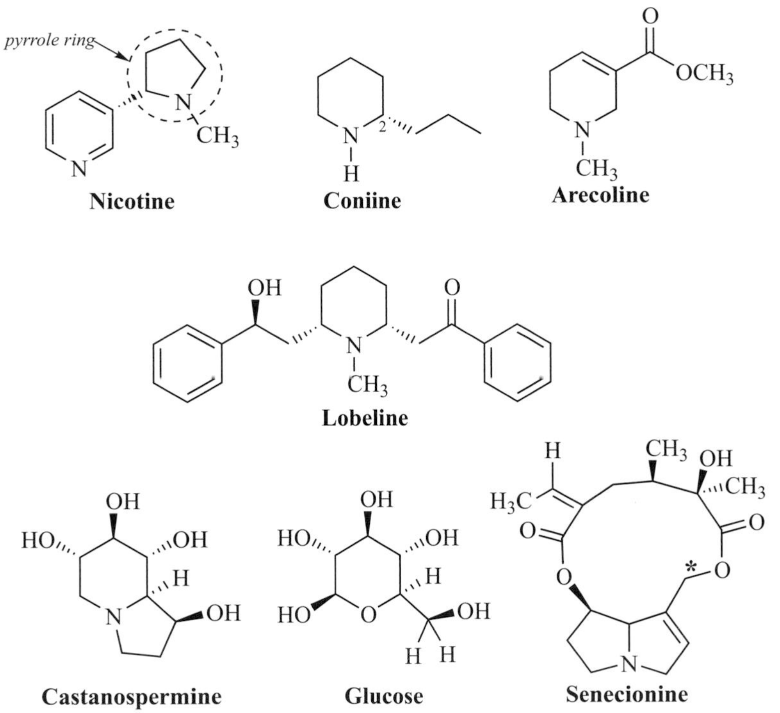

Fig. 6.57

but, as it also has a piperidine ring system, it is included in this section for convenience.

Senecionine is a member of the pyrrolizidine class of alkaloids, which have gained notoriety due to their hepatotoxic properties. These compounds possess a reactive carbon (* in Fig. 6.57), which is readily alkylated by reactive thiol groups present in many enzymes found in the liver. This accounts for the withdrawal of comfrey (*Symphytum officinale*, Boraginaceae), which has a long history of use as a medicinal plant but also contains these toxic alkaloids. Senecionine occurs in groundsel (*Senecio vulgaris*, Asteraceae), which is problematic in farms and paddocks where it can cause poisoning of livestock and horses.

PHENYLALKYLAMINE ALKALOIDS

The natural products of this group do not have a cyclic nitrogen atom but have either a free amine or an alkyl-substituted amine. In Chinese medicine, Ma Huang (*Ephedra sinica*, Ephedraceae) has a long tradition of use as a treatment for colds, asthma and other bronchial conditions. The biologically active component of this species is **ephedrine** (Fig. 6.58), which possesses CNS stimulatory, vasoconstrictive and bronchodilatory properties. These effects are similar to those of the natural hormone **adrenaline (epinephrine)**, which is structurally similar (Fig. 6.58). Ephedrine has two stereogenic (chiral) centres and, therefore, has four possible isomers. Injections of (−)-ephedrine are used for severe asthma and life-threatening anaphylactic shock. Another isomer of ephedrine, (+)-**pseudoephedrine**, is used in cough preparations such as Sudafed for its bronchodilatory properties. Herbal *Ephedra* has recently gained notoriety as 'herbal ecstasy', with a number of sources selling plant material over the Internet and in magazines. Claims of the stimulant's 'ecstasy-like' properties are not unfounded due to the high similarity in structure of ephedrine and **ecstasy (methylenedioxy-methylamphetamine, MDMA)**. These herbal preparations are dangerous and should therefore be avoided.

The indigenous peoples of central and north Mexico and the south-western USA ingest the dried heads ('buttons') of the cactus (*Lophophora williamsii*, Cactaceae) as part of their religious ceremonies. This plant material, known as **peyote**, induces vivid dreams and hallucinations; the biologically active natural product responsible is **mescaline**, a trimethoxylated phenylethylamine. Ingestion of pure

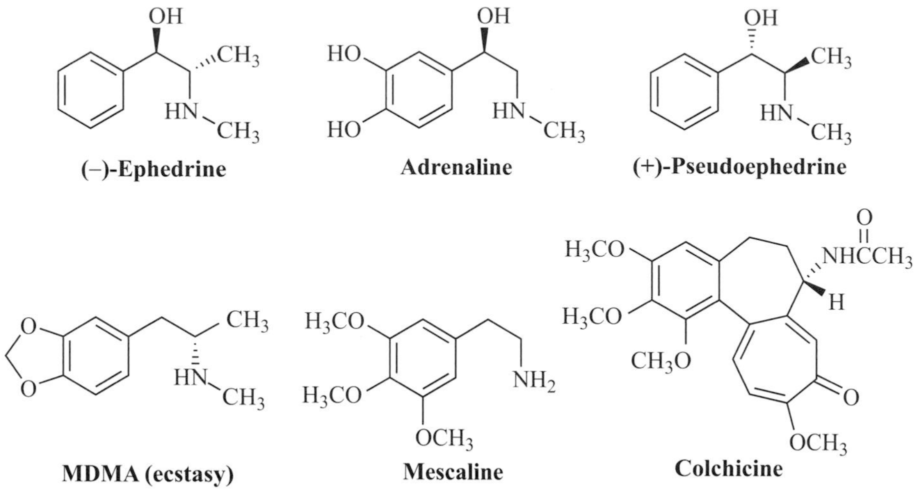

Fig. 6.58

mescaline fails to give the same response as consumption of peyote, which is possibly due to the contribution of other compounds present in the plant material.

A compound that is included in this section for convenience is **colchicine**, an alkaloidal amine from the autumn crocus (*Colchicum autumnale*, Colchicaceae). This plant was known by the Greek physician Dioscorides and has been widely used on the Arabian Peninsula for centuries in the treatment of gout and it is still used today for this purpose. However, it is highly cytotoxic and antimitotic, being an inhibitor of microtubule formation.

QUINOLINE ALKALOIDS

The Spanish conquistadors who invaded Peru in the latter part of the 16th century discovered that the indigenous Incas of this area used a preparation of the bark of a rain-forest tree to treat fevers, especially malaria. The Jesuit priests accompanying the invading force collected large amounts of this bark and used it to prevent and treat malaria. The bark was shipped back to Europe where it became known as **Jesuit bark** or Peruvian bark and gained great fame as a treatment for malaria. The trees responsible for this biological activity are of the genus *Cinchona* (Rubiaceae), which produce the quinoline alkaloid **quinine**, first isolated in 1820 by the French pharmacists Pelletier and Caventou (Fig. 6.59). The structure of this compound was not known, however, until 1908 and total synthesis was only achieved in the mid-1940s. The pure compound was used extensively as an antimalarial and was a template for synthetic antimalarials such as **quinacrine, chloroquine** and **mefloquine**. Resistance to these agents, particularly chloroquine, has become increasingly widespread, in particular through removal of the antimalarial from the cell by plasmodial membrane-bound efflux mechanisms, resulting in a low intracellular (ineffective) concentration of the drug. Interestingly, quinine is

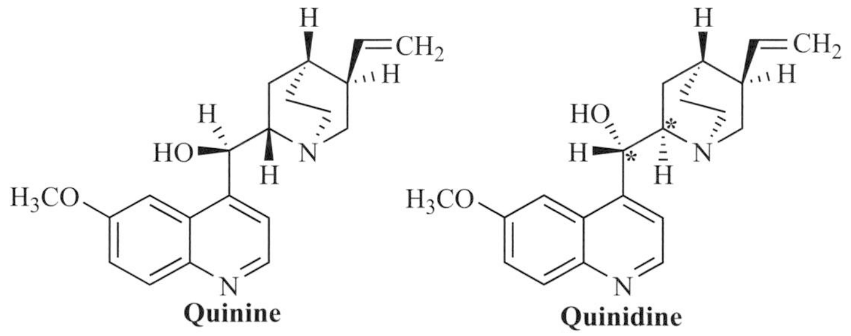

Fig. 6.59

active in many cases against chloroquine-resistant malaria and there has been increased use of this drug. It is thought that quinine and other quinoline antimalarials exert their effects by binding to haem, a degradation product of haemoglobin. This haem–quinoline conjugate is toxic and leads to death of the parasite. In the absence of quinine, haem is converted into a polymeric form known as haemozoin or malaria pigment which is non-toxic. Plasmodia are highly adaptable organisms and at present there is a need for new antimalarials to counter multidrug resistance in *Plasmodium falciparum*.

Quinine also has a use as a treatment for night cramps in the elderly and is added to Indian tonic water where it imparts a bitter taste and a brilliant fluorescence under UV light.

Quinidine is an isomer of quinine and has different configuration at the positions marked * in Fig. 6.59. It was observed that patients suffering from malaria who also had atrial fibrillation were cured of arrhythmias by quinine and quinidine. Quinidine is used to treat type I cardiac arrhythmias.

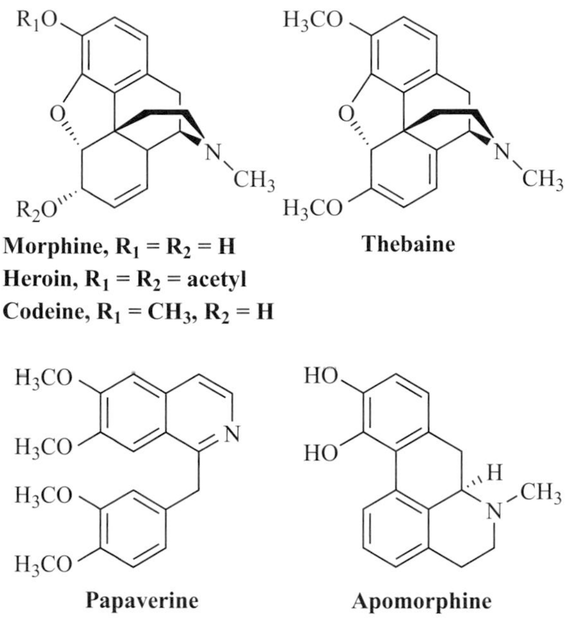

ISOQUINOLINE ALKALOIDS

Within the alkaloids as a group, the isoquinolines have had a profound effect on human society as agents for pain relief and as drugs of abuse. In particular, **opium**, which is rich in **morphinane**-type isoquinolines, has been used for millennia in the treatment of pain and as a narcotic substance and, arguably, no other substance has caused so much human misery.

Opium is the gummy exudate of the unripe capsules of the opium poppy (*Papaver somniferum*, Papaveraceae) and contains more than 30 alkaloids, of which the major components are **morphine**, **codeine**, **thebaine**, **papaverine** and **noscapine** (Fig. 6.60).

The majority of opium, which is produced for illegal drug use, now originates in Afghanistan.

When the British conquered the area of Bengal (now eastern India and Bangladesh) in the late 18th century, they discovered an area rich in opium fields and, as at that point in time there was a huge demand for Chinese tea, the opium was therefore used as a form of currency. Unfortunately, the addictive nature of opium was not well known and many Chinese became addicted through smoking the crude drug in opium dens (which were also a part of London life in the 19th century). This generated a huge social problem and resulted in war (**opium war**) between Britain and China, resulting

Morphine, $R_1 = R_2 = H$
Heroin, $R_1 = R_2 = $ acetyl
Codeine, $R_1 = CH_3$, $R_2 = H$

Thebaine

Papaverine

Apomorphine

Fig. 6.60

in China having to cede land (including Hong Kong) to the British.

Morphine, derived from the name for the Greek god of sleep *Morpheus*, possesses both a basic tertiary amine and an acidic phenol functional group. These groups allow morphine to be readily purified by acids and bases; pure morphine was produced in the 1880s and was rapidly recognized as an excellent analgesic when injected (despite its addictive properties). Morphine is readily converted into the drug of abuse, **heroin** (**diamorphine**), by acetylation of both hydroxyl groups using acetic anhydride. Much has been written on the destructive nature of heroin as a drug of abuse, but this agent is highly useful in the management of pain, particularly in patients with terminal cancer.

Why morphine should dramatically affect analgesia in humans was a mystery until the discovery that we also produce a natural **end**ogenous morphine-like substance (**endorphin**), which acts at the same site as morphine and is a pentapeptide (Tyr-Gly-Gly-Phe-Met). This molecule, named **met-enkephalin** (met being the terminal methionine residue, and enkephalin being derived from the Greek for 'in head') has a portion that shows striking similarity to morphine and explains why both molecules bind to the opiate receptor. Morphine is used as a centrally acting analgesic and as a smooth muscle relaxant.

Codeine is the phenolic methyl ether of morphine and is widely used as an over-the-counter analgesic and a cough suppressant. It is formulated with other analgesic agents such as aspirin and paracetamol. Both morphine and codeine are the most important analgesics for the management of moderate to severe pain. A number of semi-synthetic morphinanes have been produced as analgesics and cough suppressants; these include **pholcodine** and **dihydrocodeine**. Morphine was also used as a template for other analgesic agents including **pethidine**, which is one of the most widely used synthetic opiates.

Thebaine is the starting point for the synthesis of many agents, including codeine and veterinary sedatives such as **etorphine**.

Papaverine is an antispasmodic and is formulated with some analgesics such as aspirin. It is also used as a treatment for male impotence, and its activity as a Ca^{2+} channel blocker led to the development of **verapamil**. **Apomorphine** is prepared by heating morphine with concentrated hydrochloric acid and has recently been shown to be of use in the treatment of Parkinson's disease as this compound is a dopamimetic. **Papaveretum** is a total alkaloid extract of opium (containing 85% morphine, 8% codeine and 7% papaverine) from which the minor alkaloid **noscapine** has been removed as it is genotoxic. Papaveretum is used as a premedication.

Indigenous peoples of South America use a variety of arrow poisons for hunting purposes, of which **curare** is a strong muscle relaxant. This poison is prepared from plants of the family Menispermaceae, notably *Chondrodendron tomentosum*, which kills by paralysis of the muscles required to breathe. The major active component of this species is the isoquinoline alkaloid **tubocurarine**, so named because the curare poison was carried in bamboo 'tubes' prior to use (Fig. 6.61).

Tubocurarine is a quaternary salt and as a chloride has found use as a muscle relaxant in surgical procedures. The compound was also a template for the development of other muscle relaxants of which **atracurium** (**Tracrium**) is an excellent example.

Ipecac (*Caephaelis ipecacuanha*, Rubiaceae) is a shrub indigenous to Brazil and produces rhizomes (underground stems) that were used by the indigenous peoples to treat diarrhoea. The main alkaloidal components of this species are **emetine, psychotrine** and **cephaeline**. Ipecac was used to treat amoebic dysentery, but the side effects (vomiting, nausea and severe gastrointestinal disturbance) stopped its use. However, it is used as an emetic in the form of a syrup to induce vomiting after poisoning and drug overdose. In addition to its emetic and amoebicidal properties, emetine (Fig. 6.61) is an expectorant and is added to many cough medicines.

INDOLE ALKALOIDS

Like the isoquinolines, the indole alkaloids are a very important source of bioactive compounds. Snake root (*Rauvolfia serpentina*, Apocynaceae) is a shrub common to the Indian subcontinent; it has been used as a panacea in the Ayurvedic system of medicine, with uses described for the treatment of snakebite and madness. **Reserpine**, the major component of this species, was used as an antihypertensive agent, but due to side effects (neurotoxicity, cytotoxicity and depression) it is now not in use (Fig. 6.62).

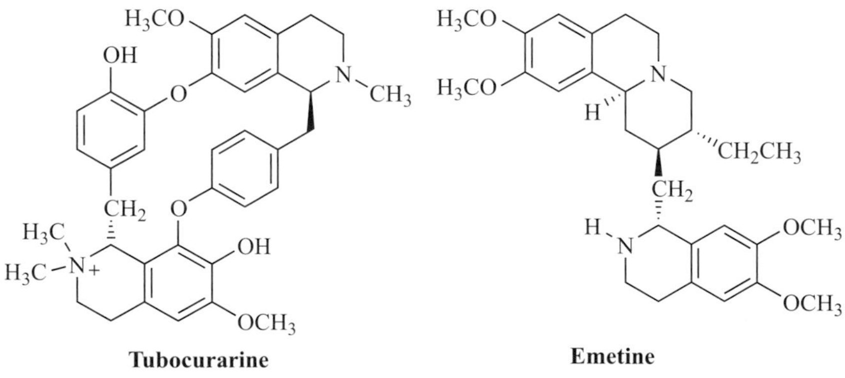

Tubocurarine

Emetine

Fig. 6.61

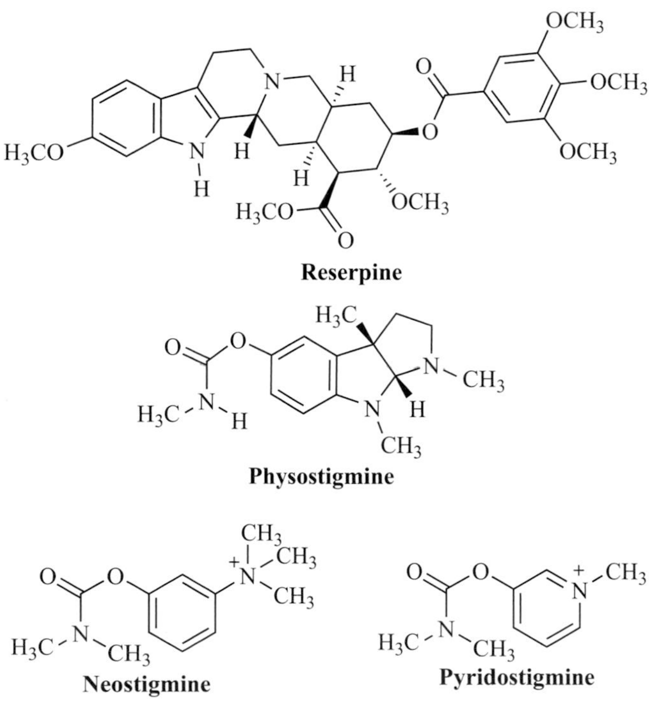

Reserpine

Physostigmine

Neostigmine

Pyridostigmine

Fig. 6.62

British missionaries working in the Calabar coast area of West Africa (Nigeria and Cameroon) reported that criminal trials were conducted using the Calabar bean (*Physostigma venenosum*, Fabaceae). The beans of this plant are highly toxic and, when an individual was accused of a crime, they were forced to consume an extract of the bean. This practice was 'trial by ordeal' and accounts for the other name for the Calabar bean, the 'ordeal bean'. Should the individual live then they were innocent of the crime, but death indicated guilt. The margin between innocence and guilt was probably a result of the completeness or incompleteness of extraction of the toxic chemicals from the plant! The toxic component of this species is **physostigmine** (Fig. 6.62), which is an inhibitor of acetylcholinesterase, resulting in an enhancement of the activity of acetylcholine (which is degraded by acetylcholinesterase). There is interest in this compound in the treatment of Alzheimer's disease in which a low concentration of acetylcholine in the brain is observed. Synthetic compounds based on physostigmine include **neostigmine** and **pyridostigmine**, which are used to treat myasthenia gravis, a rare disease characterized by severe muscle weakness.

Poisoning through contamination of rye grain by fungi, in particular by *Claviceps purpurea*, has been described since the Middle Ages. This fungus produces dark-coloured structures (sclerotia) known as **ergot** on rye plants; these structures are rich in indole alkaloids. The poisoning from ingestion of bread made from contaminated grain is highly unpleasant, with victims complaining of burning, 'fire-like' sensations throughout their extremities and of vivid highly coloured hallucinations. These poisons can cause massive constriction of blood vessels, leading to 'blackened' limbs and gangrene. This condition became known as St Anthony's fire after the saint who spent much of his life meditating in the fire-like heat of the Sinai desert. Because bread was the main staple diet in the Middle Ages, it is likely that this condition was widespread, especially as the damp surroundings in which grain was kept are conducive to the growth of the fungus. Ergot was used as an obstetric preparation in the 1500s to shorten labour during childbirth. It contains several groups of indole alkaloids such as the **ergometrine** type, which have simple amide side-chains, and the **ergotamine** group, which possess complex amino acid derived side-chains (Fig. 6.63).

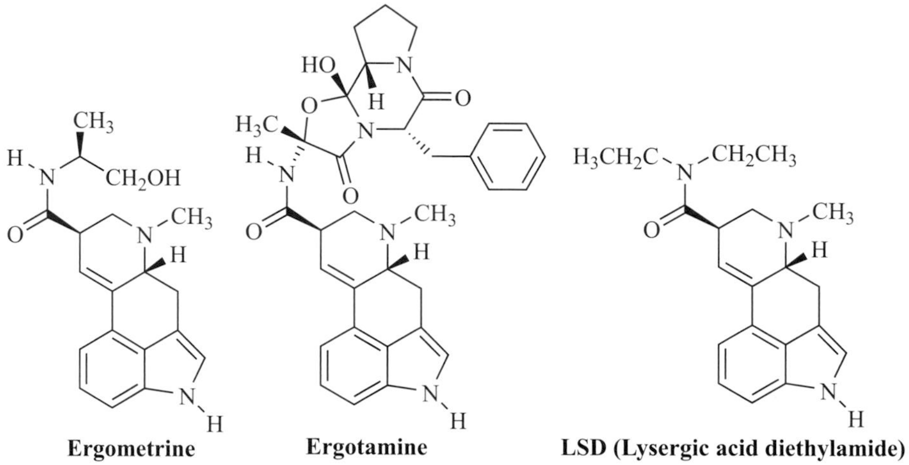

Fig. 6.63

Ergometrine is an oxytocic used to expel the placenta after childbirth or to increase contractions. This compound also acts on the pituitary as well as on the uterine muscles. Ergotamine was first used in the 1920s for the relief of migraine and is still used today. It reduces vasodilation, which can occur in throbbing migraine headache. The ergot alkaloids were used as a template for the semi-synthesis of **bromocriptine, pergolide** and **cabergolide**, which have use in neurological disorders such as Parkinson's disease. Ergot can cause hallucinations, and the hallucinogenic drug of abuse **LSD (lysergic acid diethylamide)** is structurally related to these compounds (Fig. 6.63).

Many of the psychoactive compounds (including LSD) are structurally related to **tryptamine**, as are the **harmine** and **harmaline** alkaloids from *Peganum harmala* (Syrian Rue, Nitrariaceae) and the yahé

or ayahuasca preparations (*Bansiteriopsis caapi* and *B. inebrians*, Malpighiaceae), which are prepared by Amazonian shamen. Ayahuasca is used as part of the community rituals of some Peruvian groups to preserve their traditional ways and to promote bonding and the establishment of social order. **Ibogaine**, from iboga (*Tabernanthe iboga*, Apocynaceae), is hallucinogenic and anticonvulsant, and has recently been studied as a treatment for heroin addiction. Psychoactive indole derivatives are even found in amphibia, notably in the skin of species of the genus *Bufo*, which produce **bufotenin** (Fig. 6.64).

Mushrooms of the genera *Psilocybe, Panaeolus, Conocybe* and *Stropharia* are known to produce psychoactive substances such as **psilocybin**, which is a phosphate salt in the fungi and is converted into **psilocin** *in vivo* (Fig. 6.64). The Aztecs of Mexico

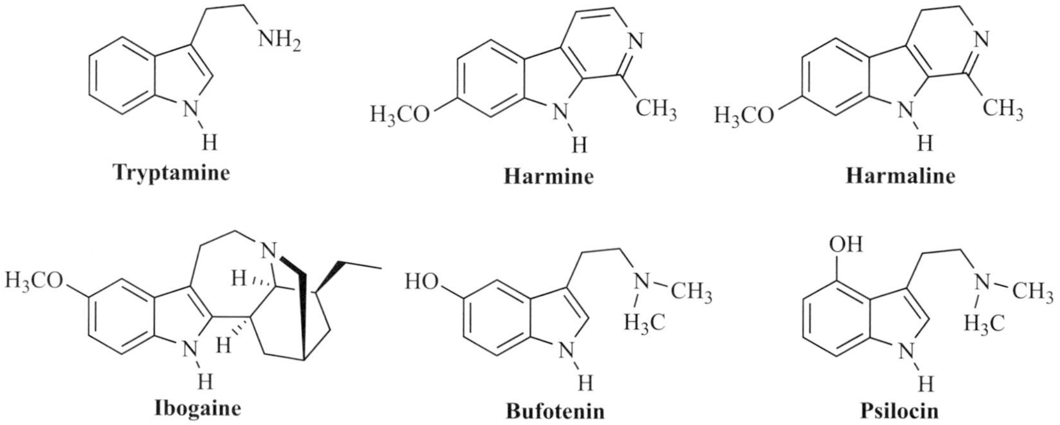

Fig. 6.64

revered certain fungi (*Psilocybe mexicana*, Strophar-iaceae) as the 'flesh of the Gods' and gave it the name Teonanactl. The reverence for these mush-rooms is presumably attributed to the profound hallucinogenic effects they exert, and, in Europe, many related species such as the liberty cap (*Psilocybe semilanceata*) are collected illegally for recreational abuse. These fungi are colloquially referred to as 'magic mushrooms', but as fungal taxonomy is highly complex there are risks of col-lecting poisonous species and the outcome may not be 'magic' at all.

The most important alkaloids of the indole group are the anticancer agents **vincristine** and **vinblas-tine** from the Madagascar periwinkle (*Catharanthus roseus*, Apocynaceae). These are complex **bisindole** (dimeric indole) natural products present in small quantities in the plant material. **Vindesine** is a semi-synthetic derivative which is also used clini-cally. These compounds are used for the treatment of Hodgkin's lymphoma, acute leukaemia and some solid tumours (Fig. 6.65) and are dealt with in further detail in Chapter 8.

Strychnine and **brucine** (Fig. 6.66) are intensely bitter indoles from the seeds of nux-vomica or 'vomiting nut' (*Strychnos nux-vomica*, Loganiaceae), which is a tree indigenous to India. Preparations of nux-vomica were used as a stimulant tonic until the middle of the 20th century. However, these compounds are highly poisonous (strychnine is used as a rodenticide) and they are responsible for

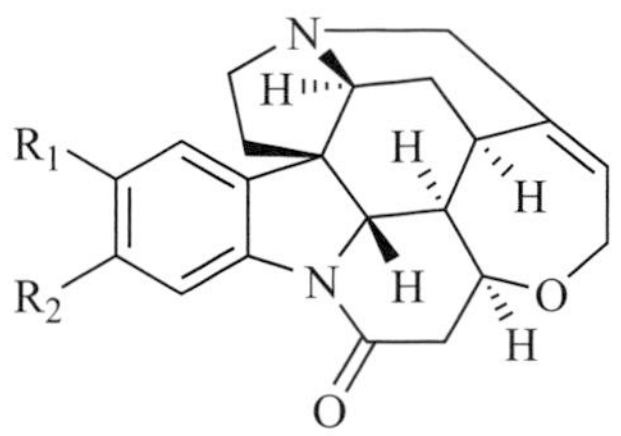

Strychnine, $R_1 = R_2 = H$
Brucine, $R_1 = R_2 = CH_3O$

Fig. 6.66

occasional poisoning incidents. They are of histori-cal interest only in pharmacy and are now used as research tools.

TROPANE ALKALOIDS

The European plant deadly nightshade (*Atropa bella-donna*, Solanaceae) produces **hyoscyamine** (Fig. 6.67), which occurs in the plant as a racemic mixture [(+) and (−) isomers, sometimes denoted (±)] at the chiral centre denoted * in Fig. 6.67. This mixture is often referred to as **atropine**. The generic name of the plant refers to Atropos, the ancient Greek Fate who, in mythology, cut the thread of life, and bella-donna, meaning beautiful lady in Italian and refers to the use of the juice of the berries of this plant by ladies in the 16th century to dilate the pupils of their eyes which was considered an attractive feature.

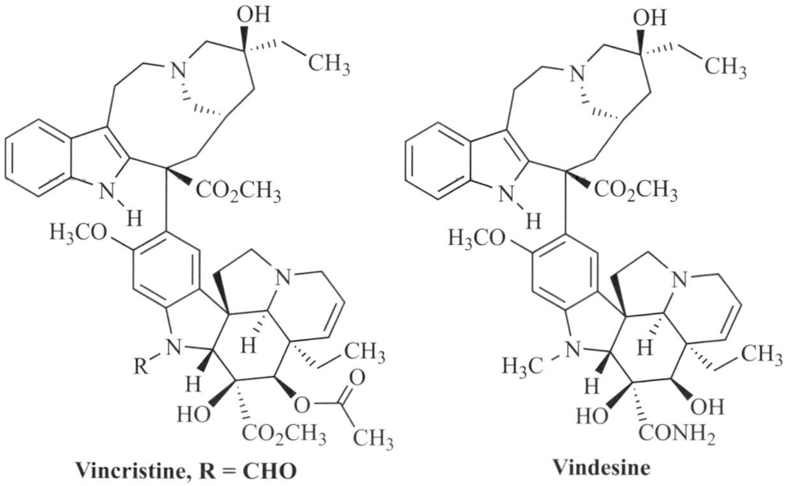

Vincristine, R = CHO
Vinblastine, R = CH$_3$

Vindesine

Fig. 6.65

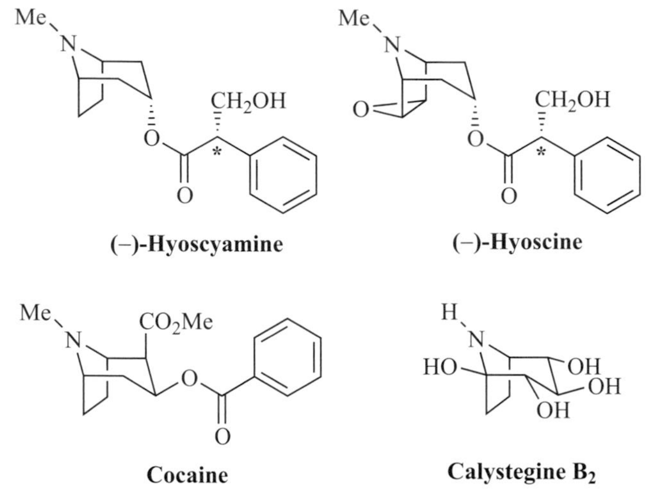

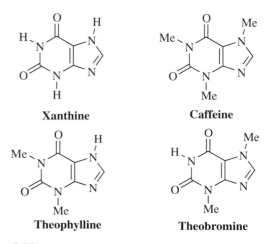

(−)-Hyoscyamine

(−)-Hyoscine

Cocaine

Calystegine B₂

Fig. 6.67

Hyoscyamine is an anticholinergic and also has been used to treat acute arrhythmias and to dilate the pupil of the eye (a mydriatic) for ophthalmic examinations. Semi-synthetic derivatives are also used (such as **tropicamide**) that are less longer-acting. Hyoscyamine also occurs in other species of Solanaceae, notably henbane (*Hyoscyamus niger*) and thornapple (*Datura stramonium*), together with **hyoscine**, also known as **scopolamine**, which is the epoxide derivative of hyoscyamine. Hyoscine is widely used as a premedication prior to operations to dry up secretions produced by inhalant anaesthetics and reduce nausea caused by the opiates. It is also a component of many travel (motion) sickness preparations.

The drug of abuse **cocaine** comes from the South American plants *Erythroxylum coca* and *E. truxillense* (Erythroxylaceae), which grow at high altitudes in the Andes in Colombia, Peru and Bolivia. As with heroin, this drug causes much misery and is a highly addictive CNS stimulant. Medicinally, cocaine has limited use as a local anaesthetic in ear, nose and throat surgery, and in the control of severe pain for patients with terminal cancer.

The calystegines, typically **calystegine B₂**, are *nor*-tropane alkaloids ('nor' meaning lacking a carbon) which lack the N-methyl group of the tropanes. These compounds are widely distributed in the plant kingdom, particularly in the plant families Solanaceae and Convolvulaceae, which include a number of fruit and vegetables (e.g. tomatoes). The calystegines are currently of interest as inhibitors of glycosidase enzymes and they may have potential toxicity when ingested.

XANTHINE ALKALOIDS

The xanthine alkaloids are probably the most widely known (and used) group of alkaloids, being constituents of popular daily beverages such as tea (*Camellia sinensis*, Theaceae) and coffee (*Coffea arabica*, Rubiaceae). Coffee contains the xanthine (or **purine**) alkaloid **caffeine** (1–2%) (Fig. 6.68); typically a cup of instant coffee contains approximately 50 mg of caffeine. The caffeine content is appreciably higher in Turkish or Arabic coffees, which are highly concentrated and may contain up to 300 mg of caffeine per cup. Caffeine is a CNS stimulant and is a component of Proplus, a highly popular product amongst students to

Xanthine

Caffeine

Theophylline

Theobromine

Fig. 6.68

counter fatigue and drowsiness. It is also a diuretic and is used in combination with analgesics.

Together with caffeine, **theophylline** and **theobromine** (Fig. 6.68) are minor components of tea; theobromine also occurs in cocoa (*Theobroma cacao*, Malvaceae). All three alkaloids differ only in the number and position of methyl substituents around the xanthine ring system. Theophylline is a diuretic and its derivatives (e.g. **aminophylline**) are used to relax the smooth muscle of the bronchi for relief of asthma.

IMIDAZOLE ALKALOIDS

The only member of this class that is of pharmaceutical merit is **pilocarpine** from jaborandi (*Pilocarpus jaborandi*, Rutaceae), a tree common to South America (Fig. 6.69). Pilocarpine is a cholinergic agent and is

Pilocarpine

Fig. 6.69

used to stimulate muscarinic receptors of the eye in the treatment of glaucoma. In the eye, this compound and derivatives (salts such as the hydrochloride and nitrate) cause pupillary constriction (miosis) and relieve eye pressure by facilitating better ocular drainage. Currently, there is interest in this class of alkaloid as muscarinic agonists in the treatment of Alzheimer's disease.

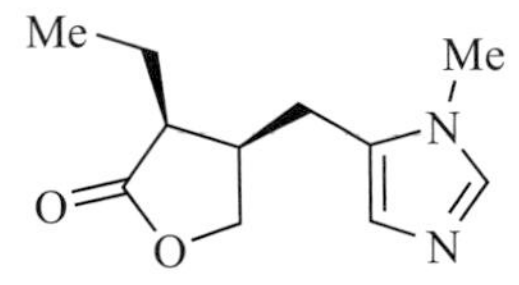

Further reading

Appendino, G., Fontana, G., Pollastro, F., 2010. Natural products drug discovery. In: Mander, L.,Lui, H.W. (Eds.), Comprehensive Natural Products II, vol. 3. Elsevier, Oxford, pp. 205–236.

Bruneton, J., 1995. Pharmacognosy, phytochemistry, medicinal plants. Springer-Verlag, Berlin.

Dewick, P.W., 2009. Medicinal natural products: a biosynthetic approach, third ed. Wiley, Chichester.

Evans, W.C., 2002. Trease and Evans' pharmacognosy, fifteenth ed. Baillière Tindall, London.

Luckner, M., 1990. Secondary metabolism in microorganisms, plants and animals, third ed. Springer-Verlag, Berlin.

Mann, J., 1994. Chemical aspects of biosynthesis. Oxford chemistry primers. Oxford University Press, Oxford.

Robbers, J.E., Speedie, M.K., Tyler, V.E., 1996. Pharmacognosy and pharmacobiotechnology. Williams & Wilkins, Baltimore.

Samuelsson, G., Bohlin, L., 2010. Drugs of natural origin: a treatise of pharmacognosy. Taylor & Francis, London.

Thadani, M.B., 1996. Medicinal and pharmaceutical uses of natural products. Cantext Publications, Winnipeg.

Torsell, K.B.G., 1997. Natural product chemistry: a mechanistic, biosynthetic and ecological approach, second ed. Swedish Pharmaceutical Press, Stockholm.

Chapter 7

Methods in natural product chemistry

In Chapter 6 we looked at the initial process in the selection of **biomass** (plant or microbe), its extraction and screening in different formats (high- and low-throughput screening), the isolation of the active components (bioassay-guided isolation) and the evaluation of the drug lead in clinical trials to the final drug. In this chapter we deal with the isolation process in more detail and cover the techniques that are used to isolate and characterize an active compound using chromatographic and spectroscopic techniques.

BIOASSAY–GUIDED ISOLATION

Bioassay-guided isolation is the physical process used to isolate biologically active chemicals from a natural source. Many of the chemicals described in Chapter 6 are from plant sources, but microbes are also an exceptionally valuable source of chemical diversity, in particular the filamentous bacteria (the Actinomycetes) of which the antibiotic-producing genus *Streptomyces* is the most widely studied for bioactive compounds. The fungi are also important and microbiologists spend time working in **biota-rich** environments such as the Amazon basin collecting, typing (identifying) and culturing samples for shipment back to the laboratory to be screened for bioactivity. As with plants, this process can be highly complicated, particularly in the identification of fungi, of which there may be potentially millions of new species waiting to be described in remote locations. This exercise is extremely worthwhile, as it is highly likely that new species will contain new chemistry that may have interesting bioactivity when fully

screened. This will be particularly relevant for the **Basidiomycetes**, a large group of fruiting fungi that produce a mushroom cap (basidium) and are sometimes difficult to grow in solution fermentation.

PREPARATION AND EXTRACTION

Whether samples are plants, microbes (**fermented** or **solid phase**), marine animals (corals, slugs, tunicates) or insects they are referred to as **biomass**. In the case of plants, following their identification and classification by a field botanist into a species and family, samples are collected from the aerial parts (leaves, stem and stem bark), the trunk bark and roots or, in the case of large trees, the heartwood (sometimes referred to as timber). These samples are then gently air-dried, although this can be problematic in highly humid environments such as rainforests and coastal regions. Better control is achieved in the laboratory using drying cabinets or lyophilizers (freeze-driers), although biomass must be dried quickly to avoid degradation of components by air or by microbes. Care must be taken with lyophilizers as they utilize a high vacuum, which can remove volatile components that may have interesting biological activities.

Once biomass has been dried, it is ground into small particles using either a blender or a mill. Plant material is milled twice, first using a coarse mill and then a fine mill to generate a fine powder. The grinding process is important as effective extraction depends on the size of the biomass particles; large particles will be poorly extracted, whereas small particles have a higher surface area and will therefore be extracted more efficiently.

Selection of the **solvent extraction** approach is very important. If a plant is under investigation from an ethnobotanical perspective, then the extraction should mimic the traditional use. For example, if an indigenous people use a specific extraction protocol such as a water extract, a cold/hot tea, alcohol or alcohol–water mixtures, then an identical or at least a very similar method should be used in the laboratory so that the same natural products are extracted. Failure to extract biomass properly may result in loss of access to active compounds. Additionally, using an inappropriate extraction method, such as strong heating of biomass with a solvent, may result in degradation of natural products and consequent loss of biological activity.

Numerous extraction methods are available, the simplest being **cold extraction** (in a large flask with agitation of the biomass using a stirrer) in which the ground dried material is extracted at room temperature sequentially with solvents of increasing polarity: first hexane (or petroleum ether), then chloroform (or dichloromethane), ethyl acetate, acetone, methanol and finally water. The major advantage of this protocol is that it is a **soft extraction method** as the extract is not heated and there is little potential degradation of natural products. The use of sequential solvents of increasing polarity enables division of natural products according to their solubility (and polarity) in the extraction solvents. This can greatly simplify an isolation process. Cold extraction allows most compounds to be extracted, although some may have limited solubility in the extracting solvent at room temperature.

In **hot percolation**, the biomass is added to a round-bottomed flask containing solvent and the mixture is heated gently under reflux. Typically, the plant material is 'stewed' using solvents such as ethanol or aqueous ethanol mixtures. The technique is sometimes referred to as **total extraction** and has the advantage that, with ethanol, the majority of lipophilic and polar compounds is extracted. An equilibrium between compounds in solution and in the biomass is established, resulting in moderate extraction of natural products. Heating the extracts for long periods may also degrade labile compounds; therefore a pilot experiment should first be attempted and extracts assessed for biological activity to ascertain whether this extraction method degrades the bioactive natural products. Care should be taken, as extraction is never truly total; for example, some highly lipophilic natural

products are insoluble in polar solvents (e.g. the monoterpenes).

Supercritical fluid extraction utilizes the fact that some gases behave as liquids when under pressure and have solvating properties. The most important example is carbon dioxide which can be used to extract biomass and has the advantage that, once the pressure has been removed, the gas boils off leaving a clean extract. Carbon dioxide is a non-polar solvent but the polarity of the supercritical fluid extraction solvent may be increased by addition of a modifying agent, which is usually another solvent (e.g. methanol or dichloromethane).

The most widely used method for extraction of plant natural products is **Soxhlet extraction** (Fig. 7.1). This technique uses continuous extraction by solvents of increasing polarity. The biomass is placed in a Soxhlet thimble constructed of filter

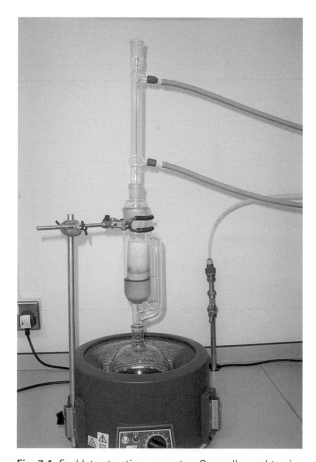

Fig. 7.1 Soxhlet extraction apparatus. Generally used to give greatest yield of extract when extracts are stable in hot solvent.

paper, through which solvent is continuously refluxed. The Soxhlet apparatus will empty its contents into the round-bottomed flask once the solvent reaches a certain level. As fresh solvent enters the apparatus by a reflux condenser, extraction is very efficient and compounds are effectively drawn into the solvent from the biomass due to their low initial concentration in the solvent. The method suffers from the same drawbacks as other hot extraction methods (possible degradation of products), but it is the best extraction method for the recovery of big yields of extract. Moreover, providing biological activity is not lost on heating, the technique can be used in drug lead discovery.

In general terms, regardless of the extraction method used, extracts are of two types: **lipophilic** ('fat-loving'), resulting from extraction by non-polar solvents (e.g. petrol, ethyl acetate, chloroform, dichloromethane), and **hydrophilic** ('water-loving'), produced by extracting biomass with polar solvents (e.g. acetone, methanol, water).

The value of using solvents of different polarities is that the chemical complexity of the biomass is simplified when taken into the extract, according to the solubility of the components. This can greatly simplify the isolation of an active compound from the extract. Additionally, certain classes of compounds may have high solubilities in a particular solvent (e.g. the monoterpenes in hexane), which again can simplify the chemical complexity of an extract and help with the isolation process.

Regardless of the extraction technique used, extracts are concentrated under vacuum using rotary evaporators for large volumes of solvent (>5 ml) or 'blown down' under nitrogen for small volumes (1–5 ml), ensuring that volatile components are not lost. Removal of solvent should be carried out immediately after extraction, as natural products may be unstable in the solvent. Aqueous extracts are generally freeze-dried using a lyophilizer. Dried extracts should be stored at –20 °C prior to screening for biological activity as this will decrease the possibility of bioactive natural product degradation.

If it is known that certain classes of compounds, such as acids or bases, are present in the biomass, they can be extracted using a tailored protocol. The most common group of natural products that are extracted in this manner are the alkaloids (see Chapter 6 and below), which are often present in plant material as salts. A brief outline of how these basic compounds may be extracted is as follows:

1. Alkaloids can be recovered from their salts by making the dry powdered plant material alkaline with aqueous ammonia. This leaves the alkaloids as **free bases** that are no longer ionic salts and are much more soluble in organic solvents such as dichloromethane or ethyl acetate.
2. This increased solubility in organic solvents allows **partitioning** of the free bases into ethyl acetate or dichloromethane, which can then be separated from the aqueous ammonia layer in a separating funnel as these solvents form immiscible layers.
3. The dichloromethane solution will contain the free bases, which can be extracted with aqueous acid, for example by extracting three times with 2 M hydrochloric acid, and the alkaloids will transfer from the organic phase to the aqueous phase as hydrochloride salts. The remaining dichloromethane layer can be tested using a specific colour test for alkaloids (e.g. Dragendorff's reagent) to ensure that all of the alkaloids have been transferred to the acidic aqueous layer.
4. The acidic layer can then be basified, which results in the precipitation of the alkaloids (which are no longer salts and therefore no longer soluble in aqueous media) and can be extracted back into an organic solvent (ethyl acetate or dichloromethane).

This extraction method generates a mixture of alkaloids that are essentially free of neutral or acidic plant components and is specific for compounds that are basic (able to form free bases). However, care should be taken with alkaloid extractions as the acids and bases employed may destroy active natural products that have functional groups which are readily susceptible to degradation (e.g. glycosides, epoxides and esters). Additionally, the stereochemistry of a molecule may be affected by the presence of these strong reagents. The most important factor to consider is: *is biological activity retained following the extraction protocol?*

ISOLATION METHODS

Once an extract has been generated by a suitable extraction protocol and activity is demonstrated in a bioassay (e.g. an antibacterial test), the next step is to fractionate the extract using a separation method so that a purified biologically active component can be isolated.

PARTITIONING

Possibly the simplest separation method is partitioning, which is widely used as an initial extract purification and 'clean up' step. Partitioning uses two immiscible solvents to which the extract is added; this can be sequential by using immiscible organic solvents of increasing polarity. Typically, this may take place in two steps: (1) water/light petroleum ether (hexane) to generate a non-polar fraction in the organic layer; (2) water/dichloromethane or water/chloroform or water/ethyl acetate to give a medium-polar fraction in the organic layer. The remaining aqueous layer will contain polar water-soluble natural products. This is a soft separation method and relies on the solubility of natural products and not a physical interaction with another medium (e.g. adsorption on silica gel in thin-layer chromatography, TLC; see below). Partitioning may give rise to excellent separations, particularly with compounds that differ greatly in solubility; for example, monoterpenes are easily separated from phenolics such as tannins.

GEL CHROMATOGRAPHY

Assuming that the extract is still active, the next step is chromatography. A procedure that is widely used as an initial clean-up is **gel chromatography**, also known as size **exclusion chromatography**. This technique employs a cross-linked dextran (sugar polymer) which, when added to a suitable solvent (e.g. chloroform or ethyl acetate), swells to form a gel matrix. The gel contains pores of a finite size that allow small molecules (<500 Da) to be retained in the matrix; larger molecules (>500 Da) are excluded and move quickly through the gel. This gel is loaded into a column and the extract is added to the top of the column. Large molecules are the first to elute, followed by molecules of a smaller size. This is an excellent method for separating out chlorophylls, fatty acids, glycerides and other large molecules that may interfere with the biological assay. Different sorts of gels are available which may be used in organic solvents (e.g. LH-20) or aqueous preparations such as salts and buffers (e.g. G-25). Therefore both non-polar and polar natural products can be fractionated using this technique. Additionally, compounds are not only fractionated according to size but there is also a small amount of adsorption chromatography occurring, as the dextran from which the gel is made contains hydroxyl groups that interact with natural products, facilitating some separation according to polarity.

This is a non-destructive 'soft' method with a high recovery (compounds are rarely strongly adsorbed) and a high quantity of extract (hundreds of milligrams to grams) may be separated. A further benefit of this technique is that many different gels are available with a variety of pore sizes that can be used to separate compounds from 500 to 250,000 Da. This is the method of choice for large molecules, in particular proteins, polypeptides, carbohydrates, tannins and glycosides, especially saponin and triterpene glycosides.

ION-EXCHANGE CHROMATOGRAPHY

The separation of small polar compounds, in particular ionic natural products, is often problematic. It is possible to separate these metabolites from larger molecules (using gels) but they are generally very strongly adsorbed with normal-phase sorbents such as silica or alumina, and, even with the use of polar solvents and modifiers (e.g. acid and base), efficient separations may not be achievable. Additionally, these compounds are not retained on reverse-phase sorbents such as C_{18} or C_8. These natural products possess functional groups, such as CO_2H, -OH, $-NH_2$, that contribute to the polarity of the molecule, and this may be used to develop a separation method using **ion-exchange chromatography**.

This technique is limited to natural products that can carry charge on their functional groups. The **sorbent** or **stationary phase** has charged groups and mobile counter ions which may exchange with ions of the functional groups present in the natural product as the mobile phase moves through the sorbent. Separation is achieved by differences in affinity between ionic components (polar natural products) and the stationary phase. These ion-exchange sorbents or resins are divided into two groups: **cation** exchangers, which have acidic groups (CO_2H, $-SO_3H$) and are able to exchange their protons with cations of natural products, and **anion** exchangers, which have basic groups ($-N^+R_3$) that are incorporated into the resin and can exchange their anions with anions from the natural product. These ion-exchange resins may be used in open column chromatography or in closed columns in applications such as high performance liquid chromatography (HPLC).

An example of the technique is shown in Fig. 7.2. **2,5-Dihydroxymethyl-3,4-dihydroxypyrrolidine** (DMDP) from *Lonchocarpus sericeus* (Fabaceae) is a nematocidal polyhydroxylated alkaloid (PHA),

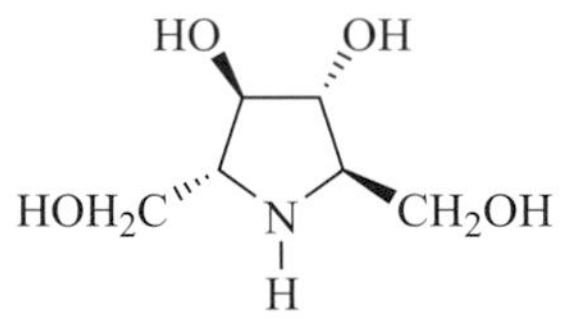

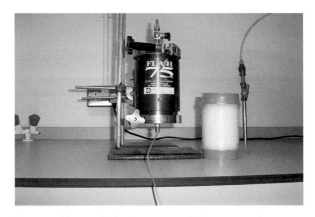

2,5-Dihydroxymethyl-3,4-dihydroxypyrrolidine (DMDP)

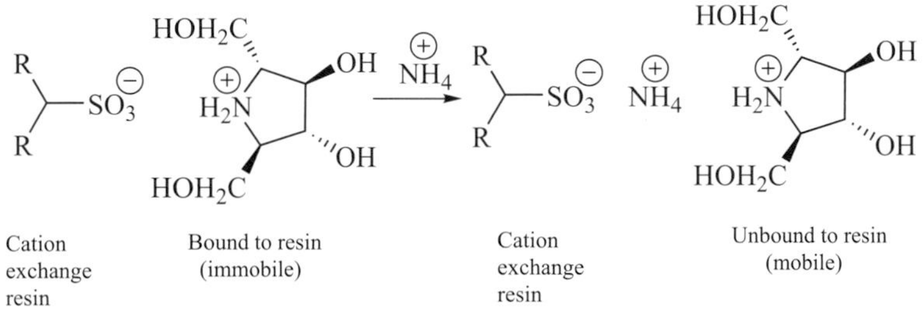

Cation exchange resin   Bound to resin (immobile)   Cation exchange resin   Unbound to resin (mobile)

Fig. 7.2

and also inhibits insect α- and β-glucosidases. Compounds of this type are bases and form cations in acidic solutions. When added to a cation exchanger [e.g. Amberlite CG-120, which has a sulfonic acid bound to the resin which can exchange its proton (cation)], the DMDP cations are retained (bound) by the cation exchanger and protons are displaced. If the cation exchanger is then eluted with a solution containing a stronger cation such as NH_4^+ (e.g. from 0.2 M NH_4OH), then the DMDP cation is desorbed from the exchanger and is unbound and mobile. This affinity can be used to separate such alkaloids from acidic (anionic) or neutral components which would not be retained by the cation exchanger and may be washed from the resin by water.

Plant extracts that contain DMDP are used as a nematocide against infected crops (bananas) in Costa Rica and are licensed by the National Institute of Biodiversity. This is an example of a renewable resource as the extracts may be prepared from the seeds of the plant and DMDP is ecologically friendly as it is biodegradable.

BIOTAGE™ FLASH CHROMATOGRAPHY

Biotage™ flash chromatography may be used for quick efficient separations. This employs pre-packed solvent-resistant plastic cartridges (Fig. 7.3), which contain the sorbent (silica, alumina, C_{18}, HP-20, or ion exchange resin). These cartridges are introduced into a **radial compression module** (the metal cylinder in Fig. 7.3), which pressurizes the

Fig. 7.3 Biotage flash chromatograph. Fast separations are achieved with good resolution.

cartridge and sorbent radially. This results in a very homogeneous packed material (sorbent), reduces the possibility of solvent channelling when the system is run and minimizes void spaces on the column head.

Using this technique, milligrams to tens of grams can be separated. The bioactive extract can be dissolved in solvent and loaded onto the column directly; solvent is then pumped through the column and fractions are collected, resulting in a rapid separation of extract components. This is a rapid method; 10 g of extract can be fractionated into 12 fractions of increasing polarity in 30 min using a step gradient solvent system. There are a number of benefits to this, particularly that speed minimizes contact with reactive sorbents (e.g. silica) and that hazardous sorbents such as silica, which when free may cause silicosis, are contained in the cartridges. Additionally, the cartridges may be re-used, reducing the cost of the bioassay-guided process. The high flow-rates employed by this technique (20–250 ml/min) retain 'band-like' movement of the components through the column, resulting in a high resolution. Compounds eluting from the column may be detected by TLC (of fractions) or the eluant may be passed through a UV detector so that compounds that absorb UV light can be detected as they elute from the column. Some laboratories run several of these flash columns simultaneously, resulting in a high number of fractionated extracts having sufficient mass for further purification of the active components.

THIN–LAYER CHROMATOGRAPHY

Thin-layer chromatography (TLC) is one of the most widely used and easiest methods for purifying a small number (2–4) of components, typically following a Biotage flash separation. This method employs glass or aluminium plates that are pre-coated with sorbent (e.g. silica gel) of varying thickness dependent on the amount of material to be loaded onto the plates. The coating on analytical plates is generally of 0.2 mm thickness; preparative plates may have a coating 1–2 mm thick. The compound mixture is loaded at 1–2 cm from the bottom edge of the plate as either a spot or a continuous band. The plate is then lowered into a tank containing a predetermined solvent which will migrate up the plate and separate the compound mixture according to the polarity of the components.

In analytical use, micrograms of material may be separated using this technique and samples such as drugs of abuse (e.g. cannabis resin) may be compared with standards (e.g. tetrahydrocannabinol) for quick identification.

Sorbent-coated plates often incorporate a fluorescent indicator (F_{254}) so that natural products that absorb short-wave UV light (254 nm) will appear as black spots on a green background. Under long-wave UV light, certain compounds may emit a brilliant blue or yellow fluorescence. Both UV absorbance and fluorescence properties may be used to monitor the separation of compounds on a TLC plate.

Preparative scale TLC has great use and loadings of 1–100 mg can readily produce enough purified material for biological assays and structure elucidation. It is rapid and cheap and has been the method of choice for separating lipophilic compounds. Preparative plates are available from suppliers as pre-coated plates of 1–2 mm thickness in silica, alumina or C_{18}. However, home-made plates offer greater flexibility by allowing the incorporation of modifying agents into the sorbents (e.g. silver nitrate for separation of olefinic compounds – known as argentation TLC), use of other sorbents (ion exchange, polyamide, cellulose) and the addition of indicators and binders.

The scale-up from analytical to preparative mode is crucial, as an increase in the sample load may drastically change the separation of the components. Normally, the method developed on the analytical scale must be modified, generally with a reduction of solvent system polarity. Preparative TLC is used as a final clean-up procedure to separate 2–4 compounds. The sample is dissolved in a small volume of solvent and applied as a thin line 2 cm from the bottom of the plate and dried. The plate is then eluted in a suitable solvent and UV-active compounds are visualized at 254 or 366 nm. Natural products that are not UV-active will need development using a suitable spray reagent such as vanillin-sulphuric acid, Dragendorff's reagent, phosphomolybdic acid or antimony trichloride. In this case, an edge of the plate is sprayed with the reagent (taking care that only a small area of the plate is covered) and separated compounds are visualized as coloured bands. The bands containing pure natural product are scraped off the plate and the natural product is desorbed from the sorbent. This desorption may be carried out by placing the compound-rich sorbent into a sintered glass funnel and washing with a suitable solvent followed by collection and concentration of the filtrate. The purified 'band' should then be assessed for purity by analytical TLC.

There are a number of advantages of this method for the analysis and isolation of biologically active natural products:

● It is cost-effective compared with instrumental methods and requires little training or knowledge of chromatography
● Easy scale-up from analytical to preparative mode with quick isolation of milligram to gram amounts of product
● Flexibility of choice of mobile and stationary phases
● A separation may be readily optimized to 'zero in' on one component and methods may be quickly developed

- Practically any separation can be achieved with the correct mobile and stationary phases
- A large number of samples may be analysed or separated simultaneously.

The major disadvantages of TLC are that:

- loading and speed are poor compared with flash chromatography
- there is poor detection and control of elution compared with high-performance liquid chromatography.

HIGH–PERFORMANCE LIQUID CHROMATOGRAPHY

The final separation technique discussed in this section is high-performance liquid chromatography (HPLC). This method is currently in vogue and is widely used for the analysis and isolation of bioactive natural products. The analytical sensitivity of the technique, particularly when coupled with UV detection such as photodiode array (PDA), enables the acquisition of UV spectra of eluting peaks from 190 nm to 800 nm. The flow-rates of this system are typically 0.5–2.0 ml/min and sample loading in the analytical mode allows the detection and separation of tens to hundreds of micrograms of material. With PDA UV detection, even compounds with poor UV characteristics can be detected. This is especially useful in the analysis of natural products such as terpenoids or polyketides which may have no unsaturation or chromophores that give rise to a characteristic UV signature.

HPLC is a highly sensitive technique when coupled to electronic library searching of compounds with a known UV spectrum. Modern software enables the UV spectra of eluting peaks to be compared with spectra stored electronically, thereby enabling early identification of known compounds or, usefully, the comparison of novel compounds with a similar UV spectrum, which may indicate structural similarity. It is also possible to increase the size of these electronic libraries and improve the searching power of the technique. HPLC is a powerful technique for **fingerprinting** biologically active extracts and comparisons can be drawn with chromatograms and UV spectra stored in an electronic library. This is currently very important for the quality control of herbal medicines for which appropriate standards in reproducibility of extract quality must be met.

HPLC can be run in fully automated mode and with carousel autosamplers it is possible to analyse tens to hundreds of samples. These HPLC systems are computer-driven and not only run samples, but may be programmed to process data and print out chromatograms and spectra automatically. Radial compressed column technology can also be made use of in HPLC and, as with Biotage flash chromatography, can access highly varied column technology, including standard sorbents such as normal phase (silica) and reverse-phase (C_{18} and C_8) and more 'exotic' stationary phases such as phenyl, cyano, C_4, chiral phases, gel size exclusion media and ion exchangers. This versatility of stationary phase has made HPLC a highly popular method for bioassay-guided isolation.

HPLC is a high-resolution technique, with efficient, fast separations. The most widely used stationary phase is C_{18} (reverse-phase) chromatography, generally employing water/acetonitrile or water/methanol mixtures as mobile phase. These mobile phases may be run in **gradient elution mode**, in which the concentration of a particular solvent is increased over a period of time, starting, for example, with 100% water and increasing to 100% acetonitrile over 30 min, or in **isocratic elution mode**, in which a constant composition (e.g. 70% acetonitrile in water) is maintained for a set period of time.

HPLC is also used preparatively and, with the aid of computer-controlled pumping systems, very accurate mixing of solvents can be achieved leading to superb control of elution power. Many preparative columns employ radial compressed column technology as these columns have a long column life, few void volumes, homogeneous column packing with little solvent channelling and excellent 'band flow' of components as they flow through the column. As with TLC, an analytical HPLC method is developed for scale-up to preparative HPLC; flow-rates of 50–300 ml/min are common. Detection in preparative HPLC generally utilizes a UV detector that has been optimized to detect the natural product of interest (e.g. at 254 nm) by knowledge of the spectra acquired by analytical PDA HPLC. A large sample loading of tens of milligrams to grams of material can be achieved and rapid isolation can be facilitated by the use of intelligent fraction collectors that can 'peak collect' compounds as they elute from the column by receiving input from the UV detector.

The technique can be used for the majority of natural products that are soluble in organic solvents and can be adapted to ion exchange for the isolation of highly polar compounds. HPLC is the method of choice for the pharmaceutical industry because of its excellent separating power, speed and reproducibility. The major disadvantage of this technique, however, is its expense, as analytical instrumentation may cost upwards of £20,000, and preparative HPLC may be £30,000. Consumables for this technique are also expensive, especially preparative columns (£2000), which may have a short life and at high solvent flow-rates there is a high cost for purchase and disposal of high-purity solvents.

ISOLATION STRATEGY

How do the isolation methods described above fit together? Figure 7.4 gives a general isolation protocol starting with selection of biomass (e.g. plant or microbe), which is then extracted using a Soxhlet apparatus, cold or hot percolation or supercritical fluid extraction. Hydrophilic extracts will then typically undergo ion exchange chromatography with bioassay of generated fractions. A further ion exchange method of bioactive fractions would yield pure compounds, which could then be submitted for structure elucidation. Lipophilic extracts could initially be partitioned to generate a further hydrophilic fraction which could be dealt with by ion exchange chromatography as described above.

The lipophilic portion may then be either subjected to gel chromatography to remove or separate large components (e.g. chlorophylls, fatty acids or glycerides), or this step skipped, and then flash chromatography used to generate a series of fractions that would undergo bioassay. Active fractions can then be further purified by using either HPLC or TLC to give pure compounds, for submission to structure elucidation. This is only a general outline for isolation of bioactive natural products; there is no tailored protocol and the physicochemical properties of natural products differ enormously, sometimes making the isolation of chemicals from nature a highly difficult and intellectually challenging problem. In very rare cases, organisms produce very simple extracts (2–4 components), which may be readily separated into pure compounds, but in the majority of cases extracts are highly complex and the active component may be present at a very low concentration or even be unstable, further contributing to the difficulty of the bioassay-guided isolation process. It is also possible that activity may even diminish during the separation process; this could be due to a synergistic effect occurring through several components working in concert in the bioassay. There is currently much interest in this area, and it is possible that the value and efficacy of certain herbal medicines (which contain tens to hundreds, or even thousands, of natural products) are due to several active components; thus the bioassay-guided isolation approach may not be appropriate for the study of these agents. The facts remain, however, that many useful pharmaceutical entities were developed using this approach and, because of the sheer number of organisms still to be investigated, it is certain that bioassay-guided isolation will yield many new medicines in the future.

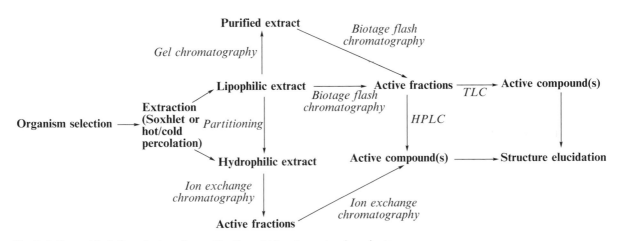

Fig. 7.4 General isolation strategy for purification of bioactive natural products.

STRUCTURE ELUCIDATION

Ideally, bioassay-guided methods should afford a pure natural product of at least 5 mg in weight. Current structure elucidation techniques are available that can determine the structures of compounds on micrograms of material, although larger quantities are of benefit for further biological assays and will save time and money in the pharmaceutical industry setting, so that valuable resources do not need to be used in the acquisition of more biomass and a potentially lengthy bioassay-guided isolation process.

Structure elucidation of natural products generally employs the classical spectroscopic techniques of **mass spectrometry** (MS) and **nuclear magnetic resonance** (NMR) **spectroscopy**. The first steps, however, should be the recording of infrared (IR) and ultraviolet-visible (UV-Vis) spectra to determine the presence of certain functional groups and conjugation in the molecule. Rather than a theoretical approach to this subject, we will use a bioactive natural product to highlight the strengths of these techniques.

In a project to isolate and characterize antibiotics from plants, *Thymus vulgaris* (thyme), a member of the mint family (Lamiaceae), was extracted with hexane and ethyl acetate. Each of these extracts was highly active in a bioassay to discover compounds with activity against methicillin-resistant *Staphylococcus aureus*. Extracts were analysed by TLC and bulked due to similarity. Biotage flash chromatography, followed by preparative HPLC, led to the isolation of the pure active natural product, compound X, which was a pale yellow volatile oil with a pungent aroma. The UV spectrum showed a maximum at 277 nm, indicative of the presence of an aromatic ring. The IR spectrum showed absorptions attributable to aromatic and aliphatic C-H groups and a broad peak at 3600 nm indicative of an hydroxyl functional group.

MASS SPECTROMETRY

This technique allows the measurement of the molecular weight of a compound and, once a molecular ion has been identified, it is possible to measure this ion accurately to ascertain the exact number of hydrogens, carbons, oxygens and other atoms that may be present in the molecule. This will give the molecular formula. A number of ionization techniques are available in MS, of which **electron impact** is widely used. This technique gives good fragmentation of the molecule and is useful for structure elucidation purposes as the fragments can be assigned to functional groups present in the compound. The disadvantage of this technique is that molecular ions are sometimes absent. Softer techniques such as **chemical ionization** (CI), **electrospray ionization** (ESI) and **fast atom bombardment** (FAB) mass spectrometry ionize the molecule with less energy; consequently, molecular ions are generally present, but with less fragmentation information for structure elucidation purposes.

Compound X was submitted to FAB-MS; the spectrum is shown in Fig. 7.5. The scale on the x-axis is the mass (m) to charge (z) ratio (m/z). As compound X readily forms single ions, m/z is in effect $m/1$ and therefore directly related to the weight of fragments and, in the case of the molecular ion, the molecular weight of the compound.

A molecular ion (M^+) is seen at m/z 150. This is supported by additional peaks where the molecule picks up a hydrogen ion at m/z 151 $[M+H]^+$ and loses a hydrogen ion at m/z 149 $[M–H]^+$. The spectrum was run using FAB ionization and little fragmentation is evident. There are some useful fragments, however, in particular at m/z 135, which is 15 mass units less than the molecular ion and almost certainly corresponds to $[M–Me]^+$, indicating that this molecule contains a methyl group (15 mass units), which is readily lost in the mass spectrometer.

Accurate mass measurement of the molecular ion at m/z 150 gave a figure of 150.104700. If a computer program is used to calculate the number of carbon, hydrogen and oxygen atoms that would be required to give this weight, a formula of $C_{10}H_{14}O$ is produced. The theoretical mass of this formula is 150.104465, which is very close to the measured accurate mass. The theoretical mass takes into account the accurate masses of carbon, hydrogen and oxygen, and the nearest 'fit' to the measured mass gives the $C_{10}H_{14}O$ formula. Interestingly, compound X has 10 carbon atoms and, as it is a volatile oil, it is likely to be a member of the monoterpene group of natural products.

At this stage it would be possible to perform a database search on this molecular formula and the producing organism (*Thymus vulgaris*) from sources such as SciFinder (**Chemical Abstracts)** or the **Dictionary of Natural Products**, although there are many natural products with this formula and therefore further structure elucidation is required.

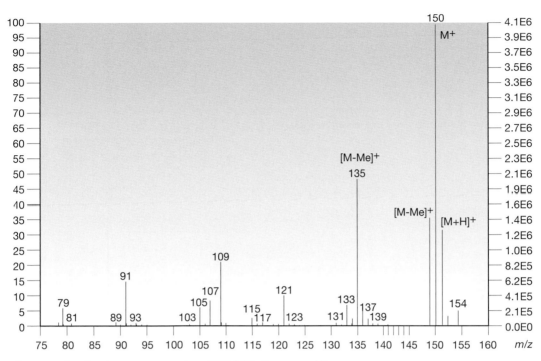

Fig. 7.5 Fast atom bombardment mass spectrum (FAB-MS) of compound X.

NMR SPECTROSCOPY

^{1}H NMR spectroscopy

The next step in this process is the recording of a ^{1}H NMR spectrum (Fig. 7.6). This will indicate the number of hydrogen atoms associated with a particular group (**integration**) and how **shielded** or **deshielded** that group is. Shielding and deshielding occur due to the presence of groups that are either electron-withdrawing (deshielding) or electron-donating (shielding).

Inspection of the ^{1}H NMR spectrum of compound X recorded in the solvent deuteron-chloroform CDCl$_3$, which has a peak at 7.27 ppm (**Z** in the spectrum), shows three deshielded peaks (**A, B** and **C**), each integrating for one proton (the figures under the x-axis are the integration and indicate how many protons are associated with each peak). These protons occur in the aromatic region (6.00–8.00 ppm) and have a particular coupling pattern. Additional signals include a broad peak (**D**), indicating that it is exchangeable and possibly an hydroxyl group, a multiplet at 2.84 ppm (**E**) integrating for one proton and a singlet at 2.23 ppm (peak **F**) integrating for three protons, which is

due to a methyl group. The last peak in the spectrum (**G**) is a doublet (two lines) integrating for six protons. This is due to two methyl groups occurring in the same position of the spectrum as they are equivalent. This equivalence occurs because they are in the same 'environment'. This signal appears as a doublet because these methyls are coupled to one proton (multiplicity $= n + 1$, where n is the number of nearest neighbouring protons), and the most likely candidate for this single proton is the multiplet at 2.84 ppm. This proton is a complex multiplet because it couples to all six of the protons of the two coincident methyl groups. This coupling system indicates that these two groups form an isopropyl group [(CH$_3$)$_2$CH-]. The one-proton multiplet at 2.84 ppm (peak **E**) and methyl group at 2.23 ppm (**F**) are slightly deshielded (higher ppm) with respect to the methyl groups at 1.23 ppm (**G**), indicating that they are attached to a group that causes electron withdrawal (possibly an aromatic ring, which is inferred by the presence of the aromatic protons).

Expansion of the aromatic region 6.6–7.1 ppm (Fig. 7.7) shows the coupling pattern of the aromatic ring. Inspection of this area allows measurement of coupling constants, referred to as *J* values. Taking

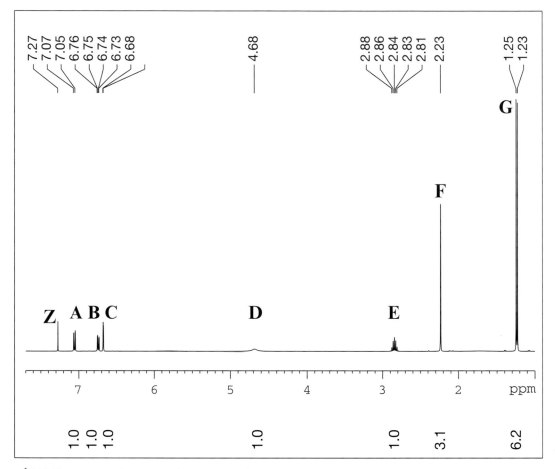

Fig. 7.6 ^{1}H NMR spectrum of compound X recorded in CDCl$_3$.

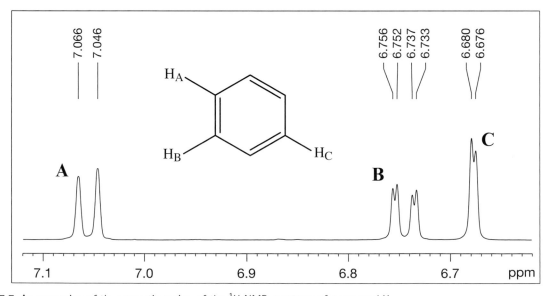

Fig. 7.7 An expansion of the aromatic region of the ^{1}H NMR spectrum of compound X.

peak **A**, which is a doublet (two lines), as an example, this is done by subtracting the lower ppm value for this peak from the higher ppm value and multiplying the difference by the field strength at which this experiment was measured (400 MHz in this case). This gives:

$$(7.066 - 7.046 \text{ ppm}) \times 400 = 8 \text{ Hz}$$

The size of this coupling constant indicates that peak A is coupled to another proton which is *ortho* to itself (*ortho* coupling constants are of the order of 6–9 Hz). Peak **B** is a double doublet (and has four lines) with two couplings (8 and 1.6 Hz), indicating that this is the proton which is *ortho* to peak **A** (it has the same coupling constant of 8 Hz) and the smaller coupling constant (1.6 Hz) is indicative of a *meta* coupling to another proton (meta coupling constants are typically 1–2 Hz). Peak **C** at 6.67 ppm is a doublet (1.6 Hz) which has the same coupling constant as one of those for peak **B**, indicating that this is the proton that is *meta* to **B**. This part of the spectrum therefore tells us that we have an aromatic ring with three protons attached to it in the 1, 2 and 4 positions (Fig. 7.7).

Taking all of the fragments from the ^{1}H spectrum into consideration, there are three aromatic protons, a broad exchangeable peak, a multiplet, a methyl singlet and a six-proton doublet corresponding to two coincident methyl groups. This total of 14 protons is identical to the number found in the molecular formula using MS.

^{13}C NMR spectroscopy

The proton spectrum has revealed much about the number of protons present and their chemical environments – i.e. whether they are shielded or deshielded by electron-donating or electron-withdrawing groups, respectively. The next step is the acquisition of a ^{13}C NMR spectrum which will give further information regarding the environment of the different groups and the number of carbons present. Two ^{13}C NMR spectra of compound X are shown in Fig. 7.8.

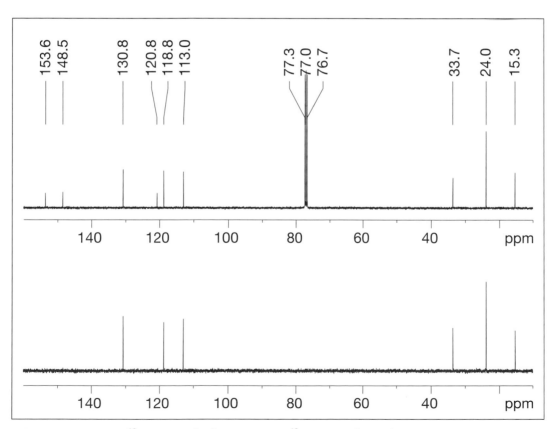

Fig. 7.8 Broadband decoupled ^{13}C spectrum (top) and DEPT-135 ^{13}C spectrum (bottom) of compound X.

The top spectrum is the **broadband decoupled** spectrum which shows all of the carbons present; the carbons appear as singlets due to proton decoupling. The top spectrum of compound X was recorded in $CDCl_3$, which occurs as three lines at 77.0 ppm. There are only nine carbons evident, which might be confusing as we know from the mass spectrum that compound X should contain 10 carbons. However, as the ^1H spectrum has two coincident methyl groups, it is possible that there are two carbons associated with the peak at 24 ppm. If both methyl groups were in the same environment (as they are in an isopropyl group), then they would occur at the same position in the spectrum. As with the proton spectrum, the carbon signals occur over a large range, which is again determined by whether the carbons are deshielded (high ppm value) or shielded (low ppm value). The lower ^{13}C spectrum has been produced by a special experiment called **DEPT-135**, which lacks the solvents signals, but, more importantly, it only shows carbons that have protons attached to them (CH, CH_2 and CH_3). As compound X does not have any CH_2 groups (there are no groups in the ^1H spectrum which integrate for two protons), only CH and CH_3 carbons are shown. This is useful as it allows quaternary carbons (carbons with no protons attached) to be identified, and it can be seen that there are three additional aromatic quaternaries in the top spectrum, at 153.6, 148.5 and 120.8 ppm. The range for aromatic carbons is 110–160 ppm. The carbon at 153.6 is highly deshielded and it is possible that this carbon is attached to an oxygen atom (from the OH group in compound X). The three peaks at 130.8, 118.8 and 113.0 are all carbons bearing one proton (CH or methine carbons); these correspond to proton peaks **A, B** and **C** in the ^1H spectrum (Fig. 7.6). The remaining peaks at 33.7, 24.0 and 15.3 are carbons associated with the multiplet (peak **E**), two coincident methyl groups (peak **G**) and a methyl singlet (peak **F**).

Homonuclear correlation spectroscopy

The next technique that can aid in the structure determination of compound X is **COrrelation SpectroscopY** (COSY), which reveals couplings between protons that are close (two, three or four bonds distant from each other). It is referred to as a **homonuclear** (same nuclei, both of which are ^1H) two-dimensional technique because the data are displayed in a matrix format with two one-dimensional

experiments (^1H spectra) displayed on the *x*- and *y*-axes (Fig. 7.9). A diagonal series of peaks correspond to the ^1H spectrum signals. Peaks that are away from the diagonal (referred to as **cross-peaks**) indicate coupling between signals.

For example, inspection of Fig. 7.9 shows a cross-peak between the signal at 1.23 ppm (coincident methyl groups, **G**) and the multiplet signal at 2.84 ppm (group **E**), confirming that they are coupled to each other (implied by the couplings in the ^1H spectrum) and that together **E** and **G** are an isopropyl group. Additionally, group **F** (a methyl singlet at 2.23 ppm) shows a coupling to proton **A**, indicating that the methyl group is *ortho* to this proton (Fig. 7.9).

Inspection of an expansion of the aromatic region (Fig. 7.10) provides further support for the coupling pattern already suggested by the ^1H spectrum. H_A has an *ortho* coupling to H_B and, in addition to coupling to H_A, H_B has a *meta* coupling to H_C and appears as a double doublet (four lines). This coupling pattern is indicative of a 1,2,4-protonated aromatic ring and confirms the data from the ^1H spectrum.

The related technique of **Nuclear Overhauser Effect SpectroscopY** (NOESY) is also useful as it shows through space correlations and through bond coupling between protons. Once the through bond correlations are determined by a COSY spectrum, the through space correlations can be seen. This allows the measurement of how close one proton is to another, which can be very useful in assigning the stereochemistry of a natural product.

Heteronuclear correlation spectroscopy

COSY spectra are referred to as homonuclear spectra as they are acquired by detecting only one type of nucleus (^1H), but it also possible to detect the interactions between two different nuclei such as ^1H and ^{13}C. This is known as **heteronuclear correlation spectroscopy**, of which two types will be discussed here: **Heteronuclear Single Quantum Coherence** (HSQC) and **Heteronuclear MultiBond Coherence** (HMBC).

HSQC shows which protons are attached to which carbons. Figure 7.11 shows an HSQC spectrum for compound X from which clear correlations can be seen for protons **A–C** and **E–G** with the carbons to which they are attached. Proton **D** is a proton attached to oxygen (an hydroxyl group), so there

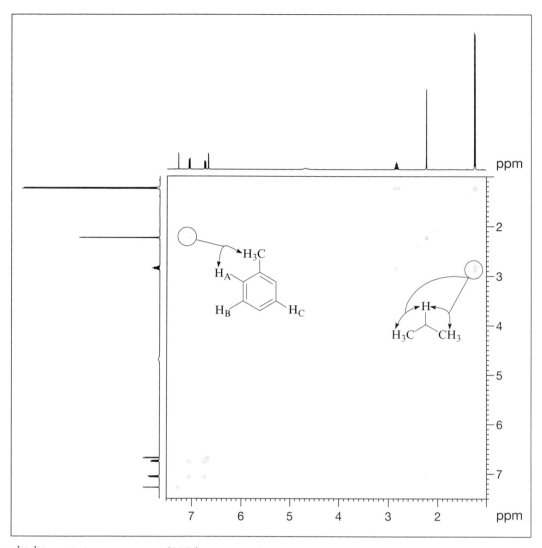

Fig. 7.9 ^{1}H-^{1}H correlation spectroscopy (COSY) spectrum of compound X.

is no carbon to correlate to (and therefore no signal). The aromatic protons all correlate to carbons at higher ppm; the aliphatic protons correlate to lower ppm carbons.

HMBC shows correlations between protons and the carbon atoms that are two and three bonds distant; these couplings are referred to as ^2J and ^3J, respectively. The experiment is set to show correlations that occur where the coupling constant between protons and carbons is of the order of 7 Hz. Two bond correlations are not always present in the spectrum as the coupling constant for ^2J correlations may be less or greater than 7 Hz. Figure 7.12 shows the HMBC spectrum for compound X.

HMBC spectra are highly informative and allow partial structure fragments to be constructed which can enable the full structure elucidation of natural products. The correlations for each proton group of compound X are given in Fig. 7.13.

It is already known from the HSQC spectrum which protons are attached to which carbons and the HMBC spectrum allows the final structure of compound X to be pieced together. For peak **A** (1 H aromatic doublet proton at 7.05 ppm) there are three correlations, one to the carbon associated with peak **F** and to two quaternary carbons.

Peak **B** (1 H aromatic double doublet proton at 6.74 ppm) correlates to the carbon to which peak **E**

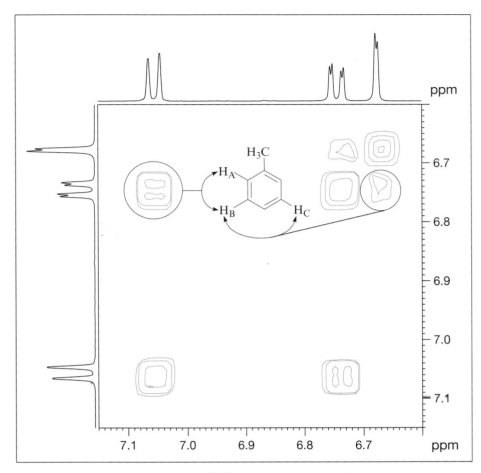

Fig. 7.10 An expansion of the aromatic region of the COSY spectrum of compound X.

is attached; this fixes the isopropyl group next to peak **B** on the aromatic ring (peak **E** is part of the isopropyl system with peak **G**). Further correlations for peak **B** include couplings to carbons that are directly attached to peak **C** and to a quaternary carbon.

Peak **C** (1 H aromatic doublet proton at 6.68 ppm) also couples to the carbon bearing the proton associated with peak **E**; this confirms the position of the isopropyl side-chain between protons **B** and **C**. Proton **C** also couples to the same quaternary carbon as **B** and to the carbon attached to proton **B**. There is also a small coupling to the most downfield carbon at 153.6 ppm.

Peak **D** (hydroxyl group, 4.68 ppm) is broad, and long-range correlations to carbons are absent. Peak **E** (1 H multiplet proton at 2.84 ppm) shows correlations to the carbons attached to peak **G** (these are the

coincident methyl groups), to both carbons attached to peaks **B** and **C** and to a quaternary carbon, which is the carbon to which the isopropyl group is directly attached.

For peak **F** (3 H singlet protons at 2.23 ppm) there are two correlations that appear equidistant at 15.3 ppm in the carbon domain and are an artifact of the HMBC spectrum (they are in fact the unsuppressed direct correlation between the protons of peak **F** and the carbon to which they are directly attached; compare with the HSQC spectrum in Fig. 7.11). There are three couplings for peak **F**: to the carbon attached to proton A, and to two quaternary carbons, one of which is the most downfield carbon (153.6 ppm).

Finally, peak **G** (6 H doublet at 1.23 ppm) shows a correlation to the neighbouring methyl carbon of the isopropyl group (and an unsuppressed one-

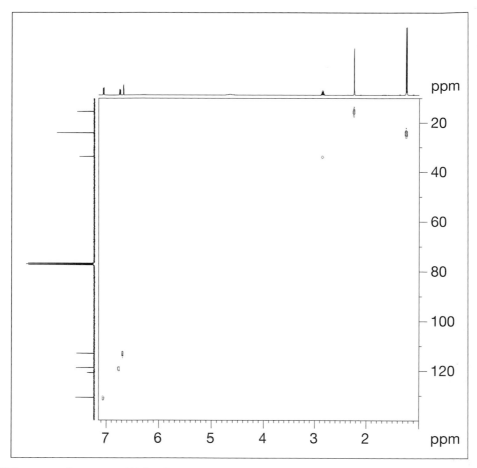

Fig. 7.11 HSQC spectrum for compound X showing correlations between protons and the carbon atoms to which they are directly attached.

bond signal equidistant about the peak **G** signal), a correlation to the carbon directly attached to peak **E** and to an aromatic quaternary carbon.

Figure 7.13 shows all of the correlations for each peak. The position of the hydroxyl group has yet to be assigned, but, as there is only one position available on the aromatic ring, the hydroxyl must be placed *ortho* to the methyl group. This is supported by the fact that the carbon to which this hydroxyl group is attached is the most downfield aromatic quaternary carbon (153.6 ppm), and heteroatoms such as oxygen are known to deshield carbon nuclei (compare the ppm value of this quaternary carbon with other quaternary aromatic carbons in compound X).

A database search indicates that compound X is **carvacrol** (Fig. 7.13), which is a common component of volatile oils, especially those from plants belonging to the mint family (Lamiaceae) of which *Thymus vulgaris* is a member.

X–RAY STRUCTURAL ANALYSIS

HMBC spectra are a very powerful way of determining the fragments and full structure of natural products and, although carvacrol is a simple example, the technique can be extended to highly complex natural products such as cardiac glycosides and polyketides. Together with simple spectroscopic techniques such as UV-visible and IR spectroscopy, NMR and MS are now the most widely used methods to determine structure.

Possibly the most comprehensive way to determine the three-dimensional structure of a

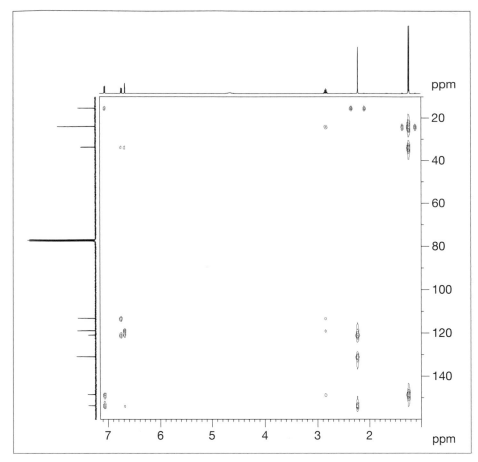

Fig. 7.12 HMBC spectrum for compound X showing correlations between protons that are two and three bonds distant from carbon atoms.

molecule is to use X-ray structural analysis. This technique requires the compound to be in the form of a crystal of suitable quality, which is then placed in the path of an X-ray source. The atoms of the crystal diffract the X-rays in a pattern that is characteristic of the arrangement and type of atoms present. The pattern can then be interpreted by computer programs to give a three-dimensional structure of the compound. Unfortunately, natural products do not always readily form crystalline substances (for example carvacrol is an oil); moreover, the amounts of material produced by some organisms are small and can make the production of crystals challenging. However, X-ray structural analysis can provide information on the stereochemistry of a molecule and, if crystals are readily available, the structure can be solved in a matter of hours.

THE INDUSTRIAL APPROACH TO NATURAL PRODUCT DRUG LEAD DISCOVERY

Industry is currently putting much emphasis on discovering drugs from synthetic rather than natural sources, which, given the rich history that natural products have in the development of new drugs is foolish. Nevertheless, the companies involved in natural product drug discovery use a highly organized approach to reduce the time taken to find a biologically active compound and put it into drug development.

CHOICE OF BIOLOGICAL TARGET

The first decision a company will make is to choose the target – i.e. for what disease state is a drug being sought. Clearly, this decision is market-driven, with

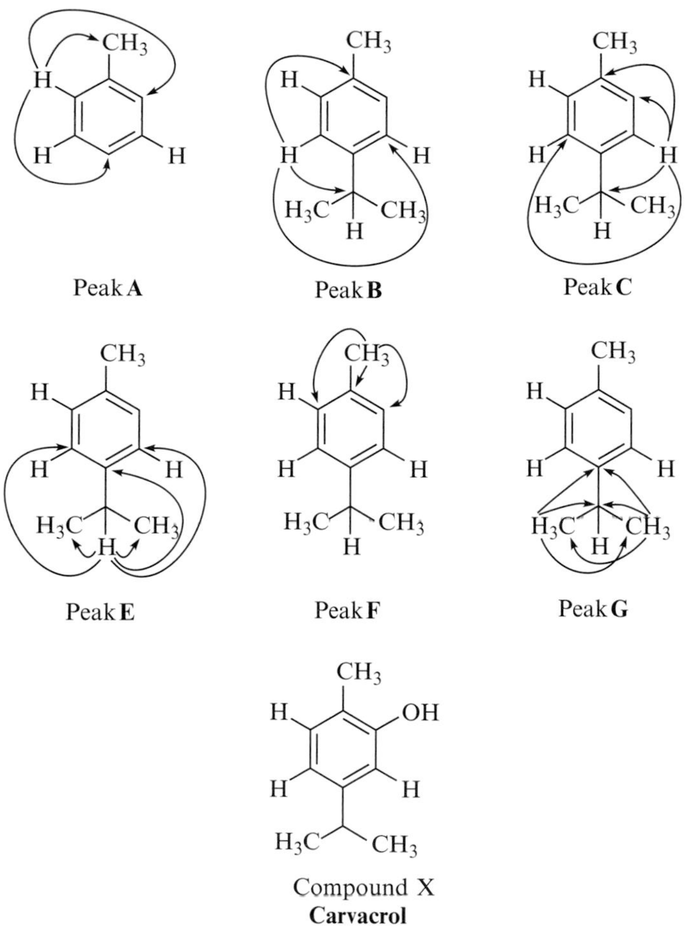

Peak A   Peak B   Peak C

Peak E   Peak F   Peak G

Compound X
Carvacrol

Fig. 7.13

many large companies preferring to look for anticancer or antiarthritis drugs, which have enormous potential markets, rather than antimalarials or antitubercular drugs, for which there is an enormous need, but among populations that are less able to pay for these drugs. Some companies have an historical association with a particular medicinal area. It is also true that the decision to work on a particular assay for a disease state is fashion-driven. For example, several companies may be working on the same target that has recently been described in the literature as being particularly important in the development of a disease state.

ASSAY SELECTION AND DEVELOPMENT

The selection of an assay is the next step. Clearly, the assay should show a good correlation with, and reflect, the particular disease state. For example, to select a target such as the inhibition of a certain enzyme is of limited use, if it later transpires that the enzyme is not key to the proliferation of the disease. The decision to look at just a cellular or a molecular assay is important; ideally, both cellular and molecular mechanisms should be investigated using several assays. The relevance to disease state, the ease and speed of performing the assay, a good response, sensitivity and insensitivity to common natural products, and the ability to perform the assay in a high-throughput screening (HTS) format are all issues that will impact on the selection of a biological assay. Development of this assay (creation, evaluation and validation for HTS) may take many months and in some cases years. As this process can be very expensive, the need for speed of assay development is vital.

can provide more information such as retention times of peaks, their UV spectra (with photodiode array) and molecular weight (and fragment) information, which is acquired as peaks elute from the UV detector into the mass spectrometer. All of these data can be built into a spectral library to allow searching of peaks with characteristic retention times, UV and mass spectra with those already acquired. This process is very powerful and enables recognition of known peaks to be made rapidly, thereby reducing costs in the discovery process.

For compounds that are lipophilic and volatile, a combination of **gas chromatography and mass spectrometry (GC-MS)** can be used to separate components to give retention times and eluting peaks which can be fed into a mass spectrometer to acquire characteristic molecular weight and fragmentation information. This technique can also be applied to polar water-soluble components such as the calystegines and other polyhydroxylated alkaloids if they are first derivatized with a suitable agent (e.g. trimethylsilyl chloride) to increase their volatility. Other more exotic dereplication processes for polar compounds include **capillary electrophoresis–mass spectrometry (CE-MS)**, which can be used for compounds that are positively or negatively charged. In capillary electrophoresis, extracts are separated in a capillary filled with buffer, which has a potential difference (voltage) applied to it. Compounds of varying charge can be separated by this technique and, when coupled to a UV detector and mass spectrometer, the technique has great utility.

NATURAL PRODUCT LIBRARIES

Traditionally, drug-lead discovery has used HTS of extracts in microtitre plates in high number to discover active extracts. Extracts are then produced in large amounts (scale-up) and compounds are isolated using the bioassay-guided route. This process is highly productive and there are many examples of drugs that have been discovered in this way. There are, however, a number of drawbacks with this process; it is expensive, time-consuming and may not lead to a drug candidate if there are problems with acquiring large amounts of the natural product or if the active component is a well-known compound with an uninteresting broad spectrum of activities. It is also true that this approach has

come under threat from other competing methods of drug lead discovery, in particular combinatorial chemistry libraries in which high numbers of compounds are synthesized and dispensed into microtitre plates and screened for bioactivity.

Natural product chemistry has had to evolve to cope with this approach, and several companies now market **natural product libraries**. These libraries are banks of microtitre plates with pure natural products in individual wells at a known concentration and, in effect, the chemistry has already been done. Organisms are selected on the basis of unknown chemistry or chemotaxonomic information, extracted with solvents, and teams of chemists isolate hundreds of compounds from the extracts. This process can be highly automated, with flash chromatography and preparative HPLC being run in parallel to separate extracts into fractions and fractions into pure compounds. There are varying levels of structure elucidation information available on pure compounds (i.e. full NMR, MS, IR, UV); this is determined by the customer, who will be the company who buys (or leases) the library from the library producer.

There are a number of benefits to this procedure over conventional HTS and synthetic libraries:

- The isolation chemistry in HTS has always been the slow bottleneck. The process is faster in the library generation which enables decisions about active natural products to be made rapidly.
- All compounds have a **defined concentration** in the microtitre plate and so the potency of the compound in the assay is known immediately; this is not true with extract screening. Most active extracts may contain one major component with poor activity or, even worse, the least-active extract may have a low concentration of a very potent compound which may be deprioritized.
- Screening a pure compound will give a better assay response, as single components have a cleaner interaction with the biological target and there are no interfering compounds present in the extract (e.g. tannins, which may mask the presence or absence of an active component).
- The dereplication process is more successful with pure compounds and a large amount of data can be acquired.
- Identification of the active compound may be total before screening and this can give useful information on any structure–activity relationships with other screened compounds.

- The whole process is now much quicker; the limiting step is now assay technology, which is itself very rapid.
- Large amounts of pure compounds can be isolated (5–10 mg), so retesting and further assays can be performed quickly without delay in further isolation.
- Most importantly, the **cost** is less than HTS as the time for discovery of a natural lead is reduced.

Several companies have adopted this approach, notably Hypha Discovery Ltd (http://www.hypha discovery.co.uk) who market a fungal natural product library produced using a novel fermentation technique. The company sells (or licences) the library for drug and agrochemical discovery to larger companies. For compounds that are of further interest to the customer, Hypha Discovery can then scale-up the extraction and purification of the compound by large-scale fermentation at their facilities.

ALTERNATIVE APPROACHES IN NATURAL PRODUCT DRUG LEAD DISCOVERY

Many fungi and bacteria do not produce natural products when fermented and it is possible that they require an external stimulus from another organism to do so (e.g. other microbes or molecules secreted into their environment by another organism). This presence of unproductive organisms results in a loss of access to chemical diversity. Additionally, only 5% of microbes may be culturable and fermentable and there is, therefore, great potential to discover new therapeutic agents if ways are discovered to tap into the genetic, and, therefore, chemical, capability of these organisms.

Some companies utilize the procedure of combinatorial biosynthesis, in which DNA is taken from uncultivable organisms or from soil to build a library of characterized DNA fragments. It is then possible to insert this DNA into a host such as *Escherichia coli* or a yeast, which are readily fermentable organisms. The importance of this technique is based on the assumption that the host may use this DNA in the biosynthesis of new natural products. The host is then fermented and screened for bioactivity; this process may also be used to generate compounds for natural product library production. This is an innovative approach and may lead to new

classes of natural products and allow full exploitation of microbial chemistry. Unfortunately, it may need much research to exploit this opportunity, especially given that many kilobases of DNA are required to produce even simple natural products. Additionally, the host may not utilize the foreign DNA, or it is possible that the DNA inserted may not code for proteins that make natural products.

WHY NATURAL PRODUCTS AS DRUGS?

In the previous sections we have briefly looked at some of the classes of compounds produced by nature and how they can be isolated and their structures elucidated; but why are natural products such an important source of drugs? There are many examples of drugs from nature and this is possibly a result of biological and chemical diversity.

In screening for new bioactive compounds, it is important to access as wide a range of diverse biological specimens as possible because it is thought that this high range of biological diversity mirrors or gives rise to a high degree of chemical diversity (i.e. a wide array of structurally unrelated molecules). Ideally, a drug discovery programme should have access to as many different species as possible from groups such as plants, fungi, filamentous bacteria, corals, sea animals and amphibia. The tropics hold a vast repository of numbers of such species, and there is, therefore, enormous potential to discover new bioactive entities in this region of the world. Using Costa Rica as an example, the Instituto Nacional de Biodiversidad (INBio) has been conducting a national inventory of plants, insects, microbes and animals, and has so far assessed almost 500,000 species. This incredible genetic resource could potentially generate millions of natural products to be assessed for biological activity. Individual species are also adept at producing not only different classes of natural product (e.g. flavonoids and monoterpenes simultaneously), but also analogues of the same natural product class (Fig. 7.14).

It is this richness in chemistry, coupled with the structural complexity of certain types of natural product (e.g. paclitaxel), that makes natural products such a valuable commodity for the discovery of new drugs. It has been estimated that 25% of all prescription medicines owe their origin to a natural source and that, in the field of anticancer drugs, almost 60% of agents are either natural products

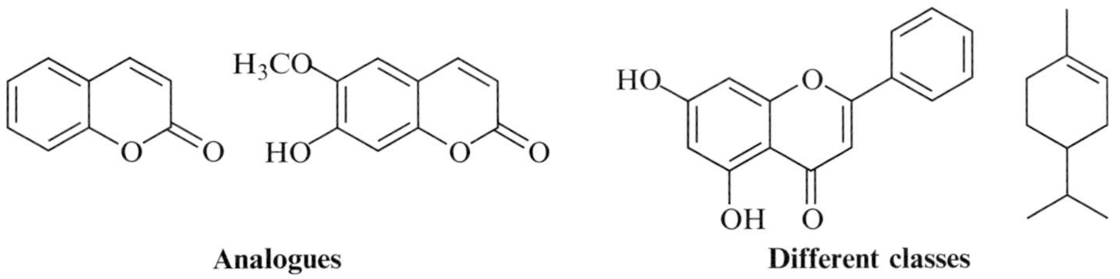

Analogues   **Different classes**

Fig. 7.14

or are derived from a natural product source. Additionally, many natural products are produced by the organism as a chemical defence (e.g. as an antimicrobial or as an antifeedant substance) against another organism; thus, in many cases, *there is already an inherent biological activity associated with natural products.*

Large pharmaceutical companies have been scaling down their interest in natural products, preferring to access their chemical diversity through synthetically produced libraries of compounds. Unfortunately, many of these libraries lack the true chemical diversity, chirality, structural complexity and inherent biological activity of natural products. It is therefore a matter of time before tried and tested natural product sources once again become widely used in drug discovery.

The **Convention on Biological Diversity** is a treaty between 182 countries to recognize the authority that countries/states have over their genetic resources (see also Chapter 5, p54-55). The treaty recognizes that access to biodiversity, be it plant, microbial or animal, is governed by the sovereign authority of that particular state. This means that it is not possible to acquire biological specimens from an area without 'prior informed consent' on 'mutually agreed terms' and that, should any commercial benefit arise from collection of biota (e.g. in the discovery of a new drug), then 'equitable sharing of benefits' should occur. This is an exceptionally important concept for profit sharing and one that can be highlighted by the example of **prostratin** (Fig. 7.15) from *Homolanthus nutans* (Euphorbiaceae).

Paul Cox, an ethnobotanist working in Samoa, became intrigued by the local use of the inner bark of *Homolanthus nutans* to treat yellow fever, which is a clinical manifestation of the viral disease hepatitis. He collected samples of these species and sent them for testing at the National Cancer Institute (NCI) for assessment of antiviral activity in anti-AIDS

Prostratin

Fig. 7.15

assays. The active component, **prostratin**, was isolated and the structure determined as a diterpene related to the phorbol ester group of natural products. Interest waned in this compound as the phorbol esters are known to be strongly tumour-promoting. However, Paul Cox was not deterred by this because of the local use of the plant and he urged the NCI to assess prostratin for tumour promotion. Interestingly, prostratin does not promote tumour growth. It appears to prolong the life of HIV-infected cells and stops infection of healthy cells by HIV. Whilst prostratin is still in development, the authorities of the village from which the discovery originated have negotiated an agreement signed by the prime minister of Samoa. The AIDS research Alliance who are developing prostratin will ensure that 20% of commercial profits that come from prostratin will go back to Samoa. In this settlement, revenues will go back to the village and to the families of the traditional healers who gave the original information on the use of *H. nutans*. This example highlights the fact that it is not only important that financial recompense is made to the originators of ethnobotanical research, but also that this traditional knowledge has value which must be preserved.

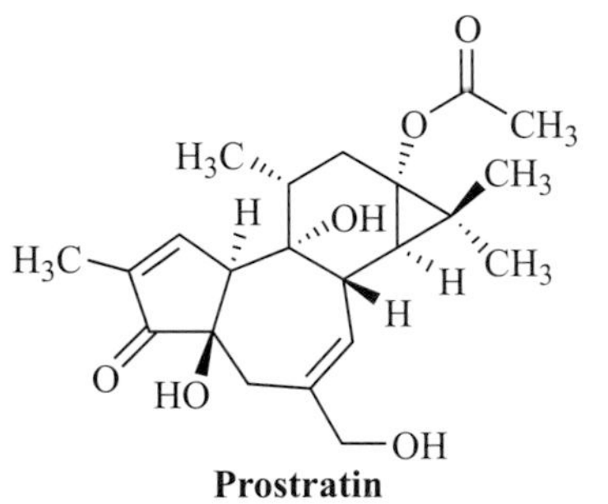

Further reading

Balick, M.J., Cox, P.A., 1996. Plants, people and culture: the science of ethnobotany. Scientific American Library, New York.

Crews, P., Rodriguez, J., Jaspars, M., 2009. Organic structure analysis, second ed. Oxford University Press, Oxford.

Hostettmann, K., Marston, A., Hostettmann, M., 2010. Preparative chromatography techniques: applications in natural product isolation, second revised ed. Springer-Verlag, Berlin.

Sarker, S.D., Latif, Z., Gray, A.I., 2010. Natural products isolation.

Methods in biotechnology, second ed. Humana Press, Totowa.

Williams, D.H., Fleming, I., 2007. Spectroscopic methods in organic chemistry, sixth ed. McGraw-Hill, London.

Chapter **8**

Anticancer natural products

Plants have been the basis of sophisticated medical systems for thousands of years, particularly in China and India, and they have an essential role in health care. The World Health Organization has estimated that 80% of the Earth's inhabitants rely on traditional medicines for primary health care, and plant products are highly important in the remaining 20% of the population (Farnsworth et al 1985). During the period 1959–1980 approximately 25% of US prescription medicines contained plant extracts, plant constituents or agents that were derived from natural sources. Over 119 chemicals from 90 plants species are important drugs in many countries and three-quarters of these were derived from studying the chemistry of traditional medicines (Farnsworth et al 1985).

Natural products have made an enormous impact on the discovery of compounds that kill cancer cells; in fact, possibly 60% of all cancer drugs that are used clinically are either natural products or owe their origin to a natural source. The most comprehensive study conducted on cytotoxic agents from nature has been carried out by the **National Cancer Institute (NCI)**, a US government agency that has invested in the identification of a number of anticancer drugs.

THE NATIONAL CANCER INSTITUTE

The **National Cancer Institute (NCI)** was established in the USA in 1937 'to provide for, foster and aid in coordinating research related to cancer'. This organization has been involved in many of the great discoveries in fundamental research of cancer and particularly in the characterization of cytotoxic natural products. During the 1950s it was realized that there was a need for screening of natural extracts in a discovery programme and the **Cancer Chemotherapy National Service Center** was set up (Cragg et al 1993). The objectives of this organization were to procure compounds and to screen and evaluate them in a preclinical and, finally, full clinical setting. This service developed into the modern organization known as the **Developmental Therapeutics Program (DTP)**.

Apart from endeavours to find anticancer agents from natural and synthetic sources, the DTP has also initiated a programme to discover and preclinically develop anti-AIDS agents. Being a US government-funded agency, the NCI accepts and screens compounds from many sources, including academics in universities and pharmaceutical companies. This philanthropic activity increases the chances of finding lead compounds with activity against the many types of cancer and against HIV. Much of the early NCI screening focused on natural products produced by fermentation of microbes, such as filamentous bacteria, and, prior to 1960, only a small numbers of plants (1500) were investigated.

Early successes to exploit plants as a source of anticancer agents included the characterization of podophyllotoxin-type lignans from *Podophyllum peltatum*, and their semi-synthetic derivatives, and vincristine and vinblastine from *Catharanthus roseus* (Fig. 8.1). These discoveries drove further interest in plants at the NCI, and collections of plant material were expanded to include 60 countries. This collection strategy was quite extensive and, between 1960

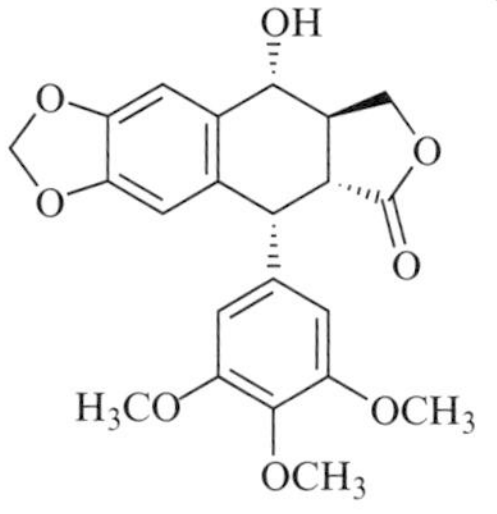

Podophyllotoxin

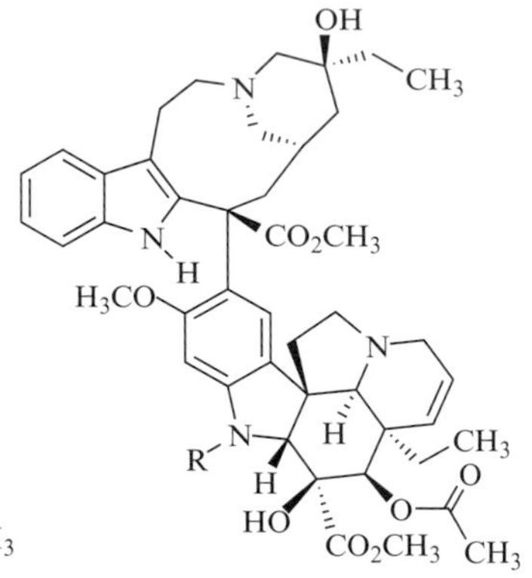

Vincristine, R = CHO
Vinblastine, R = CH₃

Fig. 8.1

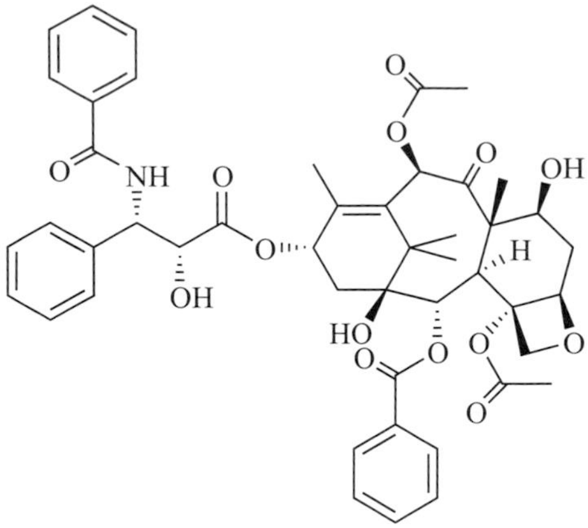

Paclitaxel (Taxol)

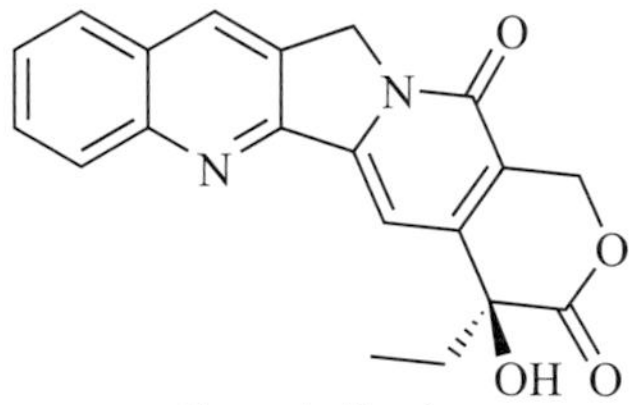

Camptothecin

Fig. 8.2

and 1982, 114,000 extracts from 35,000 plants species were screened against a number of tumour types (Cragg et al 1993).

Methods to assess antitumour activity are being continually improved and, after 1975, the P388 mouse leukaemia cell line was used to assay for the presence of compounds that are cytotoxic. Following bioassay-guided isolation of the active agents, a secondary screen known as the human xenograft mouse model was used to assess agents with significant activity. In this model, human tumour cells are introduced beneath the skin of mice lacking an immune response. The cells rapidly grow to form a tumour; compounds may then be administered to the mouse and any effects on the reduction in tumour size measured. This mouse model is still used today and cells from different tumour types may be introduced. Any compounds with broad-spectrum activity were prioritized for preclinical development and eventually clinical trials.

Bioassay-guided fractionation of active extracts led to the characterization of a large number of agents from many different natural product classes. Arguably the most significant discovery from the NCI screening programme was named **taxol**, from *Taxus brevifolia* (Taxaceae) (Fig. 8.2). The compound had been previously isolated in 1971 by Wall and co-workers and its activity against a melanoma cell line and in the human xenograft model led to its selection for preclinical development in 1977. Initially, there were problems in acquiring large amounts of the compound, but solutions to these problems and the report of its unique mode of action by promotion of tubulin polymerization and stabilization of microtubules against depolymerization increased interest. Taxol (now known as paclitaxel; see below) has excellent activity against ovarian and breast cancers and was approved in the USA by the FDA in 1993.

Another agent of note, again from the group of Wall, is **camptothecin** from the Chinese ornamental tree, *Camptotheca acuminata* (Nyssaceae) (Fig. 8.2). Chinese clinical trials were conducted on this agent, which showed promise against a number of different cancer types, including gastric, liver, head, neck and bladder cancers. However, US clinical trials of the sodium salt were terminated due to a limited number of responses. There has been much work on this class of natural product, with two companies (SmithKline Beecham and Daiichi) having developed and released two products: **topotecan** and **irinotecan**.

Between 1985 and 1990 the NCI developed a new *in vitro* screen that uses 60 human cell lines from nine cancer types representing leukaemia, lung, colon, central nervous system (CNS), melanoma, ovarian, renal, prostate and breast cancers. Synthetic or natural products are made up at concentrations ranging from 10^{-4} M to 10^{-8} M and then tested against the 60 different tumour cell lines. The data that are acquired from this test system are evaluated to decide if further investigation is warranted (Alley et al 1988, Grever et al 1992).

The results from the screening are reported in a graph format which calculates the potency of the compound against all 60 cell lines in terms of three indicators:

- GI_{50}: the concentration at which growth is inhibited by 50%
- TGI: the concentration at which cell growth is totally inhibited
- LC_{50}: the concentration at which 50% of the cells are killed.

The importance of these three factors is that a fingerprint of a compound's anticancer activity is generated which can be correlated, using a mathematical model, with test results for known anticancer drugs (Paull et al 1989). This can even give an idea of whether a compound works by a similar mechanism of action as a known anticancer agent such as vincristine. Promising compounds with interesting selective profiles of activity (e.g. activity against one particular cell line) are then retested to confirm the reproducibility of these results. In 1995 a three cell line prescreen was introduced to increase the throughput of compounds whilst not reducing the number of compounds with activity in the 60 cell line assay. These cell lines were from lung, CNS and breast tumour types.

A new acquisition programme was initiated in 1986 with contracts for the cultivation and extraction of fungi and bacteria and the collection of marine organisms and terrestrial plants (Cragg et al 1997). Marine organisms were collected from many diverse locations, including the Caribbean, Australasia, Central and South Pacific, Indian Ocean and Polynesia. Plant material was collected in over 25 countries in the tropical and subtropical regions by specialist organizations with botanical expertise such as the Missouri Botanical Garden, the University of Chicago and the New York Botanical Garden.

Collaborations with the NCI rely on working closely with qualified organizations (e.g. universities, research institutes, botanical gardens) in the source country that has access to the biological diversity. Botanists and biologists from source countries collaborate in collections, which are invaluable to the NCI, and in many cases training is provided and workshops are organized for local personnel so that there is a transfer of expertise in certain areas. The source countries send biomass back to the National Products Repository in Frederick, Maryland. In the past, invitations have been made to local scientists of source countries to visit the NCI for collaborative research in natural products (Cragg et al 1997). This fosters openness and true collaboration between the NCI and source country.

For biomass collection, dried plant material (usually in the dry weight range of 0.3–1.0 kg) and frozen marine organism samples (1 kg) are shipped to Frederick and stored at –20°C, lessening the possibility of sample degradation. Biomass is extracted with methanol/dichloromethane (1:1) and then water to give organic and aqueous extracts which are given NCI numbers and stored at –20°C until required for screening (Cragg et al 1997). The extracts are then tested in the *in vitro* human cancer cell line screen and active extracts undergo bioassay-guided fractionation to isolate pure natural products. Structure elucidation is carried out using NMR and mass spectrometry. Compounds demonstrating significant antitumour activity are selected for secondary testing in *in vivo* systems and those with good activity advance to preclinical and, finally, clinical development. During this process there is the opportunity to license compounds out to companies for development; this is the preferred route due to the large costs of conducting the development process.

Importantly, agreements ensure that any royalties that may arise are shared with the country of origin and, as previously mentioned with the Convention on Biodiversity, it is a legal requirement that the collection of organisms is only possible with the 'prior informed consent' of the authorities of the source country (see Chapter 5, p. 55).

A full review of antitumour agents is beyond the scope of this text but we will briefly cover the three main sources of anticancer agents (marine sources, plants and microbes), giving selected examples of agents and their sources. The reader is urged to consult the excellent reviews by Cragg and co-workers on this subject (Cragg & Newman 1999, 2000, Cragg et al 1993, 1997).

MARINE ANTICANCER NATURAL PRODUCTS

Marine organisms have no history of medicinal use but, because the oceans cover 70% of the Earth's surface, there is a vast reserve for the discovery of new natural product drugs. This huge environment is home to a fantastic range of diverse organisms and, of the 28 major animal classes, 26 exist in aquatic areas and eight are exclusively aquatic (Cragg et al 1997). Collection of biomass is usually carried out by diving and in some cases submersibles can give access to organisms that occur in deeper sites, although this is a highly expensive procedure.

The discipline of marine natural product chemistry is comparatively new compared to phytochemistry, with relatively small numbers of natural products having been reported. At present there is one marine natural product which is used as an anticancer drug clinically (Ecteinascidin 743, Yondelis), and a number are in clinical trials and their potent activities highlight the future importance of this source. A compound in development worth noting is **bryostatin-1**, which is a novel macrocyclic lactone derived from the marine bryozoan, *Bugula neritina*. This compound modulates protein kinase C activity and phase I studies have demonstrated activity against several tumour types. Bryostatin-1 has subsequently been investigated extensively in phase II clinical trials as a single agent and data suggest that it may have potential in combination with other cytotoxic agents. **Didemnin B** (*Trididemnum solidum*) was the first marine natural product to enter clinical trials and has recently been shown to induce apoptosis (programmed cell death) in a wide range of cell lines. **Aplidine** (Fig. 8.3) or **dehydrodidemnin B**, which is structurally related to didemnin B, is a marine **depsipeptide** obtained from the **tunicate** *Aplidium albicans*, originally found in the Mediterranean. Tunicates, which are also known as **sea squirts**, are organisms that attach themselves to submerged objects and feed by removing microscopic organisms from the water that is drawn

through them. Depsipeptides are cyclic peptides that also possess a cyclic ester functional group. Aplidine blocks the cell division cycle in human tumour cell lines and prevents the onset of DNA synthesis. Like didemnin B, it has also been shown to be an inducer of apoptosis in many cell systems. Additionally, using the xenograft assay, grafted into athymic mice, aplidine demonstrated considerable activity against colon, bladder, lung, prostate and stomach tumours, and against melanoma and lymphoma tumours. This agent is currently in clinical trials. Aplidine demonstrates some of the very best features of a natural product, being highly chiral and exhibiting great functionality. Both of these features contribute to the high cytotoxicity of this molecule, which in nature is probably produced by *Aplidium* species as a chemical defence mechanism.

One of the most promising groups of agents comes from the sea hare (*Dolabella auricularia*), an herbivorous mollusc from the Indian Ocean which produces cytotoxic linear peptides. An interesting member of this class is **dolastatin-10** (Fig. 8.4), an inhibitor of microtubule assembly, currently in clinical trials.

It is possible to synthesize these compounds; their peptide chemistry is highly amenable to the production of many analogues of the dolastatin class of which a number have been synthesized to date.

Perhaps the most interesting antitumour marine compounds and the first anti-cancer drug to come from this marvelous source is **ecteinascidin-743,** now marketed as Yondelis (Trabectidin) (Fig. 8.5), from *Ecteinascidia turbinata*, which is a tunicate found in the Caribbean and Mediterranean. Ecteinascidin-743 has very potent activity against a broad spectrum of tumour types in animal models; it binds to the minor groove of the DNA double helix and inhibits cell proliferation, leading to apoptosis

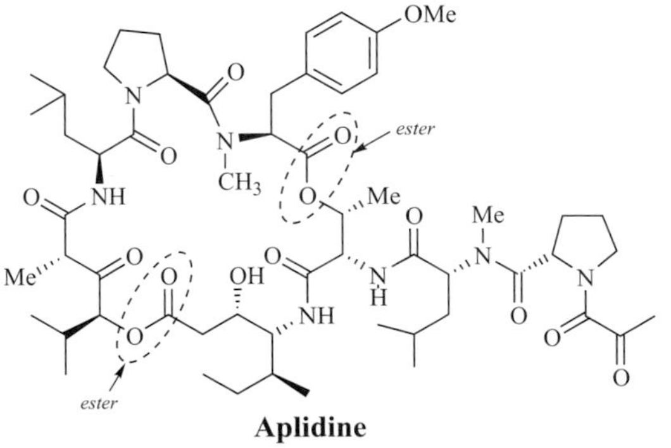

Aplidine

Fig. 8.3

Dolastatin-10

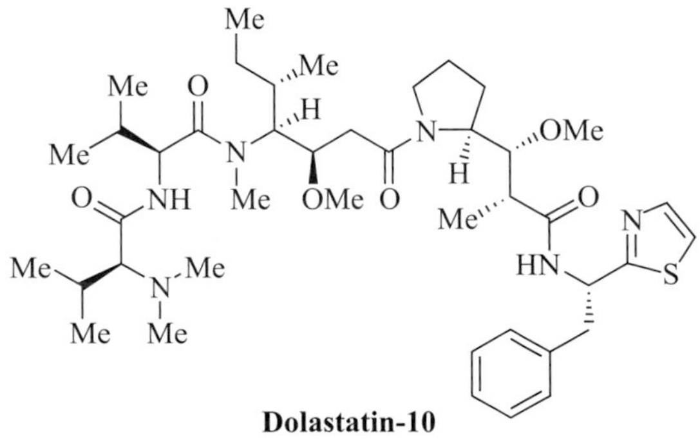

Fig. 8.4

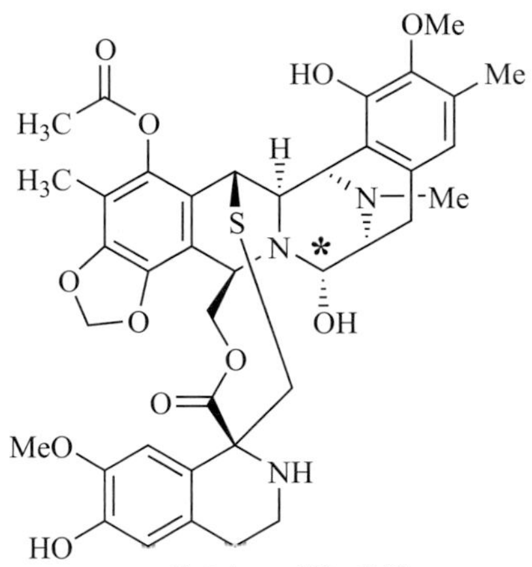

Ecteinascidin-743

Fig. 8.5

40 years some major antitumour agents derived from this source have been released onto the market: the **vinca alkaloids** (**vinblastine, vincristine** and **vinorelbine**), agents based on the **podophyllotoxin class** (**etoposide** and **teniposide**), the **taxanes** (**paclitaxel** and **taxotere**) and the **camptothecin**-derived cytotoxics (**topotecan** and **irinotecan**). Plants are, therefore, a superb source of cytotoxic agents and, given the enormous number still to be investigated, there is great potential to discover new anticancer drugs. It is also true that advances in genome biology and target selection will ensure that plants will continue to provide new anticancer leads. There is even a case to reinvestigate plant extracts which have already been evaluated against old assays to assess them in new assays based on targets recently described by elucidation of the genome.

CAMPTOTHECA ACUMINATA (NYSSACEAE)

In 1957, a small number of ethanolic plant extracts (1000) were screened at the Cancer Chemotherapy National Center (USA) and extracts of *Camptotheca acuminata* were shown to possess high activity. The late Dr Monroe Wall, who will be remembered as a leading expert in plant antitumour agents and a wonderful enthusiast for natural product research, established a natural product research group at Research Triangle Institute which conducted some research that was funded by the NCI. Dr Wall, who was later joined by Dr Mansukh Wani, became interested in the constituents of *Camptotheca*, particularly due to the high activity of these extracts. Wood and bark (20 kg) were collected for extraction and the extracts were shown to be active against a mouse leukaemia life prolongation assay in which it was unusual to find activity (Wall & Wani 1995). During the 1960s, the bioassay-guided isolation process was slow and it could take as long as 3 months to get bioassay results from the mouse life-prolongation assay back to the chemists working on the extracts (Wall & Wani 1995).

When compared with cellular assays today, in which it may only take a few days to decide if extracts and fractions are active, it is worth noting how diligent, persistent and thorough these researchers were. Extraction of the plant material was carried out first using a non-polar solvent (hot heptane) to remove very non-polar natural products. The plant material was then extracted with ethanol and this extract was treated with chloroform

of cancer cells. This binding to the minor groove of DNA allows an alkylation reaction to occur between a guanine residue of the DNA and an electron-deficient carbon on the molecule (* in Fig 8.5).

It was shown that ecteinascidin-743–DNA adducts are recognized by the nucleotide excision repair system, which is inherent to each cell and is present to protect the cell from accumulation of mutations and DNA damage. When this repair system encounters the adduct, rather than repairing the cell apoptosis occurs. Of particular interest is that ecteinascidin-743 cytotoxicity only occurs during active transcription of genes; this has obvious potential in cancer cells which rely on increased transcription and translation. Ecteinascidin-743 also inhibits the induction of the gene *MDR1*, which encodes a membrane pump responsible for multidrug resistance, which can drastically affect the potency of antitumour agents. These characteristics make ecteinascidin-743 unique and this compound was approved as an anticancer drug in combination with doxorubicin, particularly for the treatment of relapsed ovarian cancer, in the European Union in 2009.

PLANT ANTITUMOUR AGENTS

Plants have been an excellent source of antitumour agents and there is much anecdotal evidence for their use against tumours in traditional systems of medicine, particularly in the Chinese, Ayurvedic, Jamu and African systems. The track record of plant anticancer agents is excellent and over the last and aqueous ethanol to give two phases, the lipophilic chloroform phase being highly active. Additional extraction of the aqueous phase with chloroform gave a further active chloroform extract. High activity was associated with all of the chloroform extracts of the ethanolic portion, indicating that the active natural product had a degree of lipophilicity. Column chromatography was initially attempted on these active extracts using alumina as the sorbent, but what was not known at the time was that the active component binds very tightly to alumina and could not be eluted from the column. Extensive partitioning of the extract was tried in separating funnels using the quaternary system (four solvents) chloroform/carbon tetrachloride/methanol/water and each of the fractions were assayed in the mouse life-prolongation assay and *in vitro* cellular cytotoxicity assay. This partitioning system gave excellent separation and active fractions were combined to yield a yellow precipitate, which was subjected to chromatography on silica to which the active agent did not irreversibly bind. Further crystallization of active fractions led to the isolation of the active agent, **camptothecin** (Fig. 8.6). The structure elucidation of this natural product was carried out by conversion to its chloroacetate, which was then further converted to the iodoacetate salt which gave crystals of sufficient quality for X-ray structural analysis.

At the time, camptothecin had a unique structure, possessing an α-hydroxylactone, and being a highly unsaturated alkaloid (nitrogen-containing) natural product of the quinoline alkaloid group. When treated with sodium hydroxide, the lactone ring opened with the formation of a sodium salt that was much more water-soluble than camptothecin. When this salt was acidified, the lactone was again regenerated and the water solubility decreased.

Camptothecin was shown to be extremely active in the life-prolongation assay of mice treated with

leukaemia cells and in solid tumour inhibition. These activities encouraged the NCI to initiate clinical trials with the water-soluble sodium salt. Trials were conducted in a small number of patients (18) and there were five partial responses against gastrointestinal tumours of short duration (Gottlieb & Luce 1972). There were, however, toxic side effects. A phase II study was conducted but unfortunately there were only two responses to the treatment (Moertel et al 1972). The sodium salt was also studied in a much larger clinical trial in China using 1000 patients with better results against head, neck, gastric, intestinal and bladder carcinomas. These results were more promising than those of the US trial possibly due to the fact that the US patients had already been treated with other cytotoxic drugs and their tumours may have become multidrug-resistant. It is also now known that the lactone (which is absent in the lactone ring-opened sodium salt) of the compound is important for activity.

Wall and Wani continued to isolate and evaluate *Camptotheca* metabolites and found that one such product in particular, **10-hydroxycamptothecin** (Fig. 8.6), was more active than camptothecin, and this may have stimulated a number of companies to prepare further water-soluble analogues of 10-hydroxycamptothecin.

Interest in this natural product and its analogues was low until 1985 when it was discovered that camptothecin works by inhibition of topoisomerase I, which is an enzyme involved in many important cellular processes by interacting with DNA. This finding fuelled further interest in this class of compound as the mechanism by which it functioned as an inhibitor of tumour growth was understood. Much work was conducted by pharmaceutical companies on this template and two products became available as a result of this research, **irinotecan** and **topotecan** (Fig. 8.7). The structural importance of the parent natural product, 10-hydroxycamptothecin, as a template can be seen in both of these products.

Irinotecan was approved in 1994 in the USA. It is less toxic than camptothecin and is used to treat metastatic colorectal cancer; it is also effective against lung cancer and leukaemias. Irinotecan has much greater water solubility than camptothecin. It is a prodrug, being metabolized *in vivo* by hydrolysis of the carbamate ester to give the phenolic topoisomerase I inhibitor, which is 1000 times more potent than the parent compound.

Topotecan (Fig. 8.7) was approved for use in the USA in 1996. It is active against ovarian cancer.

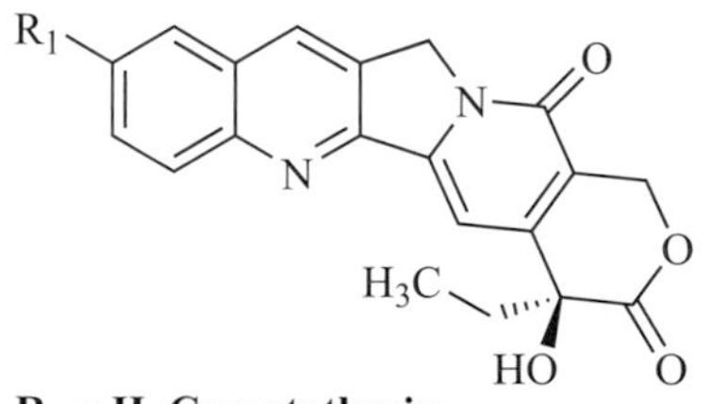

R_1 = H, Camptothecin
R_1 = OH, 10-Hydroxycamptothecin

Fig. 8.6

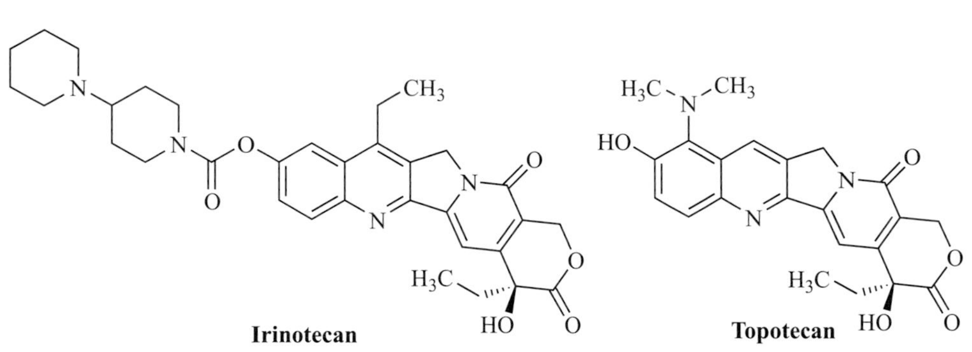

Irinotecan   **Topotecan**

Fig. 8.7

TAXUS BREVIFOLIA (TAXACEAE)

In the early 1960s a number of plants were collected from the USA and assessed for antitumour activity under an NCI-supported programme. One of these specimens was *Taxus brevifolia*. This plant, commonly known as the Pacific yew, is a member of the Taxaceae family and is related to the English yew (*Taxus baccata*), which is common in churchyards in the UK. The Pacific yew is a slow-growing tree common to the western coast of the USA. Active extracts were tested at the Research Triangle Institute in 1964 (Wall & Wani 1995).

The extraction of the plant material was conducted using a partitioning protocol similar to that employed in the isolation of camptothecin. The isolation of the active component employed a highly extensive partitioning procedure utilizing many steps between aqueous and organic solvents. The biological activity of the fractions was monitored at all stages and 0.5 g of the active compound was isolated. This was an exceptionally low yield (0.004%) from 12 kg of plant material and the name **taxol** was assigned to the active natural product. Taxol was shown to be active against solid tumours and highly active against leukaemia models in the mouse life-prolongation assay. The compound was also active against a melanoma cell line. As with camptothecin, structure elucidation was not a trivial process (it can still be difficult today!) and there were only a handful of techniques that could be used to determine the structure, including UV, IR, elemental analysis (determination of C, H and N composition) and mass spectrometry; there were not many NMR techniques available in the early 1960s, which made structure elucidation an extremely difficult task. The structure elucidation of this compound is an example of a masterful piece of natural product research and the reader is urged to consult the superb review by Wall & Wani (1995) and the book by Goodman & Walsh (2001).

^{1}H NMR spectra suggested that taxol had a number of ester groups attached to it and was possibly a diterpene natural product of the taxane group. Elemental analysis and mass spectrometry gave a molecular formula of $C_{47}H_{51}NO_{14}$ for taxol, but it was not possible to obtain crystals of the compound of sufficient quality for X-ray structural analysis. At this stage chemical degradation techniques were used to help elucidate the structure. Base-catalysed methanolysis yielded compounds that could be crystallized and submitted for X-ray structural analysis for structure elucidation. Elegant work, which included the use of further chemical degradation plus ^{1}H NMR and high-resolution mass spectrometry, was conducted to piece these fragments together to give the final structure of taxol (Fig. 8.8) (Wall & Wani 1995).

This was the first report of a taxane diterpene with cytotoxic activity. Taxol is a highly functional molecule possessing esters, epoxides, hydroxyls, amide, ketone groups and unsaturation. It has a large number of chiral centres (11) and is very difficult to synthesize; this was achieved in 1994 after 26 steps and is obviously not a feasible option for production on a large scale.

For the antitumour activity it is essential that the ester group at position C_{13} is present as the hydrolysed product is inactive. Work on taxol at RTI ended in 1971. Although Dr Wall and co-workers tried to get the NCI to assess taxol further, it was thought that the concentration in the plant was too low, the extraction and isolation were too difficult and the tree supply too limited. There were two developments which re-ignited interest in this compound, the first being its activity in a melanoma cell line and the discovery of its unique mode

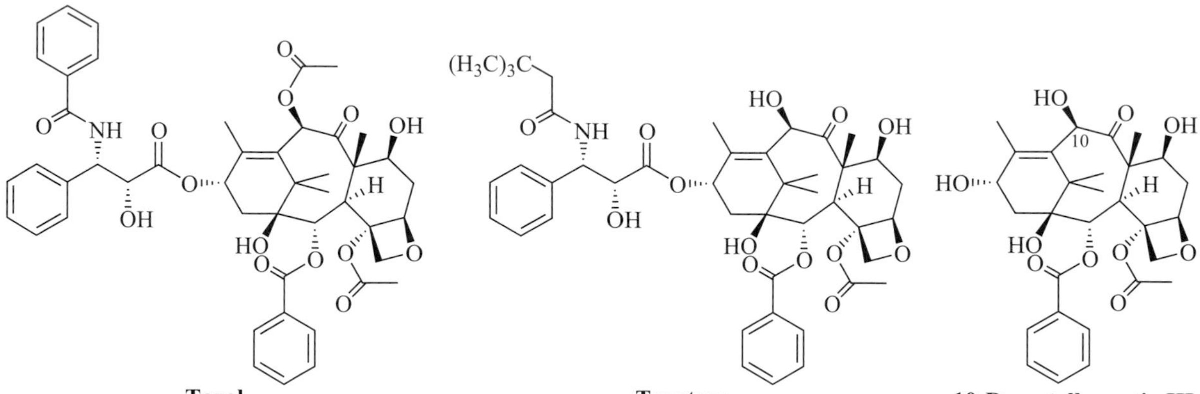

Taxol   Taxotere   10-Deacetylbaccatin III

Fig. 8.8

of action. Initial work suggested that taxol had similar activity to other agents which were 'spindle poisons' such as vincristine and colchicine. The work of Susan Horowitz's group demonstrated that, whilst taxol inhibited mitosis, it actually stabilized microtubules and inhibited their depolymerization back to tubulin, which is the exact opposite of other agents that bind to soluble tubulin and inhibit the polymerization of tubulin into microtubules.

The fact that taxol worked by a new mechanism and that it was a highly unusual and novel structure encouraged further research into this agent, resulting in clinical trials and the development of analogues such as taxotere (Fig. 8.8).

The supply issues concerning taxol were overcome with its semi-synthesis by the conversion of metabolites present in larger amounts (e.g. **10-deacetylbaccatin III**; Fig. 8.8) in the needles of the related English yew (*Taxus baccata*). As the needles are a renewable resource, there is no need to destroy trees by the removal of bark. Taxol is now commercially produced by plant cell culture by large-scale fermentation of the plant cells.

Taxol, now renamed **paclitaxel**, was approved in 1993 and marketed under the trade name **Taxol** by Bristol Myers Squibb for ovarian cancer and the secondary treatment for breast and non-small-cell lung cancers. Docetaxel is marketed as Taxotere by Rhone-Poulenc Rorer and, like Taxol, prevents the mitotic spindle from being broken down by stabilizing microtubule bundles. Docetaxel, approved for use in the USA in 1995, is slightly more water-soluble than Taxol and is also administered by the intravenous route. It is used for the treatment of breast and ovarian cancers.

BETULA ALBA (BETULACEAE)

Betulinic acid (Fig. 8.9) is a pentacyclic triterpene that occurs in several plants. It can be chemically derived from betulin, a natural product found in abundance in the outer bark of white birch trees (*Betula alba*).

There is currently interest in betulinic acid as it selectively kills human melanoma cells leaving healthy cells alive. The incidence of melanoma has been increasing at a higher rate than any other type of cancer and, therefore, the need for new anticancer agents that selectively target melanoma is great. The effectiveness of betulinic acid against melanoma cancer cells has also been evaluated in a xenograft assay with athymic (nude) mice. When mice were injected with melanoma cells, the tumour size was observed for 40 days following injections of betulinic acid. Betulinic acid effectively inhibited tumour growth in the mice, with little drug toxicity and side effects such as weight loss. This natural product has been shown to be an inducer of apoptosis (programmed cell death) in cancer cells with a high degree of specificity for melanoma cells. This unique specificity is unusual when compared to other

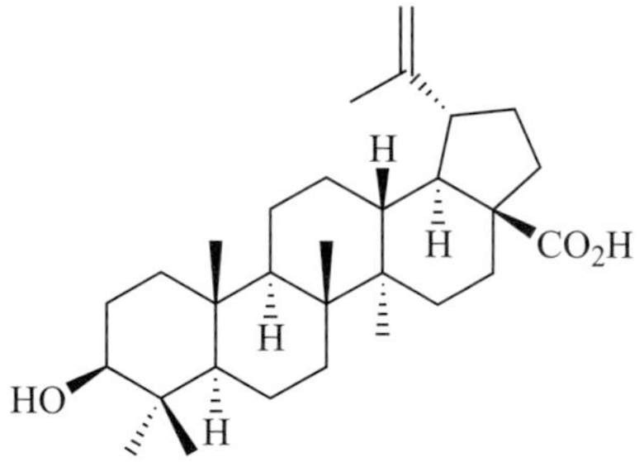

Betulinic acid

Fig. 8.9

cytotoxic agents such as camptothecin or paclitaxel, which exhibit a far broader spectrum of activity.

This natural product appears to have limited toxicity, is inexpensive and abundantly available from the bark of white birch trees in the form of betulin (the hydroxyl derivative) which can be readily converted to betulinic acid through a simple oxidation reaction. The compound is currently undergoing preclinical development.

PODOPHYLLUM PELTATUM (BERBERIDACEAE)

Podophyllum peltatum has a number of common names, including the mayapple, Devil's apple and American mandrake, and is a perennial plant found in the woodlands of Canada and eastern USA.

The plants reach 10–45 cm in height and have long, thin rhizomes which are the underground stem from which the roots grow. The rhizomes are known to be poisonous and are the most important part of the plant, containing high concentrations of **podophyllotoxin** and α- and β-**peltatin**, all of which are cytotoxic.

The closely related Asian species, *P. emodi* (syn. *P. hexandrum*), which is known as Indian podophyllum, contains these active lignan ingredients at a lower concentration. Podophyllotoxin and related lignans are also found in the rhizomes of another species *P. pleianthum*, which in Japan and China is used to make a preparation to treat snakebites and genital tumours.

The rhizomes of *P. peltatum* have a long history as a medicine among native North American tribes (Penobscot Indians of Maine). They are gathered in autumn, dried and ground to a powder, and the material is eaten or drunk as an infusion of the powder as a laxative or to get rid of intestinal worms. The powder was also used as a poultice to treat warts and skin growths. Currently, extracts of the plant are used in topical medications for genital warts and some skin cancers. However, the mayapple rhizome powder has a strong purgative action and the compounds in it are too toxic for self-medication.

Ethanolic extracts of the rhizomes are known as **podophyllin**, which is included in many pharmacopoeias for the topical treatment of warts and *condylomata acuminata*, which are benign tumours. Podophyllin resin is highly irritant and unpleasant and cannot be used systemically. The main natural product is the podophyllotoxin lignan class (see Chapter 6) of which podophyllotoxin was the first to be isolated in 1880 and the structure proposed in 1932. There are many components in podophyllin; the most important from the antitumour perspective are the lignans. **Podofilox** is a purified form of podophyllin which acts as a cell poison against cells undergoing mitosis, and, although this extract is not a systemic chemotherapeutic agent, it is used topically in creams as a treatment for genital warts.

Chemists working at the Sandoz pharmaceutical company developed the hypothesis that podophyllin resin may contain anticancer lignan glycosides that are more water-soluble and less toxic than podophyllotoxin, and several of these natural products were isolated. The compounds did, indeed, possess greater water solubility but unfortunately had less antitumour activity. Much work was done on these glycosides to make them resistant to enzymic hydrolysis, maintain their water solubility and improve their cellular uptake. This was a difficult task as, paradoxically, improving the water solubility decreased the cellular uptake (and therefore activity).

By a serendipitous event, a crude fraction of podophyllin was treated with benzaldehyde, resulting in a mixture of products that were mainly benzyl derivatives of lignan glycosides (Stähelin & von Wartburg 1991). The crude reaction mixture was highly cytotoxic and active in the mouse life-prolongation assay against a leukaemia cell line. Some of the components of this mixture were isolated but were not as active as the whole mixture. Condensation of benzaldehyde with the reaction mixture generated a series of acetals that were not hydrolysed by glucosidase enzymes and were less water-soluble. Additionally, the crude mixture worked by a different mechanism from the purified products by stopping the tumour cells from undergoing mitosis. This preparation was marketed for cancer treatment under the name of Proresid. Work on Proresid with bioassay-guided isolation against a mouse life-prolongation assay with a leukaemia cell line indicated that there was a highly active agent present. As with paclitaxel and camptothecin, in the 1960s it was very difficult to isolate and identify minor components and the process took several years to complete. The most abundant component of Proresid is **podophyllotoxin benzylidene glucoside** (1) (Fig. 8.10); a minor component is **4′-demethylepipodophyllotoxin benzylidene glucoside** (2), which was found to be the most active agent (Fig. 8.10).

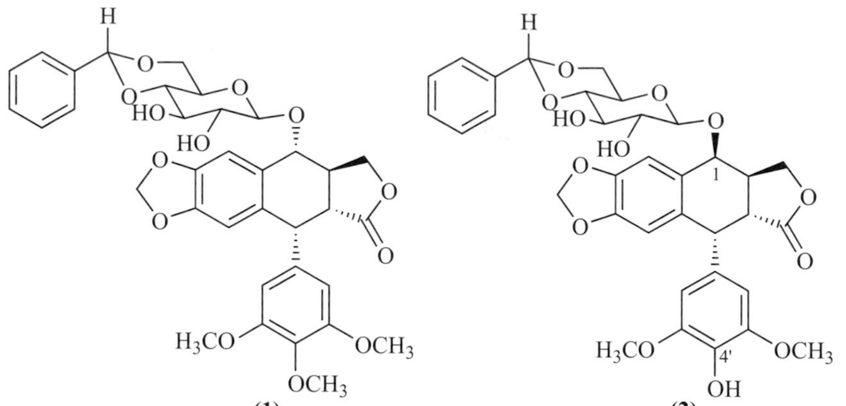

Fig. 8.10 Structures of podophyllotoxin benzylidene glucoside (1) and 4′-demethylepipodophyllotoxin benzylidene glucoside (2).

There was much synthetic work conducted to produce analogues that retain the same structural features of compound (2), which is epimeric at position 1 and lacking a methyl at position 4′ with respect to compound (1). The two most important analogues synthesized so far are **etoposide** and **teniposide** (Fig. 8.11) which have much more potency than the parent compound.

Etoposide is marketed as Vepesid for small cell lung cancer, testicular cancer and lymphomas; **teniposide** is also used in the treatment of brain tumours. Podophyllotoxin binds to tubulin and is a member of the 'spindle poison' group of agents and functions by preventing microtubule formation.

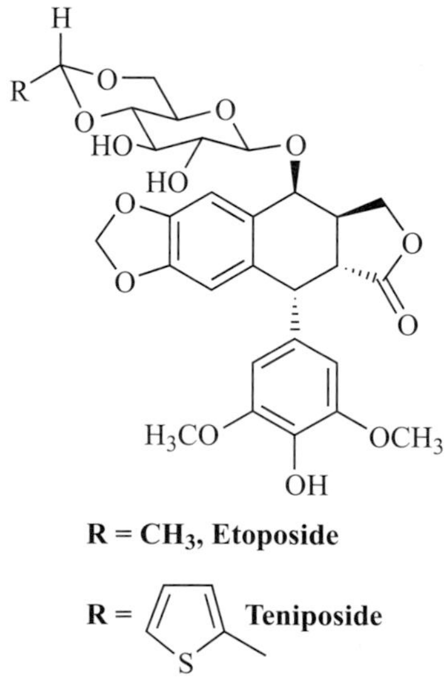

Etoposide and teniposide work via a different mechanism by inhibiting the enzyme topoisomerase II preventing DNA synthesis and replication. The difference in mechanism is attributable to the small adjustment in structure with etoposide and teniposide being 4′-demethyl compounds and having different stereochemistry at position C_1.

CATHARANTHUS ROSEUS (APOCYNACEAE)

The Madagascar periwinkle (*Catharanthus roseus*, syn. *Vinca rosea*) was originally native to Madagascar. It has been widely cultivated for hundreds of years and can now be found growing wild in most countries, including the UK. The natural wild plants are a pale pink with a purple eye in the centre but many colours have been developed by horticulturalists, ranging from white to pink and purple. The plant has had a long history of treating a wide assortment of diseases and was used as a folk remedy for diabetes in Europe for centuries. In China, the plant has been used for its astringent and diuretic properties and as a cough remedy, and in the Caribbean it is used to treat eye infections and for diabetes. Historically, the periwinkle has had a reputation as a magic plant: Europeans thought it could ward off evil spirits, and the French referred to it as 'the violet of the sorcerers'.

Jamaicans have traditionally used a tea from *C. roseus* to treat diabetes although it has not been possible to find a basis for this use. Over 150 alkaloids have been characterized in the plant, a number of which are **indole alkaloids** and include **dimeric** or **bis-indole alkaloids**. These components are

R = CH$_3$, Etoposide

R = [thiophene structure] Teniposide

Fig. 8.11

broadly referred to as **vinca alkaloids** after the name of a synonym for this plant, *Vinca rosea*.

The discovery of the vinca alkaloids from the Madagascan periwinkle is a classic example of drug discovery and, although extracts of the species had a reputation as being useful in the treatment of diabetes, a screening programme at the pharmaceutical company Eli Lilly revealed that extracts inhibited the growth of certain types of cancer cells. Bioassay-guided isolation of extracts of the plant led to the characterization of the active alkaloidal compounds **vincristine** and **vinblastine** (Fig. 8.12).

These natural products are structurally highly complex and are dimeric indole alkaloids that can be synthesized but are too expensive to produce in this way. The natural yield of the drugs in the plant is exceptionally low (0.0002% for vincristine), which makes them very expensive antitumour agents. They exert their anticancer effects by inhibiting mitosis by binding to tubulin, thus preventing the cell from making the spindles it needs to be able to move its chromosomes around as it divides. Vinblastine is marketed as Velbe by Eli Lilly and is useful for treating Hodgkin's disease, lymphomas, advanced testicular cancer, advanced breast cancer and Kaposi's sarcoma. This drug has a number of side effects, including hair loss, nausea, lowered blood cell counts, constipation and mouth sores. Vincristine is marketed as Oncovin by Eli Lilly and is used to treat acute leukaemia, Hodgkin's

disease and other lymphomas. Semi-synthetic vinca alkaloids of note include **vindesine** (marketed under the name Eldisine), used to treat leukaemia and lung cancers, and **vinorelbine** (marketed as Navelbine by GlaxoSmithKline), which is used as a treatment for ovarian cancer. Vinorelbine has a wider range of antitumour activity than the other vinca alkaloids and is used, in combination with cisplatin, in treating patients with non-small-cell lung cancers.

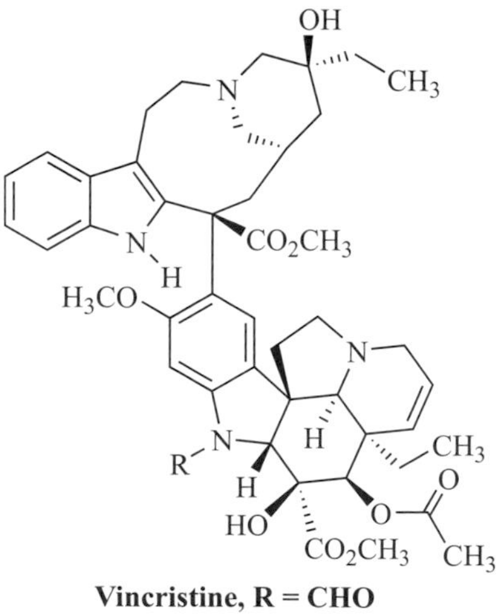

MICROBIAL ANTITUMOUR AGENTS

Microbial sources of chemical diversity are probably the most important for the pharmaceutical industry, with collection of microbes (Actinomycetes and fungi), culturing and fermentation leading to a greater ease of access to extracts with no need for re-supply of biomass from distant sources. There are, however, issues concerning refermentation, and in some instances extracts produced by fermentation of an organism may vary. An advantage of microbes as a source of chemistry is that cultures of the microbe can be stored at −135°C indefinitely, but there is still need for material collection agreements with the source country.

Like plants, microbes are an enormous source of bioactive natural products; the anticancer metabolites are a good example, with many important therapeutic groups such as the **anthracycline, bleomycin** and **actinomycin** classes. These agents have been used for quite some time and highlight the need for further investigation of microbes as a source, and there are still many species that need to be cultured, extracted and screened, particularly amongst the fungi. Microbes are also present in many harsh environments; this may give rise to unique chemistry and thus these organisms possibly have great untapped potential.

THE ANTHRACYCLINES

This group is a large complex family of antibiotics and many were investigated before a useful antitumour agent was isolated. They are structurally and biosynthetically related to the tetracyclines (Chapter 6), being derived from the polyketide pathway. One of the first agents to be described in this class was **daunorubicin** from *Streptomyces peucetius* and *Streptomyces caeruleorubidis* (Fig. 8.13).

Vincristine, R = CHO
Vinblastine, R = CH₃

Fig. 8.12

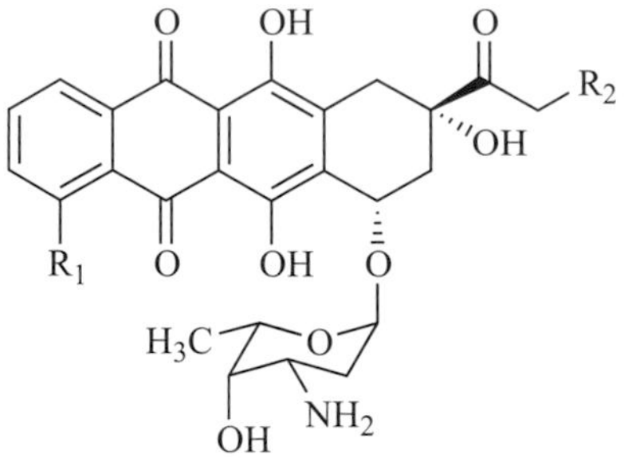

R_1 = OCH_3, R_2 = H, Daunorubicin
R_1 = OCH_3, R_2 = OH, Doxorubicin
R_1 = H, R_2 = H, Idarubicin

Fig. 8.13

This agent is active against leukaemias. One of the most widely used related antitumour agents is **doxorubicin** (Adriamycin) from *Streptomyces peucetius* var. *caesius*, discovered in the late 1960s, which is highly active against a broad spectrum of both solid and liquid tumours. A number of semi-synthetic analogues have been produced of which **idarubicin** has enhanced antitumour potency and is less cardiotoxic than doxorubicin. These compounds possess a tetracyclic linear ring system (based on **anthracene**, hence the term **anthracycline antitumour antibiotics**) to which an amino sugar is attached. These agents bind to DNA and inhibit DNA and RNA synthesis. The main antitumour action of this group is by inhibition of topoisomerase II.

THE BLEOMYCINS

This group consists of a closely related mixture of glycopeptide antibiotics from the filamentous bacterium *Streptomyces verticillus*. They were discovered in 1966 by screening of culture filtrates against tumours. The bleomycin mixture is partly resolved (purified) prior to formulation for clinical use under the name blenoxane, which consists of a mixture of **bleomycin A$_2$** (55–70%) and **bleomycin B$_2$** (30%) (Fig. 8.14). These natural products occur as blue copper chelates.

The different analogues are distinct from each other only in the terminal amine functional group and a number of unusual functional groups are present in the bleomycin skeleton, including amino acids, pyrimidine rings and sugars. The bleomycins are DNA-cleaving drugs and cause single- and double-strand breaks in DNA. The dithiazole

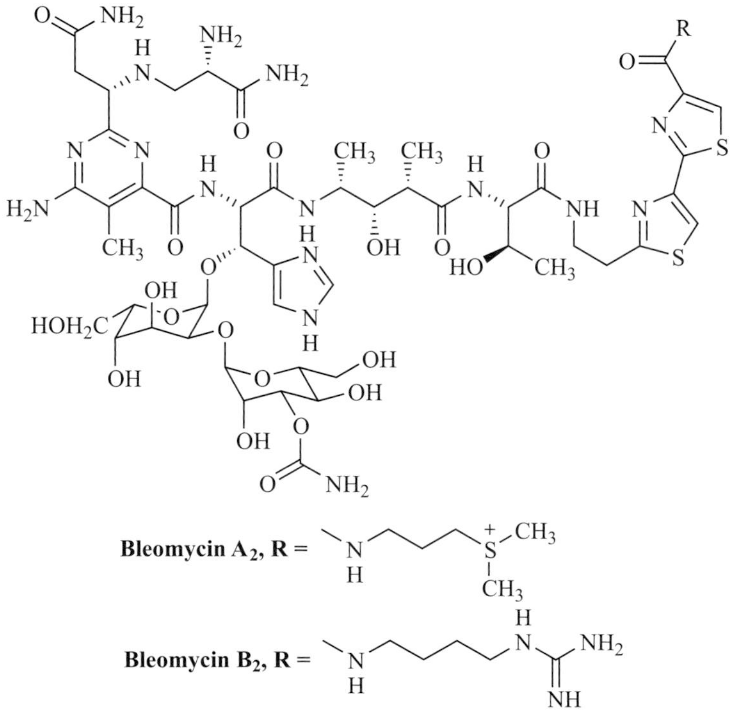

Bleomycin A$_2$, R =

Bleomycin B$_2$, R =

Fig. 8.14

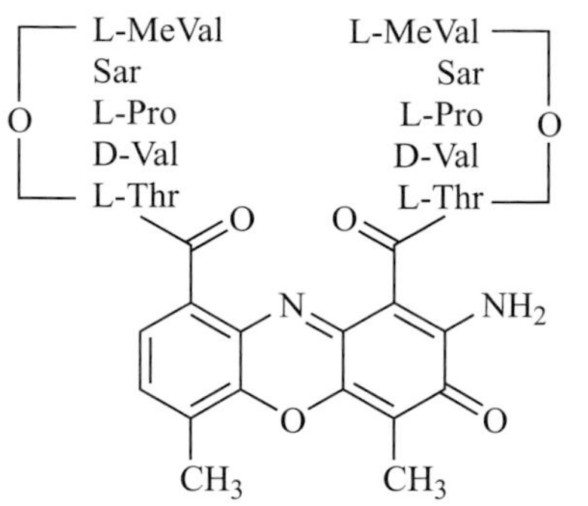

Actinomycin D

Fig. 8.15

groups are essential for activity and are believed to be important in the binding of the bleomycins to DNA. This class of drugs has use in the treatment of lymphomas, head and neck tumours and testicular cancer with very little bone-marrow toxicity.

THE ACTINOMYCINS

Actinomycin D (dactinomycin) is an antibiotic from *Streptomyces parvullus* first isolated in 1940. It is an antimicrobial compound which is toxic and has limited use as an antitumour agent. Structurally, it consists of a planar phenoxazinone dicarboxylic acid attached to two identical pentapeptides (Fig. 8.15). A number of analogues of different peptide composition are known.

The planar group of this agent intercalates with double-stranded DNA, inhibits topoisomerase II and RNA synthesis, and can also cause single-strand DNA breaks. The principal use of this group is in paediatric tumours, including kidney (Wilms) tumours, but the use is limited due to unpleasant side effects.

FURTHER STRATEGIES FOR THE DISCOVERY OF ANTITUMOUR AGENTS

There are a number of potential strategies that can be applied to attempts to discover new natural product cytotoxic agents. The most obvious is to obtain biomass in previously unexplored environments, for example the collection of marine organisms in places such as the Persian Gulf, the Red Sea and deep water collections in the Pacific. Such collections can only work with close collaboration with organizations based in the countries controlling these areas. In the marine environment, there are still many areas that could harbour extensive chemical resources, such as deep sea vents, which occur along ocean ridges of the East Pacific and the Galapagos Rift. In these areas on the sea bed, superheated water seeps up from areas of geothermal activity and the environments around these vents are rich in both microscopic and macroscopic life. These organisms are subject to extremes of pressure and heat which may have profound effects on their natural product chemistry capability.

In terms of terrestrial plants, there is still much work to be done; of the 250,000 higher plant species, only a fraction (10–15%) have been systematically investigated for chemistry and biological activity. If the correct agreements can be put in place, there are still vast tracts of rainforest that are virtually untapped as sources for chemical diversity.

Terrestrial animals, such as insects, of which there are millions of species, are to all intents and purposes practically uninvestigated for biological activity, and organizations such as the Costa Rican Instituto Nacional de Biodiversidad (INBio) have been carrying out a national inventory of species, including insects. What is needed is investment in this resource, with pharmaceutical companies developing collaborations and screening extracts from these institutes.

Further investment in research is needed to extend searches into many of the world's ecosystems, some of which may well disappear with changes in climate.

Very often access to microbially derived chemical diversity is limited to the supply of certain types of organisms (e.g. readily culturable Actinomycetes). It has been estimated that less than 1% of bacterial species and less than 5% of fungal species are currently known; thus millions of species remain undiscovered and enormous chemical diversity remains to be tapped. Research into the development of new culturing techniques will in the future give access to this chemistry.

Investment is, therefore, needed in natural product resources. At present, pharmaceutical companies are scaling down their interest in natural product drug discovery, preferring either to farm out this process to smaller companies or to investigate synthetic compounds that can be produced in-house in their thousands by combinatorial chemistry techniques. Unfortunately, the synthetic chemistry that produces these combinatorial libraries is in most cases simple, introducing limited functional group chemistry and, most importantly, little stereochemistry into the synthesized compounds. Natural products, on the other hand, are in many cases highly functional and chiral; these facets have evolved as the producing organism has evolved. In many cases it can also be demonstrated that these natural products confer an advantage on the organism, for example as antibiotic substances (e.g. the tetracyclines and macrolides).

What is more important, and what many large pharmaceutical companies seem determined to ignore, is that natural products are a tried, tested and proven route to new drugs, and that the fascination with new discovery technology is only of any value if it produces new therapeutic agents.

References

Alley, M.C., Scudiero, D.A., Monks, A., et al., 1988. Feasibility of drug screening with panels of human tumor cell lines using a microculture tetrazolium assay. Cancer Res. 48, 589–601.

Cragg, G.M., Boyd, M.R., Cardellina II, J.H., et al., 1993. Role of plants in the National Cancer Institute Drug Discovery and Development Program. In: Kinghorn, A.D., Balandrin, M.F. (Eds.), Human medicinal agents from plants. American Chemical Society, Washington, DC.

Cragg, G.M., Newman, D.J., 1999. Cancer Invest. 17, 153–163.

Cragg, G.M., Newman, D.J., 2000. Antineoplastic agents from natural sources: achievements and future directions. Expert Opin. Investig. Drugs 9, 2783–2797.

Cragg, G.M., Newman, D.J., Weiss, R.B., 1997. Coral reefs, forests and thermal vents: the world wide exploration of nature for novel antitumour agents. Semin. Oncol. 24, 156–163.

Farnsworth, N.R., Akerele, O., Bingel, A.S., Soejarto, D.D., Guo, Z., 1985. Medicinal plants in therapy. Bull. World Health Organ. 63, 965–981.

Goodman, J., Walsh, V., 2001. The story of taxol. Cambridge University Press, Cambridge.

Gottlieb, J.A., Luce, J.K., 1972. Cancer Chemother. Rep. 56, 103–105.

Grever, M.R., Schepartz, S.A., Chabner, B.A., 1992. The National Cancer Institute: cancer drug discovery and development program. Semin. Oncol. 19, 622–638.

Moertel, C.G., Schutt, A.J., Reitemeier, R.J., et al., 1972. Phase II study of camptothecin (NSC-100880) in the treatment of advanced gastrointestinal cancer. Cancer Chemother. Rep. 56, 95–101.

Paull, K.D., Shoemaker, R.H., Hodes, L., et al., 1989. Display and analysis of patterns of differential activity of drugs against human tumor cell lines: development of mean graph and COMPARE algorithm. J. Natl. Cancer Inst. 81, 1088–1092.

Stähelin, H.F., von Wartburg, A., 1991. The chemical and biological route from podophyllotoxin glucoside to etoposide. Ninth Cain Memorial Award Lecture. Cancer Res. 51, 5–15.

Wall, M.E., Wani, M.C., 1995. Camptothecin and taxol: discovery to clinic. Thirteenth Bruce F Cain Memorial Award Lecture. Cancer Res. 55, 753–760.

Further reading

Cragg, G.M., Grothaus, P.G., Newman, D.J., 2009. Impact of natural products on developing new anti-cancer agents. Chem. Rev. 109, 3012–3043.

Delgado, J.N., Remers, W.A., 1998. Wilson and Gisvold's textbook of organic medicinal and pharmaceutical chemistry, tenth ed. Lippincott-Raven, Philadelphia.

Pan, L., Chai, H., Kinghorn, A.D., 2010. The continuing search for antitumor agents from higher plants. Phytochem. Lett. 3, 1–8.

Pratt, W.B., Ruddon, R.W., 1994. The anticancer drugs, second ed. Oxford University Press, Oxford.

Newman, D.J., Cragg, G.M., 2009. Microbial antitumor drugs: natural products of microbial origin as anticancer agents. Curr. Opin. Investig. Drugs 10, 1280–1296.

Newman, D.J., Cragg, G.M., 2007. Natural products as sources of new drugs over the last 25 years. J. Nat. Prod. 70, 461–477.

Rang, H.P., Dale, M.M., Ritter, J.M., 1999. Pharmacology, fourth ed. Churchill Livingstone, London.

Section 4

Pharmaceuticals and nutraceuticals derived from plant extracts

Chapter 9

Production, standardization and quality control

Most people look at herbal medicines and the products derived from them from the perspective of the benefits they expect to receive. However, in pharmaceutical terms, aspects of production (agricultural production or wild-crafting, extraction, fractionation, formulation, quality assurance), the legal framework of their use, and clinical aspects (safety, pharmacovigilance) are of at least equal importance. Consequently, plant-derived medicines are diverse and include, for example:

- **pure compounds**, which are often isolated from botanical drugs (and which are not considered to be herbal medicines)
- **traditionally used medicinal plants**, loose or in teabags to form infusions, including 'instant teas', and tinctures, ethanolic extracts, essential oils, fatty acids and dried extracts
- **cut or powdered botanical crude drugs** (generally simply called crude drug throughout the text), used as such (i.e. unprocessed)
- **non-standardized extracts**, with varying information about quality and, consequently, sometimes uncertain information about clinical efficacy and pharmacological effects
- **standardized extracts**, generally with relatively well-established clinical and pharmacological profiles

Here a very short overview is given of the whole process, from the agricultural production of materials collected from the wild, to the processing and production of the pharmaceutical product or health-food supplement. A more detailed discussion is beyond the scope of this introduction, but can be found, for example, in Evans (2009).

In all cases, the basis for drug production is the **botanical drug** (see Chapter 2), which can be defined as:

- **dried parts of entire plants, plants organs, or parts of plant organs** for use as medicines, aromatics and spices, or as excipients used in the production of pharmaceuticals. A typical example is the flower of camomile (*Matricaria recutita*)
- **Isolated products** obtained directly from plants but which no longer have an organ structure, such as essential and fatty oils, balsams, etc. An example is the exudate of the leaves of aloe [*Aloe vera* (L.) Burm. f., or *Aloe barbadensis* Mill.], obtained by cutting the fleshy leaves and collecting the resulting liquid, which is called 'aloes' when dried.

BIOLOGICAL RESOURCES AND CONSERVATION

At least 250,000 species of higher plants are known. Of these, a large number have important uses for humans, including foods, building materials, dyes, spices and as medicinal plants. It is impossible to say how many of these are 'medicinal', since a plant may be used only locally or on a worldwide level. Fewer than 300 are truly universal or widely used and researched in detail for their pharmacological and toxicological effects. Even fewer have been tested for clinical efficacy. In Europe, at least 2000 medicinal and aromatic plant species are used on a commercial basis. About two-thirds of these are native to Europe and a large proportion of these are still collected from the wild. This fact is not detrimental in itself, but it may pose risks, including, for example:

- Problems in obtaining a consistent quality of product, including the risk of adulteration
- Over-exploitation of native populations of certain plant species.

More than half of all medicinally used species are still collected from the wild, including the less frequently used species. An example of an over-exploited resource collected from the wild has been discussed in detail by Lange (2000). Pheasant's eye (false hellebore or *Adonis vernalis* L.) is a native of Southern and Central Europe and is used there for cases of minor cardiac arrhythmias. The plant is threatened not only by its pharmaceutical use (as a phytomedicine as well as a homoeopathic remedy), but also by its use as an ornamental plant and a dye source. Exploitation of *Adonis vernalis* affects many south-eastern European countries, including Hungary, Romania and the Ukraine. Importantly, detrimental (unsustainable) harvesting techniques are still used and there is a constant risk that the exploited biomass exceeds the sustainable levels and that techniques are used which harm the population severely (Lange 2000).

Coptis teeta Wallich [Mishmi (gold thread), Ranunculaceae] is an example of a species that is under threat of extinction due to over-exploitation. It is found in the eastern Himalayan regions, particularly a small mountainous region of Arunachal Pradesh in north-eastern India. The rhizome is a prized medicinal commodity and is used for gastrointestinal complaints and malaria. However, it has been brought close to extinction by deforestation and over-exploitation. Conservation schemes have been proposed, but it is too early to be certain whether the species can be saved from extinction.

AGRICULTURAL AND BIOTECHNOLOGICAL PRODUCTION

Most important medicinal plants are now produced under controlled agricultural conditions (Franz 1999). Such production systems require certain conditions for each species with respect to:

- temperature and annual course of temperature
- rainfall (if it is not possible to irrigate the fields)
- soil characteristics and quality (edaphic factors)
- day length and sun characteristics
- altitude.

These factors are assessed in detailed studies for each species that is cultivated. Generally, it is essential that the production is based on the principles of GMP (good manufacturing practice) and/or ISO (International Organization for Standardization) certification, in this case GAP (good agricultural practice) and the subsequent processing steps (drying, cutting, grinding, storage, packaging, transport, etc., which are covered by GMP) are essential for high-quality and reproducible batches. Medicinal plants are a delicate product and in many cases inadequate storage of transport can ruin a whole year's work. For example, essential oil containing drugs will easily lose their active ingredients if the botanical drug is exposed to heat or humidity.

MOISTURE LEVELS

All drugs are at risk of decaying if the humidity in the drug material exceeds 15%. Improperly stored botanical drugs have a musty smell and often change colour (green material turning yellow or brown). However, different levels of moisture are acceptable for each drug. For example, the moisture contents given in Table 9.1 are considered to be within the normal range and do not pose any problems for these drugs.

Table 9.1	Acceptable moisture content for storage of some botanical drugs (after Franz 1999)	
BOTANICAL DRUG	**MOISTURE CONTENT (%)**
Chamomile flower (*Matricariae* flos, from *Matricaria recutita* L.)	8–10
Linseed (Lini semen from *Linum usitatissimum* L.)	5–9
Digitalis leaf (Digitalis lanatae folium, from *Digitalis lanata* Ehrh.)	8–12
Frangula bark (Frangulae cortex, from *Rhamnus frangula* L, syn. *Frangula alnus* Mill.)	5–8
Thyme herb (Thymi herba, from *Thymus vulgaris* L.)	8–11
Gentian rootstock (Gentianae radix, from *Gentiana lutea* L.)	8–15
Fennel fruit (Foeniculi fructus, from *Foeniculum vulgare* Mill. subsp. *vulgare*)	6–12

MICROBIOLOGICAL CONTAMINATION

Other specific requirements for storage and transportation of the drug have to be met and, in many cases, this is now controlled via GAP and GMP standards. A similar requirement relates to microbial contamination of botanical drugs. Each natural material naturally harbours a large number of spores and other microorganisms. The maximum number of microorganisms allowed is regulated in the European Pharmacopoeia (for details see Eur. Ph. 2002, Chapter 2.6.12):

- Up to 10^5 aerobic microorganisms per g or ml, including:
  - up to 10^3 yeast and fungi per g or ml
  - up to 10^3 enterobacteria per g or ml
- No detectable *Escherichia coli* (in 1 g or ml)
- No detectable *Salmonella* sp. (in 10 g or ml).

PESTICIDES

Pesticides are commonly used to prevent the infestation of the botanical material with large amounts of unwanted species of plants, insects or animals. These may cause harm or otherwise interfere with the production, storage, processing, transport and marketing of botanical drugs. Acceptable limits have been defined in the Eur. Ph. (Chapter 2.8.13). There is also a detailed description of the sampling methods and the relevant qualitative and quantitative methods. Importation of herbs from countries with less restrictive legislation on pesticides means that this material should be checked very carefully. Examples of relevant limits for some important pesticides are given in Table 9.2.

PLANT BREEDING

Cultivated species are normally optimized to relatively high and constant levels of active ingredients. Other important goals for breeding relate to the reproducibility of the drug. *Matricaria recutita* (the common camomile), for example, should have large and homogenous flower heads. Simple, mechanized harvesting and good storage characteristics are normally required for a botanical drug. Other desired features include high yield, high resistance to pathogens (insects, mites, fungi, bacteria and viruses), reproducibility of the yield, good adaptation to the location, low demands regarding ecological requirements, low content of water (for easier drying) and

Table 9.2	Limits of some important pesticides allowed in botanical material
PESTICIDE	**CONCENTRATION LIMIT (MG/KG)**
Aldrin and dieldrin (sum of)	0.05
Chlordane (sum of *cis*-, *trans*- and oxychlordane)	0.05
DDT (sum of various related compounds)	1.0
Endrin	0.05
Fonofos	0.05
Malathion	1.0
Parathion	0.5
Permethrin	1.0
Pyrethrins (sum of)	3.0
Source: Eur. Ph. 2002.	

stability of the plant's organs. The degree to which a certain trait is inherited from one generation to the next is important; if this cannot be assured there is a constant risk of losing high-yielding strains. This risk can be reduced by *in vitro* culture or cloning, or by propagating through cuttings, but this is not ideal for high-production systems as it is time-consuming and therefore costly.

IN VITRO CULTIVATION

In vitro culture involves the use of non-differentiated cell aggregates (submersed or callus cultures). These are most commonly used in the production of ornamental and food plants (e.g. orchids, strawberries). In the case of medicinal plants, cell cultures are used:

- as a starting point for investigating the biochemical basis of the biosynthesis of natural products and for breeding new varieties/strains
- as a basis for vegetative propagation of plants to be used as a phytomedicine or for isolating a pure natural product, especially if a consistent quality of the strains or a fungi- or virus-free culture is required. For example, high-yielding strains of *Catharanthus* and *Dioscorea* may be required, or the development and maintenance of pyrrolizidine-free strains of common comfrey (*Symphytum officinale* L.) and coltsfoot (*Tussilago farfara* L.), or virus-free *Digitalis lanata* Ehrh. cultures
- for the semi-synthetic production of some natural products (e.g. production of digoxin from digitoxin)

- for the direct synthesis of a medicinal natural product, although this is only rarely achieved by this method. Today, this process is restricted to the production of paclitaxel and its precursors (first isolated from the Pacific yew, *Taxus brevifolia* Nutt.) and shikonin (a dye and medicinal product used in Asian medicine from *Lithospermum erythrorhizon* Sieb. & Zucc.).

THE PACIFIC YEW AS AN EXAMPLE

The Pacific yew (*Taxus brevifolia* Nutt., Taxaceae) is a botanical drug which exemplifies all the various approaches for producing a medicinally used natural compound. In 1962 several samples of *Taxus brevifolia* Nutt. were collected at random for the National Cancer Institute (NCI) and the US Department of Agriculture. These samples were included in a large screening programme at the NCI. A potent cytotoxic effect was documented in one *in vitro* system. After a lengthy development process, clinical studies started 13 years later in 1984. It took a further 10 years before paclitaxel was approved for the treatment of anthracycline-resistant metastasizing mammary carcinomas. In the meantime the compound had been licensed for a variety of other cancers and semi-synthetic derivatives produced such as docetxel, which are also now employed (see also Chapter 8).

The strategy for obtaining the pure active ingredient thus moved from collection from the wild during (1962)/1975–1990 to the commercial silvicultural production of a biosynthetic precursor of paclitaxel in another species of *Taxus* (European yew, *T. baccata* L.) during 1990–2002, to the current (2003) commercial *in vitro* production using fermentation technology:

- *Taxus brevifolia* is a very slow-growing species, which produces the active ingredients only in very small amounts. Since paclitaxel was for many years isolated from the bark, trees had to be felled in order to obtain it. The requirement for paclitaxel increased dramatically with progress in the clinical development of the drug in the mid-1970s (the amount required to meet the annual therapeutic requirements of patients with ovarian cancer in the USA was estimated to be 15–20 kg). If other cancers common in the USA were to be treated with this compound, around 200–300 kg of the pure compound would have been required per year. This amount can be isolated from approximately 145,000 tons of bark. Collecting such amounts would have been completely unsustainable and would have resulted in the extinction of the species within a few years.

- In the 1990s the semi-synthetic production of paclitaxel from natural products in other *Taxus* spp. (10-desacetylbaccatin II isolated from the European yew, *T. baccata*) allowed for the production of large amounts of paclitaxel. Up to this point, a conflict of interest between conservation and medicinal use was unavoidable.

- Large-scale production using cell-culture techniques is now feasible and has been approved by the FDA. Today, most of the paclitaxel required is produced using fermentation technology (Goodman & Walsh 2001).

DRUG PREPARATION AND EXTRACTION

A number of diverse overall approaches and specific techniques are available for processing crude plant (or rarely animal) material. For phytomedicines, the general framework is relatively well circumscribed, based on European and national legislation.

EXTRACTS

According to the Eur. Ph. (2002, Chapter 01/2002-765), an *extract* is a concentrated preparation of liquid (fluid extract or tinctures) or intermediate (semi-liquid) or solid (dry extract) consistency normally produced from dried botanical or zoological material by a technique involving the use of adequate solvents for obtaining a mixture of compounds. For some preparations, the material to be extracted may undergo a preliminary treatment prior to extraction. Examples for the latter include defatting, inactivation of enzymes or most commonly simply grinding.

Extracts are prepared by maceration, percolation or other suitable, validated methods using ethanol or another suitable solvent. After extraction, unwanted material may be removed if this is deemed appropriate.

Preparation and extraction is the core process of the industrial production of phytopharmaceuticals, and require a detailed analysis of the best conditions for each plant-derived drug. An important difference is whether a plant is going to be used as a phytomedi-cine or an individual biologically active compound is to be isolated from the material. For the former purpose, the botanical drug must conform to Phar-macopoeial requirements or another process that assures reproducible quality; for the latter, optimi-zation to obtain large yields of the relevant com-pound(s) is essential.

Very often a botanical drug is gathered during the flowering period of the plant (aerial parts, leaves, flowers), during spring (bark) and at the end of the vegetative season (root and rootstock). However, there are many exceptions; for example, cloves [Caryophylli flos, *Syzygium aromaticum* (L.) Merr. & L. M. Perry] are collected prior to the opening of the flowers and the flower buds are used pharmaceu-tically. For digitalis, the leaves are collected rather late during the vegetative process (October).

Extraction (e.g. percolation, maceration, pressing of fresh plant material for expressed juice) is again specific for each drug and depends on the phy-totherapeutic product required.

There are many different types of drug prepara-tions, including:

- fresh plant material, used popularly as an infusion or decoction
- dried and cut drug material, often used in industrial production
- dried and powdered drug material, commonly used as an infusion or decoction. If such material is to be used pharmaceutically it must comply with standards as defined in the monograph for the specific botanical drug. If no such monograph exists the material has to comply with the general monograph for herbal drugs (Eur. Ph. 2002, 01/2002-1433)
- extraction and subsequent bulk production of pure natural products (e.g. morphine, digoxin, digitoxin, camptothecin) or a mixture of closely related ones (e.g. sennosides from Senna, aescin from horse chestnut, quillaia saponins from soapbark) using validated, standard phytochemical techniques (chromatography, partitioning between solvents of differing polarity, precipitation, etc.)
- unstandardized tinctures are hydroalcoholic (or alcoholic) extracts of crude drug material used as a liquid botanical drug
- an extract prepared from dried drug material using defined solvent systems is processed into a

variety of pharmaceutical products (e.g. tablets for crude extracts). Such extracts are often characterized by the drug:solvent ratio, which gives the relationship of the volume of solvent to the amount of drug extracted (e.g. 1:10) (see p. 154). In many high-quality products, these extracts are 'standardized' by mixing high- and low-yield material. By 'spiking' the extract with an enriched extract, a 'modified' extract with a defined range of active natural products is obtained (e.g. dry aloe extracts standardized to 19.0–21.0% of hydroxyanthracene derivatives calculated as barbaloin)

- a particularly interesting case is that of the so-called 'special extracts'. A special extract is prepared by first extracting the drug with a defined solvent system and then processing the extract so that a well-defined extract with specific ranges of ingredients is obtained. These extracts have a significantly reduced percentage of unwanted compounds, and an increased percentage of compounds that contribute significantly to the pharmacological activity and clinical effectiveness. In the case of ginkgo leaves (Ginkgo folium, *Ginkgo biloba* L.), for example, the desired natural products include the flavone glycosides (16–26%) and the terpene lactones (5–7%); whereas the polyphenols, polysaccharides, and especially the ginkgolic acids, are less desirable constituents (for details see p. 158–159 and 249)
- there are several special methods of extraction; for example, the cold pressed extract of the rootstock of *Echinacea* species is developed into an immunostimulant product. The fresh rootstock is used for this and the sap is processed into a commercial botanical pharmaceutical. For material to be used pharmaceutically, the process must be validated.

EFFECT OF PREPARATION METHODS ON CONTENT

Different methods of preparing botanical material and subsequent extraction result in extracts with differing composition and different concentrations of active (as well as undesired) ingredients. A wide range of factors both in relation to the production of the botanical starting material (the botanical drug)

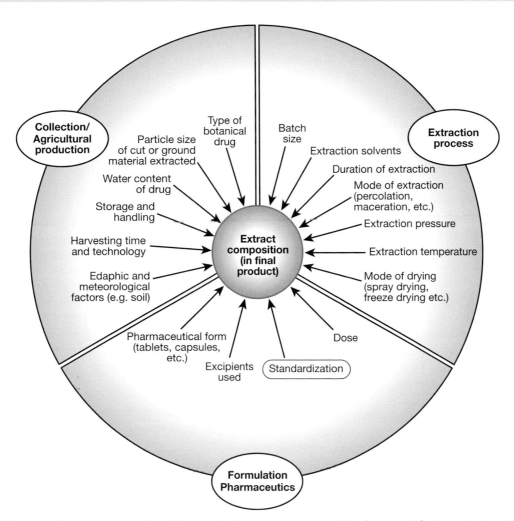

Fig. 9.1 The extraction process and selected factors that impact on the composition (and quality) of an extract and the final product.

and its processing, extraction and formulation have an impact on the chemical composition and thus the pharmacological activity of a phytotherapeutic preparation (Fig. 9.1). Strictly speaking, for an assessment of the pharmacological effect and clinical effectiveness of a botanical drug, precise data on the composition of the extract are needed. Just as importantly, pharmacological or clinical data on two products can only be compared meaningfully if the composition of the extracts is known. This implies, for example, that a meta-analysis of clinical studies is only feasible if the botanical drug materials used are similar and the resulting extracts have a comparable composition, a consideration often omitted by authors of such studies.

QUALITY CONTROL AND STANDARDIZATION

QUALITY CONTROL: GENERAL PROCEDURES

Quality-control measures vary considerably. The most relevant apply to plant extracts and unprocessed plants (the quality control of pure compounds is covered by standard pharmaceutical procedures). Quality control is a multistep process that covers all stages from the growing of the botanical material to the final control of the finished product and the evaluation of its stability and quality over time. It is essential at all stages of the production of the botanical material, including transportation, extraction and processing, storage and the elaboration of the finished pharmaceutical product. Many factors can influence the quality of the finished product, for example:

- the quality of the botanical material used, which in turn is influenced by a multitude of biogenic (e.g. infections with fungi) and climatic factors, and also includes the risk of contamination with heavy metals, pesticides, herbicides and the like (see above)
- the adequate processing of the fresh material, including drying, transportation and storage
- the use of appropriate and reproducible extraction techniques
- storage under appropriate conditions (generally dry, cool, in the dark)
- use of the material only within the generally accepted shelf-life of the botanical drug.

Specifically, quality control needs to assure:

- the correct botanical identity of the drug (i.e. the correct species and plant part) in an appropriate quality (time of collection, age)
- the purity of the material used (i.e. that other botanical drugs are only present in minimal amounts)
- contaminants such as insects, mites, bacteria, fungi, heavy metals, herbicides, fungicides, pesticides, insecticides and any other toxins are below the legal (e.g. Eur. Ph.) threshold

- that the required level of active compounds (only if a minimum level of these natural products is defined) or a defined level of biological activity (if the drug is characterized biologically or pharmacologically) is reached.

The best level of quality control can be achieved if the above requirements are defined in a monograph in a legally binding pharmacopoeia. In Europe, the relevant one is the European Pharmacopoeia (Eur. Ph.). Typically, such a monograph includes the following:

- Title (English name, Latin name used in international trade)
- Definition of the drug (plant part to be used; whether it is fresh, dried, cut or powdered, and possibly also specifying constituents typical for the drug, with minimal amounts required)
- Characteristics: i.e. organoleptic or other properties of the drug (smell, colour, other similar characteristics; taste is rarely included in the Eur. Ph. for reasons of safety)
- Identification (macroscopic and microscopic description, and in some cases thin-layer chromatographic (TLC) characteristics; see Table 9.3)
- Tests for purity (providing data on maximum amounts of foreign matter, i.e. non-acceptable substances, loss on drying, ash)
- Required level of biologically active or lead compounds
- Storage (general information about required forms of storage).

Table 9.3	Examples of botanical drugs characterized with the help of TLC		
DRUG (ENGLISH AND INTERNATIONAL TRADE NAMES)	**LATIN NAME OF PLANT SPECIES**	**REFERENCE SUBSTANCES USED**	**SUBSTANCES DETECTED VIA TLC**
Bitter fennel/Foeniculi amari fructus	*Foeniculum vulgare* subsp. *vulgare Mill.*	Anethole, fenchone	Anethole, fenchone, terpenes
Hamamelis leaf/Hamameli folium	*Hamamelis virginiana* L.	Tannic acid, gallic acid	Hamamelitannins (gallotannins), gallic acid
Peppermint leaf/Menthae piperitae folium	*Mentha* × *piperita* L.	Menthol, cineole, thymol, menthyl acetate	Monoterpenes of the essential oil (menthol, cineole, methyl acetate)
Primula (cowslip) root/Primulae radix	Primula veris L. and/or *P. elatior* (L.) Hill	Aescin[a]	Primula saponins
Senna leaf/Sennae folium	*Cassia angustifolia* Vahl and *C. senna* L.	Senna extract	Sennosides A–D, rhein-8-glucoside
Wormwood/Absinthii herba	*Artemisia absinthium* L.	Methyl red,[a] resorcinol[a]	Bitter sesquiterpene lactones, e.g. absinthin

[a]Reference substance normally not present in extracts of the species, but used because of suitability of R_F values compared with those present in the extract.

Pharmaceutical drugs have to comply with all the characteristics as they are defined in such a monograph, and material that does not comply must be rejected. In many cases, TLC methods for quality control are included, such as those given in Table 9.3.

There are several other methods in current use which help to assure a reproducible quality of the botanical material, whether it is used as a drug as such or whether it is used for preparing an (standardized) extract.

BOTANICAL (CLASSICAL PHARMACOGNOSTICAL) METHODS

One of the main tools for analysing botanical material is the microscope. Since botanical drugs have characteristic features, these can easily be used to establish the botanical identity and quality of a drug (see also Chapter 3).

A typical example is the various types of crystals formed by calcium oxalate. Several species of the family Solanaceae are used for obtaining atropine, which can be used as a spasmolytic in cases of gastrointestinal cramps and asthma, and as a diagnostic aid in ophthalmology for widening the pupil. Species with high concentrations of atropine include *Atropa belladona* (deadly nightshade or belladonna), *Datura stramonium* [thorn apple or Jimson (Jamestown) weed] and *Hyoscyamus niger* (henbane). Each is characterized by typical crystal structures of oxalate: sand, cluster crystals and microspheroidal crystals, respectively. These are subcellular crystal structures, which can easily be detected using polarized light and are thus a very useful diagnostic means, even though they are not involved in the medically relevant effects described above.

Another typical example is that of the glandular hairs, which in many species contain the essential oil. They are a very useful diagnostic feature because they have a characteristic structure. Fig. 9.2 shows glandular hairs that are typical of the Lamiaceae and Asteraceae.

A third example is the structure of the cells that form the surface of leaves and which contain the stomata (pores for the exchange of respiratory and photosynthetic gases). Form, size, number of stomata and many other features can be used to identify a certain species, or to detect untypical contaminating plant material in a drug.

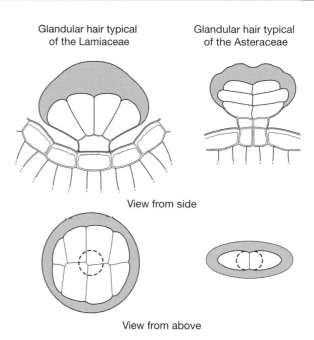

Fig. 9.2 Diagnostic features of botanical drugs that are revealed upon microscopic examination include typical glandular hair as found in the Lamiaceae and the Asteraceae. The top drawings show the lateral view; the bottom drawings show the view from above.

Other methods rely on typical properties of botanical drugs. The **bitterness value**, for example, is used for solutions of drugs that are used for their bitter(appetite stimulating) effect (Eur. Ph. 2002, Chapter 2.8.15). It is determined organoleptically (i.e. by taste) by comparison with quinine as standard. The bitterness value is important for centaury herb (Centaurii herba, *Centaurium erythraea* Rafn.), gentian root (Gentianae radix, *Gentianalutea* L.) and wormwood herb (Absinthii herba, *Artemisia absinthium* L.).

An example of a simple biophysical method is the **swelling index** (Eur. Ph. 2002, Chapter 2.8.4). This index is an indicator for the amount of polysaccharides present in a certain drug. It is defined as the volume (in ml) occupied by 1 g of a drug, including any adhering mucilage, after it has swollen in an aqueous liquid for 4 h. The drug is treated with 1.0 ml of ethanol (96%) and 25 ml water in a graduated cylinder, shaken every 10 min for 1 h and allowed to stand as specified. Some of the drugs are tested without pretreatment (e.g. fenugreek, ispaghula, linseed); others have to be powdered to a defined particle size prior to measuring the swelling index (e.g. marshmallow root). The required minimal swelling indices for a variety of

Table 9.4	Swelling indices for a variety of botanical drugs	
DRUG	SWELLING INDEX[a]
Agar (from several genera of marine algae, especially *Gelidium* and *Gracilaria*)	>10
Cetraria (Lichen islandicus, from *Cetraria islandica* (L.) Ach. s.l.)	>4.5
Fenugreek (Foenugraeci semen, from *Trigonella foenum-graecum* L.)	>6
Ispaghula husk (Plantaginis ovatae testae, from *Plantago ovata* Forssk.)	>40 (determined on 0.1 g of powder)
Ispaghula seed (Plantaginis ovatae semen)	>9
Linseed (Lini semen, whole drug from *Linum usitatissimum* L.)	>4
Linseed (Lini semen, powdered drug)	>4.5

[a]Measured as a multiple of the original volume.

botanical drugs are given in Table 9.4. If these values are not reached, it may be an indication that the botanical drug is contaminated with other drugs or that it is not of adequate quality (e.g. because it was not stored properly).

The key to modern industrial quality control is the phytochemical methods for the identification of active ingredients and their quantification. Phytochemical analysis indicates whether a sample contains the correct drug in the specified quality, whether it has been extracted in an appropriate manner and stored under the right conditions. The most commonly used analytical techniques are:

- **HPLC (high-performance liquid chromatography)**, used especially in the quantification of compounds and fingerprinting of extracts
- **GC (gas chromatography)**, used mostly for essential oils, and sometimes combined with mass spectrometry (MS)
- **TLC (thin-layer chromatography)**, which is simple and cheap and provides a good analytical tool for establishing the identity of a drug and for detecting contaminants containing similar types of compounds. The method is widely used, but not detailed, and it is not possible to quantify substances fully using TLC
- **NIR (near-infrared spectroscopy)**, used to assess the identity and quality of a botanical sample,

and also used for crude drug material. This technique is gaining in popularity

DNA-barcoding, that is the identification of a specific DNA sequence of selected genes in a species, is currently being developed to clearly identify from which species a botanical drug is derived. This method allows for the authentication of a species, but does not provide information on the purity of a botanical drug (i.e. if other plant parts were included, too) nor does it provide information on the quality of the material (e.g. its level of active constituents).

For most widely used botanical drugs, the relevant protocols can be found in the respective pharmacopoeias (see Box 9.1) or in protocols provided by the manufacturer. In the future, we may see the use of DNA-fingerprinting techniques as a novel and very sensitive tool for analysing the quality of all sorts of botanical material, including medicinal drugs.

Pulverized and other crude drug material may be sold as a medicine or health supplement, in which case there is no (chemical) quality control. In the pharmacopoeias of some EU countries a minimum amount of an ingredient, which is considered to be the active one, may be required for some crude drugs (see above). Some alternative and complementary forms of phytotherapy (e.g. Bach flower remedies) have no (or very limited) quality control. Exceptions are homoeopathic medicines (which are based on a completely different philosophical principle) and some high-quality but unlicensed herbal medicines.

DRUG: SOLVENT RATIO AND DRUG EXTRACT RATIO

Several indicators are used to describe the extract characteristics as it relates to the production process. In essence one can provide quality parameters by defining an extract in relation to the amount of a specific solvent used or by defining it in relation to the amount of starting material (plus type of solvent(s) used and the mode of extraction).

The drug:solvent ratio is calculated by dividing the amount of (dried) plant material by the amount of solvent used for extracting it. If the following information is provided 'DSR = 1:4 (EtOH, 70%) by maceration', the botanical drug was macerated with a four-fold amount of 70% ethanol.

BOX 9.1   Sample monograph from the European Pharmacopoeia (reprinted, with modifications, from European Pharmacopoeia 2002, p 1013–1014, with permission)

Devil's claw root

Harpagophyti radix

Definition

Devil's claw root consists of the cut and dried tuberous, secondary roots of *Harpagophytum procumbens* DC. [and/or *H. zeyheri* Decne]. It contains not less than 1.2% harpagoside ($C_{24}H_{30}O_{11}$; M_r 494.5), calculated with reference to the dried drug.

Characters

Devil's claw root is greyish-brown to dark brown and it has a bitter taste. It has the macroscopic and microscopic characters described in identification tests A and B.

Identification

A. It consists of thick, fan-shaped or rounded slices or of roughly crushed discs. The darker outer surface is traversed by tortuous longitudinal wrinkles. The paler cut surface shows a dark cambial zone and xylem bundles distinctly aligned in radial rows. The central cylinder shows fine concentric striations. Seen under a lens, the cut surface presents yellow to brownish-red granules.

B. Reduce to a powder (355). The powder is brownish-yellow. Examine under a microscope using *chloral hydrate* solution R. The powder shows the following diagnostic characters: fragments of cork layer consisting of yellowish-brown, thin-walled cells; fragments of cortical parenchyma consisting of large, thin-walled cells, sometimes containing reddish-brown granular inclusions and isolated yellow droplets; fragments of reticulately thickened vessels and tracheidal vessels with associated lignified parenchyma from the central cylinder; small needles and crystals of calcium oxalate are present in the parenchyma. The powder may show rectangular or polygonal pitted sclereids with dark reddish-brown contents. With a solution of phloroglucinol in hydrochloric acid, the parenchyma turns green.

C. Examine by thin-layer chromatography (*2.2.27*), using a suitable silica gel as the coating substance.

Test solution. Heat on a water-bath at 60°C for 10 min 1.0 g of the powdered drug (355) with 10 ml of *methanol R*. Filter and reduce the filtrate to about 2 ml under reduced pressure at a temperature not exceeding 40°C.

Reference solution. Dissolve 1 mg of harpagoside R in 1 ml of methanol R.

Apply to the plate as bands 20 µl of each solution. Develop over a path of 10 cm using a mixture of 8 volumes of *water R*, 15 volumes of *methanol R* and *77* volumes of *ethyl acetate R*. Dry the plate in a current of warm air. Examine in ultraviolet light at 254 nm. The chromatograms obtained with the test solution and the reference solution both show in the middle a quenching zone corresponding to harpagoside. The chromatogram obtained with the test solution shows other distinct bands, mainly above the zone corresponding to harpagoside. Spray with a 10 g/l solution of *phloroglucinol R* in *alcohol R* and then with *hydrochloric acid R*. Dry the plate at 80°C for 5–10 min. In the chromatograms obtained with the reference solution and the test solution the zone corresponding to harpagoside is green. The chromatogram obtained with the test solution also shows several yellow to brown zones below and above the zone corresponding to harpagoside.

Tests

Starch. Examine the powdered drug (355) under a microscope using *water R*. Add *iodine solution R1*. No blue colour develops.

Foreign matter (*2.8.2*). It complies with the test for foreign matter.

Loss on drying (*2.2.32*). Not more than 12.0%, determined on 1.000 g of the powdered drug (355) by drying in an oven at 100–105°C.

Total ash (*2.4.16*). Not more than 10.0%.

Assay

Examine by liquid chromatography (*2.2.29*) using *methyl cinnamate R* as the internal standard.

Internal standard solution. Dissolve 0.130 g of *methyl cinnamate R* in 50 ml of *methanol R* and dilute to 100.0 ml with the same solvent.

Test solution. To 0.500 g of the powdered drug (355) add 50 ml of *methanol R*. Shake for 1 h and filter. Transfer the filter with the residue to a 100 ml flask, add 50 ml of *methanol R* and heat under a reflux condenser for 1 h. Cool and filter. Rinse the flask and the filter with 2 quantities, each of 5 ml, of *methanol R*. Combine the filtrate and the rinsing solution and evaporate to dryness under reduced pressure at a temperature not exceeding 40°C. Take up the residue with 3 quantities, each of 5 ml, of *methanol R* and filter the extracts into a 25 ml volumetric flask. Whilst washing the filter, dilute to 25.0 ml with *methanol R*. To 10.0 ml of this solution add 1.0 ml of the internal standard solution and dilute to 25.0 ml with *methanol R*.

Continued

BOX 9.1   Sample monograph from the European Pharmacopoeia (reprinted, with modifications, from European Pharmacopoeia 2002, p 1013–1014, with permission)—cont'd

Reference solution. Dilute 0.5 ml of the reference solution described in identification test C to 2.0 ml with *methanol R.* The chromatographic procedure may be carried out using:
- a stainless steel column 0.10 m long and 4 mm in internal diameter packed with *octadecylsilyl silica gel for chromatography R* (5 μm)
- as mobile phase at a flow rate of 1.5 ml/min a mixture of equal volumes of *methanol R* and *water R*
- as detector a spectrophotometer set at *278* nm
- a 10 μl loop injector.

Inject the test solution. Adjust the sensitivity of the detector so that the height of the peak due to methyl cinnamate is about 50% of the full scale of the recorder. Determine the retention time of harpagoside using 10 μl of the reference

solution examined under the same conditions as the test solution.

Calculate the percentage content of harpagoside from the expression:

$$\frac{m_2 \times F_1 \times 7.622}{F_2 \times m_1}$$

m_1 = mass of the drug, in grams
m_2 = mass of *methyl cinnamate R*, in grams in the internal standard solution
F_1 = area of the peak corresponding to harpagoside in the chromatogram obtained with the test solution
F_2 = area of the peak corresponding to methyl cinnamate, in the chromatogram of the test solution.

Storage
Store protected from light.

Importantly, the ratio does not provide information on the quality of the plant material used or other parameters influencing the result of the extraction. In addition to this ratio, the solvent used, and the form of extraction (e.g. percolation – an extraction by moving fluids through powdered materials; maceration soaked in a liquid in order to produce an extract) needs to be included.

DEFINITIONS

Drug:extract ratio (DER): The ratio of a botanical drug to the amount of extract obtained, for example, 4 to 1 (4:1) – four units of a dried starting material (the botanical drug) yield one unit of extract (e.g. kg)

Drug:solvent ratio (DSR): The ratio of a botanical drug to the amount of solvent used in the extraction, for example, 1 to 8 (1:8) – eight units are used to extract one unit of a botanical drug. In general m/v (mass/ volume) or m/m (mass/mass) are used as units and very often a range is given (e.g. 1 to 6–10). In addition, the solvent and the type of extraction must also be stated.

The drug:extract ratio, on the other hand, gives information on *the amount of extract obtained from a botanical drug:* 4:1 (maceration, 70% ethanol). In this case 4 units (e.g. kg) of a drug yield 1 unit of dried extract. This DER is often given as a range (e.g. 3–5) and always in whole numbers. It varies considerably depending on the type of botanical drug which

is extracted and the solvents used. If chamomile flowers, for example, are extracted in water, the DER is in the range 6–8:1; if, on the other hand turmeric is extracted with 96% EtOH, the DER typically is in the range of 20–50:1. In other words, in the first case a large amount of extract can be obtained from a botanical drug (12–18%), in the second case only a very small amount (2–5%) can be obtained.

STANDARDIZATION

The concept of standardization is relatively recent for phytomedicines, but it is rapidly becoming essential to ensure that patients are provided with high-quality botanical products. Standardization can be defined as a **requirement to have a minimum amount of one or several compounds or groups of compounds in the extract**. Often a range from a minimum to a maximum amount is given. In the field of phytomedicines standardization *only* applies to extracts. For example, if an extract has to contain at least 8% of compound class X expressed as compound X1, this would indicate that the extract has to contain at least 8% of a class of compounds (e.g. flavonoids) as expressed in one specific compound of this group (as for example rutin). This quantification is normally done using HPLC or another appropriate analytical tool. An essential basis (but not a substitute) for this is the establishment of reproducible pharmaceutical quality (see previous chapter).

Why is standardization necessary and important? There are many reasons for using well-defined extracts, including, for example:

- reproducible composition and generally higher **quality** of the product. Standardization may require that the quantity of unwanted material in the extract should not exceed a certain limit, while active ingredients will have to be above a minimum concentration
- provided that the product is registered, it thus becomes a **medicine** that should comply with the basic standards required for all drugs
- standardization allows **comparison of the clinical effectiveness, pharmacological effects and side effects** of a series of products (e.g. against placebo). If a product is not standardized to active compounds, the comparison with other products derived from the same botanical drug is more problematic, since the composition may vary greatly
- such products give patients greater (objective and subjective) security and thus increase the level of trust people have in herbal products
- ensuring the quality of products sold has always been, and continues to be, a key responsibility of the pharmacist.

An example of a **standardization** in which a range (a maximum *and* minimum amount) of a certain compound or of several compounds is defined, is the extract of the leaves of *Ginkgo biloba* L. (Ginkgo folium). In this case, a standardized extract with a content of 2.8–3.4% ginkgolides, 2.6–3.2% bilobalide, 22–27% flavonoids and less than 5 ppm ginkgolic acid is commonly used. Such an extract is often called a 'special extract' and is obtained by further processing an extract in order to enrich desired compounds and reduce the amount of undesired ones. The production of ginkgo special extract is not a standardization in the strict sense, but a process of defining a range for certain compounds or classes of compounds.

TYPES OF EXTRACT

In dealing with the standardization of phytomedicines, there is a further problem. Extracts contain a mixture of active and inactive ingredients, but often it is not known which compounds contribute to the activity or the pharmacological effects of the extract. Generally, the whole herbal drug preparation (e.g. the extract) is regarded as the active pharmaceutical

ingredient. For quality control, several systems of classification have been proposed. A particularly useful one is now widely used on an EU-wide level; it has been described in a monograph of the Eur. Ph. (2003) and is thus accepted as a binding quality standard. Three classes of extracts are distinguished:

- **(Truly) standardized extracts (type A)**: extracts standardized to active constituents
- **Quantified extracts (type B1)**: extracts standardized to constituents that contribute to the activity
- **Other extracts (type B2)**: extracts standardized to lead compounds of unknown pharmacological relevance, which serve as quality markers.

This first classification heavily impacts on strategies for pharmaceutical quality control.

Standardized extracts

Truly standardized extracts are extracts for which the active constituents (single or groups) are known. They can thus be standardized to a defined content of the active constituent(s) giving a clearly defined amount of an active natural product. Examples include:

- **digitalis leaf** (Digitalis folium, foxglove)
- **senna dry extracts**: standardized to 5.5–8.0% hydroxyanthracene glycosides, calculated as sennoside B with reference to dried extract (Eur. Ph.)
- **belladonna leaf dry extract** (Belladonnae folium from *Atropa belladonna* L., deadly nightshade): standardized to 0.95–1.05% of alkaloids calculated as hyoscyamine (Eur. Ph.).

Adjustment (standardization) to a defined content is acceptable using inert excipients or preparations with a higher or lower content of active constituents. This type of extract is sometimes also referred to as 'normalized' extract, a term that is a much better description of this process of quality control (see above).

Quantified extracts

These are extracts with constituents having known therapeutic or pharmacological activity. Groups of compounds likely to have the desired pharmacological activity are unknown, but are not solely responsible for the clinical efficacy of the extract. The monograph must define a range of content of the selected constituent(s), some of which are lead compounds. This category includes special extracts, in which a certain compound or groups of compounds have been enriched and unwanted compounds have been excluded. Standardization by blending different batches of a herbal drug before extraction, or by mixing different lots of herbal drug preparation, is acceptable. Adjustment using excipients is *not* acceptable. Examples:

- *Ginkgo biloba* **L. leaf** (Ginkgo folium, ginkgo or maidenhair tree)
- *Hypericum perforatum* **L. aerial parts** (Hyperici herba, St John's wort).

Other extracts

These are extracts generally accepted to be pharmacologically active. However, the constituents responsible for this activity are not known and consequently **quality markers** have to be defined. These give information on the overall quality of the phytomedicine for control purposes and may be used to monitor good manufacturing practice, but cannot be used as evidence that the relevant active compounds are present in sufficient amounts or not. Examples:

- *Echinacea* (Echinacea radix and herba)
- *Crataegus* **aerial parts** (Crataegi folium cum flore, hawthorn)
- *Passiflora incarnata* **L. aerial parts** (Passiflorae herba, passion flower).

EXAMPLES OF DRUGS AND THEIR QUALITY CONTROL AND STANDARDIZATION

Several examples of ways to assure the identity of a botanical drug (quality control) and, if applicable, the ways extracts derived from such a drug are standardized have been discussed. Here, examples of

how a drug is characterized are given, together with some general background information and a brief discussion of the strengths and weaknesses of the various methods.

STANDARDIZED EXTRACTS

DIGITALIS PURPUREA FOLIUM (FOXGLOVE LEAVES)

Note: Digitalis purpurea folium is the botanical drug of the genus *Digitalis* and is currently monographed in the Eur. Ph. In this discussion, additional data on Digitalis lanatae folium (not monographed in Eur. Ph.) and *Digitalis* glycosides (monographed) are included.

William Withering's 'An account of foxglove and some of its medical uses' (1785) introduces foxglove as a remedy for dropsy and oedema, later additionally used for heart conditions, especially congestive heart failure. This is largely due to an inhibitory effect on Na^+/K^+-ATPase. Today, pure compounds (including semi-synthetic derivatives of digitalis glycosides, rather than standardized extracts) are used. The glycosides digoxin (the most widely used in the UK), digitoxin and lanatoside C all have monographs in the Eur. Ph. and are isolated industrially from the botanical drug using a multistep process. Therapeutically used digitalis glycosides are generally not chemically pure but may contain up to 5% (Eur. Ph.) or even 11% (USP) of other compounds. *Digitalis lanata* Ehrh. (Scrophulariaceae) is the species cultivated for obtaining the raw pharmaceutical product. Digitoxin is a degradation product of lanatoside A (from *Digitalis lanata*) [as well as of purpurea glycoside A (from *D. purpurea* L.)] (Fig. 9.3).

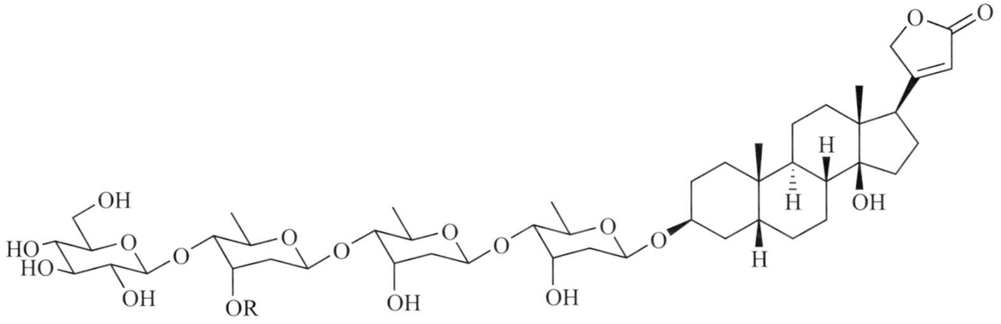

R = acetyl, **Lanatoside A**
R = H, **Purpureaglycoside A**

Fig. 9.3

Since the active constituents are known, foxglove extracts clearly fall into the category of (truly) standardized extracts. The extracts are important in the industrial production of the pure compounds and, consequently, numerous methods for quality control have been developed; these show the range of pharmacognostical tools available to assess the quality of the botanical drug and the extract derived from it.

QUALITY CONTROL

Typical microscopical characteristics of the pulverized drug (see Fig. 9.4) include:

- 2–7-celled clothing trichomes (clothing hairs) with cells often collapsed and glandular hairs composed of a characteristic gland and a unicellular stem cell (pedicel)
- characteristic structure of polygonal epidermal cells and stomata
- calcium oxalate and sclerenchyma are absent.

After the identification of the botanical drug using, for example, microscopic methods or methods described below, the material is investigated in order to quantify the active ingredients (phytochemical analysis). HPLC and TLC may be used both to establish the identity of a botanical drug and to quantify the actives.

Although these methods are generally quite reliable and offer a high degree of reproducibility, the core problem of digitalis is that the cardenolides differ widely in their pharmacological potency and

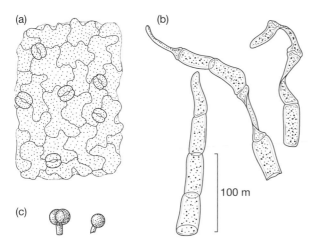

(a)

(b)

100 m

(c)

Fig. 9.4 Microscopic appearance of powdered botanical drug material from digitalis leaf (Digitalis purpurea folium), showing (a) irregularly shaped lower epidermis with stomata, (b) unusual multicellular hairs with some cells having collapsed during the drying process, (c) glandular hairs.

that the safe dose range is very narrow. Therefore, biological methods have considerable advantages over chemical analysis. The most widely used is inhibition of the activity of Na^+/K^+-ATPase in a solubilized preparation:

$$ATP \xleftarrow{\text{ATPase}} ATPaseADP + P_i$$

If the ATP is labelled radioactively (^{32}P), the resulting amount of free radiolabelled P_i can easily be determined. Alternatively, the final reaction product of two subsequent reactions can be determined:

ADP

$$+phosphoenolpyruvate \xleftarrow{\text{pyruvatekinase}} ATP + pyruvate$$

In a last step, pyruvate is metabolized by lactate dehydrogenase to yield lactate:

$$Pyruvate + NADH \xleftarrow{\text{lactate dehydrogenase}} NAD + lactate$$

Although the above methods can be used for quantifying compounds in botanical material, the exact determination of digitalis glycosides in blood and plasma is even more important. For this, radioimmunoassay (RIA) or enzyme linked immunosorbent assay (ELISA) has been shown to be the most reliable method.

- **RIA** An antigen (digoxin, etc., covalently bound to a hapten) is used to induce antibody production in a rabbit. The quantity of digitoxin is determined by co-incubating the labelled antigen–hapten (defined amount) with the unlabelled antigen (unknown); if more unlabelled antigen is present, the amount of bound antigen is reduced. The analysis of trace amounts is possible, but such a highly specific method is generally only available in specialized laboratories.
- **ELISA** The antibodies are fixed to the surface of, for example, a microtitre plate. The sample with an unknown amount of antigen (digitoxin) is then added together with hapten-bound enzyme-labelled (e.g. peroxidase) antigen (also digitoxin). Both compete for the binding positions. After washing, the read-out is the rate of production of a coloured compound, which is quantified photometrically. The amount of digoxin in a sample is calculated from the amount of labelled antigen, which is highest when the least unbound antigen is present.

Lastly, *in vivo* biological determination was used for many years (i.e. the LD_{50} in guinea pigs). This is determined using an infusion of solution with an unknown amount of digitoxin and measuring the survival time of the animals. The concentration is determined by comparison with a standard solution applied to control animals.

(TRULY) STANDARDIZED EXTRACTS

SENNAE FOLIUM (SENNA LEAF)

This is a commonly used purgative appropriate for short-term use, with well-established effectiveness and significant side effects if used over prolonged periods of time. The species used pharmaceutically are *Cassia senna* L. (syn. *C. acutifolia* Delile), also known as Alexandrian senna, and *Cassia angustifolia* Vahl, or Tinnevelly senna (Caesalpiniaceae). Both names make reference to the former ports of export of the botanical material. The name in international trade for both species is Sennae folium (=senna leaf). The following constituents are important for the pharmacological effects of the drug:

- Sennosides, including sennosides A and B (Fig. 9.5)
- Glucosides of rhein (e.g. rhein-8*O*-glucoside) and aloe-emodin.

Quality control

Some characteristic microscopic features of the drug include the unique non-lignified warty hairs up to 250 μm long, and small cluster crystals as well as prisms of calcium oxalate. Another characteristic are the stomata with two cells with the long axes parallel to the pore (diacytic stomata), the mid-rib bundle and larger veins of the leaves surrounded by a zone of lignified pericyclic fibres and a sheath of parenchymatous cells containing prisms of calcium oxalate (Fig. 9.6).

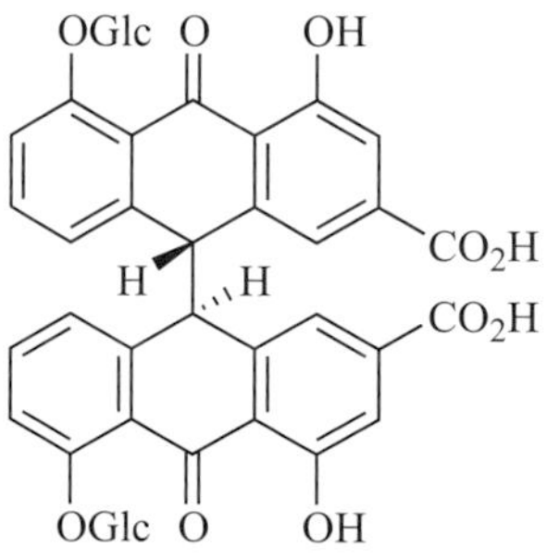

OGlc O   OH

CO_2H

H   H

CO_2H

OGlc O   OH

Sennoside A

Fig. 9.5

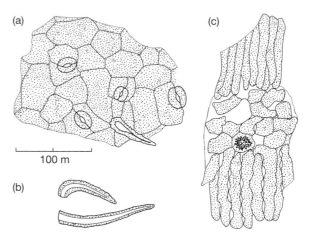

Fig. 9.6 Microscopic appearance of the lower surface of senna leaves (Sennae folium) showing (a) the epidermal cells, (b) typical bend hairs with an uneven surface, (c) cross-section of a leaf with an irregular oxalate crystal.

As regards phytochemical methods, according to the Eur. Ph., sennosides and rhein-8-glucoside should be detected using 98% acetic acid/water/ethyl acetate/1-propanol (1:30:40:40). Prior to spraying with Borntraeger reagent (potassium hydroxide), the glycosides are oxidized and hydrolysed by spraying the plate with nitric acid and subsequent heating (120°C, 10 min). In this case an extract is used as reference material. Sennosides show up as red-brown spots at R_F 0.15–0.44; sometimes, rhein-8-glucoside can also be detected as a red zone around R_F 0.40. This methods allows the detection of other anthranoid-containing drugs, but, since the material is grown commercially, adulteration or contamination with other drugs is rare. This is another clear example of a type A extract. The active constituents are well known, they are easily characterized by TLC, and quantification of the active compounds is possible (e.g. with the help of HPLC).

QUANTIFIED EXTRACTS

GINKGO BILOBA LEAVES

Ginkgo biloba leaves are used for improving cerebral and peripheral circulation in the elderly, as well as for vertigo and other complaints that involve reduced cerebral circulation. Unlike many other phytomedicines, most of the pharmaceutically relevant products are hydroalcoholic 'full' or 'special' extracts, the latter being analytically very well characterized. In this case, a relatively broad range of active ingredients are known, of which two groups of compounds are particularly relevant:

- Flavonoids (0.5–1%): flavone and flavonol glycosides, acetylated flavonol glycosides, biflavonoids
- Terpene lactones (0.03–0.25%).

Special extracts have the largest share of the market in Continental Europe. Although the two groups of compounds are important for understanding the pharmacological effects of the drug, other compounds may also be important. These extracts also have a significantly reduced level of unwanted groups of compounds (polyphenols, polysaccharides and ginkgolic acids) and an increased percentage of flavonoid glycosides (16–26%) and terpene lactones (5–7%). It is, therefore, a typical example of a type B1 extract, in which the constituents have known therapeutic or pharmacological activity. But these compounds are not solely responsible for the clinical efficacy of the extract.

Quality control

Microscopy is less useful in quality control here, so phytochemical methods are predominant.

In the case of the crude drug, TLC is only feasible for the flavonoids. The terpene lactones are only present in a small concentration and they are accompanied by substances which interfere with the analysis. The special extracts can be analysed using the following TLC methods:

- Flavonoids: ethyl acetate/formic acid/glacial acetic acid/water (100:11:11:26), detection with diphenylboryloxyethylamine.
- Biflavones: chloroform/acetone/formic acid (75:16.5:8.5), detection with diphenylboryloxyethylamine.
- Terpene lactones: toluene/acetone (70:30), detection with acetic acid reagent.

Standardization

The above methods are qualitative and, as in the previous examples, do not allow the quantification of the relevant compounds. Consequently, HPLC and GC methods are paramount for the quantification of lead substances:

- HPLC is used for the determination of the three aglycones quercetin, kaempferol and isorhamnetin (after hydrolysis of the glycosides).

- GC is used for the quantification of the terpene lactones.

No single method gives all the results required, thus complex analyses are required.

OTHER EXTRACTS

PASSIFLORAE HERBA (PASSION FLOWER)

Passion flower herb (Passiflorae herba, *Passiflora incarnata* L.) is used as a mild phytomedicine in chronic fatigue syndrome, nervousness and anxiety. Some clinical studies and other data point to the efficacy of the drug, but it is not clear which compounds are responsible.

Quality control

Microscopic analysis gives a very characteristic picture, including prominent pieces of the lower epidermis with cells around the stomata, which cannot be distinguished from the other cells of the epidermis (anomocytic), and cluster crystals below the surface. The material is also characterized by typical hairs (Fig. 9.7).

Of the known ingredients, flavone glycosides such as isovitexin are relatively abundant, and traces of essential oil and a cyanogenetic glycoside have been found. The presence of harman-type alkaloids, which was reported in earlier work, has not been corroborated in more recent studies. Clinical data confirm the usefulness of this species for the conditions mentioned above, but the compounds responsible for the activity are not definitively known. Chrysin and other flavonoids have been shown to be biologically active, and, consequently, the flavonoids are used as **markers**. Thus it is an example of a type B2 extract. In this case, quality control can only assure reproducible quality of the extract. Both qualitative and quantitative methods have been developed:

- Qualitative analysis: TLC analysis of a methanolic extract (Eur. Ph.) using rutin and hyperoside as reference; plate development with acetic acid/water/ethyl methyl ketone/ethyl acetate (10:10:30:50), detection at 365 nm (UV) after spraying with diphenylboryloxyethylamine
- Quantitative analysis: spectrophotometric or fingerprinting with HPLC.

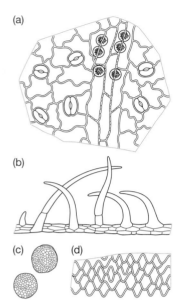

Fig. 9.7 Microscopic appearance of passion flower herb (Passiflorae herba) showing (a) typical fragment of the lower epidermis of a leaf with some calcium oxalate structures along the small veins, (b) sickle-shaped long unicellular trichomes and (c) the unusual pollen. Contrary to drugs derived from leaves, herb material contains typical elements of the flowers, such as the epidermis of the inner corolla (d) and relatively large amounts of pollen, and/or fruit and also often stem material.

ECHINACEA ROOT (*E. PURPUREA* AND *E. PALLIDA*)

Echinacea purpurea and *E. pallida* are used as immunostimulants and in the treatment of respiratory infections. Both species are employed in the preparation of pharmaceutical products and some data on efficacy are available for both. Other species are also used, but there is insufficient information available to validate their use. The active constituents are not known. Extracts of these two species on the market (and generally accepted to be pharmacologically active) can therefore be classified as type B2. Prominent constituents include caffeic acid derivatives (about 1%), especially echinacoside (*E. pallida*),

cichoric acid (*E. purpurea*), alkamides (*E. purpurea*), minor amounts of essential oil and polysaccharides (both *Echinacea* spp.).

Quality control

The drug is difficult to identify microscopically, but some botanical characteristics can be used. As a consequence, methods for quality control (identification) focus on phytochemcial techniques.

Drug identification (authentication), using phytochemical methods, is generally performed with TLC (ethyl acetate/formic acid/glacial acetic acid/water, 100:11:11:26). This method detects the caffeic acid derivatives, which thus serve as a marker for the pharmaceutical quality and also identify the plant material used for producing the phytopharmaceutical. Some good HPLC methods are available, but have not yet been systematically employed in quality control. As the active constituents are not known, they cannot, of course, be quantified.

CONCLUSION

There are many strategies for securing adequate quality. The process of quality assurance covers the whole range from the agricultural production, the extraction and formulation, to dispensing the product. The more commonly used medicinal plants are in the European Pharmacopoeia or other pharmacopoeias and the relevant technical data can be found there. Both botanical/pharmacognostical and phytochemical methods are relevant and which methods are used depends on the type of pharmaceutical product.

Standardization is a method of assuring a minimum level of active ingredients in the extract and it is becoming increasingly important as a means of ensuring a consistent composition of high-quality phytopharmaceutical products and offers opportunities to produce herbal medicines of reproducible composition.

References

European Pharmacopoeia, 2002. Council of Europe (Directorate for the Quality of Medicines), fourth ed. European Pharmacopoeia, Strasbourg.

European Pharmacopoeia, 2003. European Directorate for the Quality of Medicines and HealthCare (EDQM). Strasbourg, France.

Evans, W.C., 2009. Trease and Evans's pharmacognosy, sixteenth ed. WB Saunders, London.

Franz, C., 1999. Züchtung und Anbau von Arnzeipflanzen.

In: Rimpler, H. (Ed.), Biogene Arzneistoffe, 2 Aufl. Wissenschaftliche Verlagsgesellschaft, Stuttgart, pp. 1–19.

Goodman, J., Walsh, V., 2001. The story of taxol. Nature and politics in the pursuit of an anti-cancer drug. Cambridge University Press, Cambridge.

Lange, D., 2000. Conservation and sustainable use of *Adonis vernalis*, a medicinal plant in international trade. Plant species conservation monographs, vol. 1. Federal Agency for Nature Conservation, Bonn.

Further reading

Eschrich, W., 1999. Pulver-Atlas der Drogen der deutschsprachigen Arzneibücher. Deutscher Apotheker Verlag, Stuttgart.

Heinrich, M., Pieroni, A., Bremner, P., 2005. Medicinal plants and phytomedicines. In: Nesbitt, M., Prance, G. (Eds.), The cultural history of plants. Routledge (Taylor and Francis), New York, pp. 205–238.

Heinrich, M., Modarai, M., Kortenkamp, A., 2008. Herbal extracts used for upper respiratory tract infections: Are there clinically relevant interactions with the Cytochrome P450 enzyme system? Planta Med. 74, 657–660.

Hohmann, B., Reher, G., Stahl-Biskup, E., 2001. Mikroskopische Drogenmonographien der deutschsprachigen Arzneibücher. Wissenschaftliche Verlagsgesellschaft, Stuttgart.

Mukherjee, P.K., Mukherjee, D., Venkatesh, M., Rai, S., Heinrich, M., 2009. The sacred lotus (*Nelumbo nucifera*) – phytochemical and therapeutic profile. J. Pharm. Pharmacol. 61, 407–422.

Rahfeld, B., 2009. Mikroskopischer Farbatlas pflanzlicher Drogen. Spektrum Akademischer Verlag, Heidelberg.

Rimpler, H., 1999. Biogene Arzneistoffe. Wissenschaftliche Verlagsgesellschaft, Stuttgart.

Stewart, K.M., Cole, D., 2005. The commercial harvest of devil's claw (*Harpagophytum* spp.) in southern Africa: The devil's in the details. J. Ethnopharmacol. 100, 225–236.

Chapter 10

Toxicity of herbal constituents

Most toxic effects of herbal medicines are due to the poor quality of the product. For example, herbal medicines may be adulterated with synthetic medicines and other compounds, or there may be problems in the production of such herbal medicines. However, some toxic compounds, including the pyrrolizidine alkaloids and aristolochic acids, still pose potential serious risks for a few plant-derived products.

This chapter is not about toxic plants as such (see Nelson et al 2006), but about those plants used as herbal medicines and in therapy. Most common herbal remedies are fairly safe in clinical use; not because they are 'natural', but because the long history of use has uncovered some of the adverse effects.

Traditional use is not always a reliable indication of safety, since toxicity which results only from chronic use, or manifests after a long interval between taking the medicine and the onset of a reaction, may make the connection difficult. Many patients do not consider phytomedicines to be 'drugs', therefore an association may not have been made between the remedy and an adverse reaction, so even though a herb has been used for hundreds of years there may remain cause for vigilance. Knowledge of the chemistry and metabolism of the constituents of a herb can help to predict toxicity problems.

As with all medicines, side effects and interactions with other drugs are possible; but these are a consequence of the therapeutic use of the herb and an assessment of the usual risk:benefit ratio should be made. Problems produced by misidentification, variations in composition, which may cause overdose or underdose, and contamination with microorganisms, pesticides or heavy metals are quality issues; however, there are a number of known toxic constituents,

which confer no apparent health benefit, and herbs containing them should be avoided. Allergic reactions can be elicited by any drug, and idiosyncratic responses by definition cannot be foreseen; these are certainly not restricted to plant medicines, although some plant families (e.g. Asteraceae, Ranunculaceae) are notorious for their allergenicity.

PYRROLIZIDINE ALKALOIDS

These have only been reported in the plant families Boraginaceae, Asteraceae, Leguminosae, Apocynaceae, Ranunculaceae and Scrophulariaceae, and not in all species. Medicinal herbs that may be affected include comfrey (*Symphytum* spp.), butterbur (*Petasites hybridus* (L.) P. Gaertn., B. Mey. & Scherb.), alkanet (*Alkanna tinctoria* Tausch, Boraginaceae), coltsfoot (*Tussilago farfara*) and hemp agrimony (*Eupatorium cannabinum* L., Asteraceae). Not all pyrrolizidine alkaloids are toxic, only those that are unsaturated at the 1,2-position (e.g. senecionine; Fig. 10.1). These are liver toxins and can produce veno-occlusive disease of the hepatic vein as well as being hepatocarcinogenic, and their effects are cumulative. Several documented clinical examples can be found in the literature. Although highly toxic, they are chemically rather labile and may, therefore, not present the serious risk originally thought, at least in herbal medicines that have undergone a lengthy process involving heat. For example, when six commercial samples of comfrey leaf were tested, none of these alkaloids were detectable. However, in fresh plant material, and also root samples, they may be present in significant amounts. The total

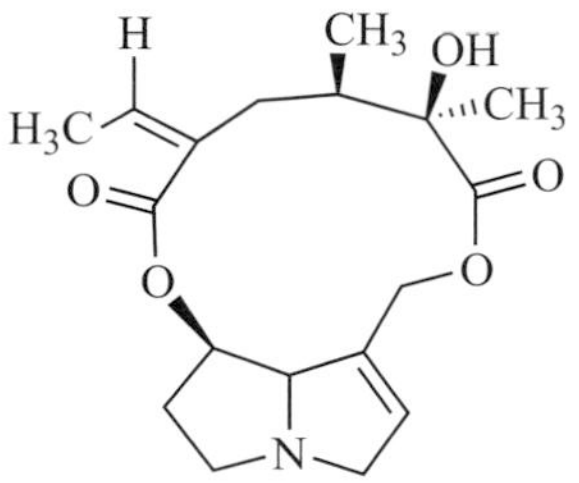

Senecionine

Fig. 10.1

recommended maximum dose of these alkaloids is less than 1 μg daily for less than 6 weeks per year. If herbal products, which may contain these, are to be employed (and some are very useful, e.g. butterbur and coltsfoot; see Chapter 16), the content must be estimated and, if necessary, the alkaloids should be removed before use.

ARISTOLOCHIC ACID

Most species of birthwort (*Aristolochia*, known as snakeroot) and related genera including *Asarum*, all from the family Aristolochiaceae, contain aristolochic acid and aristolactams. *Aristolochia* has been found as an ingredient in a slimming formula along with dexfenfluramine and in Europe, since the mid 1990s, more than one hundred cases of nephropathy caused by the systemic and long term use of Chinese snakeroot (*Aristolochia fangchi* Y.C. Wu ex L.D. Chow & S.M. Hwang), mainly in these weight-loss preparations, has highlighted the risk of using preparations which contain aristolochic acids. Aristolochic acid A (Fig. 10.2) is nephrotoxic and has been responsible for several deaths from renal failure. *Aristolochia* and other species containing these compounds are banned from sale in Europe and the USA, but may still be present in imported Chinese medicines, and *A. fangchi* has

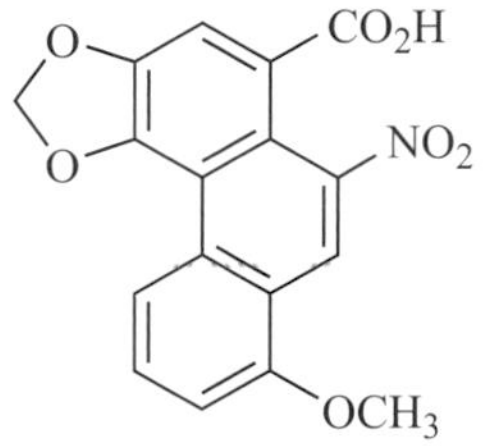

Aristolochic acid A

Fig. 10.2

been found substituted for *Stephania tetrandra* S. Moore. Herbs containing these substances must not be used. The disastrous consequences of using them have been a wake-up call for the regulatory authorities and the herbal industry. On the other hand, in many regions of the world species from the genus are widely used as local and traditional medicines especially in the treatment of gastrointestinal complaints like diarrhoea, of snake bites and poisoning, and of gynaecological conditions, including the treatment of sexually transmitted diseases (STDs) such as syphilis and gonorrhoea (Heinrich et al 2009; Nortier et al 2000).

ACONITINE AND CONTROVERSIAL CLAIMS ABOUT 'DETOXIFICATION'

Aconitum species (Ranunculaceae) are widely distributed throughout the northern hemisphere and have been used medicinally for centuries. They provide a fascinating example of a highly toxic botanical drug, which, according to claims made by some practitioners, can be detoxified by means of its method of preparation. The tubers and roots of *Aconitum* species such as *Aconitum kusnezoffii* Reichb. and *Aconitum japonicum* Thunb. are commonly used in Traditional Chinese Medicine in the treatment of conditions including syncope, rheumatic fever, painful joints, gastroenteritis, diarrhoea, oedema, bronchial asthma, various types of tumour and even some endocrinal disorders like irregular menstruation. However, the cardio- and neurotoxicity of this drug is potentially lethal, and the improper use of *Aconitum* in China, India, Japan and some other countries still results in a high risk of severe intoxication Singhuber et al 2009.

Based upon the regulations stipulated by the State Food and Drug Administration of China (SFDA), only the processed (i.e. 'detoxified') tubers and roots of *Aconitum* are allowed to be administered orally or adopted as raw materials for pharmaceutical manufacturing. To date, more than 70 traditional and modern techniques are applied for processing *Aconitum* roots for medicinal use. In China, only two assays are accepted for the quantitative determination of the alkaloid content in *Aconitum* species in the *Chinese Pharmacopoeia 2005*, and these allow a maximum of 0.15% and 0.20% respectively of alkaloids, calculated as aconitine. Botanical drugs which are below this threshold can be used medicinally in China but this position is not accepted in Europe.

MONOTERPENES AND PHENYLPROPANOIDS

Most mono- and sesquiterpenes found in essential oils are fairly safe, apart from causing irritation when used undiluted and allergic reactions in susceptible individuals. However, some have been shown to be carcinogenic, for example safrole (from *Sassafras* bark) and β-asarone (from *Acorus calamus* L.) (Fig. 10.3). They do not appear to give cause for concern when present in minute amounts in other oils. Methysticin, from nutmeg, is toxic in large doses, and has been postulated as being a metabolic precursor of the psychoactive drug methylene dioxymethamphetamine. Thujone (Fig. 10.3), which is present in wormwood (*Artemisia absinthium* L.) and in the liqueur absinthe, is also toxic and hallucinogenic in large doses.

SESQUITERPENE LACTONES

These compounds are present in many Asteraceae plants, and are often responsible for the biological activity of the herb. Some are cytotoxic and some are highly allergenic, which can cause problems if misidentification occurs of, for example, mayweed (*Anthemis cotula*) for one of the chamomiles (*Anthemis nobilis* L. or *Matricaria recutita* L.). Anthecotulide (Fig. 10.4) is one such allergen and is present in several species of the Asteraceae (the daisy family, Compositae).

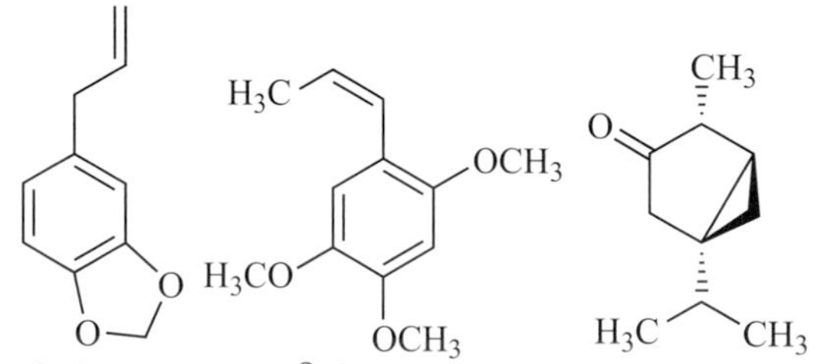

Safrole   **β-Asarone**   **Thujone**

Fig. 10.3

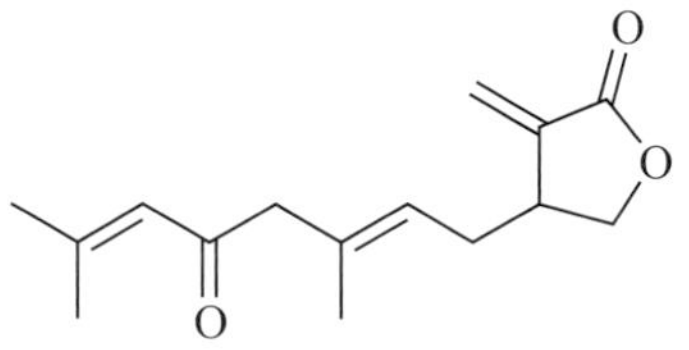

Anthecotulide

Fig. 10.4

DITERPENE ESTERS

The phorbol, daphnane and ingenol esters are found in plants of the Euphorbiaceae and Thymeliaceae. Some are highly pro-inflammatory and are known to activate protein kinase C, as well as having tumour-promoting (co-carcinogenic) activity. The most important is tetradecanoyl phorbol acetate (formerly known as phorbol myristate acetate; Fig. 10.5), which is an important biochemical probe used in pharmacological research. Some of these plants were formerly used as drastic purgatives (e.g. croton oil, from *Croton tiglium* L., Euphorbiaceae) but should now be avoided in herbal products.

PLANT LECTINS AND AGGLUTININS

Castor beans, which are used to produce castor oil for use in medicines and cosmetics, contain a toxic lectin, ricin. This is denatured during manufacture of the oil, but the oil, and the seed cake remaining (which is used as animal feed), should not be used without heat processing. Pokeweed (*Phytolacca americana* L.), which is sometimes used as an anti-inflammatory herb, contains phytoagglutinins called pokeweed mitogens. These have been known to cause gastrointestinal upset when taken in the fresh herb, but as they are heat-labile they may denature on processing. They are also used as biochemical tools in immunology research, for example in blood grouping, erythrocyte polyagglutination, and lymphocyte subpopulation studies.

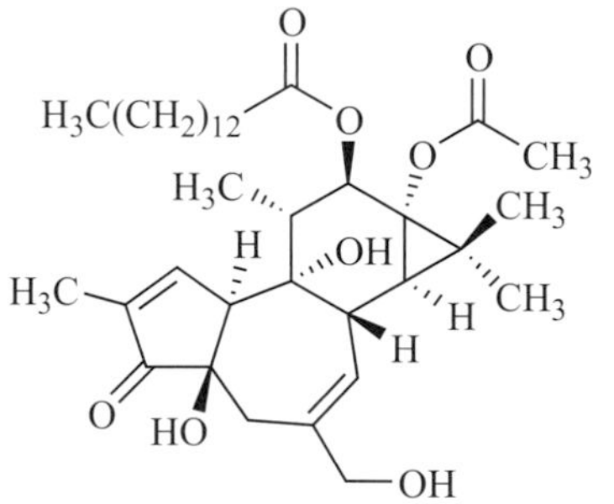

Tetradecanoyl phorbol acetate (TPA)

Fig. 10.5

FURANOCOUMARINS

Some furanocoumarins (e.g. psoralen, xanthotoxin and imperatorin), which are found in giant hogweed (*Heracleum mantegazzianum* Sommier & Levier) and other umbelliferous plants, as well as in some citrus peels, are phototoxic and produce photodermatitis and rashes on contact. They have a minor legitimate use in PUVA therapy (psoralen plus UV-A radiation) in the treatment of psoriasis, but this is an uncommon therapy used only in specialist hospital clinics. These compounds are known to form adducts with DNA, as shown in Fig. 10.6.

URUSHIOL DERIVATIVES

The urushiols (Fig. 10.7), anacardic acids and ginkgolic acids are phenolic compounds with a long side-chain. The uroshiols are found in poison ivy (*Toxicodendron radicans* (L.) Kuntze) and poison oak [*T. quercifolium* (Michx.) Greene] and cause

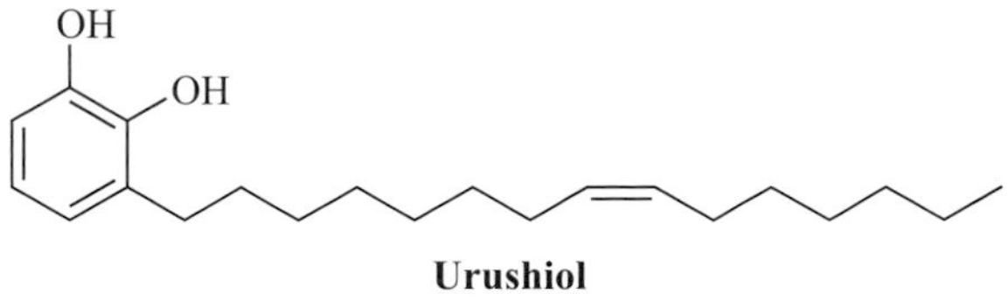

Urushiol

Fig. 10.7

severe contact dermatitis. This is a major problem in the USA, but less so in Europe where the plants are not native. The anacardic acids, which are found in the liquor surrounding the cashew nut (*Anacardium occidentale* L.), are less toxic. The ginkgolic acids are reputed to cause allergic reactions; however, they are present in the Ginkgo biloba seed more than in the leaf, which is the medicinal part. Ginkgo rarely causes this sort of reaction so in practice it is not regarded as a health hazard.

The examples above are not comprehensive but highlight some core problems and how this can be controlled with appropriate pharmaceutical measures.

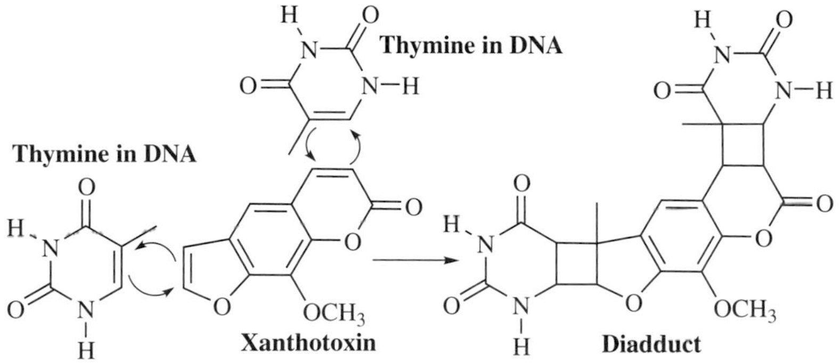

Fig. 10.6

References

Heinrich, M., Chan, J., Wanke, S., Neinhuis, Ch., Simmonds, M.S.S., 2009. Local uses of *Aristolochia* species and content of aristolochic acid 1 and 2 – a global assessment based on bibliographic sources. J. Ethnopharmacol. 125, 108–144.

Nelson, L.S., Shih, R.D., Balick, M., 2006. Handbook of poisonous and injurious plants, second ed. NY and Springer Heidelberg, The New York Botanical Garden.

Nortier, J.L., Martinez, M.C., Schmeiser, H.H., et al., 2000. Urothelial carcinoma associated with the use of a Chinese herb (Aristolochia fangchi). N. Engl. J. Med. 342, 1686–1692.

Singhuber, J., Zhu, M., Prinz, S., Kopp, K., 2009. Aconitum in traditional Chinese medicine – a valuable drug or an unpredictable risk? J. Ethnopharmacol. 126, 18–30.

Chapter 11

What makes phytomedicines unique?

Phytomedicines have particular attributes, which are not encountered when using synthetic drugs or single compounds. Although many natural products have been isolated and are used therapeutically as single ingredients, for example most alkaloids (morphine, hyoscine), cardiac glycosides (digoxin), anticancer agents (paclitaxel, vincristine) and other highly potent drugs. Many more are used in the form of herbal remedies or phytomedicines. Either the whole herb or an extract of the plant is prepared, and may be combined with other herbs or extracts.

Also, there is a continuum between products which are a (health) food and those which are a potent herbal medicine (called the food–medicine interface). In the area of food research, considerable efforts have been put into understanding the benefits of a 'balanced diet' and thus a diet which is composed of a complex combination of mixtures. However, in medicines research in general and specifically in research on herbal medicines systematic research has only been developed since the start of this century (Williamson 2001).

Generally, highly toxic drugs are used as single entities since the dose needs to be very precise, but the natural mixture found in a plant extract may have benefits conferred by some form of interaction between the components. Conversely, there may be toxic ingredients present that do not contribute to the therapeutic efficacy and which are, therefore, undesirable. If the toxic component is also one of the active principles, then the usual assessment of risk:benefit profile applies, but quite often the toxic compound serves no useful purpose and must either be removed or some form of limit test applied. Some examples are discussed in Chapter 10.

Phytomedicines often take a while to produce a measurable improvement and appear to have a cumulative effect; for this reason, long-term therapy is routine. This is not a unique property of natural products but is also found in conventional medicines (e.g. the antidepressants, where several weeks of treatment may be necessary before a clinical improvement is seen). The use of drug combinations is also not confined to herbal products; for example, cancer chemotherapy and the treatment of HIV and hypertension routinely use drug combinations. In addition, although many phytomedicines may have been characterized phytochemically, their mechanism of action is still unknown, which makes isolation of one constituent impossible.

PROPERTIES OF MIXTURES

Herbal practitioners have always argued that the effects of combinations of ingredients, such as those found in herbal medicines, contribute to the efficacy of phytomedicines, but until recently there has been little evidence to demonstrate that this is the case. In the absence of direct (i.e. clinical) evidence to demonstrate that combination effects are taking place, indirect evidence may be useful, for example, instances where it appears that the dose of supposed active constituents, calculated on the basis of the amount of a known constituent, is too low to have an effect, but clinical and pharmacological evidence has shown that the preparation is in fact effective. This is the case with willow bark, which will be discussed later. In general, synergistic and other interactions within herbal mixtures are considered to be positive, enabling lower doses of potent compounds to be used and reducing the incidence and severity of side effects. The properties of mixtures described below apply to all types of combinations between two or more drugs, whether of herbal or synthetic origin. They also apply to drug interactions, which are also a form of synergistic, antagonistic or additive effect, and the mechanisms of interaction are the same. The body does not know or care where a therapeutic agent originated; it deals with them all in the same way, and with the same mechanisms and the same enzymes!

SYNERGISTIC, MULTI-FACTORIAL AND POLYVALENT EFFECTS

Synergy and other forms of interaction between the constituents of herbal extracts is expected, and widely cited as a fundamental tenet of phytotherapy, but it is still poorly documented, despite a great deal of interest. Interactions may result in enhancement of a therapeutic effect, reduction of toxicity or preservation of stability. Synergy is a specific type of interaction, and needs to be proven experimentally; however, although it may take place, it actually may not be the most important type of interaction occurring in herbal mixtures. Not only may two or more components of a mixture interact with each other, but also single constituents may interact with different pharmacological targets. Thus, the various interaction mechanisms involved in the action of phytomedicines are now mainly referred to as **multi-factorial effects** (also known as **polyvalent action**) and may include the following:

- **Several compounds affecting a single target, either directly or indirectly:** this may include synergy, the metabolism of one active altered by the presence of others in the extract, or the bioavailability of a component changed by the presence of another. These are true interactions and may include pharmacokinetic and pharmacodynamic interactions
- **A single compound affecting multiple targets:** this is not an interaction between components of a mixture of course, but it helps to explain why a particular herbal medicine (or any drug, for that matter) can be used for different purposes

- **Multiple compounds affecting multiple related targets:** these are not necessarily interactions, but the result of a number of constituents acting in different ways; however, interactions could certainly also be taking place. There may be cases where the effect of one compound cancels out the effect of another by antagonism and this would not be known unless fractionation of an extract before testing had been carried out.

Several or all of these mechanisms may be taking place at the same time, and the overall effect is, therefore, the result of a complex interaction between different components of a mixture and different targets which may all be relevant in the treatment of a particular condition. There may be unwanted interactions in or between phytomedicines, such as the presence of high levels of tannins in a herbal drug, which may complex with and inhibit the absorption of proteins and alkaloids. As with conventional medicines, interactions may be mediated via the induction or inhibition of cytochrome P450 enzymes or P-glycoprotein, and these are discussed below. It must also be remembered that herbalists use preparations and mixtures not necessarily intended to target a particular enzyme or biochemical system. The use of phytomedicines has been described as the 'herbal shotgun' approach, as opposed to the 'silver bullet' method of conventional medicine. This approach would not only encompass synergy in a herb, but would even include routine practices such as adding a laxative to a formula for haemorrhoids.

While here we focus on the unique characteristics of complex mixtures, novel concepts and approaches in pharmacology show 'the other side of the coin'. **Network pharmacology** and **systems biology** are used to represent the different types of relationships between biological entities such as genes, proteins, chemical compounds, and transcription factors. In essence, the single drug single target view is giving way to a more complex understanding of networks within an organism affected by a medicine and the complexity of the intervention (Pujol et al 2010).

MECHANISMS OF INTERACTION

Interactions can also be classified as:

- *pharmacodynamic*: where the effects of one drug are altered or added to by the presence of another at the site of action (so-called 'pharmacological' interactions)
- *pharmacokinetic*: processes involving absorption, distribution, metabolism and excretion.

An example of both is provided by Ayurveda, where an ancient combination formula known as 'Trikatu' contains black pepper (*Piper longum*). Pepper contains the alkaloid piperine, which has many useful pharmacological activities (anti-inflammatory, anti-allergic, digestive), which add to the desired effects of the other ingredients in the formula. These could be considered to be pharmacodynamic interactions. However, piperine is also known to increase the bioavailability of a number of drugs by enhancing absorption. Piperine modulates the multidrug transporter P-glycoprotein and influences the efflux of other compounds, both herbal and synthetic drugs, from cells (Najar et al 2010). P-gp (the 'permeability protein') is a trans-membrane ATP-binding cassette transporter or pump, which transports various molecules across intra- and extra-cellular membranes, especially in the gut, kidney, liver and blood–brain barrier. It regulates the distribution and bioavailability of many drugs by blocking or facilitating entry into cells. Thus, increased intestinal expression of P-gp will reduce absorption of drugs that are substrates, reducing bioavailability, lowering drug plasma concentrations, and, therefore, reducing efficacy. Inhibition of P-gp will conversely increase plasma concentrations, which may lead to enhanced efficacy, but also, possibly, drug toxicity. Many other natural products are also known to modulate P-gp, and these include curcumin, quercetin, hesperidin and epigallocatechin gallate. They affect the bioavailability of not only other herbal components, but also 'conventional' drugs, and this is an untapped therapeutic area which remains to be explored. Inhibition of P-gp by non-toxic, common elements of the diet may even help to delay or inhibit resistance to, for example, antibiotics and anti-cancer drugs.

Piperine, along with many other natural compounds, also inhibits both constitutive and inducible cytochrome P450 (CYP-450) drug metabolizing enzymes. Inhibition reduces the metabolism (and, therefore, rate of clearance from the body) of any other substance metabolized by the same enzymes, whether of herbal or other origin, and thus enhances its blood levels. The opposite can occur: CYP enzymes can be induced, enhancing the clearance of any drug metabolized by the same enzymes.

MEASURING SYNERGY

The general understanding of synergy is that it is an effect seen by a combination of substances that is greater than would have been expected from a consideration of individual contributions. It does,

however, have a precise mathematical definition, which may depend on the method used to prove it. Such methods have been discussed extensively (Berenbaum 1989, Spelman et al 2006, Wagner 2009, Wagner and Ulrich-Merzenich 2009, Williamson 2001) and the isobole method is generally accepted as the method of choice. It is independent of the mechanism of action and applies under most conditions; it makes no assumptions as to the behaviour of each agent and is, therefore, applicable to multiple component mixtures. An isobole is an 'iso-effect' curve, in which a combination of ingredients (d_a, d_b) is represented by a point on a graph, the axes of which are the dose axes of the individual agents (D_a and D_b). If there is no interaction, the isobole (the line joining the points representing the combination to those on the dose axes representing the individual doses with the same effect as the combination) will be a straight line. If synergy is present, the dose of the combination needed to produce the same effect will be less than that for the individual components and the curve will be 'concave up'. The opposite applies for antagonism, which produces a 'concave down' isobole, as shown in Fig. 11.1.

It is quite possible to have synergy at one dose combination and antagonism at another, with the same substances; this would give a complicated isobole with a wave-like or even elliptical appearance. Therefore, for complex multicomponent mixtures, a method

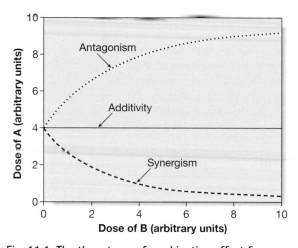

Fig. 11.1 The three types of combination effect for a mixture of an effective agent A and an ineffective compound B. If there is no interaction between A and B, the isobole is a straight line parallel to the dose axis of B (additivity). If there is a synergistic interaction, an isobole deviating towards the B axis is seen: i.e. in the presence of B, smaller doses of A are sufficient to produce the predetermined effect. When there is antagonism, the isobole deviates away from the B axis.

using deviation from predictions can be more suitable; here, predicted responses are plotted and compared with actual values obtained experimentally.

There are only a few examples of synergy available from the literature, mainly because it is so difficult to prove it conclusively. To do so would necessitate first testing the individual constituent(s) and comparing the activity with an equivalent dose in the mixture. In addition, different dose combinations would be needed to construct the relevant isoboles for proof. It is an immense undertaking and prohibitively expensive in terms of time and money.

Antagonism is a much easier concept to define, being a reduced effect from that expected, and tends to be more easily demonstrated regardless of the mathematical derivation. We, therefore, tend to use the term 'polyvalent action' to denote a combination effect, without necessarily qualifying it. This can apply to either an increased therapeutic effect, a reduced profile of side effects or, preferably, both.

MULTIPLE PHARMACOLOGICAL EFFECTS IN A SINGLE PLANT

Ispaghula, *Plantago ovata*

Ispaghula, or psyllium husk, is (paradoxically) effective in both constipation and diarrhoea. The laxative effect is achieved principally through its fibre content, but the reason why it is more effective in chronic constipation than other types of fibre may be due to the fact that the seed also contains constituents with gut stimulatory properties, mediated partly through cholinergic activation, which is likely to enhance the laxative effect. Interestingly, it also contains gut inhibitory constituents, which could provide a scientific explanation for the traditional use of ispaghula in diarrhoea. In addition to gut stimulatory and inhibitory constituents, ispaghula also contains anti-amoebic constituents explaining its traditional use in amoebic dysentery, thus demonstrating multiple effects, some supporting and some opposing a particular activity, in one medicinal plant (Gilani and Rahman 2005).

Liquorice, *Glycyrrhiza glabra*

In Traditional Chinese Medicine (TCM), liquorice (*Glycyrrhiza glabra*) is added to many formulae as a synergistic agent, to enhance activity and detoxify, and it demonstrates a number of instances of synergism not only with its own constituents, but also with other herbs. For example, blood levels of glycyrrhizin are lower, due to reduced absorption, if it is taken as part of an extract or mixture rather than as an isolated compound. Whole extracts of liquorice inhibit angiogenesis, granuloma formation and fluid exudation in inflammation, as does isoliquiritin, whereas glycyrrhizin and glycyrrhetinic acid tend to promote angiogenesis (reviewed in Williamson 2001). The mechanism of the antiinflammatory effect has recently been further investigated on both cyclooxygenase (COX) and lipoxygenase (LOX) products, using models of lipopolysaccharide (LPS)-induced prostaglandin E_2 (PGE_2), calcimycin-induced thromboxane (TXB_2), and leukotriene (LTB_4) release, in murine macrophages and human neutrophil cells. The whole plant extract, and isolated glabridin, inhibited the release of PGE_2 and TXB_2 (COX products) and LTB_4 (a LOX product), while isoliquiritigenin exerted an inhibitory effect only against COX products and failed to suppress LOX products (Chandrasekaran et al 2010). Glycyrrhizin failed to exhibit any inhibitory effects on both COX and LOX products in this model, although it has previously shown antiinflammatory activity by inhibiting the generation of reactive oxygen species by neutrophils. However, glycyrrhizin has also recently been shown to attenuate LPS-induced acute lung injury by inhibiting cyclooxygenase-2 (COX-2) and inducible nitric oxide synthase expression. In this case, the elevated concentrations of pro-inflammatory cytokines interleukin 1β and tumour necrosis factor (TNF)-α in bronchoalveolar fluid, caused by LPS administration, were significantly inhibited by glycyrrhizin pre-treatment, as was the concentration of nitric oxide (NO) in lung tissues (Ni et al 2011). These examples illustrate the complexity of the effects involved in even a single herbal extract, and it may be that this is found much more commonly than has been previously thought. Liquorice has many other beneficial effects, and is still the subject of intensive research for its potential use as an anticancer, antiviral, smooth-muscle relaxant, antipsoriatic and even memory enhancing agent, and it is likely that even more mechanisms and interactions will be discovered.

CLINICAL EXAMPLES OF SYNERGY AND POLYVALENT ACTION

Ginkgo, *Ginkgo biloba*

The ginkgolides are known to be platelet-activating factor (PAF) antagonists, a mechanism of antiinflammatory activity, and a synergistic interaction between ginkgolides A and B has been shown using an *in vitro* platelet aggregation test. A positive interaction was shown by an isobole curve using a 50% mixture of the two. Furthermore, the presence of the other ginkgolides and the ginkgoflavones also had an effect on the overall activity: a mixture of ginkgolides A, B and C, at a dose of 100–240 mg, generated a PAF-antagonizing effect in humans which was equivalent to a dose of 120 mg of a standardized ginkgo extract containing only 6–7 mg of ginkgolides, together with bilobalide and flavonol glycosides (Wagner 1999). However, the ginkgo flavones are also anti-inflammatory, the combination being considered additive and possibly synergistic in effect as well as increasing blood circulation to the brain, and a total ginkgo extract acts as an antioxidant activity in brain preparations. Clinical studies have shown ginkgo to be effective in improving cognitive function as well as the early stages of dementia; the preparation used being a total extract not just the flavonoids. This suggests polyvalent as well as synergistic activity

Ginkgo, taken in combination with other herbs, also shows synergistic-like interactions: a double-blind, cross-over trial using 20 young, healthy volunteers tested ginseng (*Panax ginseng*) with ginkgo extract and found it to be more effective in improving cognitive function than either alone. Cognitive performance was assessed in three studies, using 'serial threes' or 'serial sevens', which are arithmetic tests involving subtracting from a random number. Although single treatments showed improvements, the combination produced a significant and sustained improvement, especially in the 'serial sevens' test (Scholey and Kennedy 2002).

Cannabis, *Cannabis sativa*

Cannabis has potential as a therapeutic agent in chronic conditions such as rheumatoid arthritis, HIV infection and multiple sclerosis. Documented reports of interactions within the herb include the fact that levels of tetrahydrocannabinol (THC) in the brain can be elevated by cannabidiol, and it is known that THC taken alone can induce anxiety, which can be attenuated by the presence of cannabidiol in the herb. There is additional evidence to show that the effect of the herb is both qualitatively and quantitatively different to that of isolated THC (Wilkinson et al 2003). The herb extract is a better antispastic agent than THC alone, as measured in an immunogenic model of multiple sclerosis (Fig. 11.2). The graph shows that the extract acts more rapidly than isolated THC. The rest of the extract has no effect in this system, suggesting that in this case, the effect of THC is enhanced by the presence of other compounds in the extract, but there is no additive effect.

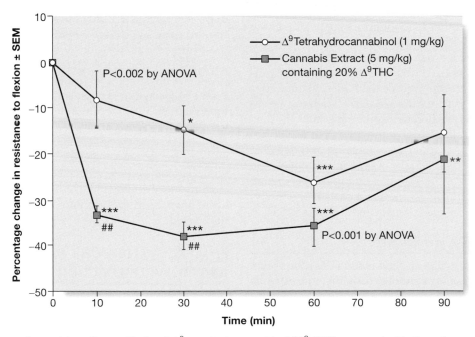

Fig. 11.2 The anti-spasticity effects of isolated Δ^9-tetrahydrocannabinol (Δ^9-THC) compared with that of a cannabis extract containing a matched dose of Δ^9-THC, in a mouse model of multiple sclerosis.

Willow bark, *Salix alba*

A randomized, placebo-controlled trial of the efficacy of a standardized extract of willow bark, for osteoarthritis of the hip and knee, was carried out recently mainly in elderly patients. The level of pain was assessed by both the patient and physician and efficacy was confirmed. However, the results also suggested the involvement of some form of synergy. Firstly, the gastrointestinal side effects commonly encountered with non-steroidal anti-inflammatory drugs, including aspirin, were not seen at the doses used, although it is usually assumed that willow bark is effective due to its salicin (and therefore salicylic acid) content. Furthermore, when the amount of salicin in the study preparation was taken into account, the dose used (equivalent to 240 mg of salicin daily) was insufficient to explain the activity. Investigations were then carried out to see if another mechanism might be operating. The effect on COX-1 (a cyclooxygenase isoenzyme) was examined and no involvement found (despite the fact that COX-1 is inhibited by aspirin). COX-1 is responsible for many of the side effects, especially those on the digestive system. However, COX-2 and lipoxygenase, which are also involved in pain and inflammation, were both inhibited. This shows that phytomedicines do not necessarily work in the same way as isolated constituents, and indicated that interactions were taking place in the willow bark preparation, but further clinical studies are needed for confirmation.

IMPLICATIONS OF SYNERGY

Bioassay–led isolation of actives

Scientists often investigate and extract medicinal plants with a view to finding the single chemical entity responsible for the effect, but this may lead to inconclusive results. If a combination of substances is needed for the effect, then the bioassay-led method of investigation, narrowing activity down first to a fraction and eventually to a compound, is doomed to failure, and this has led to the suggestion that some widely used plants are in fact devoid of activity. An example would be the investigation into the 'sausage tree' (*Kigelia pinnata*), where fractionation destroyed the previously noted cytotoxic effect. In a similar case, evidence of interaction between herbs was provided by a clinically successful formulation of Chinese herbs used to treat eczema. However,

when investigated phytochemically and pharmacologically, the activity was lost during the fractionation procedure and was only present within the mixture. The possibility of polyvalent action should, therefore, be taken into account, and, if activity appears to be lost during purification, interactions should be suspected and a search for synergy could be instigated.

ESTABLISHING THE ACTIVE PHARMACEUTICAL INGREDIENT (API) OF A PRODUCT

There are many examples of multifactorial effects in a single plant due to several constituents acting at multiple targets, as described above, and consequently many herbal medicines can be used for several different disorders. This presents an opportunity for developing specific extracts, or combinations for particular purposes, based on the same plant (and perhaps in different combinations with other herbs), for different therapeutic indications. Once the optimum composition of a product has been determined by pre-clinical and clinical studies, this specific extract should be considered the 'active pharmaceutical ingredient' (API). For a manufacturer, this provides an opportunity for patent protection. It also means that all extracts are not necessarily equivalent in therapeutic effect, or bioavailability.

OTHER REASONS FOR NOT ISOLATING INDIVIDUAL CONSTITUENTS

The most important reason for not isolating an individual component is the presence of multifactorial or polyvalent effects in a mixture, and the enhanced therapeutic benefit that such effects are expected to produce. However, there are issues of cost, and also the following should be taken into account:

- **Unstable constituents:** Sometimes the presence of all of the components isolated from the plant material, which may include antioxidants for example, may 'protect' the actives from decomposition. Examples of herbs in which this is thought to take place include valerian (*Valeriana* spp.), garlic (*Allium sativum*), ginger (*Zingiber officinalis*) and hops (*Humulus lupulus*).

- **Unknown active constituents:** For some herbs, even those which are widely used, the actives may not have been completely identified. This is in fact very common, and as can be seen from the example of liquorice discussed earlier, even for a herb with a very long history, new effects for old compounds are continually being discovered. Other examples include raspberry leaf (*Rubus idaeus*), chasteberry (*Vitex agnus castus*), passion flower (*Passiflora incarnata*), hawthorn (*Crataegus* spp.) and many others.

- **A range of actives identified:** It is unusual for a plant to contain only one active constituent. Even for cannabis, where there is only one significant psychoactive ingredient, tetrahydrocannabinol, other constituents of the herb may enhance its activity, as shown in Fig. 11.2. Other examples include *Echinacea*, devil's claw (*Harpagophytum procumbens*), artichoke (*Cynara scolymus*), St John's wort (*Hypericum perforatum*), liquorice (*Glycyrrhiza glabra*) and many others.

Of course, more than one of these situations may apply within a single herb.

METABOLOMICS AND THE FUTURE OF RESEARCH ON PHYTOMEDICINES

Solving such challenges posed by complex mixtures has preoccupied scientists for decades. Since the early 1990s hyphenated techniques have allowed scientists to identify many of the metabolites in an extract in a relatively short period of time. A range of novel approaches, and, most importantly, **metabolomics,** now offer unique opportunities for understanding such complex mixtures, and their effects. Metabolomics has been defined as 'both the qualitative and quantitative analysis of all metabolites in an organism', or: *the metabolome represents the collection of all metabolites in a biological organism, which are the end products of its gene expression* (Daviss 2005). In essence, this allows an understanding of the complete profile of extractable metabolites from an organism or in this case a phytomedicine. It is intricately linked with **multivariate data analysis** – a technique for analysing data sets with a large number of variables. In case of NMR of crude extracts, patterns can be visualized and interpreted. This can be done in a comparative manner distinguishing, for example, between differences between relatively similar extracts or it can be linked with, for example, a specific (generally *in vitro*) biological activity. Ultimately this enables the construction of a complex database of the metabolome (cf. Verpoorte et al 2007). For example, Harris et al (2007) developed a method for the analysis of *Vaccinium angustifolium* Ait. (lowbush blueberry), used as an over-the-counter treatment of diabetic symptoms. Using such an approach that focused on phenolic metabolites, the major metabolites found in the ethanol extracts of leaf, stem, root and fruit were analysed and compared. This allowed a detailed understanding of the complex characteristics of these blueberry extracts.

References

Berenbaum, M., 1989. What is synergy? Pharmacol. Rev. 41, 93–141.

Chandrasekaran, C.V., Deepak, H.B., Thiyagarajan, P., Kathiresan, S., Sangli, G.K., Deepak, M., et al., 2010. Dual inhibitory effect of *Glycyrrhiza glabra* (GutGard™) on COX and LOX products. Phytomedicine [Epub ahead of print 2010 Sep 21].

Daviss, B., 2005. Growing pains for metabolomics. The Scientist 19, 25–28.

Gilani, A.H., Rahman, A.U., 2005. Trends in ethnopharmacology. J. Ethnopharmacol. 100, 43–49.

Harris, C.S., Burt, A.J., Saleem, A., et al., 2007. A single HPLC-PAD-APCI/MS method for the quantitative comparison of phenolic compounds found in leaf, stem, root and fruit extracts of *Vaccinium angustifolium*. Phytochem. Anal. 18, 161–169.

Najar, I.A., Sachin, B.S., Sharma, S.C., Satti, N.K., Suri, K.A., Johri, R.K., 2010. Modulation of P-glycoprotein ATPase activity by some phytoconstituents. Phytother. Res. 24, 454–458.

Ni, Y.F., Kuai, J.K., Lu, Z.F., et al., 2011. Glycyrrhizin treatment is associated with attenuation of lipopolysaccharide-induced acute lung injury by inhibiting cyclooxygenase-2 and inducible nitric oxide synthase expression. J. Surg. Res 165, e29–e35 [Epub 2010 Nov 10].

Scholey, A.B., Kennedy, D.O., 2002. Acute, dose-dependent cognitive effects of Ginkgo biloba, Panax ginseng and their combination in healthy young volunteers: differential interactions with cognitive demand. Hum. Psychopharmacol. 17, 35–44.

Spelman, K., Duke, J.A., Bogenschutz-Godwin, M.J., 2006. The synergy principle at work with plants, pathogens, insects, herbivores and humans. In: Cseke, L.J., Kirakosyan, A., Kaufman, P.B., Warber, S., Duke, J.A., Brielman, H.L. (Eds.), Natural products and plants. CRC Press, New York.

Pujol, A., Mosca, R., Farrés, J., Aloy, P., 2010. Unveiling the role of network and systems biology in drug discovery – review article. Trends Pharmacol. Sci. 31, 115–123.

Verpoorte, R., Choi, Y.H., Kim, H.K., 2007. NMR-based metabolomics at work in phytochemistry. Phytochem. Rev. 6, 3–14.

Wagner, H., 1999. New targets in the phytopharmacology of plants. In: Herbal medicine, a concise overview for healthcare professionals. Butterworth-Heinemann, Oxford, pp. 34–42.

Wagner, H., 2009. Synergy research: a new approach to evaluating the efficacy of herbal mono-drug extracts and their combinations. Nat. Prod. Commun. 4, 303–304.

Wagner, H., Ulrich-Merzenich, G., 2009. Synergy research: approaching a new generation of phytopharmaceuticals. Phytomedicine 16, 97–110.

Wilkinson, J.D., Whalley, B.J., Baker, D., et al., 2003. Medicinal cannabis: is Δ-9 THC responsible for all its effects? J. Pharm. Pharmacol. 55, 1687–1694.

Williamson, E.M., 2001. Synergy and other interactions in phytomedicines. Phytomedicine 8, 401–409.

Further reading

Schmid, B., Lüdtke, R., Selbmann, H. K., et al., 2001. Efficacy and tolerability of a standardised willow bark extract in patients with osteoarthritis: a randomised, placebo-controlled, double-blind trial. Phytother. Res. 15, 344–350.

Ulrich-Merzenich, G., Panek, D., Zeitler, H., Wagner, H., Vetter, H., 2009. New perspectives for synergy research with the "omic"-technologies. Phytomedicine 16, 495–508.

Section 5

Medicinal plants in selected healthcare systems

SECTION CONTENTS

Chapter 12

Traditional systems of herbal medicine

INTRODUCTION

All modern medicine is derived originally from ancient herbal traditions. These have evolved to produce the conventional medicine known in the West, which uses both synthetic drugs and isolated natural compounds. Plant extracts are now rarely used by physicians or in hospitals, although herbal remedies are popular with the public and improvements in their formulation have resulted in a new generation of phytomedicines that are more potent than before and also chemically standardized. There is, however, a resurgence of interest in the older Oriental systems; this is due partly to dissatisfaction with conventional treatments and partly to the constantly growing interest in all things natural, environmentally friendly and biodegradable. These older types of medicine are philosophically based, and are holistic in that they treat the patient as a whole rather than as the 'owner' of a disease or malfunctioning organ. They also have much in common with traditional medical herbalism as it was, and still is, practised in Europe and America. Whether or not pharmacists, doctors and other healthcare professionals accept the validity of these older medical systems, it is necessary for them to know about their basic principles for two main reasons. First, to be in a position to advise patients who may wish to consult an alternative practitioner and, second, because traditional use is a common starting point in the ongoing search for new drugs.

It is necessary to consider the cultural environment in which traditional remedies are being used to make our expectations more reasonable, put these

treatments in the context of Western thinking and widen the criteria of selection of remedies for our own use within modern medicine.

Three types of traditional medicine have been chosen as an illustration:

> **Traditional medicine** can be defined as: Medical practice that includes diagnosis, prevention and treatment, relying on practical experience and observations handed down from generation to generation, whether verbally or in writing.

- Traditional Chinese Medicine (TCM)
- Ayurveda
- Traditional African medicine (TAM) or traditional African medical systems (TAMS).

TAM is an example of a mainly oral tradition, which applies to many types of indigenous medicine. TCM and Ayurveda are popular and highly sophisticated and have evolved through the ages whilst keeping their philosophy intact. All three systems use herbs as well as other forms of treatment. Discussion here, however, will be restricted to herbs since they have pharmacological activities and are, therefore, within the remit of this book. Before doing so, it would be useful to identify some aspects of the general approach of traditional medical systems to health, disease and treatment that affect our perception of them.

In the context of the systems discussed in this chapter, diseases can be considered as minor or self-limiting disorders, or chronic or serious disorders.

MINOR OR SELF-LIMITING DISORDER

Such ailments include aches and pains, diarrhoea, wounds or injuries for which a common remedy will be usually offered; in addition the facilitation of childbirth will also be considered. The remedy would usually be an indigenous plant or herb, or something that is obtainable from a local market, and would be well known within the community.

CHRONIC OR SERIOUS DISORDERS

These may be fatal, life-threatening or debilitating conditions, or those that cannot be diagnosed by indigenous healers; they are often considered to have a 'supernatural' component. Examples include forms of cancer, and some genetic or metabolic diseases where obvious lesions may not be seen. Plant remedies will certainly be used, but they may be used as part of a ritual, and treatment will often also involve practices such as divination to find out which gods or ancestors have been offended and what sacrifices may be necessary to appease the supernatural entity. Naturally, the rationale behind the first type of common usage is more logical to Western thought, and scientists would therefore look, for example, for antipyretic or analgesic compounds in a herb known as a cure for fever, or for haemostatic substances in a plant used to staunch bleeding. It may even be possible to speculate, with some knowledge of chemotaxonomy, on the types of compounds that are present (e.g. tannins in a haemostatic plant, salicylates or sesquiterpene lactones in an antipyretic plant). However, if ritual is more often involved in the use of a particular plant, it is almost impossible to surmise what compounds may be present; this approach is therefore much less useful. The plant may be a treasure trove of useful compounds, but the traditional use will not provide any information about it.

THE DOSE

In traditional medicine, this usually means a lack of specific dose. Typically, a calabash, seashell or a tumbler of a decoction may be taken from time to time. Traditional medicine is more concerned with *how* to take the remedy rather than *how much*. This aspect of traditional medicine is very important indeed because it means that highly potent plants are rarely part of a traditional pharmacopoeia – pure compounds, accurate balances and volume measurements are not part of such cultures – and some plants which we now find useful were considered dangerous. For example, the foxglove, a source of the cardiac glycoside digoxin, has no historical documentation as a herbal medicine, and it was not until the 1800s that Withering used it for cardiac dropsy (congestive heart failure). Due to the narrow therapeutic index of the drug, it was necessary to develop a standardized preparation, which was powdered leaf, assayed biologically, and compressed into a tablet, before the drug gained widespread acceptance.

CORRELATION OF TRADITIONAL USE WITH SCIENTIFIC EVIDENCE

There may be a correlation between traditional usage and pharmacological action, such as the isolation of antipyretic principles from a 'fever' remedy, but, even so, it may turn out different to our expectations. A classic example is 'fever bark' (*Cinchona*), which was traditionally used in South America for fever, but in many tropical countries 'fever' really means 'malaria'. Quinine is actually antipyretic to some extent, but it has a much more relevant property, which is to kill the malaria parasite *Plasmodium*. Therefore, extracts of plants based on traditional usage should not only be tested for the activity expected, but be put through a battery of tests, since some important modern drugs have been developed from plants used for a different purpose entirely. For example:

- in the Caribbean the periwinkle *Catharanthus* (*Vinca*) *rosea* was used traditionally for treating diabetes, but on further investigation it yielded the powerful anticancer alkaloids vincristine and vinblastine
- *Fagara xanthoxyloides*, which is used in Nigeria as a chewing stick for cleaning the teeth, has been found not only to be antimicrobial, but also to have antisickling activity, and this finding has sparked off further work into this painful and chronic genetic condition.

Despite the reservations mentioned, traditional medicines have yielded many useful modern drugs, although not as many as poisonous species. Although toxic plants are only occasionally used as medicines, they are well known to the healers and may also be used for nefarious purposes, witchcraft or as 'ordeal' poisons, as, for example, Calabar bean (*Physostigma venenosum*), which is the source of the anticholinesterase physostigmine (eserine).

ASIAN AND ORIENTAL MEDICINE

The more systematic forms of traditional medicine arose in the East, particularly in India and China, and from there spread to other parts of the world where they influenced Greek, Arab and other highly sophisticated cultures. Ayurveda originated in India, and TCM in China, but in both cases they have evolved as they were incorporated into local customs; for example, **Jamu** arose in Indonesia and **Kampo** in Japan. These medical systems were (and still are) complicated and structured, and had a philosophical and religious aspect far removed from the primitive magic, superstition, divination and sacrifice that are characteristic of African, South American, Pre-Islamic Arabian and other cultures where medical knowledge was an oral (rather than written) tradition. **Tibb-I-Islam** is Islamic medicine and, therefore, practised by Muslims throughout Asia and the rest of the world, but it is more of a cultural way of looking at health (as dictated by the Koran) than a type of medicine, although of equal impact.

TRADITIONAL CHINESE MEDICINE

The study of TCM is a mixture of myth and fact, stretching back well over 5000 years. At the time, none of the knowledge was written down, apart from primitive inscriptions of prayers for the sick on pieces of tortoise carapace and animal bones, so a mixture of superstition, symbolism and fact was passed down by word of mouth for centuries. TCM still contains very many remedies, which were selected by their symbolic significance rather than proven effects; however, this does not necessarily mean that they are all 'quack' remedies! There may even be some value in medicines such as tiger bone, bear gall, turtle shell, dried centipede, bat dung and so on. The herbs, however, are well researched and are becoming increasingly popular as people become disillusioned with Western medicine. Again, Chinese medicine is philosophically based, and as an holistic therapy the concept of balance and harmony is supremely important. The relevant records and documents were discussed earlier (Chapter 2), but additional historical milestones will be included here to show the evolution of TCM into what it is today.

THE DEVELOPMENT OF TCM

Shen Nong, the legendary Chinese Emperor, is credited with the discovery of herbal medicine in around 2800 BCE, and he is also reputed to have defined the opposing yet complementary principles eventually known as **yin** and **yang**. **Confucius** (551–479 BC) is celebrated as China's greatest sage. He established a code of rules and ethics based on the premise that there is an order and harmony of the Universe resulting from a delicate balance of yin and yang forces. Humans should cultivate the five virtues of benevolence, justice, propriety, wisdom and sincerity, in order to exert their own life force in this cycle. **Lao Zi** extended the Confucian doctrine and taught that man can only achieve personal harmony by bowing to the inevitable. His followers invented a spiritual destination to the mythical 'Island of the Eastern Sea' where a herb with the power to bestow immortality was thought to grow. The way (or path) within this natural order of things is called the **Tao** and the religion is now called **Taoism**. Along this path, the two basic expressions of **yin** (negative and passive) and **yang** (positive and active) are interlocked. This philosophy was refined and extended by **Dong Zhongshu** to include the inner reaches of man himself, i.e. man as the universe on a small scale, containing within himself the locked cycle of yin and yang. It, therefore, follows that Taoist principles apply to the well-being of man, and extend to diet and medicine as factors in ensuring a balance between physical and mental health.

Food and medicine became inter-related. Herbal medicine was initially the domain of shamans and mountain recluses, who believed that the mountain mists contained high concentrations of **qi**, the vital essence of life. They practised the 'way of long life', which involved a herbal diet and medicine combined with martial arts – a link that continues today. The principles of TCM became consolidated and a search for the 'elixir of life' began to obsess the Chinese aristocracy. In TCM, drugs to rejuvenate and increase longevity are still prized.

The **Han dynasty** (206 BC to 220 AD) saw remedies (including veterinary) recorded in handy booklets or **Gansu**, which were strips of bamboo or wood bound together. All herbal medicines were collected together in *the Shen Nong Ben Cao Jing* (the pharmacopoeia of Shen Nong) and classified into three categories:

- **Upper**: drugs that nurture life
- **Middle**: drugs that provide vitality
- **Lower**: 'poisons' used for serious disease.

The most noted physician of these times was **Zhang Zhogjing**, who divided diseases into six types: three 'yin' and three 'yang'. His prescriptions aimed to correct any imbalances of these forces. He also contributed to acupuncture by drawing a map of meridians along which the body's vital energy (qi) is said to flow. During this period, the theory of the circulation of the blood was described, and anaesthetics were used, based mainly on *Datura*. By the end of the Han dynasty all the elements we regard as vital to TCM were in place, and refinement went on throughout the Tang, Song and Ming dynasties.

During the **Ming dynasty**, **Li Shizhen** (1518–1593 AD) produced the classic herbal encyclopaedia *Ben Cao Gang Mu*. It took 27 years to compile and consists of 52 volumes containing 1892 medicines. It was translated into Japanese, Korean, English, French, German and others, and is said to mark the beginning of a cultural exchange between Chinese and Western medicine.

In the **20th century**, TCM came under attack from Western influences. Missionary doctors translated Western medical journals into Chinese, and Chinese doctors who had studied abroad turned against traditional herbal medicine. However, after the 1949 communist revolution, the government of the new People's Republic of China reinstated TCM and set up new medical colleges, intended to break China's dependence on the West. The 3rd (or Cultural) Revolution of 1966–1976 brought culture to a standstill, and 'barefoot doctors' with no more than 6 months of training were sent to rural areas to replace the denounced 'intellectual' Westerners. Today, both systems coexist and even Western-style medical schools teach students TCM and acupuncture.

CONCEPTS IN TCM

QI, THE ESSENTIAL LIFE FORCE

Qi (or **chi**) permeates everything. It is transferable. For example, digestion extracts qi from food and drink and transfers it to the body; and breathing extracts qi from the air and transfers it to the lungs. These two forms of qi 'meet' in the blood and form 'human qi', which circulates through the body. It is the quality, quantity and balance of qi that determines your state of health and lifespan. Obviously, therefore, food and air affect health, so diet and breathing exercises are very important. These aspects

of treatment will be considered first, before herbs are introduced. It is considered that the original vital energy, **yuan qi**, is gradually dissipated throughout life, so it is important to conserve it using diet, kung fu, breathing exercise and herbal medicine.

YIN AND YANG

These have already been mentioned as central to Taoism, and the theory of yin and yang still permeates all aspects of Chinese thought. Attributes of both are:

- **yin**: negative/passive/dark/female/water
- **yang**: positive/active/bright/male/fire.

Yin is considered to be the stronger: fire is extinguished by water, and water is 'indestructible'. So yin is always mentioned before yang; however, they are always in balance. Consider the well-known symbol (Fig. 12.1): where yin becomes weak, yang is strong and vice versa. Both contain the seed of each other: their opposites within themselves.

THE FIVE ELEMENTS

The earth is divided into wood, fire, earth, metal and water. They dominate everything on earth, and each is associated with a vital organ of the body:

- Heart: fire
- Liver: wood
- Spleen: earth
- Lungs: metal
- Kidneys: water.

THE VITAL ORGANS

These do not correspond to our organs exactly. Exact anatomy was not considered important since it was the relationship between the organs, the five

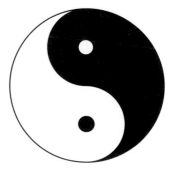

Fig. 12.1 The yin-yang symbol.

elements, qi and yin and yang that mattered. Also, until the 20th century, cutting up a human body (dead or alive) was considered a grave insult to the ancestors. An example of the relationship between them all and its treatment is that of a person with a red complexion (fire colour) and who laughs a lot (fire sound) may have an over-fired heart; in this case, herbs to sedate the heart will be given.

The organs are also considered to be yin or yang and are paired. Coupled organs are connected by meridians, or energy channels, through which qi flows. Meridians are not associated with the nervous system and cannot be seen physically. They are stimulated with herbs and by acupuncture and will have a direct effect on a particular organ as well as a toning effect on the system.

CAUSES OF DISEASE

Bacteria, viruses and chemicals are not considered to be causes. If an organ is weak, it may be attacked, and, therefore, the weakness is the cause and must be rectified. It may be the result of external forces and internal emotional factors. The external 'cosmological' forces are called the **six excesses:**

- Wind
- Cold
- Summer heat
- Dampness
- Dryness
- Fire.

Most people, if healthy, are not affected by the six excesses but, if the body is deficient in qi or weather conditions are abnormal (i.e. not what is expected), then this may cause problems.

THE SEVEN EMOTIONS

These are considered to be the major internal causes of disease. Excessive emotional activity causes a severe yin/yang imbalance, blockage of qi in the meridians and impairment of vital organ function. This leads to damage of the organs and allows disease to enter from outside, or a minor weakness from inside to develop. The seven emotions are:

- joy
- anger
- anxiety
- concentration
- grief

- fear
- fright.

Once physical damage has occurred, by whatever cause, it will need more than emotional factors to cure it and herbs will be used. There are a few other causes, which are not emotional or external excesses. These are the exception not the rule, and include epidemics, insect and animal bites, worm infestation and hereditary diseases.

DIAGNOSIS

Various methods are used:

- **Examination of the tongue**: a very important aspect
- **Pulse diagnosis**: more than one pulse will be taken, depending on the pressure exerted
- **Palpation of internal organs**: carried out to determine consistency and tone
- **Massage**: used to detect temperature and knotted muscles or nerves
- **Interviewing**: vital; questions are asked about sleep patterns, tastes in food and drink, stool and urine quality, fever, perspiration and sexual activity.

TREATMENT

The purpose is to rectify harmony, restore qi and the yin/yang balance. For example 'cold' diseases, such as cold in the lungs, coughs, vomiting and nausea are considered to be a deficiency of yang and treatment would be with a warming herb such as ginger (see examples in Table 12.1). A list of common herbs and their indications is given in Table 12.2. Once the prescription has been formulated, the patient may be given a crude herb mixture with written instructions on how to prepare it at home, perhaps as an infusion or tea. Pastes and pills are prepared by the herbalist and may take several days to complete. Slow-release preparations are made using beeswax pills; tonic wines, fermented dough (with herbs in) and external poultices are also common.

AYURVEDA

Ayurveda is considered to be the most ancient of all medical disciplines. It is a system of sacred Hindu medicine, originating in India, and as well as being an oral tradition, is also fairly well documented.

Table 12.1   Treatment of disease in traditional Chinese medicine according to the nature of disease and the remedy

TYPE OF DISEASE	EXAMPLE OF DISEASE	NATURE OF DISEASE	NATURE OF REMEDY	EXAMPLE OF REMEDY	DESIRED EFFECT
Cold	Nausea, vomiting	Yin	Yang	*Zingiber officinale*	Warming
Hot	Malaria, fever	Yang	Yin	*Artemisia annua*	Cooling
Empty	Fatigue, diabetes	Yin, yang, qi deficiency	Tonic	*Panax ginseng*	Nourishing
Full	Congestion in chest	Yang	Yin	*Scutellaria baicalensis*	Cooling
Internal	Weak pulse	Yin	Yang	*Aconitum carmichaeli*	Warming
External	Psoriasis	Yang	Yin	*Arctium lappa*	Cooling

Table 12.2   Some important herbs in traditional Chinese medicine and their uses

BOTANICAL NAME/ENGLISH NAME	CHINESE NAME	NATURE	MEDICAL USE
Aconitm carmichaeli			
Aconitum	Chuan wu tou	Very pungent and hot, yang	Heart tonic, diarrhoea, analgesic
Angelica sinensis			
Chinese angelica	Dang gui	Sweet, pungent, warm, yang	Menstrual disorders, analgesic
Arctium lappa			
Great burdock	Niu bang zi	Pungent, bitter, cold, yin	Sore throat, pneumonia, psoriasis
Artemisia annua			
Sweet wormwood	Qing hao	Bitter, cold, yin	Malaria, fever
Cinnamomum cassia			
Chinese cinnamon	Rou gui	Pungent, sweet, very hot, yang	Diarrhoea, tonic, dysmenorrhoea
Coix lacrima jobi			
Job's tears	Yi yi ren	Sweet, plain, slightly cold, yin	Dysentery, painful joints, diuretic
Cyperus rotundus			
Nut grass	Xiang fu	Pungent, sweet, neutral	Liver disorders, amenorrhoea, sedative
Ephedra sinica			
Ephedra	Ma huang	Pungent, slightly bitter, warm, yang	Bronchial asthma, hayfever
Glycyrrhiza uralensis			
Chinese liquorice	Gan cao	Sweet, neutral	Asthma, bronchitis, ulcers, steroid activity
Lonicera japonica			
Japanese honeysuckle	Jin yin hua	Sweet, cold, yin	Fever, throat infections, ulcers
Paeonia lactiflora			
Chinese white peony	Bai shao yao	Bitter, slightly cold, yin	Fever, haemostatic anti-inflammatory
Panax ginseng			
Ginseng	Ren shen	Sweet, neutral	Tonic, aphrodisiac, appetite stimulant
Perilla frutescens			
Beefsteak plant	Zi su	Pungent, warm, yang	Allergic reactions, fever
Rheum palmatum			
Rhubarb	Da huang	Bitter, cold, yin	Constipation, burns, diarrhoea, jaundice

Continued

BOTANICAL NAME/ENGLISH NAME	CHINESE NAME	NATURE	MEDICAL USE
Table 12.2 Some important herbs in traditional Chinese medicine and their uses—cont'd			
Salvia miltiorrhiza			
Salvia	Dan shen	Bitter, cold, yin	Menstrual disorders, chest pain, blood clots
Schisandra chinensis			
Schisandra	Wu wei zi	Sour, warm, yang	Diarrhoea, thirst, asthma, coughs
Scutellaria baicalensis			
Baical skullcap	Huang qin	Bitter, cold, yin	Dysentery, jaundice
Sophora japonica			
Pagoda tree	Huai hua	Bitter, slightly cold, yin	Blood disorders, clots, reduces cholesterol
Terminalia chebula			
Myrobalan	He zi	Bitter, sour, neutral	Chronic diarrhoea, dysentery, haemostatic
Tribulus terrestris			
Caltrops	Ci ji li	Sweet, warm, yang	Liver and kidney tonic, lumbago, tinnitus
Zingiber officinale			
Ginger	Gan jiang	Pungent, sweet, very hot, yang	Nausea, vomiting, colds, diarrhoea
Ziziphus jujuba			
Chinese jujube	Suan zao ren	Sweet, sour, neutral	Liver and heart tonic

Different parts of the plant, whether fresh or dried, and the type of preparation will affect the nature and medical uses of a herb, so the above are only examples. Many of the plants are the same as those used in Ayurvedic medicine, sometimes for different purposes but mainly for the same indications.

Over 5000 years ago, the great seers (or 'rishis') organized the 'fundamentals of life' into what became known as Ayurveda, and this has evolved and adapted over the years whilst still retaining the philosophical basis on which it was founded. It now accommodates modern science, especially in relation to the testing of medicines, and research and adaptation are actively encouraged. Like other forms of holistic medicine, Ayurveda considers the patient as an individual and 'normality' as what is appropriate for that particular person. The patient is viewed as unique, and is, therefore, subject to unique imbalances. This is in contrast to Western medicine, where populations are generalized and 'normal' means what is applicable to the majority. However, unlike the difficulties with homoeopathy, for example, it is perfectly possible to evaluate Ayurvedic medicines using conventional clinical trials, and this is increasingly being carried out. Another important difference is that Eastern thought greatly values subjectivity, and

even considers it to be a vital addition to objectivity, which is the goal in Western medicine.

There are only a few Ayurvedic practitioners ('vaid') in the West at present, but popularity is growing rapidly and Ayurvedic medicines are now being exported from India to many other countries. It is worthy of study for this reason, not only because it is the most ancient system of medicine still in use today, but also because it has influenced so many other types. Many ethnic populations from India and Pakistan continue to use their own traditional remedies while living in Europe, Australia or the USA, and it is important that healthcare professionals should have some knowledge of the background and remedies that they are using.

Philosophically, Ayurveda has similarities with traditional Chinese medicine, in that the concept of humanity as a microcosm within the macrocosm of the universe is accepted. There is a life force, which can be nourished, protected, and of course dissipated, as well as opposing forces or 'humors' whose balance is vital to health. In TCM there are two (yin and yang), and in Ayurveda there are three (the tridosha). There are five elements in both, but they are slightly different and will be outlined in the appropriate section. Many remedies are common to both systems, although the philosophical rationale for their application may be a little different.

CONCEPTS IN AYURVEDA

PRANA, THE LIFE ENERGY

Prana is the vital energy, activating both body and mind. Nutrient prana from the air gives energy to the vital prana in the brain, via respiration, and is thus the equivalent of qi in Chinese medicine. In the body it is seated in the head, and governs emotions, memory, thought and other functions of the mind. Prana kindles the bodily fire (**agni**) and governs the functioning of the heart, entering the bloodstream from where it controls the vital organs or **dhatus**.

BHUTAS, THE FIVE ELEMENTS

The ether (space), air, fire, water and earth are considered to be the basic elements, which are manifestations of cosmic energy. They are related to the five senses (hearing, touch, vision, taste and smell) and from them to resultant actions. As an example, ether is related to hearing, since sound is transmitted through it, and from there to the ear, the associated sense organ, leading to speech, from the organs of action which are the tongue and vocal cords. Likewise, fire is associated with the eyes as sense organs, leading to an action such as walking, by an organ of action, such as the feet.

TRIDOSHA: VATA, PITTA AND KAPHA – THE THREE HUMORS

Ether, air, fire, water and earth (the five basic elements) are manifest in the human body as three basic principles or humors known as the 'tridosha', which is unique to Ayurveda. The three humors, known as **vata, pitta** and **kapha** (individually called **doshas**), govern all biological, psychological and physiopathological functions of the body and mind. The primary requirement for the diagnosis and treatment of disease is to understand the relationship between these. Some similarities can be drawn with the ancient Greek system of medicine in which the humoral theory considers the body to consist of four fluids (phlegm, blood, yellow bile and black bile) and disease is thought to occur when these fluids are out of balance. Similarly, when the tridosha works in harmony and functions in a balanced manner, the result is health and a feeling of well-being in the individual. However, in cases of imbalance and disharmony, the result is illness or disease. The tridosha affects the creation, maintenance and destruction of bodily tissues and the elimination of toxins (**ama**) from the body. It is also responsible for psychological phenomena, including basic human emotions such as fear, anger and greed, and more complicated sentiments such as understanding, compassion and love, and as such is the foundation of the psychosomatic nature of man.

The tridosha (vata, pitta and kapha) has recently been redefined as an equilibrium, balance and coordination between the three vital body systems: the central nervous system (CNS) corresponding to vata, the endocrine system to pitta and the immune axis to kapha, operating with both positive and negative feedback. To try and correlate this ancient philosophy with modern science is difficult, but some analogies can be drawn. The tridosha can be considered to govern all metabolic activities: catabolism (vata), metabolism (pitta) and anabolism (kapha). When vata is out of balance, the metabolism will be disturbed, resulting in excess catabolism, which is the breakdown or deterioration process in the body; excess would, therefore, induce emaciation. When anabolism is greater than catabolism (excess kapha), there is an increased rate of growth and repair of organs and tissues. Excess pitta disturbs metabolism generally. The tridosha can be described further:

- **Vata**, affiliated to air or ether (space), is a principle of movement. It can be characterized as the energy controlling biological movement and is thus associated with the CNS, and governs functions such as breathing, blinking, all forms of movement, heartbeat and nervous impulses.
- **Pitta** is affiliated to fire and water, and governs bodily heat and energy. It, therefore, controls body temperature, is involved in metabolism, digestion, excretion and the manufacture of blood and endocrine secretions, and is also involved with intelligence and understanding.
- **Kapha** is associated with water and earth. It is responsible for physical structure, biological strength, regulatory functions, including that of immunity, the production of mucus, synovial fluid and joint lubrication and assists with wound healing, vigour and memory retention.

PRAKRUTI, THE HUMAN CONSTITUTION

Humans can also be divided into personality types, and the constitution of an individual (prakruti) is determined by the state of the parental tridosha at conception (unlike astrology, which depends on time of birth). Most people are not completely one type or another, but can be described as vatapitta or pittaka-pha, for example. People of vata constitution are generally physically under-developed with cold, rough, dry and cracked skin. People with pitta constitution are of medium height with moderate muscle development. Kapha people have well-developed bodies. Table 12.3 can be used to indicate constitution in a superficial way, but it is not a tool for self-diagnosis!

As well as the vata, pitta and kapha type of personalities, three attributes provide the basis for distinctions in human temperament, individual differences, and psychological and moral dispositions. These basic attributes are satva, rajas and tamas. In brief, **satva** expresses essence, understanding, purity, clarity, compassion and love; **rajas** describes movement, aggressiveness and extroversion; and **tamas** manifests in ignorance, inertia, heaviness and dullness. In Ayurveda, a state of health exists when the digestive fire (**agni**) is in a balanced condition and the bodily humors (vata-pitta-kapha) are in equilibrium. The three waste products (**mala**), which are urine, faeces and sweat, should be produced at usual levels, the senses functioning normally, and the body, mind and consciousness working in harmony. When the balance of any of these systems is disturbed the disease process begins.

AGNI, THE DIGESTIVE FIRE

Agni governs metabolism and is essentially pitta in nature. An imbalance in the tridosha will impair agni and, therefore, affect metabolism. Food will not be digested or absorbed properly, and toxins will be produced in the intestines, and may find their way into the circulation. These toxins are known as ama and are the root cause of disease. Overactive ama is also detrimental in that over combustion of nutrients may occur, leading to vata disorders and emaciation.

MALAS, THE THREE WASTE PRODUCTS

These are, as may be expected, the faeces, urine and sweat, and production and elimination of these are vital to health. Their appearance and properties can give many indications of the state of the tridosha and, therefore, health. As an example,

Table 12.3	Determining the human constitution according to the tridosha		
ASPECT OF CONSTITUTION	VATA CHARACTER	PITTA CHARACTER	KAPHA CHARACTER
Bodyweight	Low	Moderate	Overweight
Skin	Dry	Soft	Thick
	Rough	Oily	Oily
	Cool	Warm	Cool
Eyes	Small	Sharp	Large
	Dark	Green	Blue
	Dull	Grey	
Hair	Dry	Oily	Oily
	Dark	Fair	Thick
	Curly		Dark or fair
Appetite	Poor	Good	Steady
	Variable	Excessive	
Thirst	Variable	Excessive	Scanty
Mind	Restless	Aggressive	Calm
	Active	Intelligent	Slow
Emotional temperament	Insecure	Irritable	Calm
	Unpredictable	Aggressive	Greedy
Speech	Fast	Penetrating	Slow
Physical activity	Very active	Moderate	Lethargic
Sleep	Interrupted	Little sound	Heavy
			Long

To find the Ayurvedic constitution, just tick the most relevant description, and count up the ticks in each column to determine the dominant type. It may not just show one pure type, but, for example, vata-pitta or pitta-kapha. Then the best diet for a particular constitution can be found. Foods which aggravate a particular dosha should not be taken in excess by a person of that type; for example, a vata person should not take excessive amounts of lamb, cabbage, potatoes or dried fruits. However, eggs, rice, cooked vegetables and sweet fruits would be beneficial to someone of vata constitution. It can also be used to decide which type of food to eat in different seasons. For example, in summer, pitta predominates, and those foods that aggravate pitta should be avoided; but winter is the season of kapha, so seafood, melon and cows milk products are not recommended then. Autumn is the season of vata, and spring is kapha-pitta.

the colour of urine depends on the diet, and, if the patient has a fever or jaundice (pitta disorders), it may be darker. Substances such as coffee and tea, which stimulate urination, also aggravate pitta and render the urine dark yellow.

DHATUS, THE SEVEN TISSUES

The human body consists of seven basic tissues or organs (constructing elements) or dhatus. When there is a disorder in the balance of the tridosha, the dhatus are directly affected. Health can be maintained by taking steps to keep vata-pitta-kapha in balance through a proper diet, exercise and rejuvenation programme. The dhatus do not correspond to our definition of anatomy, but are more a tissue type than an individual organ.

GUNAS, THE ATTRIBUTES

Ayurveda encompasses a subtle concept of attributes or qualities called gunas. Caraka, the great Ayurvedic physician, theorized that organic and inorganic substances, as well as thought and action, all have definite attributes. These attributes contain potential energy while their associated actions express kinetic energy. Vata, pitta and kapha each have their own attributes, and substances having similar attributes will tend to aggravate the related bodily humor. The concepts governing the pharmacology, therapeutics and food preparation in Ayurveda are based on the action and reaction of the attributes to and upon one another. Through understanding of these attributes, the balance of the tridosha may be maintained. The diseases and disorders ascribed to vata, pitta and kapha are treated with the aid of medicines, which are characteristic of, but possessing the opposite attribute, to try and correct the deficiency or excess. Vata disorders are corrected with the aid of sweet (**madhur**), sour (**amla**) or saline and warm (**lavana**) medicines. The excitement or 'aggravation' of pitta is controlled by sweet (madhur), bitter (**katu**) or astringent and cooling (**kashaya**) herbs. Kapha disorders are corrected with pungent (**tikta**), bitter (katu) or astringent and dry (kashaya) herbs. The use of herbs in correcting any imbalance is of extreme importance and is essential for proper functioning of the organism. There is often little distinction between foods and medicines, and controlling the diet is an integral part of Ayurvedic treatment. Foods are also described according to their properties, such as their taste (**rasa**) and physical and chemical properties (**guna**); these affect the tridosha (see Table 12.4).

APPLICATION OF AYURVEDA

DIAGNOSIS

Taking the case history involves astrological considerations, as well as a thorough medical examination where the appearance of the tongue, properties of the urine, sweat and sputum will also be examined.

Karma, the good and bad effects across reincarnations, is also taken into account.

TREATMENT

This may involve diets, bloodletting, fasting, skin applications and enemas used to cleanse the system. There is a programme consisting of five types of detoxification, known as **panchkarma**. Drugs may then be given to bring the dhatus into balance again. These include herbal treatments as well as minerals, and there are thousands in use. In addition, yogic breathing and other techniques are used. All will have their properties described: rasa, guna and their karma, as well as which doshas they affect. Some of the most popular herbes of Ayurveda are shown in Table 12.5.

In modern Indian herbal medicine the Ayurvedic properties are described together with the conventional pharmacological and phytochemical data. Drugs are prepared as tinctures, pills, powders and some formulae unique to Ayurveda (see Table 12.6). Ayurveda is very metaphysical, too much so for many Westerners to grasp, and practitioners view it as a way of life as opposed to a career.

RASAYANA

Rasayana are remedies considered to have diverse action and, therefore, affect many systems of the body, leading to a positive effect on health – panaceas in other words. The most important are *Asparagus racemosa* (**shatavari**), *Emblica officinalos* (**amla**), *Piper longum* (**pimpli**), *Terminalia chebula* (**haritaki**), *Tinospora cordifolia* (**guduchi**) and *Withania somnifera* (**ashwagandha**). They are included in many recipes and are used to strengthen the tissues of the body. In general, modern research has found them to have antioxidant, immunomodulating and various other activities.

Acceptance of Ayurveda in Europe and other regions of the world is growing, but often its main role is in uses associated with 'wellness' and spa treatments, resulting in a dilution of traditional Ayurvedic concepts.

TRADITIONAL AFRICAN MEDICAL SYSTEMS

Very little about plant use in Africa has been written down. It is an important tradition passed on orally and many of the features of traditional African

Table 12.4 Effect of different foods on the tridosha

DOSHA	VATA		PITTA		KAPHA	
Food type	Aggravates	Balances	Aggravates	Balances	Aggravates	Balances
Meat	Lamb, pork, venison	Beef, eggs, turkey (white meat), chicken	Beef, lamb, pork, egg yolk	Chicken, turkey, egg white	Beef, lamb, pork, seafood	Chicken, turkey (dark meat), rabbit, eggs
Cereals	Rye, barley	Oats (cooked), rice, wheat	Barley, oats (cooked), brown rice, eggs	White rice, wheat, barley, oats (cooked)	Oats (cooked), rice, wheat	Barley, rye, corn
Vegetables	Raw veg, cauliflower, sprouts, cabbage, aubergine, lettuce, mushrooms, onion (raw), peas, potatoes	Cooked veg, carrots, garlic, green beans, cucumber, avocado, courgettes	Carrots, aubergine, garlic, onion, spinach, tomatoes, hot peppers	Broccoli, sprouts, lettuce, peas, cauliflower, mushrooms, courgettes	Cucumber, tomatoes, courgettes	Cauliflower, sprouts, cabbage, carrots, aubergine, lettuce, mushrooms, onions, peas, potatoes
Fruit	Dried fruit, apples, pears, water melon	Sweet fruits, apricots, peaches, bananas, cherries, grapes, citrus	Sour fruits, peaches, bananas, grapes, lemons, oranges, pineapple	Sweet fruits, apples, melon, coconut, raisins, prunes	Bananas, coconut, grapefruit, grapes, lemon, orange, melon, pineapple	Apples, apricots, peaches, pears, cherries, raisins, prunes
Dairy	All OK	All OK	Buttermilk, cheese, yogurt,	Butter, milk	None	Goats milk
Oils	All OK	All OK	Corn, sesame, almond	Sunflower, soya, olive	None	None
Condiments	All OK	All OK	Most	Coriander, fennel, turmeric	All	Salt

Table 12.5 Some important herbs of Ayurveda and their uses

BOTANICAL NAME	AYURVEDIC NAME	EFFECT ON DOSHA	MEDICAL USE
Acorus calamus			
Sweet flag	Vacha	Pacifies vata and kapha	Nerve stimulant, digestive
Adhatoda vasica			
Malabar nut	Vasaka	Pacifies pitta and kapha	Respiratory disorders, fevers
Aegle marmelos			
Bengal quince	Bael, bel	Promotes pitta	Antidysenteric, digestive, tonic
Andrographis paniculata	Kalmegh	Pacifies kapha and pitta	Liver protectant, jaundice
Green chiretta			
Eclipta alba			
Trailing eclipta	Bhringarajah	Pacifies kapha and pitta	Skin and hair disorders
Embelia ribes			
Embelia	Viranga	Pacifies kapha and vata	Vermifuge, contraceptive
Nigella sativa			
Black cumin	Kalonji	Pacifies vata and kapha	Digestive, antiseptic
Ocimum sanctum			
Holy basil	Tulsi	Pacifies kapha and vata	Expectorant, febrifuge, immunomodulator

Continued

Table 12.5   Some important herbs of Ayurveda and their uses—cont'd

BOTANICAL NAME	AYURVEDIC NAME	EFFECT ON DOSHA	MEDICAL USE
Phyllanthus emblica			
Indian gooseberry	Amla	Balances tridosha	Improves memory and intelligence, tonic
Phyllanthus niruri			
Stone breaker	Bhumyamlaki	Pacifies kapha and pitta	Diabetes, jaundice, liver protectant
Picrorrhiza kurroa			
Kutki, yellow gentian	Katurohini	Pacifies kapha and pitta	Hepatoprotective, immunomodulator
Piper nigrum			
Black pepper	Kalmirch	Pacifies vata and pitta	Digestive, respiratory disorders
Swertia chirata			
Chiretta	Chirayita	Balances tridosha	Appetite stimulant, liver disorders
Terminalia arjuna			
Arjun myrobalan	Arjuna	Pacifies pitta and kapha	Heart tonic, angina, hypertension
Terminalia chebula			
Black myrobalan	Haritaki	Balances tridosha	Digestive, blood tonic, antiasthmatic
Tribulus terrestris			
Caltrops	Gokhru	Pacifies vata and pitta	Digestive, diuretic, aphrodisiac
Withania somnifera			
Winter cherry	Ashwagandha	Pacifies kapha and vata	Analgesic, sedative, rejuvenator

Table 12.6   Methods of preparing Ayurvedic medicines

FORMULATION	METHOD OF PRODUCTION
Juice (swaras)	Cold-pressed plant juice
Powder (churna)	Shade-dried, powdered plant material
Cold infusion (sita kasaya)	Herb/water 1:6, macerated overnight and filtered
Hot infusion (phanta)	Herb/water 1:4, steeped for a few minutes and filtered
Decoction (kathva)	Herb/water 1:4 (or 1:8, 1:16 then reduced to 1:4), boiled
Poultice (kalka)	Plant material pulped
Milk extract (ksira paka)	Plant boiled in milk and filtered
Tinctures (arava, arista)	Plant fermented, macerated or boiled in alcohol
Pills or tablets (vati, gutika)	Soft or dry extracts made into pills or tablets
Sublimates (kupipakva rasayana)	Medicine prepared by sublimation
Calcined preparations (bhasma)	Plant or metal is converted into ash
Powdered gem (pisti)	Gemstone triturated with plant juice
Scale preparations (parpati)	Molten metal poured on leaf to form a scale
Medicated oils or ghee (sneha)	Plant heated in oil or ghee
Medicated linctus/jam (avaleha)	Plant extract in syrup

medical systems (TAMS) are similar to those of cultures in other parts of the world, and, like them, many practitioners were illiterate. The term 'medical system' is used to describe the complexity of medical practices in a society. The cultural diversity in Africa has resulted in a variety of different TAMS, although these often share important elements. TAMS as a whole tends to be empirical rather than theoretical, but it does assume the existence of supernatural forces in the cause of disease to a greater extent than some other systems and has been described as 'non-scientific' as a result of this. These general observations apply to TAMS in several different African societies; similar principles are involved, although details and some of the plants will be different.

CONCEPTS IN TRADITIONAL AFRICAN MEDICAL SYSTEMS

The causes of disease, as they are defined culturally, are essential for an understanding of TAMS. In African thought, all living things are connected to each other and to the gods and ancestral spirits. If harmony exists between all of these then good health is enjoyed, but, if not, misfortune or ill-health will result. Forces can be directed at humanity by displeased gods, ancestors and also by witches, resulting in disharmony, which must be resolved before good health can be restored. Treatment may also involve much more than medicine; practices such as divination and incantation may be carried out to help with diagnosis, and sacrifices may be needed to placate the supernatural entity. The traditional healer is likely also to be a religious leader, since health and spirituality are closely intertwined in TAMS.

Apart from physical examination, the diagnosis may also involve several other forms of diagnosis and treatment:

● **Confessions** may be extracted. These are thought to be both healing and prophylactic. In the case of a child, the mother may need to examine her previous behaviour, since the sins of the mother can be visited on the child (this compares with ideas in Christianity and other religions).
● **Divination** may be required, and may involve throwing objects and interpreting the pattern in which they fall. This is a consistent feature of many cultures and still persists in Europe in such forms as the 'reading of tea leaves'.

Serious illness is considered to be due to supernatural causes much more than minor aches and pains are, and treatment will correspondingly be more concerned with ritual, incantation and sacrifice than it would for minor disorders. Herbal medicines will be part of the ritual and less likely to lead to expected or anticipated pharmacological or therapeutic activity. The treatment of disease is based on mind–body dualism and is, therefore, holistic; it is concerned with the whole lifestyle of the patient. This spiritual emphasis is important and can be rationalized with respect to modern life to some extent. If **stress** is caused by a breakdown in relationships with neighbours, family or work colleagues, or to immoral behaviour and the resulting guilt, or sins due to disobedience of religious laws, lowered immune resistance and ill-health may ensue. We now recognize the importance of psychosomatic factors and the

placebo effect demonstrates this very well. Although we are at present looking at TAMS mainly as a source of new drugs, it may well be that the practices of making amends, sorting out your life and living according to a reasonable moral code has as many lessons for modern medicine as testing medicinal plants for pharmacological activity!

In TAMS, medicinal plants are used in two ways, only one of which corresponds to our perception of drug therapy. When we talk of research into traditional medicines, we are really talking about the scientific analysis of medicinal plants. Some of the most commonly used African ones are listed in Table 12.7. The traditional healer will, however, use medicinal plants not only for their pharmacological properties but their power to restore health as supernatural agents. This is based on two important assumptions:

● Plants are living and it is thought that all living things generate a vital force, which can be harnessed.
● The release of the force may need special rituals and preparations such as incantations to be

Table 12.7	Examples of common and widely used African medicinal plants and the main conditions for which they are used
SPECIES	**INDIGENOUS USE**
Rauvolfia vomitoria (Apocynaceae) *Holarrhena wulfsbergii* (Apocynaceae)	Mental illness (especially schizophrenia)
Xylopia aethiopica (Annonaceae) *Piper guineense* (Piperaceae) *Pycnanthus kombo* (Myristicaceae) *Aframomum latifolium* (Zingiberaceae) *Harpagophytum procumbens*[a] (Pedaliaceae)	Oedema Pain, inflammation, lumbago
Plumbago zeylanica (Plumbaginaceae) *Cassia alata* (Caesalpiniaceae)	Skin diseases
Elaeophorbia drupifera (Euphorbiaceae) *Picralima umbellata* (Apocynaceae)	Worms
Ricinus communis (Euphorbiaceae) *Carica papaya* (Caricaceae)	Contraceptive
Diospyros mespiliformis (Ebenaceae) *Ficus elegans* (Moraceae)	Dysentery, diarrhoea
Prunus africana[a] (Rosaceae)	Male urinary problems

[a]Developed into phytomedicines used in Europe and North America.

effective. This belief is rather similar to the concept held by some people nowadays that uncooked vegetables, particularly things such as sprouting beans, somehow contain a 'life-force' which is beneficial to health.

The method of application is essential for understanding TAMS. In conventional medicine, some form of absorption of the drug must take place. It can be orally, rectally, parenterally, topically or by inhalation. In TAMS, this is not necessarily important (although it will happen in many instances) as ingredients can be encapsulated and worn as an amulet, necklace or around the wrist or ankle. They may not even come into contact with the patient at all; perhaps being placed above the door, or under a mat or pillow. These practices are to ward off the evil spirits, which may be causing the disease.

In some cases, the choice of a species has been made on a basis that has no bioscientific rationale; for example, a plant that bears many fruits may be used to treat infertility. This is rather like the ancient 'Doctrine of Signatures', where the plant was thought to display features indicating to the healer what it should be used for. It is a recurrent theme in the history of medicine. For example, walnuts were thought to be good for the brain because they resemble the cerebellum, and in Chinese medicine the use of animal parts is thought to endow the person consuming them with the properties of the animal. Tigers' bones are taken to imbue strength and courage, and the horn of the rhinoceros to increase sexual vigour. These observations show that plants used in these ways may *not* necessarily lead us to new drugs, except as a random result.

Further reading

Govindarajan, R., Vijayakumar, M., Pushpangadan, P., 2005. Antioxidant approach to disease management and the role of Rasayana herbs of Ayurveda. J. Ethnopharmacol. 99, 165–178.

Lad, V., 1990. Ayurveda the science of self-healing. Lotus Press, Wisconsin.

Mukherjee, P.K., Mukherjee, D., Venkatesh, M., Rai, S., Heinrich, M., 2009. The sacred lotus (Nelumbo nucifera) – phytochemical and therapeutic profile. J. Pharm. Pharmacol. 61, 407–422.

Neuwinger, H.D., 2000. African traditional medicine. Medpharm, Stuttgart.

Okpako, D.T., 1999. Traditional African medicine: theory and pharmacology explored. Trends Pharmacol. Sci. 20, 482–485.

Sairam, T.V., 2000. Home remedies, vols. I–III. Penguin, India.

Sofowara, A. (Ed.), 1979. African medicinal plants: Proceedings of a conference. University of Life Press, Nigeria.

Thomas, O.O., 1989. Perspectives on ethno-phytotherapy of Yoruba medicinal herbs and preparations. Fitoterapia 60, 49–60.

Williamson, E.M. (Ed.), 2002. Major herbs of Ayurveda. Churchill Livingstone, Edinburgh.

Chapter 13

Complementary and Alternative medicine

In addition to rational phytotherapy, which is a science-based, empirical approach to the use of medicinal plants in the treatment and prevention of disease, in developed countries there are other healthcare approaches involving the use of plants. The most popular of these non-conventional approaches are discussed in this chapter (Box 13.1 and 13.2).

Therapies labelled as *Complementary and Alternative Medicines* (CAM) are in fact a highly diverse group of approaches to health care and are based on philosophies towards health and illness that are fundamentally different from the approach of conventional, scientific medicine (biomedicine) and pharmacy. These therapies are also called complementary therapies and complementary health care. These forms of treatment are simply grouped together on the basis of them being an alternative to established healthcare systems.

MEDICAL HERBALISM

HISTORY

In the UK, medical herbalism traces its historical traditions partly to Galen's (a Greek physician of the 2nd century AD) model of 'bodily humours' (blood, black bile, yellow bile, phlegm), their 'temperaments' (e.g. hot, cold, damp) and the belief that illness resulted from an imbalance in these humours. Herbs were used to correct the imbalance and were often described as, for example, 'heating' or 'cooling'; a 'cooling' herb, such as peppermint, would be used to treat a 'hot' condition, such as fever. In the UK, herbalism has also drawn on other traditions, such as the use of herbs in North America after Samuel Thomson, although Thomson was himself influenced by herbalism in Europe.

MODERN HERBALISM

Today, medical herbalism, practised by medical herbalists, draws on traditional knowledge, but, increasingly, this is interpreted and applied in a modern context. For example, herbalists use current knowledge of the causes and consequences of disease as well as some of the diagnostic tools, such as blood pressure measurement, used in conventional medicine. Also, there is an increasing emphasis on using evidence from modern randomized controlled clinical trials to support the traditional use of herbal preparations. Some other aspects of modern-day herbalism as seen by the herbalists are listed below:

- A patient's psychological and emotional wellbeing, as well as physical health, is considered, resulting in the claim that a holistic therapy is offered.
- Herbalists select herbs on an individual basis for each patient (in line with the holistic approach), thus it is likely that even patients with the same physical symptoms will receive different combinations of herbs.
- Herbalists also aim to identify the underlying cause (e.g. stress) of a patient's illness and to consider this in the treatment plan.
- Herbs are used to stimulate the body's healing capacity, to 'strengthen' bodily systems and to 'correct' disturbed body functions rather than to treat presenting symptoms directly.

BOX 13.1   Complementary and alternative medicines (CAM)

Many of these therapies involve the administration (internally or externally) of plant-derived preparations, such as herbal tinctures or essential oils. In case of homoeopathy other substances are also used (e.g. minerals) and they are administered in a highly diluted form ('potentiation'), an approach which as such differentiates homeopathy from biomedicine. Several of these approaches, such as **medical herbalism** and **homoeopathy**, are described as 'holistic' or complete systems of healing in that they proffer a philosophy for health and illness, together with a distinct approach to the diagnosis and treatment of a wide range of complaints and disorders. In addition to the therapies listed above, CAM includes acupuncture, chiropractic, massage, osteopathy, reflexology and other therapies. It should be noted that individuals with a scientific interest in herbal medicines do not consider the rational use of herbal preparations (i.e. science-based phytotherapy) to be part of CAM.

- Herbs may be used, for example, with the aim of 'eliminating toxins' or 'stimulating' the circulation. The intention is to provide long-term relief from the particular condition.

Importantly, different constituents of a medicinal plant are seen as acting together in some (undefined) way that has beneficial effects. For example, the constituents may have additive effects, or interact to produce an effect greater than the total contribution of each individual constituent (known as 'synergy'), or the effects of one constituent reduce the likelihood of adverse effects due to another constituent. Similarly, it is also believed that some combinations of different herbs interact in a beneficial way. There is some experimental (but little clinical) evidence that such interactions occur, although it cannot be assumed that this is the case for all herbs or for all combinations of herbs. Synergy is discussed in detail in Chapter 11.

CONDITIONS TREATED

Medical herbalists treat a wide range of acute (e.g. infections) and, more usually, chronic conditions. Very often the chronic conditions are those that are difficult to treat, including irritable bowel syndrome, premenstrual syndrome, eczema, acne and other skin conditions, cystitis, arthritis, depression, chronic fatigue syndrome or migraine.

HERBALISTS' PRESCRIPTIONS

A first consultation with a herbalist may last for an hour or more, during which the herbalist will explore the detailed history of the illness. Generally, a combination of several different herbs (usually four to six) is used in the treatment of a particular patient. Some examples of such combinations are given in Table 13.1, although there are no 'typical' prescriptions for specific conditions; as stated above, even patients with the same condition are likely to receive

---

BOX 13.2   Core characteristics of some important forms of complementary and alternative medicine which make use of medicinal plants

Medical herbalism is embedded in the European traditions of medicine and by understanding a patient's psychological, emotional and physical health a herbalist selects herbs on an individual basis.

Homoeopathy also focuses on understanding a patient's psychological, emotional and physical health, but treatment with specially prepared highly diluted ('potentiated') is used ('like cures like' or in Latin, *similia similibus curentur*). Thus its philosophical basis and therapeutic approaches are completely different from approaches where biologically active preparations are used.

Anthroposophical medicine also focuses on a holistic understanding of illness in terms of how the four 'bodies' and the functional systems interact with each other. Diagnosis involves conventional tools, the patient's life story and social context, and even bodily expressions. It uses an integrated therapeutic programme including diet, therapeutic movement (eurythmy), artistic therapies and massage, and anthroposophic medicines.

Aromatherapy is the therapeutic use of essential oils generally distilled from plants and used for therapeutic purposes generally or in order to increase a person's wellbeing.

Flower remedies of various types are obtained using a very simple extraction procedure used on the flowers of a range of common plant species and they are widely available for self-treatment.

Table 13.1	Examples of herbal prescriptions
PLANT	**PLANT PART**
Menopausal symptoms	
Cimicifuga racemosa (black cohosh)	Roots, rhizome
Leonorus cardiaca (motherwort)	Aerial parts
Hypericum perforatum (St John's wort)	Aerial parts
Alchemilla vulgaris (Lady's mantle)	Aerial parts
Stress	
Passiflora incarnata (passion flower)	Aerial parts
Valeriana officinalis (valerian)	Root
Verbena officinalis (vervain)	Aerial parts
Leonorus cardiaca (motherwort)	Aerial parts

Table 13.2	Comparison of herbalism and rational phytotherapy	
HERBALISM	**RATIONAL PHYTOTHERAPY**	
Assumes that synergy or additive effects occur between herbal constituents or between herbs	Seeks evidence that synergy or additive effects occur between herbal constituents or between herbs	
Holistic (individualistic) prescribing of herbs	Not holistic; uses symptom- or condition-based prescribing	
Preparations mainly formulated as tinctures	Preparations mainly formulated as tablets and capsules	
Mainly uses combinations of herbs	Single-herb products used mainly	
Some opposition towards tight standardization of preparations	Aims at using standardized extracts of plants or plant parts	
Not scientifically evaluated	Science-based approach	

different prescriptions. Sometimes, a single herb may be given, for example, *Vitex agnus-castus* (chasteberry) for premenstrual syndrome and dysmenorrhoea. Each patient's treatment is reviewed regularly and is likely to be changed depending on whether or not there has been a response.

Herbalists usually prescribe herbal medicines as tinctures, although sometimes more concentrated formulations (fluid extracts) are used. Where a prescription requires several herbs, tinctures and fluid extracts are blended into a mixture. Some herbalists will prepare their own stock material, others purchase it from specialist suppliers and most dispense their own herbal prescriptions. Other oral formulations (tablets, capsules) and topical preparations of herbs may also be prescribed.

COMPARISON OF HERBALISM WITH RATIONAL PHYTOTHERAPY

Herbalism contrasts with rational phytotherapy in several ways (Table 13.2). Importantly, the herbalist's approach has not been evaluated in controlled clinical trials, whereas there are numerous controlled clinical trials of specific phytotherapeutic preparations. Another important difference is that, although many of the same medicinal plants are used in each of the two approaches, the formulations of those herbs are often very different. For example, St John's wort (*Hypericum perforatum L.*) is used in both rational phytotherapy and by herbalists. However, in rational phytotherapy, the preparations used are likely to be extracts of *H. perforatum* herb (leaves and tops) standardized on hypericin content and formulated as tablets. By contrast, herbalists are likely to use a tincture of *H. perforatum* herb that is not standardized on its content of any particular constituent.

The terminology is often confusing. Herbalism is sometimes also referred to as phytotherapy, and both herbalism and rational phytotherapy are sometimes described as 'herbal medicine'. Likewise, preparations used in rational phytotherapy and in herbalism may both be referred to as 'herbal medicines' or 'phytomedicines'.

In some ways, herbalism is similar to Western medicine. For example, both use drug intervention (herbs and conventional drugs, respectively) to counteract disease, although herbalism is focused on correcting disturbed function rather than treating symptoms. Both use material doses (in contrast to homoeopathy, which uses highly dilute preparations, not all of plant origin). Herbal medicine in the UK covers a wide spectrum of practice: there are traditional herbalists who refer mainly to the older traditions and philosophy, those whose view is aligned more closely with 'modern' rational phytotherapy, and those whose practice is somewhere between the two approaches.

EVIDENCE OF EFFICACY AND SAFETY

There is a significant body of clinical evidence on the potential benefits and potential risks associated with the use of specific herbal medicines (for the most important species see Part B). The vast majority of this information relates to the use of specific herbal medicines formulated as phytopharmaceuticals and used in the same manner as conventional pharmaceuticals, usually under the supervision of a physician, to treat symptoms of disease. There has been very little investigation of the efficacy and safety of herbal medicines and combinations of herbal medicines used by herbal medicine practitioners. Furthermore, the efficacy and safety of herbalism as a treatment approach has not yet been evaluated scientifically.

HOMOEOPATHY

HISTORY

Homoeopathy was developed around 200 years ago by Samuel Hahnemann, a German physician and apothecary. His development of the principles of this controversial approach to treatment needs to be considered against the background of medical practice at the time, when the use of leeches, bloodletting, strong purgatives and emetics, and preparations containing toxic heavy metals, such as arsenic and mercury, was widespread. It is reported that Hahnemann was dissatisfied with these harsh therapeutic strategies and that this led him to give up the practice of medicine. During this period, he was stimulated to experiment with cinchona bark (which was used to treat malaria) and found that, while taking high doses of the substance, he experienced symptoms that were similar to those of malaria. Hahnemann then used this approach (which he called a 'proving') with healthy volunteers who were given many other substances in order to build up a 'symptom picture' for each substance. On the basis of his findings from these experiments, Hahnemann outlined three basic principles of (classical) homoeopathy:

1. A substance which, used in large doses, causes a symptom(s) in a healthy person can be used to treat that symptom(s) in a person who is ill. For example, Coffea, a remedy prepared from the coffee bean (a constituent, caffeine, is a central nervous system stimulant) would be used to treat insomnia. This is the so-called 'like cures like' concept (in Latin, similia similibus curentur).
2. The minimal dose of the substance should be used in order to prevent toxicity. Initially, Hahnemann used high doses of substances, but this often led to toxic effects. Subsequently, substances were diluted in a stepwise manner and subjected to vigorous shaking ('succussion') at each step. This process is called potentization.

It is claimed that the more dilute the remedy, the more potent it is. This completely opposes current scientific knowledge.
3. Only a single remedy or substance should be used in a patient at any one time.

MODERN HOMOEOPATHY

Despite of all controversies, homeopathy has spread widely and is a very popular form of health care in many European, Asian and American countries. Hahnemann's principles of homoeopathy still form the basis of modern homoeopathic practice, with the exception of the single remedy rule, which is ignored by many homoeopaths in favour of multiple prescribing. Today, around 1200 homoeopathic remedies are commonly used. For many of these, homoeopaths rely on Hahnemann's provings and, therefore, guidance on which symptoms the remedies can be used to treat. Modern-day provings involving healthy volunteers are sometimes undertaken, and several have involved rigorous study design (randomized, double-blind, placebo-controlled). However, Hahnemann did not use rigorous study design, although he did specify certain criteria; for example, subjects were not permitted to have coffee during the course of a proving.

In addition to the key principles of homoeopathy outlined above, homoeopaths also claim:

- illness results from the body's inability to cope with challenging factors such as poor diet and adverse environmental conditions
- the signs and symptoms of disease represent the body's attempt to restore order
- homoeopathic remedies work by stimulating the body's own healing activity (the 'vital force') rather than by acting directly on the disease process
- the 'vital force' is expressed differently in each individual, so treatment must be chosen on an individual basis and thus needs to be holistic

In choosing a remedy for a particular patient, a homoeopath will consider the patient's physical, mental and emotional symptoms, as well as personal characteristics, likes and dislikes. This information is then used to select the homoeopathic remedy with a 'symptom picture' that most closely matches that of the patient. Computerized repertories (databases of homoeopathic remedy symptom pictures) are now available which facilitate this process.

HOMOEOPATHIC REMEDIES

Homoeopathic remedies and herbal medicines are often confused and/or deemed to be similar. The fundamental differences between the two types of preparation are:

- Homoeopathic remedies are (mostly) highly dilute whereas herbal medicines are used at material strengths. However, since homeopathic preparations are first extracted from, for example, plant material and then diluted, there is a borderline group including mother tinctures and lower potencies (i.e. less diluted) which still may contain biomedically relevant amounts of active ingredients.
- Many homoeopathic remedies (around 65%) originate from plants, whereas by definition all herbal medicines originate from plants (for examples of plant-based homeopathic preparations see Table 13.3).

Many of the species used for preparing homoeopathic remedies have a history of medicinal use; others are poisonous if used undiluted. Other types of material used in the preparation of homoeopathic remedies include animal, insect, biological, drug/chemical and mineral.

The starting point for the production of most homoeopathic remedies is a mother tincture, usually an alcohol/water extract of crude plant material, such as dried arnica flowers. The mother tincture is then diluted according to either the decimal (dilution steps of 1 in 10; denoted by D or X) or centesimal (dilution steps of 1 in 100; denoted by C or cH) scale to form homoeopathic remedies or potencies. For example, on the decimal dilution scale, a 1X (or D1) remedy is prepared by taking one part mother tincture and adding it to nine parts diluent (dilute alcohol) and succussing the resulting 1 in 10 dilution. A 2X remedy is prepared by taking one part 1X remedy and adding it to nine parts diluent and succussing the resulting dilution, which is now a dilution of 1 in 100, and so on. The centesimal scale uses the same procedure except that each step involves adding one part mother tincture to 99 parts diluent so that the first step produces a 1 in 100 dilution (1C or 1cH), the second step a 1 in 10,000 dilution (2C) and so on. The centesimal scale goes as far as M (1 in 10^{2000} dilution, i.e. 2000 centesimal dilution steps) and 10M (1 in $10^{20,000}$) dilutions. These potencies are usually prepared robotically. There are also LM potencies which involve serial dilutions of 1 in 50,000 at each step.

Potencies at the lower end of the decimal (i.e. 1X, 2X,3X to around 6X) and centesimal scales (usually up to 3C) still contain reasonable quantities of starting material and, depending on the nature of the starting material, may elicit pharmacological or toxicological effects. For this reason, some homoeopathic remedies at these lower dilutions are classified as prescription-only medicines (POM) in the UK. Some examples of plant-derived homoeopathic remedies and the potencies below which they are POM include:

- Aconite (*Aconitum napellus*, monkshood), 3C or 6X
- Belladonna (*Atropa belladonna*, deadly nightshade), 2C or 3X
- Croton (*Croton tiglium*), 3C or 6X
- Hyoscyamus (*Hyoscyamus niger*, henbane), 2C or 3X
- Nux vomica (*Strychnos nux-vomica*), 3C or 6X.

Potencies of 24X and 12C and above are diluted beyond Avogadro's number; thus it is highly unlikely that even a single molecule of the original starting material is present.

Table 13.3 Examples of homoeopathic remedies originating from plant material

COMMON REMEDY NAME	PLANT SOURCE	COMMON PLANT NAME(S)	PLANT PART
Aconite	*Aconitum napellus*	Monkshood	Whole plant
Arnica	*Arnica Montana*	Arnica, leopard's bane	Dried flowers
Allium cepa	*Allium cepa*	Red onion	Whole fresh plant
Belladonna	*Atropa belladonna*	Deadly nightshade	Whole fresh plant
Bryonia	*Bryonia alba*	White bryony	Root
Euphrasia	*Euphrasia officinalis*	Eyebright	Whole plant
Hydrastis	*Hydrastis canadensis*	Goldenseal	Fresh root
Rhus tox	*Rhus toxicodendron*	Poison ivy	Fresh leaves
Staphisagria	*Delphinium staphisagria*	Stavesacre	Seeds
Stramonium	*Datura stramonium*	Thorn apple, Jimson weed	Fresh plant

Quality control needs to be carried out on the source materials, and the manufacturing process for homoeopathic preparations needs to adhere to the principles of good manufacturing practice to ensure that contamination does not occur.

POTENTIZATION

According to Hahnemann's second principle (but in opposition to modern pharmacological principles), the more dilute the preparation, the more potent it is. So, for example, a 6X remedy is claimed to be 'stronger' (more potent) than a 2X remedy, and a 12C remedy more potent than a 6C remedy. Also, although 2X and 1C preparations are the same concentration, a 2X is considered to be more potent because it has undergone two steps involving succussion, whereas 1C preparations have undergone only one succussion step.

Homoeopaths have put forward several arguments in an attempt to explain how highly dilute homoeopathic remedies could work. One of the most well-known of these is the 'memory of water' theory. Proponents of this theory claim that the process of succussion somehow alters the solvent molecules such that they become rearranged to form 'imprints' of molecules of the original starting material. Research exploring this theory has drawn on the disciplines of physics and biology, and has involved investigation of the physicochemical principles of homoeopathic remedies. It has been reported for some homoeopathic remedies that their physicochemical principles are different to those of the relevant solvent alone. However, these preliminary findings have had a negligible impact on the wider scientific community.

EVIDENCE OF EFFICACY

Homoeopathic treatment has been investigated in over 100 clinical trials, and the results of these studies have been subject to systematic review and meta-analysis. A meta-analysis of data from 89 placebo-controlled trials of homoeopathy indicated that the effects of homoeopathy are not completely due to placebo. Restricting the analysis to high-quality trials only reduced, but did not eliminate, the effect found. However, there was insufficient evidence to demonstrate that homoeopathy is clearly efficacious in any single clinical condition (Linde et al 1997). Many trials, particularly those with negative results for homoeopathy, have been criticized by proponents of homoeopathy because participants received the

same homoeopathic treatment rather than individualized treatment. So, another meta-analysis considered all placebo-controlled trials ($n=19$) of 'individualized' homoeopathy (i.e. where patients are prescribed the remedy most appropriate for their particular symptoms and personal characteristics; Linde and Melchart 1998). The study found that individualized homoeopathy was significantly more effective than placebo, but, when the methodologically best trials only were considered, no effect over that of placebo was seen for homoeopathy. Further work has provided strong evidence that, in homoeopathy, clinical trials of better methodological quality tend to yield less positive results. There have been several high-quality trials published since Linde et al's original meta-analysis which report negative results, and it seems likely that the original meta-analysis 'at least overestimated the effects of homoeopathic treatments' (Linde et al 1999).

SAFETY

It is unlikely that highly dilute homoeopathic remedies can lead to serious adverse drug reactions. However, the potential for toxicity with homoeopathic remedies at low dilutions should be considered, since such preparations can still contain reasonable quantities of starting material. This view is supported by the provisions of the European directive 92/73/EEC which became law in the UK in 1994 and which provides regulations for homoeopathic medicinal products. The directive required member states to set up a simplified registration procedure based on quality and safety, but not efficacy, for homoeopathic medicinal products that met certain criteria, including:

- oral or external use only
- minimum dilution of 4X
- no claims for therapeutic efficacy.

There are isolated reports in the literature of suspected adverse effects, usually allergic reactions, following the use of homoeopathic remedies (Barnes 1998a), although a causal association has not been established. There are also isolated reports of adulterated homoeopathic remedies.

Pooled data from placebo-controlled clinical trials involving homoeopathic remedies indicate that adverse effects occur more frequently with homoeopathy than with placebo, but that adverse effects are mild and transient, and the types (e.g. headaches, tiredness, skin reactions, dizziness and diarrhoea) are similar for both homoeopathy and placebo.

ANTHROPOSOPHICAL MEDICINE

HISTORY

Anthroposophical medicine is a philosophical vision of health and disease based on the work of Austrian philosopher and esoceritist Rudolf Steiner (1861–1925). Steiner's work explored how human beings and the natural world could be described, not only in physical terms, but also in terms of soul and spirit. He called this philosophy 'anthroposophy'. Its relevance in medicine, education and agriculture became an increasing part of Steiner's work, and resulted in what is now known as anthroposophic medicine.

Steiner believed that consciousness could not be defined in physical terms, as in conventional medicine, and explored how human's soul and spiritual nature relate to the health and function of the body. Nevertheless, he aimed anthroposophic medicine to be an extension, not an alternative, to conventional medicine. Steiner viewed each person as having four 'bodies' or 'forces':

- A physical body
- An etheric body, or life force
- An astral body, or conscious awareness
- A spiritual body, or self-awareness or ego.

And he considered the human-being to be made of three functional systems:

- The 'sense-nervous' system (the head and spinal column), focusing on 'cooling' and 'hardening' processes (e.g. the development of arthritis).
- The 'reproductive-metabolic' system, which includes parts of the body that are in constant motion (e.g. the limbs and digestive system) and which focuses on warming and softening processes (e.g. fevers).
- The 'rhythmic' system (the heart, lungs and circulation), which balances the other two systems. Steiner believed that health is maintained by harmonious interaction of the three systems, and that cacophonous (inharmonious) interactions between the systems result in illness.

MODERN ANTHROPOSOPHIC MEDICINE

Anthroposophic medicine today is still based on Steiner's philosophy. Practitioners of anthroposophy aim to understand illness holistically in terms of how the four 'bodies' and the functional systems interact with each other. Diagnosis involves not only several conventional tools, such as history-taking, physical examination and laboratory investigations, but also the patient's life story, social context and even body shape, movements, social behaviour and modes of artistic expression. Anthroposophic practitioners may use a range of therapies, including diet, therapeutic movement (eurythmy), artistic therapies and massage, as well as anthroposophic medicines, in an integrated therapeutic programme.

Anthroposophic medicine is particularly well-developed in Austria, Germany, Switzerland and The Netherlands, where there are hospitals specializing in anthroposophic medicine, as well as many general practitioners who practise an anthroposophical approach. In the UK there are only a few medically qualified practitioners who practise anthroposophic medicine.

CONDITIONS TREATED

Several hospitals in Germany specializing in anthroposophic medicine provide a range of treatments that are also provided by general hospitals. Anthroposophic medicine is used as a therapeutic approach, under medical supervision, for several serious conditions, including supportive treatment in cancer. There is also a wide range of over-the-counter (OTC) medicines (both general sales list and pharmacy only) used for the symptomatic relief of conditions suitable for OTC treatment, such as indigestion, constipation, coughs, colds, sore throat, catarrh, sleeplessness, muscular pain and certain skin conditions.

ANTHROPOSOPHIC MEDICINES

Steiner believed that the sizes of different parts of plants, such as flowers, leaves and roots, are disproportionate in plants with medicinal properties. Usually, the disproportionately sized part would be used therapeutically. For example, nettle (*Urtica dioica*) produces an abundance of green leaves, whereas the flowers and fruit are insignificant in terms of size. Therefore, from an anthroposophic perspective, nettle leaves are deemed to have medicinal properties. However, sometimes, the whole plant, or a part of the plant other than the disproportionately sized part would be used therapeutically. In addition, in anthroposophic medicine, it is believed that the specific part of a medicinal plant relates to one of the three different 'systems' of the body (see above): roots relate to the 'sense-nervous system', flowers and fruit relate to the 'reproductive-metabolic system' and leaves act on the 'rhythmic system'. Continuing to use nettle as an example, nettle leaves are used to stimulate the assimilation of iron (e.g. in anaemia), which is important in blood circulation.

Anthroposophic medicines are derived mainly from plants and minerals, such as calcium, iron and copper. Many products are combinations of herbal ingredients, and some products contain both herbal and mineral ingredients. Herbal and mineral ingredients are usually described by their Latin binomial name together with the plant part for herbs. For example:

- *Aconitum napellus*, planta total (=aconite, whole plant)
- *Natrium carbonicum* (=sodium carbonate).

Ingredients of anthroposophical medicines are sometimes 'potentized' using the X or D potency series (steps of 1 in 10 dilution) rather than the C potency series (steps of 1 in 100 dilution) (see above). Thus, an ingredient with a potency of 1X (or D1) has a concentration of 1 in 10 or 10%, a 2X potency has undergone two steps of 1 in 10 dilution so is 1 in 100 or 1%. As with homoeopathic remedies, at each dilution stage for an anthroposophical ingredient, the liquid is rhythmically succussed, which is claimed to 'release' the therapeutic properties of the substance. In anthroposophical medicines, ingredients are usually used at potencies below 6X (or D6). These are low dilutions, so reasonable quantities of plant constituents will be present. Thus, anthroposophical medicines containing plant-derived ingredients at dilutions below 6X can, from a pharmaceutical perspective, be considered to be herbal medicines.

Another group of products derived from the anthroposophical approach are mistletoe (*Viscum album*) preparations. Mistletoe is a semi-parasite, extracting water and mineral salts from the host trees. The preparations contain a specially processed fermented aqueous mistletoe extract growing on a range of host trees, such as apple (*Malus domestica*), pine (*Pinus* sp), or oak (*Quercus* spp.).

The three types are also available formulated with low concentrations (10^{-8} g per 100 mg fresh plant extract) of certain metal salts, such as those of copper and mercury. A lectin-standardized extract, also prepared according to the anthroposophic approach, is available, although this formulation does not include metal salts. Lectin-standardized mistletoe extracts, which are distinct from anthroposophical mistletoe preparations, are also available, particularly in Germany. Mistletoe products prepared from different host trees are prescribed for patients with different types of cancer. Treatment is usually given by subcutaneous injection, although the intravenous injection route is sometimes used, and oral formulations are also available.

In the preparation of anthroposophical medicines, particular attention is paid to the source and methods of farming used in growing plant raw materials. Plant materials are grown according to the principles of biodynamic farming, which is similar to organic farming. Pharmaceutical manufacturing companies exist that are dedicated to the production of anthroposophical medicines.

AROMATHERAPY

HISTORY

Aromatic plants and their extracts have been used in cosmetics and perfumes and for religious purposes for thousands of years, although the link with the therapeutic use of essential oils is weak. One of the foundations of aromatherapy is attributed to Rene-Maurice Gattefosse, a French perfumer chemist, who first used the term aromatherapy in 1928 (Vickers 1996). Gattefosse burnt his hand while working in a laboratory and found that lavender oil helped the burn to heal quickly with little scarring. Jean Valnet developed Gattefosse's ideas of the benefits of essential oils in wound healing, and used essential oils more widely in specific medical disorders. Marguerite Maury popularized the ancient uses of essential oils for health, beauty and wellbeing and so played a role in the modern renaissance of aromatherapy.

MODERN AROMATHERAPY

Aromatherapy is the therapeutic use of essential oils. These are obtained from plant material (e.g. roots, leaves, flowers, seeds) usually by distillation, although physical expression (using compression and pressure) is the method used to obtain some essential oils, mainly those from the skin of citrus fruits. Some of the key aspects of the use of essential oils in aromatherapy are described below:

- Aromatherapists believe that essential oils can be used not only for the treatment and prevention of disease, but also for their effects on mood, emotion and wellbeing.

- Aromatherapy is claimed to be an holistic therapy: an essential oil, or a combination of essential oils, is selected to suit each client's symptoms, personality and emotional state, and treatment may change at subsequent visits.
- Essential oils are described both with reference to reputed pharmacological properties (e.g. antibacterial, anti-inflammatory) and to concepts not recognized in conventional medicine (e.g. 'balancing', 'energizing'). There is often little agreement among aromatherapists on the 'properties' of specific essential oils.
- Aromatherapists claim that the constituents of essential oils, or combinations of oils, work synergistically to improve efficacy or to reduce the occurrence of adverse effects (described as 'quenching') associated with particular (e.g. irritant) constituents.

CONDITIONS TREATED

Aromatherapy is widely used as an approach to relieving stress, and many essential oils are claimed to be 'relaxing'. Many aromatherapists also claim that essential oils can be used in the treatment of a wide range of conditions. Often, many different properties and indications are listed for each essential oil, and conditions range from those that are relatively minor to those considered serious. For example, indications for peppermint leaf oil (*Mentha* × *piperita*) listed by one text include flatulence, ringworm, skin rashes, cystitis, indigestion, nausea, gastritis and sciatica, as well as migraine, hepatitis, jaundice, cirrhosis, bronchial asthma and impotence (Price & Price 1995). Many users self-administer essential oils either as a beauty treatment, as an aid to relaxation, or to treat specific ailments, many of which may not be suitable for self-treatment. Aromatherapy is also used in a variety of conventional healthcare settings, such as in palliative care, intensive care units, mental health units and in specialized units caring for patients with HIV/AIDS, physical disabilities and severe learning disabilities.

On a first appointment and before treating a client, an aromatherapist will take a case history, including gathering details of the client's medical history, lifestyle, diet and moods/emotions. Information gathered during the consultation is used to select essential oils thought to be appropriate for the individual concerned. The most common method used by aromatherapists for the application of essential oils is by massage, where drops of (usually) two to three essential oils are diluted in a vegetable carrier (or base) oil, such as grapeseed oil, jojoba oil, wheatgerm oil, sweet almond oil or sesame oil. The resulting 'blend' is then applied either during a full-body massage or localized massage. Other methods of applying essential oils used by aromatherapists or in self-treatment include:

- addition of essential oils to baths and footbaths (water should be agitated vigorously to aid dispersion)
- inhalations
- compresses
- use in aromatherapy equipment (e.g. burners and vaporizers).

Some practitioners advocate the oral administration of essential oils, described as 'aromatology'. However, essential oils should never be taken internally without medical supervision. Some aromatherapists also suggest that essential oils can be administered vaginally (e.g. via tampons or a douche) or rectally, but administration by these routes may cause mucosal membrane irritation and is not recommended.

ESSENTIAL OILS

Typically, an essential oil contains around 100 or more chemical constituents, mostly present at concentrations below 1%, although some constituents are present at much lower concentrations. Some essential oils contain one or two major constituents, and the therapeutic and toxicological properties of the oil can largely be attributed to those constituent(s). However, other constituents present at low concentrations can be important. The composition of an essential oil will vary according to the plant's environment and growing conditions, the plant part used and on methods of harvesting, extraction and storage. The major constituents of an essential oil can also vary in different chemotypes of the same species of plant. The constituents of essential oils are largely volatile compounds which are sensitive to the effects of light, heat, air and moisture and should, therefore, be stored in a cool place in tightly closed, darkened bottles. Even when stored correctly, the composition of essential oils can change during storage, so qualitative and quantitative analyses relate only to the composition of the oil at the time of testing. There is also the possibility of adulteration and contamination occurring during processing. Gross adulteration can be detected using established analytical techniques such as gas chromatography–mass spectrometry (GC-MS).

Essential oils should be referred to by the Latin binomial name of the plant species from which a particular oil is derived. The plant part used should be specified and, sometimes, further specification is necessary to define the chemotype of a particular plant; for example, *Thymus vulgaris* CT thymol describes a chemotype of a species of thyme that has thymol as a major chemical constituent (Clarke 2002).

EFFICACY AND SAFETY

Essential oils are believed to act both by exerting pharmacological effects following absorption into the circulation and via the effects of their odour on the olfactory system. There is evidence that essential oils are absorbed into the circulation after topical application (i.e. massage) and after inhalation, although amounts entering the circulation are likely to be very small (Vickers 1996).

Certain essential oils have been shown to have pharmacological effects in animal models and in *in vitro* studies, but there is little good-quality clinical research investigating the effects of essential oils and aromatherapy as practised by aromatherapists. Most of the clinical trials that have been conducted do not show that massage with essential oils is significantly better than massage with carrier oil alone (Barnes 1998b). There is evidence that tea tree oil applied topically is effective in the treatment of certain skin infections, but these studies have not tested aromatherapy as practised by aromatherapists.

Data regarding the safety of essential oils as used in aromatherapy are limited. Few adverse effects associated with aromatherapy treatment have been reported; most reports relate to cases of contact dermatitis in patients or aromatherapists. Minor transient adverse effects, such as drowsiness, headache and nausea, can occur after aromatherapy treatment. The increasing use of essential oils during pregnancy and labour is of concern. Because of uncertainties about the safety of essential oils during these periods, general advice is that the use of essential oils should be avoided during pregnancy, particularly during the first trimester. The use of certain essential oils should also be avoided by patients with epilepsy.

FLOWER REMEDY THERAPY

Bach (pronounced 'batch') flower remedies are probably the most well-known of this type of preparation, although there are many other types of flower remedies (also known as flower essences). Different types are usually derived from native plants of the particular region or country, such as Australian bush flower essences, rain forest essences (Brazil), Alaskan flower essences.

HISTORY

Bach flower remedies were developed by Dr Edward Bach (1886–1936), a physician and homoeopath. Bach believed that negative states of mind caused physical illness, and his approach to maintaining health was focused on the patient's psychological state. His theory was that by treating patients' emotional and mental responses to their illness, physical symptoms would then be relieved. He identified 38 negative psychological states (e.g. jealousy, hopelessness, guilt, indecision) and sought natural remedies that could be used to 'correct' these negative states of mind. It is claimed that to do this Bach visited the countryside, concentrated on these specific emotional states and was intuitively drawn towards particular wild flowers that he believed could relieve them.

MODERN FLOWER REMEDY THERAPY

Flower remedies of various types are widely available for self-selection and self-treatment. In addition some individuals undertake training to become a flower-remedy practitioner; this includes some healthcare professionals, such as some general practitioners, who use flower remedies alongside their day-to-day conventional medical practice.

FLOWER REMEDIES

Bach developed 38 flower remedies, 37 of which are based on single wild flowers and tree blossoms, and one (rock water) which is made from natural spring water. He intended each remedy to be used for a specific emotional or mental state. Some examples are:

- Gentian (*Gentiana amarella*) for despondency
- Holly (*Ilex aquifolium*) for jealousy
- Impatiens (*Impatiens glandulifera*) for impatience

- Pine (*Pinus sylvestris*) for guilt
- Rock rose (*Helianthemum nummularium*) for terror.

Bach also developed a preparation termed Rescue Remedy, which is a combination of five of the other remedies: impatiens (*Impatiens glandulifera*), star of Bethlehem (*Ornithogalum umbellatum*), cherry plum (*Prunus cerasifera*), rock rose (*Helianthemum nummularium*) and clematis (*Clematis vitalba*). Bach recommended this preparation to be used in difficult and demanding situations, such as shock, terror, bereavement.

Bach flower remedies are prepared from mother tinctures which are themselves made from plant material and natural spring water using either an infusion ('sun') method or a 'boiling' method (Kayne 2002). The infusion method is used to prepare mother tinctures for 20 of the Bach remedies: flower heads from the appropriate plant are added to a glass vessel containing natural spring water and are left to stand in direct sunlight for several hours, after which the flowers are discarded and the infused spring water retained. The boiling method involves the addition of plant material to natural spring water, which is then boiled for 30 minutes, cooled and strained. With both methods, the resulting solution is diluted with an equivalent volume of alcohol (brandy) to make the mother tincture. Flower remedies are then prepared by adding two drops of the appropriate mother tincture to 30 ml of grape alcohol. It is claimed that the resulting solution is equivalent to a 1 in 100,000 dilution. This is the same dilution as a 5X potency in homoeopathy, but preparation of flower remedies does not involve serial dilution and succussion. Thus, in material terms, flower remedies and 5X potencies can be considered equal, although from a homoeopathic perspective they are not.

Flower remedies are usually taken orally (2–4 drops added to a cold drink and sipped), although, in some cases, drops are placed directly under the tongue and even on the wrist or temples. Rescue Remedy is also available as a cream for external use.

EFFICACY AND SAFETY

Although there are many anecdotal reports of the benefits of flower remedies, there is a lack of both experimental and clinical research into their reputed effects (Barnes 1998c) and while this form of self-treatment is very popular, it remains highly controversial.

Flower remedies are widely claimed to be completely free from adverse effects. Adverse effects are unlikely to occur, given that the preparations contain only highly dilute material. However, as flower remedies contain alcohol, they may be unsuitable for some individuals. Excessive use of a flower remedy could be of concern if an individual was relying on self-treatment with flower remedies for conditions such as anxiety or depression, for which medical treatment and other professional support may be required.

GENERAL CONCLUSION

The traditions presented here are part of European medical traditions and while evidence for their clinical usefulness is very limited they remain a popular healthcare choice and one which often involves the use of plant-derived medicines. Consequently, these products are – in pharmaceutical terms – as important as other medications.

References

Barnes, J., 1998a. Homoeopathy. Pharmaceutical Journal 260, 492–497.

Barnes, J., 1998b. Aromatherapy. Pharmaceutical Journal 260, 862–867.

Barnes, J., 1998c. Complementary medicine. Other therapies. Pharmaceutical Journal 261, 490–493.

Clarke, S., 2002. Essential chemistry for safe aromatherapy. Churchill Livingstone, Edinburgh.

Kayne, S.B., 2002. Complementary therapies for pharmacists. Pharmaceutical Press, London.

Linde, K., Clausius, N., Ramirez, G., et al., 1997. Are the clinical effects of homeopathy placebo effects? A meta-analysis of placebo-controlled trials. Lancet 350 (9081), 834–843.

Linde, K., Melchart, D., 1998. Randomized controlled trials of individualized homeopathy: a state-of-the-art review. J. Altern. Complement. Med. 4 (4), 371–388.

Linde, K., Scholz, M., Ramirez, G., et al., 1999. Impact of study quality on outcome in placebo-controlled trials of homeopathy. J. Clin. Epidemiol. 52 (7), 631–636.

Price, S., Price, L., 1995. Aromatherapy for health professionals. Churchill Livingstone, Edinburgh.

Vickers, A., 1996. Massage and aromatherapy. A guide for health professionals. Chapman & Hall, London.

Further reading

Astin, J.A., 1998. Why patients use alternative medicine. Results of a national study. JAMA 279, 1548–1553.

Barnes, J., Ernst, E., 1998. Traditional herbalists' prescriptions for common clinical conditions: a survey of members of the National Institute of Medical Herbalists. Phytother. Res. 12, 369–371.

Bellavite, P., Ortolani, R., Pontarollo, F., Piasere, V., Benato, G., Conforti, A., 2006. Immunology and homeopathy. 4. Clinical Studies—Part 1 eCAM 3, 293–301.

Commission of the European Communities, 2002. Proposal for amending the directive 2001/83/EC as regards traditional herbal medicinal products. European Commission, Brussels, 2002/0008.

Dantas, F., Rampes, H., 2000. Do homeopathic medicines provoke adverse effects? A systematic review. Br. Homeopath. J. 89 (Suppl. 1), S35–S38.

Department of Health, 2001. Government response to the House of Lords Select Committee on Science and Technology's report on complementary and alternative medicine. The Stationery Office, London.

Eldin, S., Dunford, A., 1999. Herbal medicine in primary care. Butterworth-Heinemann, Oxford.

Evans, W.C. (Ed.), 2009. Trease and Evans pharmacognosy, sixteenth ed. Saunders Ltd., (Elsevier), Edingburgh.

Fulder, S., 1996. The handbook of alternative and complementary medicine, third ed. Oxford University Press, Oxford.

Giovannini, P., Schmidt, K., Canterb, P.H., Ernst, E., 2004. Research into complementary and alternative medicine across Europe and the United States. Forsch. Komplementärmed. Klass. Naturheilkd. 11, 224–230.

House of Lords Select Committee on Science and Technology, 2000. Session 1999–2000, 6th report. Complementary and alternative medicine. The Stationery Office, London.

Ipsos, MORI., 2008. Public Perceptions of Herbal Medicines. General Public Qualitative & Quantitative Research. Ipsos Mori & MHRA, London.

Kayne, S., 1997. Homoeopathic pharmacy. An introduction and handbook. Churchill Livingstone, Edinburgh.

Kennedy, J., Wang, C.C., Wu, C.H., 2008. Patient disclosure about herb and supplement use among adults in the US. Evid. Based Complement. Alternat. Med. 5, 451–456.

Mills, S.Y., Bone, K., 2000. Principles and practice of phytotherapy. Churchill Livingstone, Edinburgh.

Sandhu, D.S., Heinrich, M., 2005. The use of health foods, spices and other botanicals with the Sikh community in London. Phytother. Res. 19, 633–642.

Tisserand, R., Balacs, T., 1995. Essential oil safety. A guide for health professionals. Churchill Livingstone, Edinburgh.

Williamson, E.M., Driver, S., Baxter, K. (Eds.), 2009. Stockley's herbal medicines interactions. Pharmaceutical Press, London.

PART B

Important natural products and phytomedicines used in pharmacy and medicine

This part is devoted to plant-derived medicines arranged in therapeutic categories in a manner analogous to that of the British National Formulary (BNF), although the classification differs in some ways. For example, there is no section on immunological products and vaccines, or anaesthesia, since plant medicines are not used for these purposes and are, therefore, not represented in these categories, and natural anticancer drugs are covered in Chapter 8. A miscellaneous category of supportive, adaptogenic, tonic or cancer chemopreventive herbs has been included: these are often of Oriental or Asian origin, but are becoming important throughout the rest of the world. Examples include ginseng, ashwagandha, reishi, schisandra and green tea.

This section is not a prescribing guide, herbal compendium or pharmacopoeia, but a summary of the most important drugs obtained from plant sources and their uses. Entries are not necessarily consistent in length or the amount or nature of the information included, with more emphasis being given to the most important or those not covered extensively elsewhere. Inclusion in Part B is not a recommendation, but an acknowledgement that they are in use and so information on them is needed. Both pure compounds and herbal medicines are included; isolated natural products are used mainly in conventional medicine and are treated in the same way as any other drug, and examples given include morphine, codeine, digoxin, pilocarpine, atropine and

colchicine. Many plant drugs are used as extracts, either in crude form, or modified and standardized in some way, and these are normally described as herbal products or phytomedicines. The preparation of such extracts has been discussed in Chapter 9.

Many of these herbal drugs have now been incorporated into the European Pharmacopoeia (Eur. Ph.) and, if so, they are marked with the European symbol **EU✷** and the official Latin name is given. In these cases the Eur. Ph. should be consulted for definitions and analytical and quality-control procedures. The information in each monograph has been taken from reviews, primary references and reputable textbooks. The textbooks are standard, well-referenced works which give more details of the herbs described. Some (e.g. Barnes et al 2007, Ross 1999, 2000; Williamson et al 2009) are very detailed about the constituents, evidence and literature citations of a smaller number of herbs, others give a briefer overview of a much larger number (e.g. Williamson 2003), whereas others approach the subject from a prescribing point of view (Mills and Bone 2001, Schultz et al 1998). There are pharmacognosy reference books (Evans 2009, Haensel and Sticher 2010), Ayurvedic reference books (Williamson 2002), Chinese herbal medicine books (Tang and Eisenbrand 1992) and specialist literature on essential oils (Tisserand and Balacs 1995).

Standard references consulted for the preparation of monographs

Barnes, J., Phillipson, J.D., Anderson, L.A., 2007. Herbal medicines, third ed. Pharmaceutical Press, London.

British National Formulary, British Medical Association and the Royal Pharmaceutical Society London (published biannually)..

Evans, W.C., 2009. Trease and Evans's pharmacognosy, sixteenth ed. WB Saunders, London.

Hänsel, R., Sticher, O. (Eds.), 2010. Pharmakognosie – phytopharmazie. Springer, Berlin.

Mills, S., Bone, K., 2000. Phytotherapy. Churchill Livingstone, Edinburgh.

Ross, I., 1999. Medicinal plants of the world, vols. I and II. Humana Press, Totawa, NJ, I and II.

Schultz, V., Haensel, R., Tyler, V., 1998. Rational phytotherapy. Springer-Verlag, Berlin.

Tang, W., Eisenbrand, G., 1992. Chinese drugs of plant origin. Springer-Verlag, Berlin.

Tisserand, R., Balacs, T., 1995. Essential oil safety. Churchill Livingstone, Edinburgh.

Williamson, E. (Ed.), 2002. Major herbs of Ayurveda. Churchill Livingstone, Edinburgh.

Williamson, E., 2003. Potter's herbal cyclopedia. CW Daniels, Saffron Walden.

Williamson, E.M., Driver, S., Baxter, K., 2009. Stockley's herb–drug interactions. Pharmaceutical Press, UK.

Chapter 14

The gastrointestinal and biliary system

Gastrointestinal (GI) and liver disorders account for minor, everyday complaints as well as major health problems. Dietary measures can improve symptoms that are caused, for example, by poor eating habits, but, if these are not successful, phytomedicines are also useful. In fact, natural products are still the most commonly used remedies in cases of constipation, diarrhoea and flatulence. Plants and their derivatives also offer useful treatment alternatives for other problems such as irritable bowel syndrome, motion sickness and dyspepsia. In the case of some liver diseases, phytotherapy provides the only effective remedies currently available.

DIARRHOEA

Diarrhoea of sudden onset and short duration is very common, especially in children. It normally requires no detailed investigation or treatment, as long as the loss of electrolytes is kept under control. However, chronic serious cases of diarrhoea caused by more virulent pathogens are still a major health threat to the population of poor tropical and subtropical areas. The World Health Organization (WHO) has estimated that approximately 5 million deaths are due to diarrhoea annually (2.5 million in children under 5 years).

The first line treatment is oral rehydration therapy using sugar-salt solutions, often with added starch, and the use of gruel rich in polysaccharides (e.g. rice or barley 'water') is an effective measure. The polysaccharides of rice (*Oryza sativa*) grains are hydrolysed in the GI tract; the resulting sugars are absorbed because the co-transport of sugar and Na^+ from the GI lumen into the cells and mucosa is unaffected. Rice suspensions thus actively shift the balance of Na^+ towards the mucosal side, enhance the absorption of water and provide the body with energy, and the efficacy of rice starch has been demonstrated in several clinical studies. The treatment of diarrhoea in adults, particularly for travellers, may also include opiates or their derivatives, to reduce gastrointestinal motility. Many classical anti-diarrhoeal preparations contain opium extracts, or the isolated alkaloids morphine and codeine (e.g. kaolin and morphine mixture, codeine phosphate tablets), although these are controlled by law in some countries. Opioid derivatives such as loperamide, which have limited systemic absorption and, therefore, fewer central nervous system side effects, have superseded these agents to some extent but the natural substances are still used and are highly effective. Dietary fibre, including that found in bulk-forming laxatives (qv) can also be used to treat diarrhoea; in this case, the fibre is taken with only a small amount of water. There are other plant drugs which act in varying ways (for review see Palumbo 2006).

STARCH (AMYLUM) EU⁎

Starch is used for rehydration purposes and may be derived from rice (*Oryza sativa* L.), maize (*Zea mays* L.) or potato (*Solanum tuberosum* L.). Giving starch-based foods (like gruels) has been shown to be therapeutically beneficial and is a first line treatment in minor self-limiting cases. These are also used as excipients for tablet production. Starch particles give a very characteristic microscopic picture, which can be used to differentiate the various types, but chemical analysis is rarely carried out.

TANNIN-CONTAINING DRUGS

Tannins are astringent, polymeric polyphenols, and are found widely in plant drugs. The most important herbs used in the treatment of diarrhoea include Greater Burnet, *Sangisorba officinalis* L., Black Catechu, *Acacia catechu* Willd., Oak bark, *Quercus robur* L., Tormentil, *Potentilla erecta* (L.) Rausch , and even tea and coffee; however, many others are used in different countries (Palumbo 2006). Tannin-containing drugs are generally safe, but care should be taken with concurrent administration of other drugs since tannins are not compatible with alkalis or alkaloids, and form complexes with proteins and amino acids.

CONSTIPATION

Constipation is often due to an inappropriate diet and lack of physical activity, for example while being confined to bed during illness, or the result of taking other medication (especially opioids). It is characterized by reduced and difficult bowel movements, and is said to be present when the frequency of bowel movements is less than once in 2 or 3 days. Although the causes are not usually serious in nature, continuous irregularity in bowel movements should be investigated in case there is a risk of malignant disease. The subjective symptoms (straining heavily, hard stools, painful defecation and a feeling of insufficient evacuation) make it one of the most commonly reported health problems. Constipation is often associated with other forms of discomfort such as abdominal cramps, dyspepsia, bloating and flatulence. Alternating diarrhoea and constipation is a symptom of irritable bowel syndrome.

Various types of plant-derived laxative are used: stimulant laxatives (purgatives), which act directly on the mucosa of the GI tract; bulk-forming laxatives, which act mainly via physicochemical effects within the bowel lumen; and osmotic laxatives, which act by drawing water into the gut and thus softening the stool. Osmotic laxatives may be mineral in origin, for example magnesium salts, or derived from natural products such as milk sugars.

Patients generally require rapid relief from constipation, and the immediate effect of stimulant and saline purgatives is very well known. Although there is no problem using them occasionally, or on a short-term basis (less than 2 weeks), or prior to medical intervention such as X-ray (Roentgen) diagnostics, long-term use should be discouraged. The exception is for patients taking opioids for pain management, who may need to use stimulant laxatives routinely. The most important adverse effect of the long-term use of the stimulant laxatives and saline purgatives is electrolyte loss. Hypokalaemia, pathologically reduced levels of potassium (K^+), may even worsen constipation and cause damage to the renal tubules. The risk of hypokalaemia is increased with administration of some diuretics and hypokalaemia exacerbates the toxicity of the cardiac glycosides (e.g. digoxin), which are often prescribed for elderly patients. Hyperaldosteronism, an excess of aldosterone production, which leads to sodium (Na^+) retention, and again to potassium loss and hypertension, is also a risk. In general, the use of bulk-forming or osmotic laxatives is preferred, unless there are pressing reasons for using a stimulant laxative.

BULK-FORMING LAXATIVES

These are bulking agents with a high percentage of fibre and are often rich in polysaccharides, which swell in the GI tract. They influence the composition of food material in the GI tract, especially via the colonic bacteria, which are thus provided with nutrients for proliferation. This in turn influences the composition of the GI flora and the metabolism of the food in the tract (including an increase in gas, or flatus). Fibre-rich food is part of a healthy diet, but processed food and modern life styles have generally reduced fibre intake. Bulk-forming laxatives are generally not digested or absorbed in the GI tract, but pass through it largely unchanged.

Bulking agents can be distinguished from swelling agents in that bulking material contains large amounts of fibre, whereas swelling material is generally composed of plant material (seeds) with a dense cover of polysaccharides on the outside. Both types of medicinal drugs may swell to a certain degree by the uptake of water, but swelling agents in the strict sense include only medicinal plants that form mucilage or gel. The **swelling factor** (which compares the volume of drug prior to and after soaking it in water) is an indicator of the amount of polysaccharides present in the drug and is generally used as a marker for the quality of bulk-forming laxatives. The European

Table 14.1 Swelling factors of various bulk-forming laxatives			
COMMON NAME	BOTANICAL SOURCE	SWELLING FACTOR (EUR. PH.)	NOTES
Ispaghula seed	Plantago ovata	≥9 (seed) ≥40 (testa of the seed)	
Psyllium seed	Plantago psyllium and P. arenaria	≥10	
Linseed	Linum usitatissimum	≥4 (entire seed) ≥4.5 (ground seed)	Also rich in fatty acids (in endosperm of seed)
Wheat bran	Triticum aestivum	–	Rich in fibre

Pharmacopoeia requires a minimal value of the swelling factor for each agent, and the swelling factors of the phytomedicines detailed below are shown in Table 14.1. Preparations of bulk-forming laxatives are always taken with plenty of water. They can, paradoxically, be used to treat diarrhoea if given with very little fluid; they then absorb the fluid from the lumen and increase the consistency of the stool.

LINSEED (FLAX), *LINUM USITATISSIMUM* L. (LINI SEMEN) EU✲

Linseeds are the ripe, dried seeds of flax (*Linum usitatissimum*, Linaceae), a plant grown for its fibre (used in the clothing industry) and for the seed oil, which is used in paints and varnishes, and to make oil cloth ('linoleum'). Flax, with its characteristic blue flowers, is an annual, and has long been under human cultivation. The dark brown (less often yellowish-white) seeds are oblong or ovate with a characteristically pointed end. They are tasteless but slowly produce a mucilaginous feel when placed in the mouth. The outer layer of the seed (testa) is rich in polysaccharides, while the inner part of the seed, which contains the endosperm and the cotyledons, is rich in fatty oil. If the seeds are taken whole, the inner layer of the testa is only partially digested in the GI tract and they will be excreted in the entire form, and the fatty acids will not be released. The swelling factor should at least be 4 (entire seeds) or 4.5 (powdered drug). Linseed also possesses cholesterol-lowering properties, and contains phytoestrogenic lignans.

PLANTAGO SPECIES

Ispaghula, *Plantago ovata* Forssk. (Plantaginis ovatae semen) EU✲

The dark brown, glossy seeds from *Plantago ovata* (Indian fleawort, blond psyllium, Plantaginaceae) are useful in the treatment of chronic constipation. They are broadly elliptical in shape, up to 3.5 mm long, and are practically tasteless, becoming mucilaginous when chewed. They can help to maintain or achieve a regular bowel movement and are also useful in irritable bowel syndrome. The swelling factor should be >9 for the entire seeds and >40 for the seed husk, which is the most widely used part. The usage is similar to that of psyllium (fleawort, below).

Psyllium, *Plantago psyllium* L. and *P. arenaria* L. (Psyllii semen) EU✲

The brown, shiny, elliptical to ovate seeds (2–3 mm long) are obtained from two species of the plantain family (Plantaginaceae). *Plantago psyllium* (=*Plantago afra* L., fleawort, black or dark psyllium, plantain) and *P. arenaria* (=*P. indica*, fleawort, plantain) yield useful and commonly used emollients and bulk laxatives which help in maintaining a regular bowel movement. The seeds are narrower and somewhat smaller than ispaghula seeds. An essential characteristic of high-quality material is a high swelling factor.

Wheat bran, *Triticum aestivum* L.

Bran is less useful as a laxative (except when taken as a natural part of the diet, e.g. in breakfast cereal), since it contains phytic acid, which in high concentrations can complex with and, therefore, reduce the bioavailability of vitamins and minerals taken at the same time. However, in some patients, wheat bran (the husk from the grains of *Triticum aestivum*) is more effective than other swelling agents, and preparations containing it are available for prescribing. These are taken in water.

OSMOTIC LAXATIVES

Osmotic laxatives, such as lactulose or lactose, which are dimeric sugars derived from milk, are a useful and widely used approach to the treatment of long-term constipation. Lactose is split in the GI tract into glucose and galactose, and galactose is not generally resorbed well. Consequently, the bacteria of the colon metabolize this sugar. The resulting acids, including lactic acid and acetic acid, have an osmotic effect, and the bacteria in the colon multiply more rapidly. This results in softening and increasing in the amount of faeces, with a subsequent increase in GI peristalsis.

STIMULANT LAXATIVES

Stimulant laxatives are derived from a variety of unrelated plant species, which only have in common the fact that they contain similar chemical constituents. These are anthraquinones such as emodin (Fig. 14.1) and aloe-emodin, and related anthrones and anthranols. Anthraquinones are commonly found as glycosides in the living plant. Several groups are distinguished, based on the degree of oxidation of the nucleus and whether one or two units make up the core of the molecule. The anthrones are less oxygenated than the anthraquinones and the dianthrones are formed from two anthrone units (Fig. 14.2). Studies using dianthrone glycosides such as sennosides A and B suggest that most of these compounds pass through the upper GI tract without any change; however, they are subsequently metabolized to rhein anthrone in the colon and caecum by the natural flora (mainly bacteria) of the GI tract. Anthranoid drugs act directly on the intestinal mucosa, influencing several pharmacological targets, and the laxative effect is due to increased peristalsis of the colon, reducing transit time and, consequently, the re-absorption of water from the colon. Additionally, the stimulation of active chloride secretion results in an inversion of normal physiological conditions and a subsequent increased excretion of water. Overall, this results in an increase of the faecal volume with an increase in the GI pressure. These actions are based on the well-understood effects of chemically defined constituents; consequently, phytomedicines containing them are usually standardized to specified anthranoid content (see Chapter 9).

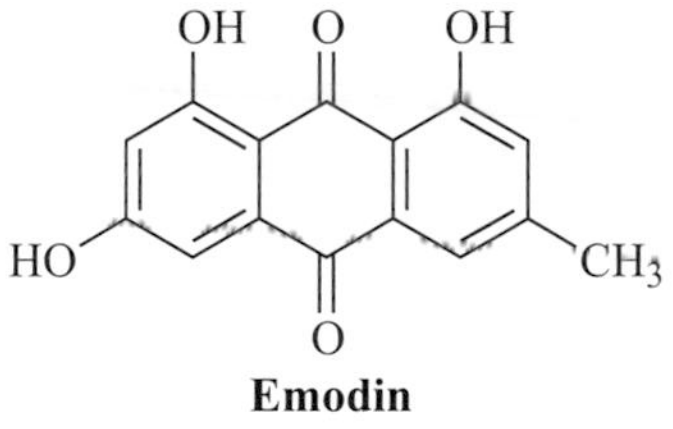

TOXICITY OF ANTHRANOID DRUGS

The monomeric aglycones (especially emodin and aloe-emodin) have been shown to have genotoxic and mutagenic effects using bacterial and *in vitro* systems such as the Ames test, and in mammalian cell lines. The long-term use of anthranoids may result in a (reversible) blackening of the colon (*Pseudomelanosis coli*), which is due to the incorporation of metabolites of the anthranoids and is thought to be associated with an increased risk of colon carcinoma. In practice, few toxic effects have been described, apart from those involving electrolyte loss described above. More immediate effects of anthranoid-containing drugs are colic and griping pains due to increased spastic contractions of the smooth musculature of the GI tract. Aloes and senna leaves are particularly prone to produce these. A synthetic derivative, danthrone (also known as dantron; not to be confused with the naturally occurring dianthrone), has been developed and, although effective, it is used only in palliative care due to its carcinogenic potential.

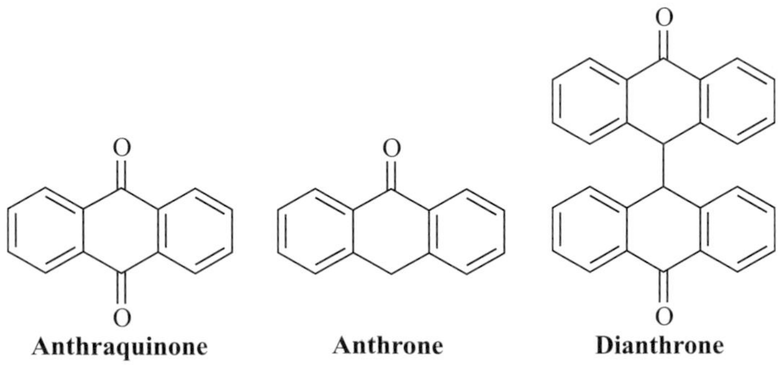

Emodin

Fig. 14.1

Anthraquinone   **Anthrone**   **Dianthrone**

Fig. 14.2

FRANGULA, *RHAMNUS FRANGULA* L. (FRANGULAE CORTEX); BUCKTHORN, *R. CATHARTICA* L. (RHAMNI CATHARTICI CORTEX) AND CASCARA, *R. PURSHIANA* DC. (RHAMNI PURSHIANI CORTEX) EU✷

The barks of several species of Rhamnaceae are used for their strong purgative effects. *Rhamnus frangula* (glossy buckthorn, frangula) has a milder action than *R. cathartica* (European buckthorn) and the berries are used in veterinary medicine. (The fruit also yields a dye, the colour of which depends partly on the ripeness.) The bark of *R. purshiana* (American buckthorn, known in commerce as Cascara sagrada) is the other main species used medicinally.

R. frangula is a densely foliated, thornless bush or tree, reaching a height of 1–7 m, common in damp environments such as bogs and along streams in North and Central Europe, as well as northern Asia. The cut bark is grey-brown with numerous visible grey-white lenticels. The leaves are broadly elliptical to obovate, about 3.5–5 cm long. The black, pea-sized berries develop from small greenish-white flowers.

Buckthorn (*R. cathartica*) is a thorny shrub with toothed leaves and a reddish brown bark; the berries are black and globular.

Cascara (*R. purshiana*) is native to the Pacific coast of North America but grows widely elsewhere. It is found in commerce in quilled pieces, often with epiphytes (lichen and moss) attached.

Constituents

R. frangula. Glucofrangulin A (Fig. 14.3) and B, which are diglucosides differing only in the **type of sugar at C6.**

R. cathartica. Emodin, aloe-emodin, chrysophanol and rhein glycosides, frangula-emodin, rhamnicoside, alaterin and physcion.

R. purshiana. Cascarosides A (Fig. 14.3), B, C, D, E and F (which are stereoisomers of aloin and derivatives), with minor glycosides including barbaloin, frangulin, chrysaloin, palmidin A, B and C and the free aglycones.

The anthrone and dianthrone glycosides, which are present in the fresh bark of these species, have emetic effects and may result in colic. In order to oxidize these compounds to anthraquinones with fewer undesirable side effects, the drug has either to be kept for a year or it is 'aged artificially' by heating it for several hours to 80–100°C.

SENNA, *CASSIA SENNA* L. AND *C. ANGUSTIFOLIA* VAHL (SENNA) (SENNAE FRUCTUS, SENNAE FOLIUM)EU✷

The genus *Cassia* (Caesalpiniaceae) is very large, with about 550 species, mostly occurring in warm temperate and tropical climates. The species are not native to Europe and were an important drug of early trading; the name 'Senna' is of Arabic origin and was recorded as early as the 12th century. Two shrubs from the genus *Cassia* (formerly called *Senna*) yield the drugs senna leaves and senna fruit: *Cassia senna* L. (syn. *C. acutifolia* L., Alexandrian senna) and *C. angustifolia* Vahl (Tinnevelly senna). The common names were derived from their original trade sources and are only applied to the fruits (pods). The second species is considered to be the milder in activity. Both the leaves and the fruits have typical microscopic characteristics, including the highly diagnostic, single-celled warty trichomes and the

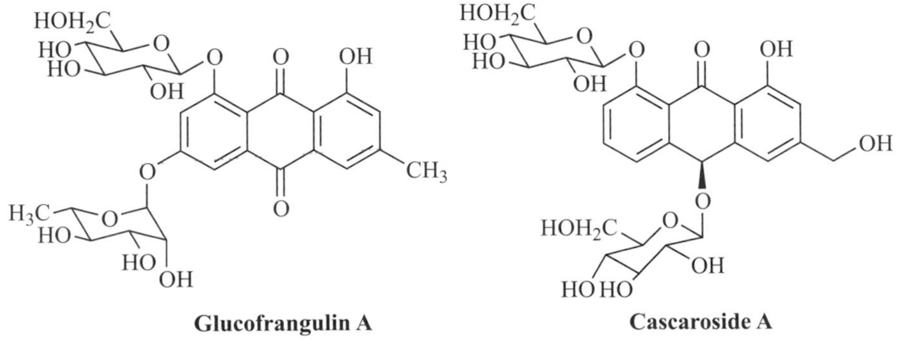

Glucofrangulin A

Cascaroside A

Fig. 14.3

crystal sheath of calcium oxalate prisms around the fibres, but it is possible to distinguish the two species microscopically.

Constituents

Leaf. Sennosides A and B (Fig. 14.4), which are based on the aglycones sennidin A and sennidin B; sennosides C and D, which are glycosides of heterodianthrones of aloe-emodin and rhein; palmidin A, rhein anthrone and aloe-emodin glycosides and some free anthraquinones. *C. senna* usually contains greater amounts of the sennosides.

Fruit. Sennosides A and B and a related glycoside sennoside A1. The sennosides, which are dianthrones, differ in their stereochemistry at C_{10} and $C_{10'}$, as well as in their substitution pattern. *C. senna* usually contains greater amounts of the sennosides.

The structure of sennoside B is given in fig. 14.4. The Eur. Ph. standard is for a glycoside content of not less than 2.5% for the leaf, 3.5% for *C. senna* fruit and 2.2% for *C. angustifolia* fruit, calculated as sennoside B. Other secondary metabolites such as flavonoids, tannins and bitter compounds are also present but not defined in the standard. The way in which the plant material is dried has a strong influence on the amount of glycosides and accordingly on the quality of the product (see above).

The other main botanical anthranoid drugs are aloes *Aloe vera*, *A. barbadensis* and other species) and rhubarb (*Rheum raponticum* and others). These are used to a lesser extent nowadays.

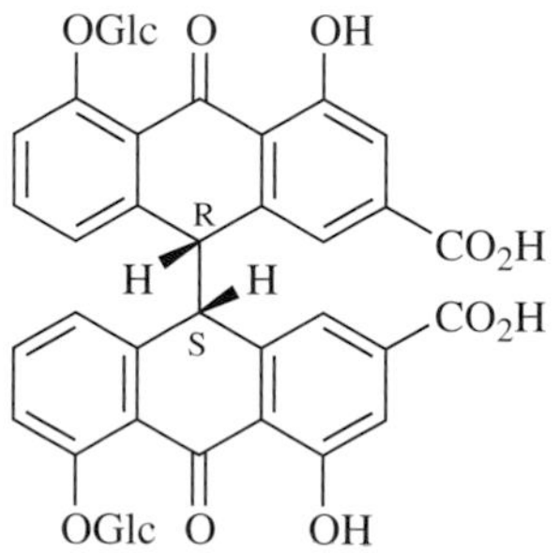

Sennoside B

Fig. 14.4

INFLAMMATORY GI CONDITIONS: GASTRITIS AND ULCERS

Inflammation of the gastric mucosa, or gastritis, is an acute inflammatory infiltration of the superficial gastric mucosa, predominantly by neutrophils. It is generally treated with antacids (magnesium and aluminium salts) and emollients (alginate, mucilages), but other phytomedicines are still occasionally used (e.g. chamomile and liquorice). These agents, especially liquorice, were used to treat gastritis and ulceration until superseded by the synthetic H_2-receptor-blocking agents (cimetidine, ranitidine, etc. and proton pump inhibitors (omeprazole, lansoprazole). Now that infection with *Helicobacter pylori* is known to be a causal factor in ulceration, antibiotic therapy is the first-line treatment of choice. Most pharmaceuticals for mild gastric inflammation contain a mixture of an emollient, to line and soothe the mucosa (e.g. an agar suspension), an antacid and possibly a carminative such as peppermint or anise oil (see section on dyspepsia).

ALGINATE EU✷

Alginate, or alginic acid, is an anionic polysaccharide distributed widely in the cell walls of brown algae including *Laminaria*, and *Ascophyllum nodosum*. Raw or dried sea weed is washed with acid to remove cross-linking ions that cause the alginate to be insoluble. It is then dissolved in alkali, typically sodium hydroxide, to produce a viscous solution of alginate. The solution is filtered to remove the cell wall debris and leave a clear alginate solution. Alginate binds with water to form a viscous gum and acts as a protective coating over the walls of the stomach and oesophagus.

CHAMOMILE *MATRICARIA RECUTITA* L. (MATRICARIAE FLOS) EU✷

German (syn. Hungarian) chamomile flowers are derived from *Matricaria recutita* (syn. *Chamomilla recutita*, *Matricaria chamomilla*, Asteraceae, the daisy family). They have a pleasant aromatic odour. The flower heads have a diameter of approximately 10 mm and are composed of many minute flowers (called florets) which are either tongue-shaped ('ligulate florets', found at the margin) or tubular ('disk' florets, found in the disk-like centre). True chamomile has a hollow receptacle (the part of the stalk where the flower parts are attached) and is devoid of the small leaf-like structures (stipules) that are common with the non-medicinal members of this genus. Chamomile is grown on a large scale, especially in Eastern Europe, Spain, Turkey, Egypt and Argentina, and has been known as a medicinal plant for several thousands of years. It is used internally for spasmodic and inflammatory illnesses of the GI tract.

Constituents

The flower heads are rich in essential oil. Two types of essential oil are recognized: one rich in bisabolol (levomenol) (Fig. 14.5) and the other in bisabolol oxides. Both contain other terpenoid compounds, including guaianolides such as matricin which are only found in the crude drug. The characteristic, dark blue azulenes (e.g. chamazulene; Fig. 14.5) are produced during steam distillation and only found in the essential oil. Flavonoids (up to 6%), especially apigenin and apigenin-7O-glycoside, caffeic acid derivatives and spiro ethers are also present. The components of the essential oil levomenol (α-bisabolol), its oxides, chamazulene, some unusual spiro ethers and the flavonoids (especially apigenin) are all essential for the pharmacological effects of the drug. The minimum amount of essential oil required by the Eur. Ph. is 0.4%.

Therapeutic uses and available evidence

Anti-inflammatory, spasmolytic, antibacterial and antifungal effects are well established both pharmacologically and clinically (see McKay and Blumberg 2006a). Chamomile is relatively safe, although allergic reactions can occur as with all plants of the family Asteraceae.
Note. The flower heads of *Chamaemelum nobile* (L.) All. (syn. *Anthemis nobilis* L., English chamomile, Roman chamomile) have a pharmacological profile similar to that of *Matricaria recutita*, and are included in the Eur. Ph. However, there is much less scientific and clinical evidence to support their use than for *M. recutita*.

LIQUORICE, *GLYCYRRHIZA GLABRA* L. (LIQUIRITIAE RADIX) EU

Liquorice (licorice) root is derived from the inner part of the root and underground stem (rhizome) of *Glycyrrhiza glabra* (Fabaceae, the bean family). The peeled drug is of much higher quality than the root with the bark, and is produced in several south-eastern European countries, Turkey, China and Russia. It has a very characteristic taste and smell, and is used in confectionery. The sweet taste also makes the identification of the drug relatively easy and so adulteration is uncommon. Microscopic identification is possible and uses characteristic crystals of oxalate, especially in the form of a sheath of parenchyma surrounding the phloem fibres, as well as the structure of the parenchyma. Liquorice is used to relieve gastric inflammation, specifically in the case of peptic ulcers and duodenal ulcers, but its use as a GI remedy is controversial because of its mineralocorticoid action. The dose should not exceed 200–600 mg of glycyrrhizin daily and the duration of treatment should be at most 4–6 weeks. More potent synthetic pharmaceuticals are now available, and it is now rarely used for this purpose. Liquorice and its preparations are contraindicated in cholestatic liver disorders, liver cirrhosis, hypertension, hypokalaemia, severe renal failure and pregnancy. With excessive use, liquorice-containing confectionery may result in similar undesired side effects. Liquorice is also used in respiratory complaints as an expectorant, mucolytic and antitussive agent.

Constituents

The most important bioactive secondary metabolite is glycyrrhizic acid (also known as glycyrrhizin; Fig. 14.6), a water-soluble pentacyclic triterpene

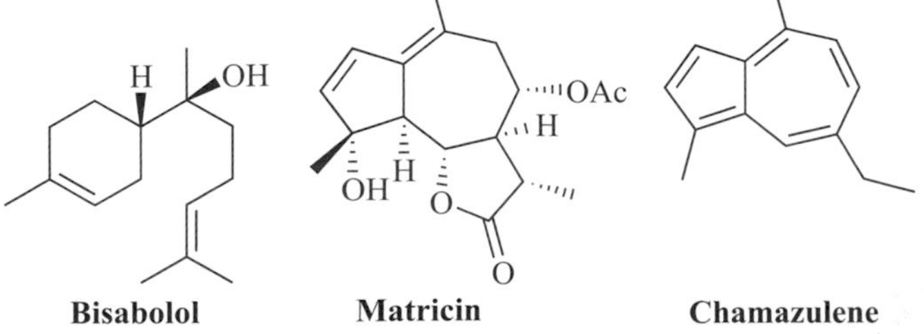

Bisabolol   Matricin   Chamazulene

Fig. 14.5

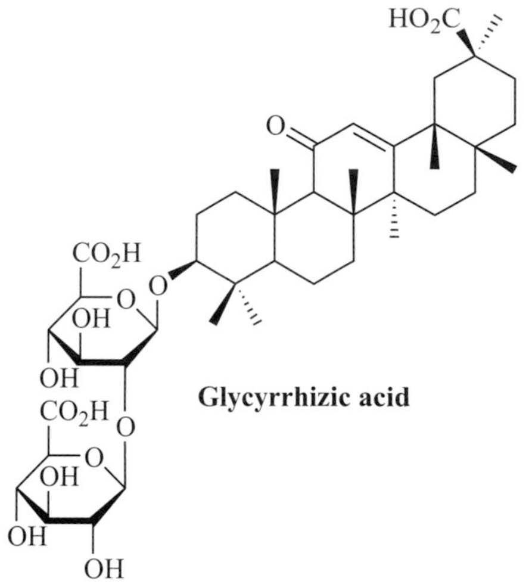

Fig. 14.6

saponin which gives the drug its characteristic sweet taste (it is about 50 times sweeter than sucrose). The genin (glycyrrhetinic acid or glycyrrhetin), on the other hand, is not sweet but very bitter. Liquorice also contains numerous flavonoids (chalcones and isoflavonoids), coumarins and polysaccharides, which contribute to the activity.

DYSPEPSIA AND BILIOUSNESS

Dyspepsia and 'biliousness' are closely associated with eating habits and are very common complaints. Patients describe the symptoms as nausea, pain and cramps, distension, heartburn and the 'inability to digest food', often experienced after rich meals. The condition is treated either with cholagogues or with bitter stimulants. A cholagogue is an agent that stimulates bile production in the liver, or promotes emptying of the gallbladder and bile ducts. Although clinical evidence is largely lacking, plant-based cholagogues are frequently prescribed by family doctors in Germany based on observational evidence and a long tradition of use, but they should not be used in cases of bile duct obstruction or cholestatic jaundice.

Liver disease is not treated as such by conventional medicine, but herbal medicine has a number of clinically proven treatments which help to protect the liver from damage and reverse some of the indicators of liver malfunction. The most important of these is silymarin, but other herbs are widely used for liver disease, although mainly with much less clinical evidence in support.

Phytomedicines used as bitter stimulants, such as Gentian and Wormwood, act directly on the mucosa of the upper part of the GI tract and especially of the bitter receptors on the tongue, stimulating the secretion of saliva and gastric juices and influencing the secretion of gastrin. An aperitif containing 'bitters', taken about half an hour before eating, stimulates gastric and biliary secretion; however, it is not known whether these effects are restricted to patients with a reduced secretory reflex, or whether an increase also occurs in healthy people.

ARTICHOKE, *CYNARA SCOLYMUS* L. (CYNARAE FOLIUM) EU

This well-known member of the Asteraceae yields the globe artichoke (a food common in French cuisine), which is the large flower head of the plant. The medicinal part is the leaf, which is used to treat indigestion and dyspepsia, and to lower cholesterol levels.

Constituents

The leaf contains the bitter sesquiterpene lactone cynaropicrin, several flavonoids and derivatives of caffeoylquinic acid, including cynarin (Fig. 14.7).

Therapeutic uses and available evidence

Antihepatotoxic effects, cholagogue activity and a reduction of cholesterol and triglyceride levels have been reported, and are now known to be due to inhibition of cholesterol biosynthesis. Clinical studies have shown that artichoke leaf extract can improve parameters such as fat intolerance, bloating, flatulence, constipation, abdominal pain and vomiting, and increase bile flow, at a daily mean dose of 1500 mg. For further details, see Bundy et al 2008, and Wider et al 2009. Artichoke extract is also useful in irritable bowel syndrome (Walker et al 2001).

GENTIAN, *GENTIANA LUTEA* L. (GENTIANAE RADIX) EU

The yellow gentian (G. lutea, Gentianaceae) is, after ethanol, the most important ingredient of the Alpine beverage *Enzianschnaps*, used as a digestive stimulant, taken after a large meal. Most medicinal products are made using the rapidly dried and non-fermented drug.

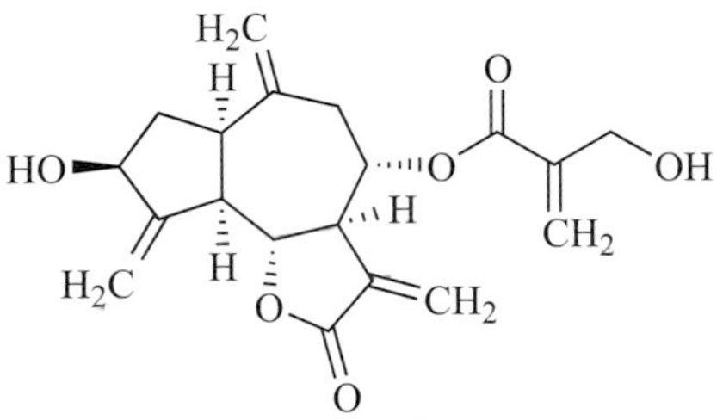

Cynaropicrin 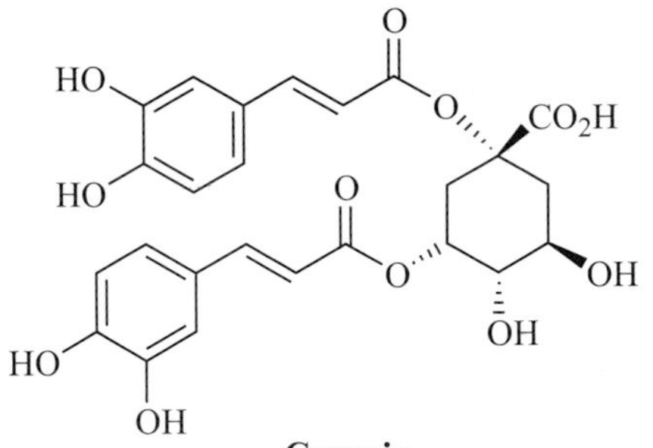   Cynarin

Fig. 14.7

The species is rare (but locally abundant) and distributed in the alpine regions of Europe and western Asia. It is a perennial herb up to 1.4 m high with showy yellow flowers. Because of the high risk of overexploitation (for use as an ornamental and as a medicine) the species is now protected throughout most of its range and attempts are being made to cultivate it. Gentian root in commerce consists of the dried rhizomes and roots of the species. The rhizome is cylindrical and may have a diameter of up to 4 cm, with long roots attached.

Constituents

The compounds responsible for the highly bitter taste are monoterpenoid compounds (Fig. 14.8) such as gentiopicroside – a seco-iridoid with a bitter value of 12,000 – and amarogentin – with a bitter value of 58,000,000, which is only present in minute amounts. The normally white inner part of the rootstock turns yellow during fermentation, due to the formation of xanthones, including gentisin.

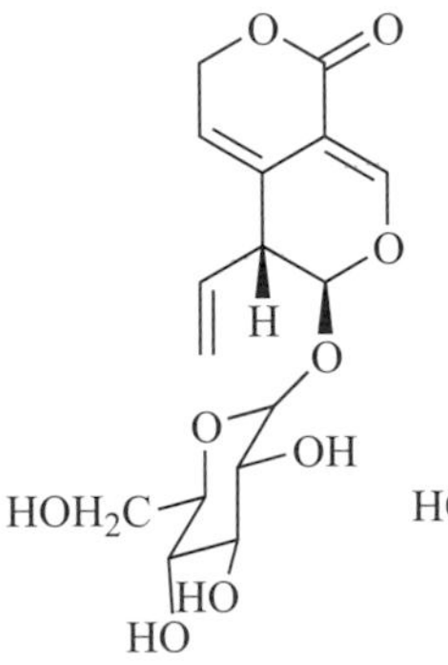

Gentiopicroside 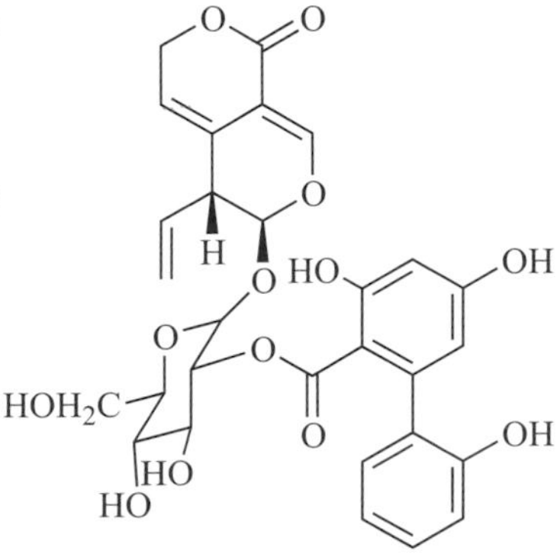   Amarogentin

Fig. 14.8

Chemical analysis is carried out following the method of the Eur. Ph., but the 'bitter value' test is also useful. This is a simple and useful measure for establishing the quality of bitter-tasting (botanical) drugs. It is the inverse concentration of the dilution of an extract (or a pure compound) which can still be detected as being bitter to testers with normal bitter taste receptors. In the case of gentian, it should at least be 10,000 (i.e. an extract that has been diluted 10,000 times should still leave a bitter taste).

Therapeutic uses and available evidence

Gentian is indicated for poor appetite, flatulence and bloating, although clinical trial evidence is lacking. Extracts stimulate gastric secretion in cultured rat gastric mucosal cells and gentiopicroside has been shown to suppress chemically and immunologically induced liver damage in mice.

WORMWOOD, *ARTEMISIA ABSINTHIUM* L. (ABSINTHII HERBA) EU

Wormwood is a bitter stimulant derived from the aerial parts of *Artemisia absinthium* (Asteraceae) and is popularly used as a tea. It is a commonly cultivated garden plant. The liqueur was a popular stimulant in many European countries during the latter part of the 19th century and early part of the 20th century, and gave rise to the condition known as absinthism, a form of mental disorder, reputed to affect the artist Van Gogh. The plant is still commonly grown in Mediterranean gardens. The leaves and young stems are densely covered with characteristic greyish-white hairs, which give the species its typical appearance.

A large number of related species are also used as a food (estragon – A. dracunculus) or medicine (*A. annua* L. – the source of artemisinine)

Constituents

The essential oil contains β-thujone (Fig. 14.9) as the major components, as well as thujyl alcohol, azulenes, bisabolene and others. Sesquiterpene lactones are also present, especially absinthin, anabsinthin, artemetin, artabsinolides A, B, C and D, artemolin and others, and flavonoids. During the process of distillation, the intensively blue chamazulene is formed, which together with the other constituents gives oil of absinth its characteristic green-blue colour. The sesquiterpene lactone absinthin is responsible for the intensive bitter taste, which according to the Eur. Ph. should be at least 10,000 (Deutsches Arzneibuch 15,000) for the crude extract (see 'Gentian' for explanation of bitter value). β-Thujone, a monoterpene, is also partly responsible for the bitterness. The essential oil content should be at least 0.2% and the bitter sesquiterpenoids 0.15–0.4%, according to the Eur. Ph. where the methods are described.

Therapeutic uses and available evidence

It is commonly used as a bitter tonic, a choleretic and also as an anthelmintic. Although its use in the form of a tea is considered safe, the essential oil, and the liqueur 'absinthe' distilled from this plant, are harmful in large doses due to the thujone content, and are not now used except where the thujone has been removed. Most of the evidence is empirical and clinical evidence is limited.

Toxicological risks

Thujone, a major component of the essential oil, is neurotoxic and hallucinogenic in large doses and can produce epileptic fits and long-lasting psychiatric disturbances. These are considered to be a problem only with the distilled ethanolic beverage (absinthe). Thujone is found in the essential oil of many unrelated species, including sage (*Salvia*

Thujone

Fig. 14.9

officinalis) and thuja (*Thuja occidentalis*), and is still used medicinally with few ill-effects. There is also some dispute as to whether 'absinthism' is anything more than plain alcoholism, since thujone levels are not always high enough to be considered as causing such severe damage.

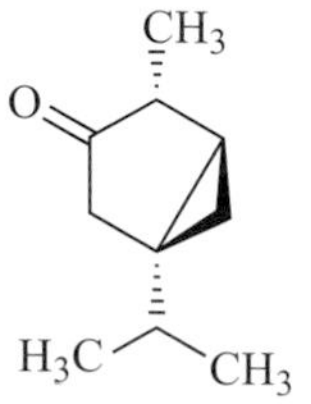

NAUSEA AND VOMITING

'Travel sickness' or 'motion sickness' is particularly common in children and is caused by the repetitive stimulation of the labyrinth of the ear. It is most common when travelling by sea, but also happens in cars, aeroplanes and when horse-riding. Vomiting, nausea, dizziness, sweating and vertigo may occur. Prophylactic treatment includes the use of antihistamines (mainly phenothiazines) and cinnarizine, and natural compounds such as the antimuscarinic alkaloid hyoscine, found the Solanaceae family. Morning sickness of pregnancy is also common but few (if any) synthetic drugs are licensed for such a use because of fears of toxicity to the unborn child. Ginger can be a useful anti-emetic for this condition, as well as for travel sickness.

GINGER, *ZINGIBER OFFICINALE* ROSCOE (ZINGIBERIS RHIZOMA) EU

Ginger (Zingiberaceae) is one of the most commonly used culinary spices in the world and has a variety of medicinal uses. The odour and taste are very characteristic, aromatic and pungent. Ginger is cultivated in moist, warm tropical climates throughout south and south-eastern Asia, China, Nigeria and Jamaica. The rhizome is the part used and is available commercially either peeled or unpeeled. African dried ginger is usually unpeeled, and the fresh rhizome, which is widely available for culinary purposes, is always unpeeled. The medicinal use of ginger in Europe has an ancient history and can be traced back to Greek and Roman times. The plant has also been mentioned in Ayurvedic and other religious scriptures dating back to 2000 BC, where it was recognized as an aid to digestion and for cases of rheumatism and inflammation.

Constituents

The rhizome contains 1–3% essential oil, the major constituents of which are zingiberene and β-bisabolene. The pungent taste is produced by a mixture of

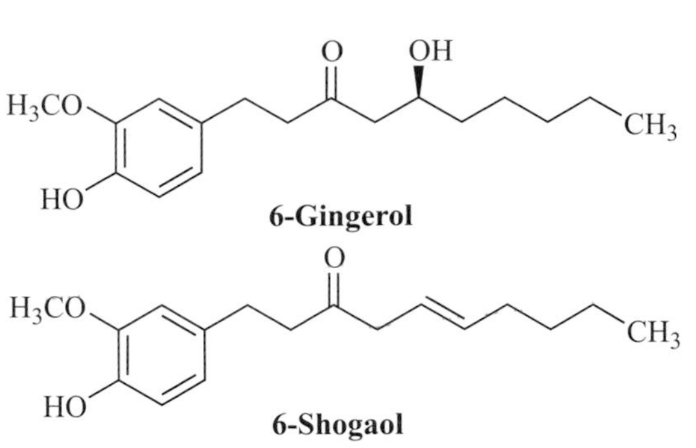

Fig. 14.10

phenolic compounds with carbon side-chains consisting of seven or more carbon atoms, referred to as gingerols, gingerdiols, gingerdiones, dihydrogingerdiones and shogaols (see Fig. 14.10). The shogaols are produced by dehydration and degradation of the gingerols and are formed during drying and extraction. The shogaols are twice as pungent as the gingerols, which accounts for the fact that dried ginger is more pungent than fresh ginger.

Therapeutic uses and available evidence

Modern uses of ginger are diverse and include as a carminative, anti-emetic, spasmolytic, antiflatulent, antitussive, hepatoprotective, antiplatelet aggregation and hypolipidaemic. Some of these actions are substantiated by pharmacological *in vivo* or *in vitro* evidence. Of particular importance is the use in preventing the symptoms of motion sickness and postoperative nausea, as well as vertigo and morning sickness of pregnancy, and there is some clinical evidence for the efficacy of ginger in these conditions (Matthews et al 2010). Ginger consumption has also been reported to have a beneficial effect in alleviating the pain and frequency of migraine headaches, and studies on the action in rheumatic conditions have shown a moderately beneficial effect. Anti-ulcer activity has been described in animals and attributed to the volatile oil, especially the 6-gingesulfonic acid content, and hepatoprotective effects have been noted in cultured hepatocytes, with the gingerols being more potent than the homologous shogaols found in dried ginger. Both groups of compounds are antioxidants and possess free radical scavenging activity. Ginger is well known to produce a warming effect when ingested, and the pungent principles stimulate thermogenic receptors. In addition, zingerone induces catecholamine secretion from the

adrenal medulla (for review, see Ali et al 2008). In Oriental medicine, ginger is so highly regarded that it forms an ingredient of about half of all multi-item prescriptions. A distinction is made between the indications for the fresh rhizome (vomiting, coughs, abdominal distension and pyrexia) and the dried or processed rhizome (abdominal pain, lumbago and diarrhoea). This is probably justifiable since the constituents are present in different proportions in the different preparations. Ginger, both in the fresh and dried form, is generally regarded as safe.

HYOSCINE (SCOPOLAMINE) EU✦

The alkaloid hyoscine (Fig. 14.11) is usually isolated from *Datura* or *Scopolia* spp., although, as the name suggests, it has originally been found in *Hyoscyamus niger*. It is a popular remedy for motion sickness, given at an oral dose of 400 μg or, more recently, as a transdermal patch containing 2 mg of the alkaloid, which is delivered through the skin over 24 h. Hyoscine is also used as a premedication, usually in combination with an opiate, to relax the patient and dry up bronchial secretions prior to administration of halothane anaesthetics.

IRRITABLE BOWEL SYNDROME, BLOATING AND FLATULENCE

Irritable bowel syndrome (IBS) is characterized by pain in the left iliac fossa, diarrhoea and/or constipation. Symptoms are usually relieved to some extent by defecation or the passage of wind, and can be treated successfully by the use of bulk laxatives with or without antispasmodic (carminative) drugs. Natural remedies include peppermint oil and other essential oil carminatives, and some of the tropane alkaloids. Atropine has been replaced

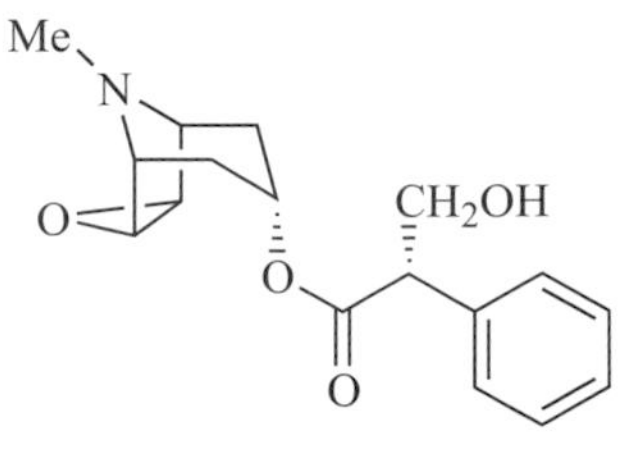

(–) Hyoscine

Fig. 14.11

by hyoscine, in the form of the N-butyl bromide, which, as a quaternary ion, is poorly absorbed from the GI tract and, therefore, has fewer anti-muscarinic side effects. Artichoke extract is also useful in irritable bowel syndrome (Walker et al 2001); see under dyspepsia and biliousness.

Flatulence, which is the passage of excessive wind from the body, is a condition for which phytotherapy offers useful therapeutic approaches. Carminatives are usually taken with food; they produce a warm sensation when ingested and promote postprandial elimination of gas. Plant-based carminatives are usually rich in essential oil, such as the fruits ('seeds') of species of the Apiaceae (celery family) and some members of the Lamiaceae (mint family). Many condiments such as cumin and caraway have carminative effects and are used as spices because of their taste *and* their pharmacological effect. The clinical validity of carminatives is based on long historical observation and is well established. The effect of many of these botanical drugs is due to their spasmolytic action, for which some *in vitro* evidence exists (Ford et al 2008), but the precise mechanism of action is unclear. It seems likely that not only is the essential oil responsible for the effect, but that the other components (e.g. the flavonoids) also contribute.

MINT LEAVES AND OILS: *MENTHA* SPECIES

Members of the mint family are widely used for their digestive effects and flavouring qualities. They contain similar compounds, but in differing proportions, which results in subtle differences in their taste and properties.

PEPPERMINT, *MENTHA × PIPERITA* L. (MENTHAE PIPERITAE FOLIUM) EU

Peppermint is a hybrid of *Mentha aquatica* and *M. spicata*, which originated spontaneously and has been known for over 2500 years; the first records are from old Egyptian graves (2600–3200 BC). Peppermint has a very characteristic, strongly aromatic and penetrating smell and taste. All species of the genus *Mentha* (the mints) have quadrangular (square) stems and decussate, elongated, dentate leaves with a pointed apex, and pinkish-blue flowers up to 5 mm long, and microscopical characteristics include glandular hairs, which are typical of the Lamiaceae. Both the leaves, in the form of a tea, and the oil are used for digestive problems.

Constituents

Peppermint leaf is rich in essential oil (0.5–4%), the main components being (–)-menthol, menthone, menthylacetate and menthofuran. The plant also contains the non-volatile polyphenolics rosmarinic acid and derivatives, flavonoids and triterpenes.

Peppermint oil is derived from the fresh plant by steam distillation and contains approximately 50% (–)-menthol (Fig. 16.4).

Therapeutic uses and available evidence

Peppermint is often taken in the form of a tea, which provides a refreshing beverage as well as a mild digestive soothing effect (see McKay and Blumberg 2006b). The oil can be given well-diluted with water or as an emulsion (2%, v/v, dispersed in a suitable vehicle) for treating colic and GI cramps in both adults and children, and in the form of enteric-coated capsules for IBS, where it is released directly into the intestine and bowel. The antispasmodic effect of peppermint oil has been well established using a series of *in vitro* models, the effect being marked by a decline in the number and amplitude of spontaneous contractions, and due at least in part to Ca^{2+}-antagonistic effects. Peppermint oil has also been shown clinically to enhance gastric emptying. Peppermint water (or emulsion) is generally safe, although must be used with care. A tragic incident with peppermint water caused the death of a young baby, although the toxicity was due to the excipient rather than to the peppermint oil (by adding concentrated chloroform water rather than the diluted form, two pharmacists inadvertently produced a lethal medication).

JAPANESE MINT, *MENTHA ARVENSIS* L.

Japanese mint is rich in menthol (about 80% of the total volatile oil, see below) and is employed as a cheaper substitute for peppermint or for extraction of menthol.

SPEARMINT, *MENTHA × SPICATA* L., SYN. *M. CRISPA*, *M. SPICATA* SUBSP. *CRISPA*

Spearmint gives toothpaste, mouthwash and chewing gum their typical taste and smell. It is an important flavouring agent, but is of limited pharmaceutical importance. Material from this species is easily identifiable from the taste and odour.

UMBELLIFEROUS FRUITS

The fruits (not 'seeds' as they are commonly known) of several members of the celery family (Apiaceae or Umbelliferae) are used as carminatives as they are rich in essential oil and have an antispasmodic effect. Many of these species are also important as spices. Flower heads of these species are umbels of white or pinkish flowers, which produce the characteristic schizocarp (double) fruits, in which two mericarps are united to form an easily separated fruit on a carpophor (a stalk which means 'carrier of fruit').

CARAWAY, *CARUM CARVI* L. (CARVI FRUCTUS) EU⁎

Caraway is the fruit of a mountain herb common in many regions of Europe and Asia.

Constituents

The essential oil (3–7%) consists mainly of (+)-Carvone and (+)-limonene, accounting for 45–65% and 30–40%, respectively, of the total oil. Carvone (Fig. 14.12) is considered to be the main component responsible for the spasmolytic action.

Therapeutic uses and available evidence

The fruits are used in cases of dyspepsia, minor GI cramps and flatulence. Little modern clinical evidence is available but caraway has long been used in products such as infant gripe water. The aqueous extract, and even more so the essential oil, acts as a spasmolytic and has antimicrobial activity.

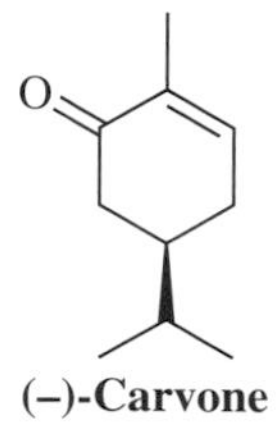

FENNEL, *FOENICULUM VULGARE* MILLER (FOENICULI FRUCTUS) EU⁎

The common fennel is a perennial herb yielding fruit and oil that are used for stomach and abdominal discomfort, as well as a spice in sweets and liqueurs. Other varieties yield the commonly used vegetable fennel. Two pharmaceutically important varieties are distinguished: *Foeniculum vulgare* var. *dulce* (sweet fennel), which is richer in anethole and has a sweet and aromatic taste, and *F. vulgare* var. *vulgare* (bitter fennel), which is rich in fenchone, resulting in a bitter taste. The two varieties are nearly impossible to distinguish microscopically; consequently, taste and smell differentiation, as well as thin layer chromatography (TLC) analysis, are essential for differentiating the two.

Constituents

All of the aerial parts of fennel are rich in essential oil, with bitter fennel fruit containing 2–6%, mostly *trans*-anethole (>60% of the oil) and fenchone (>15%) (Fig. 14.13), and sweet fennel containing 1.5–3%, composed of *trans*-anethole (80–90%) but with very little fenchone (<1%). Fatty oil and protein are also found in fennel fruit.

Therapeutic uses and available evidence

Fennel is used empirically as a carminative, for indigestion and colic in children. It is considered to be a very safe drug and is widely used as a health-food supplement as well as a spice. Fennel oil (the distilled essential oil of both varieties of fennel) is used for the same indications and has been shown to be bacteriostatic.

Other fruit drugs used for these indications are anise (Anisi fructus) from *Pimpinella anisum*, star anise (Anisi stellata fructus) from *Illicium verum*

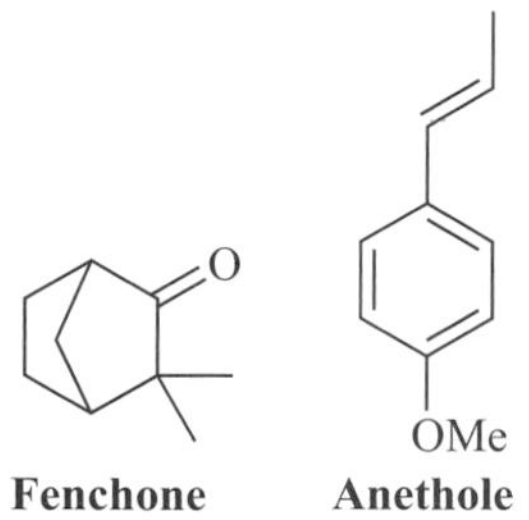

(–)-Carvone

Fig. 14.12

Fenchone   Anethole

Fig. 14.13

and coriander (Coriandri fructus) from *Coriandrum sativum*. These agents are all in the Eur. Ph.

The oils of all of these fruits are the subject of monographs in the Eur. Ph. where quantification of compounds is achieved after separation by gas chromatography. Differentiation between the two types of fennel is possible using the TLC method described in the Eur. Ph. where bitter fennel shows an additional yellow zone after spraying with sulphuric acid.

LIVER DISEASE

Liver damage, cirrhosis and poisoning should only be treated under medical supervision. There is, however, a useful phytomedicine derived from the milk thistle, *Silybum marianum* (L.) Gaertn. (Asteraceae), in the form of an extract known as silymarin. Other herbs, as shown below, are widely used for liver disease, although with less clinical evidence in support. Herbs used for 'biliousness' (see section on Dyspepsia and Biliousness) are also used in mild liver disease.

ANDROGRAPHIS, *ANDROGRAPHIS PANICULATA* NEES (ANDROGRAPHIS HERBA) EU*

Andrographis is widely used in many Asian systems of medicine to treat jaundice and liver disorders. There are few clinical studies available to support these uses, although numerous *in vitro* experiments have shown it has liver protective effects against a variety of hepatotoxins. 14-deoxyandrographolide, a constituent, desensitizes hepatocytes to TNF-alpha-induced signalling of apoptosis (Roy et al 2010). It appears to be well-tolerated but caution should be exercised when given in conjunction with antithrombotic drugs. In the West, it is more often used as an immune stimulant (see Chapter 16, Respiratory System, for more detail, including constituents).

BERBERIS SPECIES AND OTHER BERBERINE-CONTAINING DRUGS

Berberine (Fig. 14.14) is contained in *Berberis* species, for example *B. vulgaris* L., *B. aristata* DC, in Blood root, *Sanguinaria canadensis* L., Goldenseal, *Hydrastis canadensis* L., Gold Thread, *Coptis chinensis* Franch, and Greater Celandine, *Chelidonium majus* L.

Berberine has antibacterial and amoebicidal properties and is used either in the form of the pure

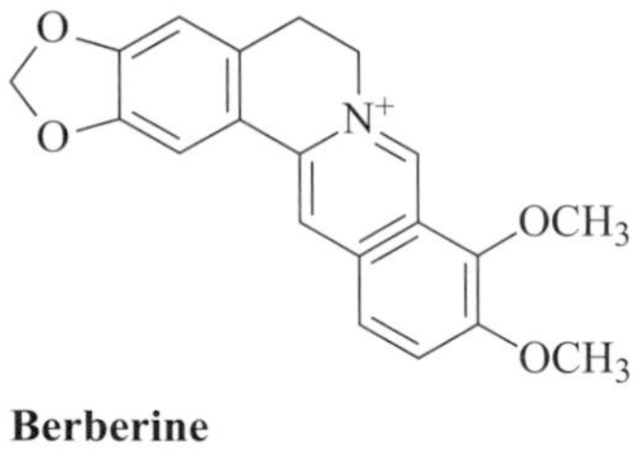

Berberine

Fig. 14.14

compound or as a component of plant extracts, to treat dysentery and liver disease (Imanshahidi and Hosseinzadeh 2008). Care should be taken when given together with anticancer drugs and with ciclosporin, since theoretical drug interactions have been described for these combinations, and berberine is known to be a substrate of P-glycoprotein and to affect expression of cytochrome P(CYP) 450 enzymes 3A4 and others.

MILK THISTLE, *SILYBUM MARIANUM* (SILYBI MARIANAE FRUCTUS) EU*

The seeds of the milk thistle, *Silybum marianum* (L.) Gaertn. (Asteraceae), yield a flavolignan fraction known as silymarin.

Constituents

The active constituents of the extract silymarin are flavolignans, mainly silybin (=silibinin), with isosilybin, dihydrosilybin, silydianin, silychristin and others.

Therapeutic uses and available evidence

In many parts of Europe, silymarin is used extensively for liver disease and jaundice. It has been shown to exert an antihepatotoxic effect in animals against a variety of poisons, particularly those of the death cap mushroom *Amanita phalloides*. This fungus contains some of the most potent liver toxins known (the amatoxins and the phallotoxins), both of which cause fatal haemorrhagic necrosis of the liver. Silymarin has been used at doses of 420 mg daily to treat patients with chronic hepatitis and cirrhosis; it is also partially active against hepatitis B virus, is hypolipidaemic and lowers fat deposits in the liver in animals. This extract can be used not only for serious liver disease, but also for general biliousness and other digestive disorders (see Saller et al 2008).

SCHISANDRA, *SCHISANDRA CHINENSIS* K. KOCH (SCHISANDRAE CHINENSIS FRUCTUS) EU⁺

Schisandra (Schizandra) berries are the fruit of the Magnolia Vine, and are very important in traditional Chinese medicine where they are used to treat liver disorders and many other conditions of general debility. Related species are also used.

Constituents

The active constituents are dibenzocyclooctene lignans, known as schisandrins (schizandrins) and gomisins. The nomenclature is confused and, for example, 'schisandrin' is sometimes referred to in the literature as 'schisandrol A', and 'gomisin A' as 'schisandrol B'.

Therapeutic uses and available evidence

A great deal of research has been carried out on the pharmacology of this plant (see review by Panossian and Wikman 2008), and liver protectant effects have been observed in animals, but clinical studies are lacking

TURMERIC, *CURCUMA DOMESTICA* VAL. (CURCUMAE DOMESTICAE RHIZOMA) EU⁺

Turmeric is used in Asian medicine to treat liver disorders and well as inflammatory conditions. For details regarding the drug and its constituents, see Chapter 21 (Musculoskeletal system). Related species include Javanese turmeric (*Curcuma xanthorrhiza* Roxb., Eur. Ph.), which is mostly used for dyspepsia and other gastrointestinal problems. Turmeric and the curcuminoids are hepatoprotective against liver damage induced by various toxins, including paracetamol (acetaminophen), aflatoxin and cyclophosphamide; they protect against stomach ulcers in rats, and have antispasmodic effects. Turmeric is also hypoglycaemic in animals, and hypocholesterolaemic effects have been observed both in animal and human clinical studies, although clinical studies for liver disease are lacking. In addition, turmeric is antibacterial and antiprotozoal *in vitro*. Turmeric is well tolerated but the bioavailability is poor and daily doses of at least 2g are normally used. For reviews see, Rivera-Espinoza and Muriel (2009) and Epstein et al (2010).

References

Ali, B.H., Blunden, G., Tanira, M.O., Nemmar, A., 2008. Some phytochemical, pharmacological and toxicological properties of ginger (*Zingiber officinale* Roscoe): a review of recent research. Food Chem. Toxicol. 46, 409–420.

Bundy, R., Walker, A.F., Middleton, R.W., Wallis, C., Simpson, H.C., 2008. Artichoke leaf extract (*Cynara scolymus*) reduces plasma cholesterol in otherwise healthy hypercholesterolemic adults: a randomized, double blind placebo controlled trial. Phytomedicine 15, 668–675.

Epstein, J., Sanderson, I.R., Macdonald, T.T., 2010. Curcumin as a therapeutic agent: the evidence from in vitro, animal and human studies. Br. J. Nutr. 103, 1545–1557.

Ford, A.C., Talley, N.J., Spiegel, B.M., et al., 2008. Effect of fibre, antispasmodics, and peppermint oil in the treatment of irritable bowel syndrome: systematic review and meta-analysis. BMJ 337, a2313.

Imanshahidi, M., Hosseinzadeh, H., 2008. Pharmacological and therapeutic effects of *Berberis vulgaris* and its active constituent, berberine. Phytother. Res. 22, 999–1012.

Matthews, A., Dowswell, T., Haas, D.M., Doyle, M., O'Mathúna, D.P., 2010. Interventions for nausea and vomiting in early pregnancy. Cochrane Database Syst. Rev 2010 Sep 8:CD007575.

McKay, D.L., Blumberg, J.B., 2006a. A review of the bioactivity and potential health benefits of chamomile tea (*Matricaria recutita* L.). Phytother. Res. 20, 519–530.

McKay, D.L., Blumberg, J.B., 2006b. A review of the bioactivity and potential health benefits of peppermint tea

(*Mentha piperita* L.). Phytother. Res. 20, 619–633.

Palumbo, E.A., 2006. Phytochemicals from traditional medicinal plants used in the treatment of diarrhoea: modes of action and effects on intestinal function. Phytother. Res. 20, 717–724.

Panossian, A., Wikman, G., 2008. Pharmacology of *Schisandra chinensis* Bail.: an overview of Russian research and uses in medicine. J. Ethnopharmacol. 118, 183–212.

Rivera-Espinoza, Y., Muriel, P., 2009. Pharmacological actions of curcumin in liver diseases or damage. Liver Int. 29, 1457–1466.

Roy, D.N., Mandal, S., Sen, G., Mukhopadhyay, S., Biswas, T., 2010. 14-Deoxyandrographolide desensitizes hepatocytes to tumour necrosis factor-alpha-induced apoptosis through calcium-dependent tumour necrosis factor receptor superfamily member 1A release via the NO/cGMP pathway. Br. J. Pharmacol. 160, 1823–1843.

Saller, R., Brignoli, R., Melzer, J., Meier, R., 2008. An updated systematic review with meta-analysis for the clinical evidence of silymarin. Forsch. Komplementmed. 15, 9–20.

Walker, A.F., Middleton, R.W., Petrowicz, O., 2001. Artichoke leaf extract reduces symptoms of irritable bowel syndrome in a post-marketing surveillance study. Phytother. Res. 15, 58.

Wider, B., Pittler, M.H., Thompson-Coon, J., Ernst, E., 2009. Artichoke leaf extract for treating hypercholesterolaemia. Cochrane Database Syst. Rev. Oct 7 (4): CD003335.

Chapter 15

The cardiovascular system

Cardiovascular (CV) disorders are responsible for many deaths in the Western world, and are a consequence of lifestyle and diet, as well as being hereditary to some extent. Serious conditions such as heart failure should be treated only under the guidance of a qualified physician, but some minor forms of CV disease respond well to changes in diet and taking more exercise, as well as phytotherapy. Cardiology has benefited greatly from the introduction of some newer semi-synthetic drugs based on natural products, including aspirin, an antiplatelet agent derived from salicin, and warfarin, an anticoagulant derived from dicoumarol. Others have been developed using a natural product as a template, for example, verapamil, a calcium channel antagonist used to treat hypertension and angina, is based on the opium alkaloid papaverine, and nifedipine, a calcium channel antagonist and amiodarone, an anti-arrhythmic, were both developed from khellin, the active constituent of *Ammi visnaga*. Cocaine has cardioactive as well as central nervous system effects, and was the starting material for the development of the anti-arrhythmics procaine and lignocaine, which are more effective and without the unwanted stimulant activity (Hollmann 1992).

Cardiovascular conditions discussed here include heart failure, venous insufficiency, thrombosis and atherosclerosis. Other conditions such as hypertension and cardiac arrhythmias are rarely treated with phytomedicines, although there are some natural products used in their treatment which will be mentioned briefly. Synthetic diuretics are widely used as antihypertensives, but phytomedicines are not suitable for this purpose as they are not sufficiently potent to reduce blood pressure. Instead, they are often incorporated into remedies for urinary tract complaints (see Chapter 20) or to reduce bloating (mild water retention, for example pre-menstrual).

HEART FAILURE AND ARRHYTHMIAS

These conditions can be treated with cardiac glycosides (cardenolides and bufadienolides) such as digoxin, isolated from the foxglove. Lily of the valley (*Convallaria majalis*) contains convallotoxin (a mixture of cardenolides), and squill (*Drimys maritima*) contains the bufadienolides scillaren A and proscillaridin, but these are rarely used now. Ouabain, isolated from *Strophanthus* spp., has been used in emergency cases. The cardiac glycosides have a positive inotropic effect, meaning that they increase the force of contraction of the heart. They are emetic and toxic in large doses and have a cumulative effect and are, therefore, unsuitable for use in the form of herbal extracts. Single isolated compounds for which the pharmacokinetics can be monitored are used instead.

There are, however, other herbal drugs that have beneficial effects upon the heart, the most important of which are hawthorn (*Crataegus*) and motherwort (*Leonurus cardiaca*). Hawthorn has anti-arrhythmic activity, and will be discussed briefly below. There is not enough evidence available at present to justify the inclusion of motherwort. In general, however, arrhythmias are treated with isolated compounds, most of which are synthetic, although quinidine (an alkaloid from *Cinchona* spp.; Fig. 15.1) is still

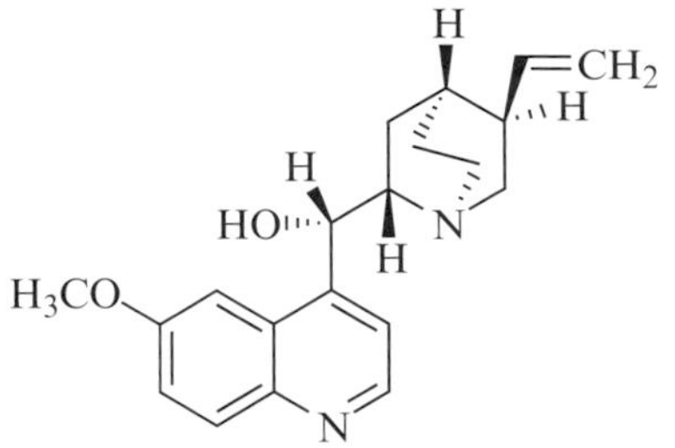

Quinidine

Fig. 15.1

used occasionally. Ajmaline, from *Rauvolfia* spp., is used as an anti-arrhythmic in some parts of the world; sparteine, from broom (*Cytisus scoparius*), was formerly employed. Both of these compounds are alkaloids.

FOXGLOVE (DIGITALIS) LEAF, *DIGITALIS PURPUREA* L. (DIGITALIS PURPUREAE FOLIUM) EU*

The purple foxglove (*Digitalis purpurea*) and its close relative the woolly foxglove (*D. lanata* L., Scrophulariaceae), yield cardiac glycosides. These plants are very common: they are indigenous to Europe and cultivated elsewhere. They do not have a long history of herbal use because of their toxicity, although the famous surgeon William Withering described their use for 'dropsy' (an old term for congestive heart failure) in 1870, and this was the first time an effective treatment for this condition had been found. The leaves are the source of the drug and are usually gathered in the second year of growth.

Constituents

Both species contain cardenolides, which are glycosides of the steroidal aglycones digitoxigenin, gitoxigenin and gitaloxigenin. There are very many cardiac glycosides, but the most important is digoxin (Fig. 15.2) and to a much lesser extent digitoxin, and the purpurea glycosides A and B. *Digitalis lanata* contains higher concentrations of glycosides, including digoxin and lanatosides, and is the main source of digoxin for the pharmaceutical industry.

Therapeutic uses and available evidence

Digoxin increases the force of myocardial contractility and reduces conductivity within the atrioventricular node. It is used primarily in the treatment of supraventricular tachycardia and heart failure and is given as a once-daily dosage in the range 62.5–250 µg. Digitalis glycosides increase the force of contraction of the heart without increasing the oxygen consumption, and slow the heart rate when atrial fibrillation is present. Due to their cumulative effect, the glycosides can easily give rise to toxic symptoms, such as nausea, vomiting and anorexia, especially in the elderly, thus blood levels should be monitored.

HAWTHORN, *CRATAEGUS* SPP. (CRATAEGI FOLIUM CUM FLORE, CRATAEGI FRUCTUS) EU*

Hawthorn is a common plant found in hedgerows and gardens throughout Europe and elsewhere; it is sometimes known as mayflower or whitethorn. The flowers, leaves and berries of at least two species are used: *Crataegus oxycanthoides* Thuill. and

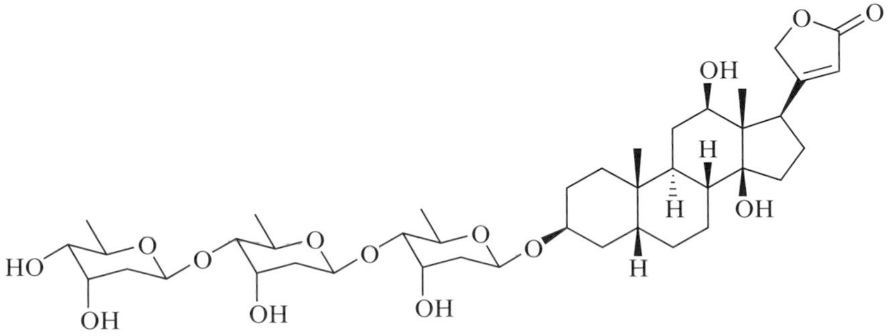

Digoxin

Fig. 15.2

C. monogyna Jacq. (Rosaceae). These are hairless, thorny, deciduous shrubs with 3–5 lobed leaves, bearing white, dense clusters of flowers, followed by deep red fruits containing one seed (in *C. monogyna*) or two seeds (in *C. oxycanthoides*). The flowers appear in early summer and the berries or 'haws' in early autumn. Jams and wines are often made from the fruit.

Constituents

The main constituents of the leaf are flavonoids, including vitexin, vitexin-4-rhamnoside, quercetin and quercetin-3-galactoside, hyperoside, rutin, vicentin, orientin; the fruit contains flavonoids, procyanidins, catechins and epicatechin dimers, as well as phenolic acids such as chlorogenic and caffeic acids. Amines such as phenethylamine and its methoxy derivative, as well as dopamine, acetylcholine and tyramine, have also been isolated. It is thought that a mixture of active constituents may be necessary for the therapeutic effect. The drug prepared from hawthorn is often standardized to contain 4–30 mg of flavonoids, calculated as hyperoside, or 30–160 mg of procyanidins, calculated as epicatechin. In the Eur. Ph., the leaf and flower, and also the berries, are identified using thin layer chromatography (TLC) with the hyperoside, rutin and chlorogenic acid as reference standards. The assays are different, however; whereas the leaf and flower use the flavonoid content, the berries are assayed for anthocyanin content.

Therapeutic uses and available evidence

Hawthorn is used as a cardiac tonic, hypotensive, coronary and peripheral vasodilator, anti-atherosclerotic and anti-arrhythmic. Animal studies have shown beneficial effects on coronary blood flow, blood pressure and heart rate, as well as improved circulation to the extremities (Alternative Medicine Review (Crataegus) 2010). Hawthorn extract inhibits myocardial Na^+, K^+-ATPase and exerts a positive inotropic effect and relaxes the coronary artery. It blocks the repolarizing potassium current in the ventricular muscle and so prolongs the refractory period, thus exerting an anti-arrhythmic effect. It seems to protect heart muscle by regulating Akt and HIF-1 signalling pathways (Jayachandran et al 2010), and reducing oxidative stress (Bernatoniene et al 2009, Swaminathan et al 2010). There are as yet few clinical trials of the drug, although a recent double-blind pilot study indicated a promising role for hawthorn extract in mild essential hypertension (Walker et al 2002). However,

other studies have found that tolerance to exercise was not improved in patients with class II congestive heart failure (Zick et al 2009). It seems likely that hawthorn can be used as an adjunct or sole treatment only in milder cases of heart disease. The usual recommended dose of standardized extract (see Constituents, above) is 160–900 mg daily. Few side effects have been observed, and both patients and physicians rated the tolerance of the drug as good, although nausea and headache have been reported infrequently.

VENOUS INSUFFICIENCY AND CIRCULATORY DISORDERS

Improvements in circulatory disorders arise from a number of different pharmacological effects, particularly those involving anti-inflammatory and antioxidant activity. Plant drugs with these actions are important in the treatment of haemorrhoids, varicose veins, impaired visual acuity and even in memory enhancement, when blood flow to the brain may be affected. They usually contain saponins with anti-inflammatory activity, or anthocyanidins and other antioxidants. The most important are bilberry, butcher's broom, horse chestnut, ginkgo and garlic.

BILBERRY, *VACCINIUM MYRTILLUS* L. (MYRTILLI FRUCTUS) EU✶

The bilberry, also known as the huckleberry or blueberry (*Vaccinium myrtillus* L., Vacciniaceae), grows on acid soil in hilly and mountainous regions of Europe, Asia and North America. It is cultivated extensively for its delicious fruit, which ripen from July to September. The soft blue-black berries, about 0.51 cm in diameter, have a persistent calyx ring at the apex and contain numerous small oval seeds. Both the ripe fruit and the leaves are used medicinally.

Constituents

The fruit contains anthocyanosides (Fig. 15.3), mainly galactosides and glucosides of cyanidin, delphidin and malvidin, together with vitamin C and volatile flavour components such as *trans*-2-hexenal and ethyl-2- and -3-methylbutyrates. Unlike other *Vaccinium* spp., bilberry does not contain arbutin or other hydroquinone derivatives. The anthocyanins can be estimated using their absorption at 528 nm, as described in the Eur. Ph.

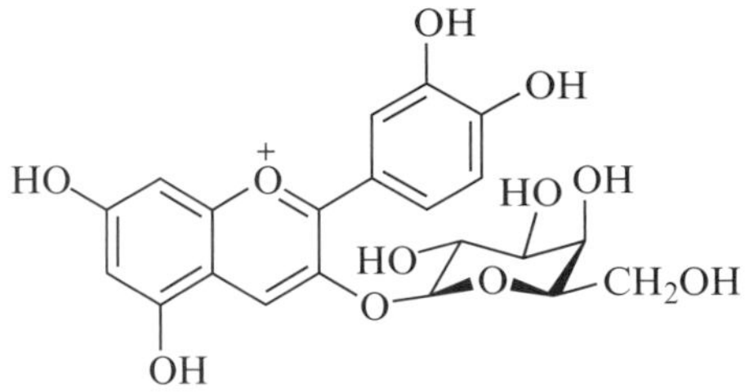

Cyanidin-3-O-galactoside

Fig. 15.3

Therapeutic uses and available evidence

The berries were traditionally used as an antidiabetic, and an astringent and antiseptic for diarrhoea. However, bilberry is now more important as an agent to improve blood circulation in venous insufficiency, especially for vision disorders such as retinopathy caused by diabetes or hypertension. The anthocyanosides are mainly responsible for these properties, due to their antioxidant and free radical scavenging properties. Other cardiovascular benefits include antiplatelet and anti-atherosclerotic effects. Bilberry extracts have a spasmolytic action on the gut and inhibit certain proteolytic enzymes. Anti-inflammatory, antiulcer effects have also been noted, and many of these have been supported by clinical studies (e.g. Christie et al 2001), although the quality of the trials for improving vision have been criticised for their methodology (Canter and Ernst 2004). The usual daily dose of a standardized anthocyanoside extract of bilberry is 480 mg, taken in divided doses. Few side effects have been observed, as would be expected of a widely consumed food substance.

BUTCHER'S BROOM, *RUSCUS ACULEATUS* (RUSCI RHIZOMA) EU*

Butcher's broom (*Ruscus aculeatus* L., Liliaceae) is an evergreen shrub native to Europe, and is found in dry woods and among rocks. It is often cultivated for its tough, spiky twigs and 'leaves', which can be preserved and used for decoration. The true leaves are reduced to small scales and the stems flattened at the ends into oval 'cladodes' which resemble leaves, each bearing a small white flower in the centre, followed by a round scarlet berry, and ending in a sharp spine. The rhizome or whole plant can be used.

Constituents

Actives are saponin glycosides, including ruscine and ruscoside, aculeosides A and B, which are based on ruscogenin (1β-hydroxydiosgenin) and neoruscogenin.

Therapeutic uses and available evidence

Butcher's broom has anti-inflammatory effects and is used mainly for diseases of venous insufficiency, such as varicose veins and haemorrhoids. The ruscogenin constituents have been shown to reduce vascular permeability and improve symptoms of retinopathy and lipid profiles of diabetic patients. The extract is either taken internally as a decoction or, more often, applied topically in the form of an ointment (or a suppository in the case of haemorrhoids). The saponins inhibit elastase activity *in vitro* and for this reason extracts are widely used in cosmetic preparations (Redman 2000). When applied topically, few side effects have been observed, apart from occasional irritation.

GINKGO, *GINKGO BILOBA* (GINKGO FOLIUM) EU*

See Chapter 17 for more detail about the plant. *Ginkgo biloba* can also be used in cases of peripheral arterial occlusive disease and other circulatory disorders. Although probably less potent than some synthetic drugs, it has the advantage of being well tolerated. Ginkgo improves blood circulation and can alleviate some of the symptoms of tinnitus, intermittent claudication and altitude sickness. Ginkgo extracts have complex effects on isolated blood vessels. The ginkgolides are specific platelet-activating factor (PAF) antagonists and inhibit effects produced by PAF, including platelet aggregation and cerebral ischaemia. The usual dose is 120–160 mg of extract daily.

HORSE CHESTNUT, *AESCULUS HIPPOCASTANEUM* L. (HIPPOCASTANI SEMEN) EU*

Aesculus hippocastaum (syn. *Hippocastanum vulgare*, Gaertn., Hippocastanaceae) is native to western Asia, but is now cultivated and naturalized in most temperate regions. It is a large tree, bearing large sticky leaf buds, which open in early spring. The leaves are composed of 5–7 large oval leaflets; the flowers have a candle-like appearance and are white or pink in colour. The bark is thick, rough, grey or brown on the external surface and pinkish-brown and finely striated on the inside. The fruits are spiny capsules, each with two to four compartments containing the well-known large shiny brown seeds or 'conkers'. The seeds, and occasionally the bark, are used.

Constituents

Both contain a complex mixture of saponins based on protoescigenin and barringtogenol-C, which is sometimes known as 'aescin' (or 'escin'), although this term refers more properly to the isomeric compound aescin (see Fig. 15.4). More than 30 saponins have been identified, including α- and β-escin, together with escins Ia, Ib, IIa, IIb, IIIa, etc. Sterols and other triterpenes such as friedelin, taraxerol and spinasterol are present, as well as coumarins (e.g. esculin=aesculin) and fraxin, flavonoids and anthocyanidins.

Therapeutic uses and available evidence

Extracts of horse chestnut, or, more usually, extracts standardized to the escin content, are used particularly for conditions involving chronic venous insufficiency (CVI), bruising and sports injuries. They can be taken internally or applied topically. A number of clinical studies have shown benefits in CVI (Pittler and Ernst 2006), deep vein thrombosis (DVT), including after surgery, varicose veins (including those of pregnancy) and for the prevention of oedema during a long (15 h) aeroplane flight. It was found to be beneficial in the treatment of cerebral oedema following road accidents. Venotonic effects, and an improvement in capillary resistance, have also been noted in healthy volunteers (Suter et al 2006). Escin has been shown to reduce oedema, decrease capillary permeability and increase venous tone, and horse chestnut extract to contract both veins and arteries *in vitro*, with veins being the more sensitive. The extract also significantly reduced ADP-induced human platelet aggregation, and these effects appear to be at least partly mediated through 5-HT(2A) receptors (Felixsson et al 2010). Horse chestnut extract also antagonizes some of the effects of bradykinin and produces an increase in plasma levels of adrenocorticotrophin, corticosterone and glucose in animals. Escin is widely used in cosmetics. The usual dose is 600 mg of extract daily, which corresponds to about 100 mg of escin. Extracts are well tolerated at therapeutic doses, but higher amounts can cause gastrointestinal upset with internal use, and occasional irritation with external application.

RED ROOT SAGE, *SALVIA MILTIORRHIZA* L. (SALVIAE MILTIORRHIZAE RADIX)

The root and rhizome of *Salvia miltiorrhiza* Bunge, also known as Danshen, are widely used in traditional Chinese medicine to treat many types of cardiovascular diseases, including ischaemic and circulatory disorders such as angina, after stroke and atherosclerosis. The root has a characteristic bright red colour, which is due to the active constituents, the tanshinones.

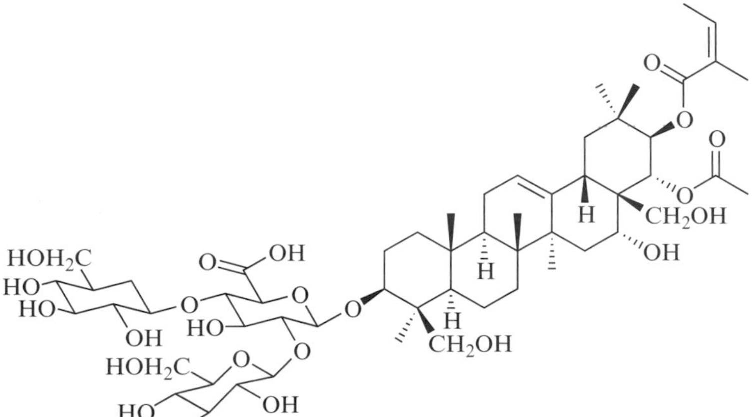

Aescin

Fig. 15.4

Constituents

The main active constituents are diterpene quinones, known as tanshinones (one of the transliterations of *danshen* is *tan-shen*, hence the quinones were called tanshinones). Tanshinone I, tanshinone II, cryptotanshinone are the major constituents, although nearly 40 variants of the basic tanshinone structures have been found in the roots. The total tanshinone content of the roots is about 1%, with tanshinone I and II and cryptotanshinone being the major components.

Therapeutic uses and available evidence

Animal studies have shown many relevant effects, such as protecting heart muscle from ischaemia and improving microcirculation. The isolated tanshinones have been shown to reduce fever and inflammation, inhibit platelet aggregation, dilate the blood vessels and aid urinary excretion of toxins. *Salvia miltiorrhiza* has a mild vasodilatory effect but does not increase cardiac output. Clinical studies carried out in China have shown benefit to patients with heart and circulatory diseases, including ischaemic stroke and acute myocardial infarction, but many of these do not fulfil the criteria required for acceptance in the West, and the efficacy has, therefore, not been accepted there (Wu et al 2007, Wu et al 2008, Yu et al 2009). In general, *Salvia miltiorrhiza* seems to be safe and well-tolerated at the usual dose of 2–6 g day for the dried root, or equivalent in the form of an extract, but there is a potential for drug interactions, especially with other cardiovascular drugs (Williamson et al 2009).

RED VINE LEAF, *VITIS VINIFERA* L. (VITIS VINIFERAE FOLIUM)

Certain varieties of grape vine (*Vitis vinifera* L., a plant which needs no description) produce red leaves which are used in the treatment of CVI and, in particular, varicose veins. Unusually, however, the definition of the botanical drug not only covers the species and a certain plant part, but also the use of a specific prominently coloured variety.

Constituents

Grape leaves contain a wide range of polyphenols including quercetin-3-O-beta-D-glucuronide and isoquercetrin (the main flavonoids), anthocyanins, oligomeric proanthocyanidins, catechin, epicatechin monomers and dimers, gallic acid and astilbine. The phytoalexin trans-resveratrol, another polyphenolic substance belonging to the stilbene group, can also be found in grape vine, organic acids, mainly malic and oxalic acid. The dried leaves of red vine should contain at least 4% of total polyphenols and 0.2% of anthocyanins.

Therapeutic uses and available evidence

Clinical studies have shown that the extract can improve objective symptoms of CVI and that it may prevent further CVI deterioration (Kalus et al 2004). Red vine leaf extracts are also used to improve the microcirculation and aid wound healing (Wollina et al 2006). *In vitro* studies indicate that they have antioxidant and anti-inflammatory properties, and that they inhibit platelet aggregation and hyaluronidase, and reduce oedema, possibly by reducing capillary permeability. Preclinical *in vivo* experiments demonstrated anti-inflammatory and capillary wall thickening effects.

Red vine leaf extract can be applied topically and taken internally, and is well-tolerated, although minor gastrointestinal effects have been reported. Commercial products are usually standardized to 90% polyphenols and 5% astilbine, with a daily dose of 360 mg red vine leaf extract being the recommended internal dose.

ANTIPLATELET AND ANTI ATHEROSCLEROTIC DRUGS

Thrombosis and atherosclerosis are the result of a sedentary lifestyle and high sugar and fat consumption. Their incidence is rising and the age at which patients show signs of these conditions is getting younger. These conditions are closely related in that atherosclerosis predisposes to thrombus formation, and can result in peripheral arterial disease, myocardial infarction and stroke. As well as improving diet and taking regular exercise, preventative drugs can be taken, many of which are natural products of some kind. Antiplatelet drugs are used prophylactically to decrease platelet aggregation and inhibit thrombosis. The standard antiplatelet drug is aspirin, which is used in doses that are lower (75–300 mg daily) than for pain relief (300 mg to 1 g, up to four times daily).

Many items of diet also have antiplatelet effects, for example the flavonoids and anthocyanidins, as well as garlic, which is used as a food supplement for this and other purposes (e.g. as an antimicrobial). Garlic also has anti-atherosclerotic effects and is part of the 'Mediterranean diet' or the 'French paradox', in which there is a generally lower incidence of heart disease despite a cuisine rich in cream and butter. Other elements of this diet include olive oil, which contains monounsaturated fatty acids, which also lower blood cholesterol levels, and red wine, which contains anthocyanidins (see bilberry, above).

Ginkgo has antiplatelet activity and is used to improve peripheral blood circulation; this has a beneficial effect on memory and cognitive processes and will be discussed in more detail in Chapter 25. Generally these medicines are very safe, but care should be taken if they are used in conjunction with anticoagulants or prior to surgery. High-fibre phytomedicines, also used as bulk laxatives such as ispaghula and psyllium husk, lower plasma lipid levels and can be used as adjuncts to a low-fat diet. Oat bran (*Avena sativa*) and guar gum (*Cyamopsis tetragonolobus*; see also Chapter 19) lower cholesterol levels; these are thought to act by binding to cholesterol Weinmann et al 2010.

GARLIC, *ALLIUM SATIVUM* L. (ALLII SATIVI BULBUS) EU✦

The garlic bulb (*Allium sativum*, Liliaceae) is composed of a number of small bulbs or 'cloves', covered with papery, creamy-white bracts. Garlic is cultivated worldwide and is used in many forms of cooking. The drug in commerce is the powder prepared from the cut, dried or freeze-dried bulb.

Constituents

Garlic contains a large number of sulphur compounds which are responsible for the flavour and odour of garlic, as well as the medicinal effects. The main compound in the fresh plant is alliin, which on crushing undergoes enzymatic hydrolysis by alliinase to produce allicin (S-allyl-2-propenthiosulphinate; Fig. 15.5). This in turn forms a wide range of compounds such as allylmethyltrisulphide, diallyldisulphide, ajoene and others, many of which are volatile. Sulphur-containing peptides such as glutamyl-*S*-methylcysteine, glutamyl-*S*-methylcysteine sulphoxide and others are also present.

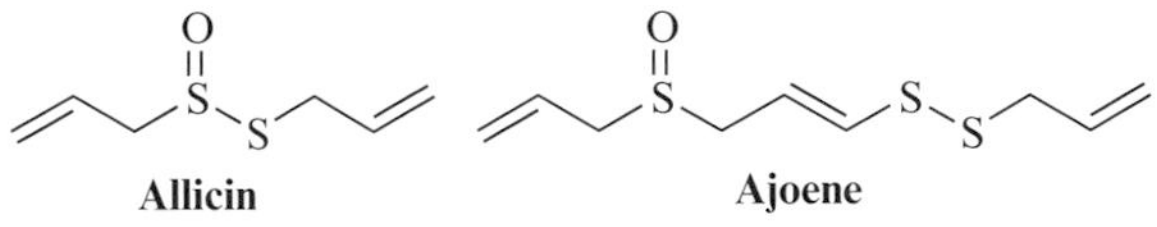

Allicin   Ajoene

Fig. 15.5

Therapeutic uses and available evidence

Different types of garlic preparations are available, such as standardized allicin-rich extracts, aged garlic extracts (particularly in the Far East) and capsules containing the oil (older products). All have different compositions, but it is recognized that the sulphur-containing compounds must be present for the therapeutic effect. Deodorized products, except for those containing the precursor allicin, are ineffective. Hypolipidaemic activity has been observed in animals with garlic extract; this has been attributed to *S*-allylcysteine which is regarded as important in this activity. *S*-Allylcysteine inhibits NF-kB synthesis and low-density lipoprotein (LDL) oxidation, which are both implicated in atherosclerosis. Allicin is also antioxidant, and garlic extracts protect endothelial cells from oxidized LDL damage. It is known that ajoene (Fig. 15.5) is a potent antithrombotic agent, as well as 2-vinyl-4*H*-1, 3-dithiin to a lesser extent. Cardiovascular benefits are supported by the antithrombotic activity, which has been shown in several studies, and an antiplatelet effect demonstrated by aged garlic extracts in humans.

Other health benefits attributed to garlic are antibacterial, antiviral and antifungal effects, and, more importantly, chemopreventative activity against carcinogenesis in various experimental models. Diallylsulphide is thought to inhibit carcinogen activation via cytochrome P450-mediated oxidative metabolism, and epidemiological evidence suggests that a diet rich in garlic reduces the incidence of cancer. Hepatoprotection against paracetamol (acetaminophen)-induced liver damage has been described and attributed to similar mechanisms. The evidence for the health benefits of taking garlic is generally good despite the poor quality of some trials (Aviello et al 2009). The usual dose of garlic products is equivalent to 600–900 mg of garlic powder daily. Garlic has few side effects, but due to the antiplatelet effects, care should be taken if given in combination with other cardiovascular drugs.

References

Altern. Med. Rev. (Crataegus), 2010. 15 (2), 164–167.

Aviello, G., Abenavoli, L., Borrelli, F., et al., 2009. Garlic: empiricism or science? Natural Product Communications 4, 1785–1796.

Bernatoniene, J., Trumbeckaite, S., Majiene, D., et al., 2009. The effect of crataegus fruit extract and some of its flavonoids on mitochondrial oxidative phosphorylation in the heart. Phytother. Res. 23, 1701–1707.

Canter, P.H., Ernst, E., 2004. Anthocyanosides of *Vaccinium myrtillus* (bilberry) for night vision – a systematic review of placebo-controlled trials. Surv. Ophthalmol. 49, 38–50.

Christie, S., Walker, A.F., Lewith, G.T., 2001. Flavonoids – a new direction for the treatment of fluid retention? Phytother. Res. 15, 467–475.

Felixsson, E., Persson, I.A., Eriksson, A.C., Persson, K., 2010. Horse chestnut extract contracts bovine vessels and affects human platelet aggregation through 5-HT(2A) receptors: an in vitro study. Phytother. Res. 24, 1297–1301.

Hollmann, A., 1992. Plants in Cardiology. BMJ Books, London.

Jayachandran, K.S., Khan, M., Selvendiran, K., Devaraj, S.N., Kuppusamy, P., 2010. *Crataegus oxycantha* extract attenuates apoptotic incidence in myocardial ischemia-reperfusion injury by regulating Akt and HIF-1 signaling pathways. J. Cardiovasc. Pharmacol. 56, 526–531.

Kalus, U., Koscielny, J., Grigorov, A., Schaefer, E., Peil, H., Kiesewetter, H., 2004. Improvement of cutaneous microcirculation and oxygen supply in patients with chronic venous insufficiency by orally administered extract of red vine leaves AS 195: a randomised, double-blind, placebo-controlled, crossover study. Drugs R D 5 (2), 63–71.

Pittler, M.H., Ernst, E., 2006. Horse chestnut seed extract for chronic venous insufficiency. Cochrane Database Syst. Rev. 25 (1). Jan CD003230.

Redman, D.A., 2000. *Ruscus aculeatus* (butcher's broom) as a potential treatment for orthostatic hypotension, with a case report. J. Altern. Complement. Med. 6, 539.

Suter, A., Bommer, S., Rechner, J., 2006. Treatment of patients with venous insufficiency with fresh plant horse chestnut seed extract: a review of 5 clinical studies. Adv. Ther. 23, 179–190.

Swaminathan, J.K., Khan, M., Mohan, I.K., et al., 2010. Cardioprotective properties of *Crataegus oxycantha* extract against ischemia-reperfusion injury. Phytomedicine 17, 744–752.

Walker, A., Marakis, G., Morris, A.P., Robinson, P.A., 2002. Promising hypotensive effect of hawthorn extract: a randomized double-blind pilot study of mild, essential hypertension. Phytother. Res. 16, 48–54.

Weinmann, S., Roll, S., Schwarzbach, C., Vauth, C., Willich, S.N., 2010. Effects of Ginkgo biloba in dementia: systematic review and meta-analysis. BMC Geriatr. 10 (14).

Williamson, E.M., Driver, S., Baxter, K., 2009. In: Stockley's herb–drug interactions. Pharmaceutical Press, London.

Wollina, U., Abdel-Naser, M.B., Mani, R., 2006. A review of the microcirculation in skin in patients with chronic venous insufficiency: the problem and the evidence available for therapeutic options. Int. J. Low. Extrem. Wounds 5, 169–180.

Wu, B., Liu, M., Zhang, S., 2007. Dan Shen agents for acute ischaemic stroke. Cochrane Database Syst. Rev. 2, CD004295.

Wu, T., Ni, J., Wu, J., 2008. Danshen (Chinese medicinal herb) preparations for acute myocardial infarction. Cochrane Database Syst. Rev. 2:CD004465.

Yu, S., Zhong, B., Zheng, M., Xiao, F., Dong, Z., Zhang, H., 2009. The quality of randomized controlled trials on DanShen in the treatment of ischemic vascular disease. J. Altern. Complement. Med. 15, 557–565.

Zick, S.M., Zick, S.M., Vautaw, B.M., Gillespie, B., Aaronson, K.D., 2009. Hawthorn Extract Randomized Blinded Chronic Heart Failure (HERB CHF) trial. Eur. J. Heart Fail. 11, 990–999.

Chapter 16

The respiratory system

Minor common disorders of the respiratory system can often be successfully treated with phytotherapy and it can be helpful as a supportive measure in more serious diseases, such as bronchitis, emphysema and pneumonia. For severe infections, antibiotic therapy may be needed and, although most antibiotics are natural products, their study is a separate issue and will not be dealt with here. However, for colds and flu-like virus infections, decongestants (e.g. menthol and eucalyptus), broncholytics and expectorants (including ipecacuanha, thyme and senega), demulcents (e.g. mallow), antibacterials and antivirals (e.g. linden and elder flowers, pelargonium) and immune system modulators (e.g. echinacea, andrographis) are popular and effective. Allergic conditions such as hay fever can be treated with butterbur, *Petasites* and, traditionally, a compound of garlic and echinacea is used for allergic and infective rhinitis. Asthma is becoming more prevalent for reasons as yet unknown, but is best treated aggressively with inhaled steroids and bronchodilators. Many bronchodilators are either of natural origin (e.g. theophylline and ephedrine) or have been developed from natural products. Although isolated ephedrine and pseudoephedrine are theoretically contraindicated in asthma because they can precipitate an attack, ephedra herb has a long history of use without apparent ill-effects; this is attributed to other constituents in the whole extract. Antimuscarinic drugs (e.g. atropine), which have bronchodilator effects and also dry up secretions, have largely been superseded by derivatives such as ipratropium. An important compound, sodium cromoglycate, is an anti-allergic drug developed from khellin, which stabilizes mast cells and is used in the form of an inhaler to treat asthma. Platelet-activating factor antagonists (e.g. the ginkgolides) have anti-allergic effects, which may be useful in asthma but are not yet employed clinically. Ginkgo is covered in Chapter 16. Leukotriene antagonists have recently been introduced for asthma therapy and, although no plant products are yet in use, there are several natural compounds (e.g. quercetin) with this property and they may become available in the future. Cough suppressants are very popular, although there is some controversy as to whether they are clinically effective. The most important antitussives are codeine and other opiate derivatives obtained from the opium poppy.

BRONCHODILATORS AND DECONGESTANTS

SYSTEMIC DRUGS

EPHEDRA, *EPHEDRA* SPP. (EPHEDRAE HERBA) EU✷

Ephedra, also known as Ma Huang (*Ephedra sinica* Stapf. and other species of the family Ephedraceae) is an ancient Chinese medicine, which is now used worldwide. It was the original source of ephedrine, a useful decongestant and bronchodilator. Traditionally, it is used to treat asthma and nasal congestion, in the form of nasal drops. Pseudoephedrine is now used more widely for respiratory congestion as it has fewer central nervous system (CNS) stimulatory properties. The plant has slender green stems, which are jointed in branches of about 20 tufts about 15 cm long, and terminate in a sharp, recurved point. These are the medicinal part. The leaves are reduced to sheaths surrounding the stems.

Constituents

Alkaloids, up to about 3%, but widely varying; the major alkaloid is (–)-ephedrine (Fig. 16.1), together with many others. These include (+)-pseudoephedrine, norephedrine, norpseudoephedrine, ephedroxane, N-methylephedrine, maokonine, transtorine and the ephedradines A–D. Other components are catechin derivatives, and diterpenes, including ephedrannin A and mahuannin A, have been isolated from other species of *Ephedra*.

Therapeutic uses and available evidence

Ephedra has been used since ancient times in China for asthma and hay fever, as a bronchodilator, sympathomimetic, CNS and cardiac stimulant. Herbalists also use it to treat enuresis, allergies, narcolepsy and other disorders, and anti-inflammatory activity has been observed in extracts. Ephedrine is used in the form of elixirs and nasal drops, and has an additional use as a heart rate accelerator in the treatment of some types of bradycardia. Pseudoephedrine, the D-isomer of ephedrine produced by chemical synthesis, is usually the compound of choice for isolated alkaloid preparations. Ephedra herb, ephedrine and pseudoephedrine are all the subject of European Pharmacopoeia (Eur. Ph.) monographs. Ephedra herb is used as an anti-allergic agent; this is supported by evidence that it induces immunoglobulin A in Peyer's patches and blocks complement activation by both the classical and alternative pathways.

Toxicological risks

The herb has been abused as a slimming aid, and an ergogenic aid in sports and athletics, but this is dangerous (Fleming 2008). For example, hypertension and other cardiovascular events, and a case of exacerbation of hepatitis, have been noted with high doses.

The absorption of ephedrine and pseudoephedrine is slower after ingestion of the herb than for isolated alkaloid preparations, and the other constituents, the ephedradins, mahuannins and maokonine, are mildly hypotensive; but both the herb and the isolated alkaloids should be avoided by hypertensive patients as well as in cases of thyrotoxicosis, narrow-angle glaucoma and urinary retention. Therapeutic doses of the herb are calculated to deliver up to 30 mg of the alkaloids, calculated as ephedrine.

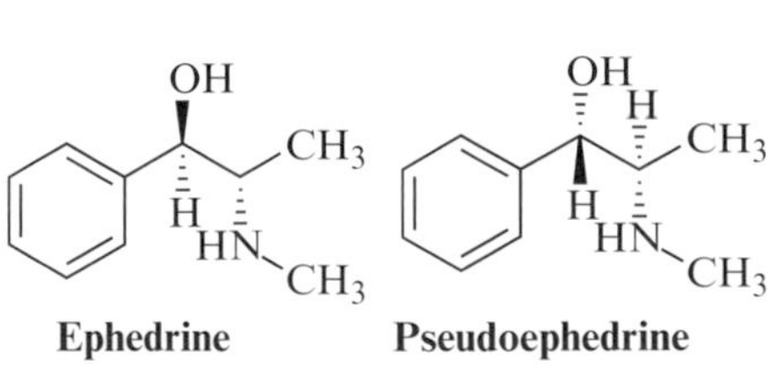

THEOPHYLLINE EU

Although a natural xanthine, theophylline (Fig. 16.2), which is found in cocoa (*Theobroma cacao*), coffee (*Coffea* spp.) and tea (*Camellia sinensis*), is almost invariably used as the isolated compound. It is indicated in reversible airways obstruction, particularly in acute asthma. Because of the narrow margin between the therapeutic and the toxic dose, and the fact that the half-life is highly variable between patients, especially smokers and in heart failure or with concurrent administration of other drugs, care must be taken. The usual dose is 125–250 mg in adults, three times daily, and half of that in children.

Side effects include tachycardia and palpitations, nausea and other gastrointestinal upsets. These can be reduced using sustained-release preparations, and this is the usual form of theophylline products.

INHALATIONS

Essential oil containing drugs are often used with aromatic compounds (especially camphor) as chest rubs, steam inhalations or nasal sprays, for their decongestant properties. They are particularly useful for infants, children, asthmatics and pregnant women for whom systemic decongestants may not be appropriate. They may also be used orally, in pastilles, lozenges, or 'cough sweets'. Oils distilled from the aerial parts of members of the pine family

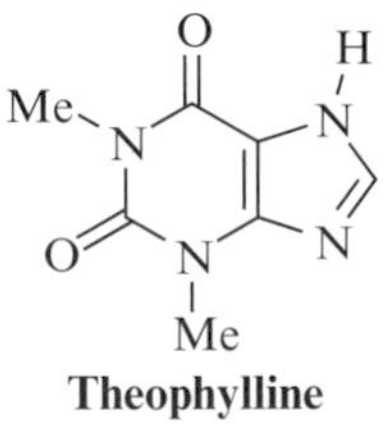

Ephedrine   **Pseudoephedrine**

Fig. 16.1

Theophylline

Fig. 16.2

[e.g. the common Pumilio (Alpine) pine (*Pinus mugo*), the European larch (*Larix decidua*) and the fir tree (*Abies* spp.)] and the Australian Myrtaceae (e.g. eucalyptus and tea-tree oil) are used frequently. These oils can also be used in steam baths.

CAMPHOR EU✱

Camphor (Fig. 16.3), a pure natural product, is derived from the Asian camphor tree (*Cinnamomum camphora* T. Nees & Eberm., Lauraceae). It is often combined with the essential oil containing drugs as an aromatic stimulant and decongestant.

Camphor has antiseptic, secretolytic and decongestant effects. Small doses were formerly taken internally for colds, diarrhoea and other complaints, but it is now used only externally.

Toxicological risks

Camphor has been in use for many years; however, 'camphorated oil' was recently taken off the market since, in large quantities, camphor may be absorbed through the skin causing systemic toxicity. Overdose causes vomiting, convulsions and palpitations, and can be fatal. However, when used externally in therapeutic doses it is generally well tolerated.

EUCALYPTUS OIL, *EUCALYPTUS* SPP. (EUCALYPTI AETHEROLEUM) EU✱

The blue gum tree, *Eucalyptus globulus* Labill., and other species (Myrtaceae) yield a highly characteristic oil which is widely used as a decongestant and solvent. The leaves are scimitar-shaped, 10–15 cm long and about 3 cm wide, shortly stalked and rounded at the base, with numerous transparent oil glands.

Constituents

The oil contains 1,8-cineole (eucalyptol; see Fig. 16.4) as the major component, with terpineol, α-pinene, *p*-cymene and small amounts of ledol, aromadendrene and viridoflorol, aldehydes, ketones and alcohols.

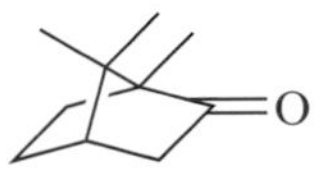

Camphor

Fig. 16.3

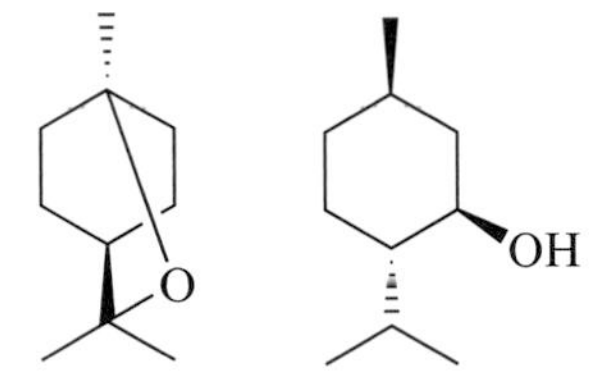

1,8-Cineole   (–)-Menthol

Fig. 16.4

Therapeutic uses and available evidence

The oil is antiseptic, antispasmodic, expectorant, stimulant and insect repellent. It is a traditional Australian Aboriginal remedy for coughs, colds and bronchitis. It may be taken internally in small doses (0.05–0.2 ml), as an ingredient of cough mixtures, sweets and pastilles, or as an inhalation; it is applied externally in the form of a liniment, ointment or 'vapour rub'. The leaf extract and oil have well-defined antiseptic effects against a variety of bacteria and yeasts. The oil is also insect-repellent and larvicidal, and is used in pharmaceutical products for these properties as well as for its antiseptic and flavouring properties in dentifrices and cosmetics. It is widely used in Menthol and Eucalyptus Inhalation BP for steam inhalation as a decongestant. Eucalyptus oil is irritant and, although safe as an inhalation, caution should be exercised when taken internally as fatalities have been reported.

MENTHOL EU✱

Menthol is a monoterpene (Fig. 16.4) extracted from mint oils, *Mentha* spp. (especially *M. arvensis*) or it can be made synthetically. Whole peppermint oil is used in herbal combinations to treat colds and influenza (as well as for colic, etc.; see Chapter 14), but isolated menthol is an effective decongestant used in nasal sprays and inhalers. Menthol can be irritant and toxic in overdose, but is generally well tolerated in normal usage.

ANTI-ALLERGICS

Most antihistamines are synthetic in origin and, although many flavonoids have anti-allergic properties, they are nowhere near as potent as, for example, cetirizine, desloratidine, fexofenadine or chlorpheniramine. Recently, however, an extract of the herbal drug butterbur (see below) was found to be equivalent in activity to cetirizine. There is a problem with toxic alkaloids in this plant, which if present must be removed from the product; thus it is not suitable as a home remedy without expert advice. Smooth muscle relaxant drugs have been used widely in asthma, and one of these, khellin (used particularly in the Mediterranean region, and isolated from *Ammi visnaga*), was investigated as a lead compound for development. One derivative, sodium cromoglycate, was discovered to have antiallergic effects (see below).

BUTTERBUR, *PETASITES HYBRIDUS* L.

Petasites hybridus (syn. *P. vulgaris, Tussilago petasites*, Compositae) is a downy perennial, common in damp places throughout Europe, with very large heart-shaped leaves and lilac-pink brush-like flowers which occur in early spring before the leaves appear. The root and herb are used.

Constituents

Butterbur contains sesquiterpene lactones (eremophinolides), including a series of petasins and isopetasins, neopetasin, petasalbin, furanopetasin, petasinolides A and B, and flavonoids including isoquercetin glycosides. However, toxic pyrrolizidine alkaloids (senecionine, integerrimine, senkirkine, petasitine and neopetasitine) may be present, usually in higher concentrations in the root.

Therapeutic uses and available evidence

Butterbur is traditionally used as a remedy for asthma, colds, headaches and urinary tract disorders. It is used as an antihistamine for seasonal allergic rhinitis, and a recent randomized, double-blind comparative study using 125 patients over 2 weeks of treatment showed that butterbur extract is as potent as cetirizine. The anti-inflammatory activity is due mainly to the petasin content. Extracts inhibit leukotriene synthesis and are spasmolytic, and reduce allergic airway inflammation and AHR by inhibiting the production of the Th2 cytokines IL-4 and IL-5, and RANTES (Brattström et al 2010), thus supporting its use in asthma. Use as prophylactic treatment for migraine has also been suggested but further evidence of efficacy is needed (Agosti et al 2006). The usual dose is an extract equivalent to 5–7 g of herb or root. Internal use is not recommended unless the alkaloids

are present in negligible amounts or have been removed from preparations, as is the case with the commercially available product, which is a 'special extract'. Maximum intake of the alkaloids should be less than 1 µg daily for fewer than 6 weeks per year.

KHELLA, *AMMI VISNAGA* (L.) LAM.

Also known as the 'toothpick plant', as the woody pedicels can be used for this purpose, khella (Apiaceae) is an herbaceous annual reaching 1.5 m in height, with divided filiform leaves and typically umbelliferous flowers. The botanical drug is the fruits, which are very small, broadly ovoid and usually found as separate greyish-brown merocarps. The drug has a long history of use in the Middle East, especially Egypt, as an antispasmodic in renal colic, for asthma and as a coronary vasodilator for angina.

Constituents

Key active principles are furanocoumarins, the most important being khellin (Fig. 16.5), together with visnagin, visnadin and khellol glucoside.

Therapeutic uses and available evidence

Khellin, visnadin and visnagin are vasodilators, with calcium channel blocking and spasmolytic activity. Khellin was the starting material for the development of several important semi-synthetic derivatives such as sodium cromoglycate, which is widely used as a prophylactic treatment for asthma, hay fever and other allergic conditions, often in the form of an inhaler or eyedrops. It was also the basis for the development of nifedipine (a calcium channel antagonist and vasodilator) used in heart disease, and amiodarone, a cardiac antiarrhythmic.

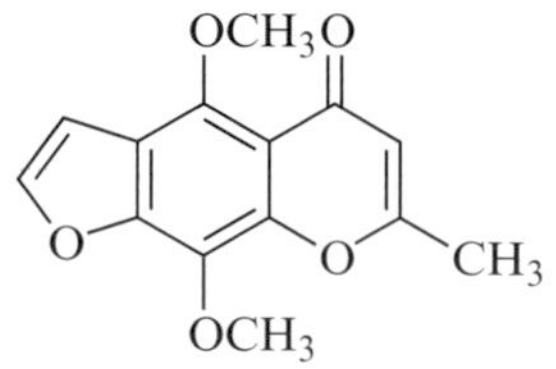

Khellin

Fig. 16.5

EXPECTORANTS AND MUCOLYTICS

The purpose of these drugs is to reduce the viscosity of mucus in the respiratory tract to enable expectoration of phlegm in cases of chest and throat infection. Frequently, essential oils are used with expectorant aromatic compounds such as camphor. Many expectorants are included in cough mixtures and, although efficacy is difficult to demonstrate, these products are very popular with patients in the absence of other treatments. All are used for coughs and colds, bronchitis and sinusitis, usually in conjunction with other decongestants, demulcents, analgesics and, occasionally, antibiotics. Some of these drugs contain essential oils and salicylates (e.g. poplar buds, thyme), and may also include the decongestants mentioned above (eucalyptus, menthol); others contain saponins (e.g. senega, ivy).

BALM OF GILEAD (POPLAR BUDS), *POPULUS* SPP.

Poplar buds (from various *Populus* spp., including *P. candicans* Ait., *P. gileadensis Rouleau*, *P. balsamifera* L. and *P. nigra* L., Salicaceae) are collected in the spring before they open. *P. gileadensis* and *P. nigra* are cultivated in Europe; the others are North American. The buds of all species are similar, being about 2 cm long and 0.5 cm wide, with narrow, brown, overlapping scales; the inner scales are sticky and resinous. The bark of these species is also used.

Constituents

All contain the phenolic glycosides salicin (salicyl alcohol glucoside), populin (benzoyl salicin) and a volatile oil containing α-caryophyllene, with cineole, bisabolene and farnesene. Flavonoids (pinocembrin and pinobanksin) and, in *P. nigra* at least, lignans, based on isolariciresinol, have been isolated.

Therapeutic uses and available evidence

Balm of Gilead is an expectorant, stimulant, antipyretic and analgesic. It is a common ingredient of herbal cough mixtures, and also ointments used for rheumatic and other muscular pains. The phenolic glycosides (e.g. salicin) and the volatile oil constituents have antiseptic and expectorant activity. Little evidence is available for efficacy, but the drug

has a long history of traditional use. The bark of poplar species is used in a similar way to willow bark, as an antirheumatic.

Balm of Gilead is generally non-toxic, except for patients who are allergic to salicylates. If excessive amounts of these drugs are taken, adverse effects such as stomach upset and tinnitus are possible, due to the salicylate content.

THYME AND WILD THYME, *THYMUS VULGARIS* L. AND *THYMUS SERPYLLUM* L. (THYMI HERBA AND SERPYLLI HERBA) EU✱

Thymus vulgaris (known as garden or common thyme) and wild thyme (*T. serpyllum*, mother of thyme or serpyllum, Lamiaceae) are indigenous to Europe, especially the Mediterranean region, and are cultivated extensively. They are small, bushy herbs, with small, elliptical, greenish-grey, shortly stalked leaves. Those of thyme are up to about 6 mm long and 0.5–2 mm broad, with entiren recurved margins. The leaves of wild thyme are a little broader and the margins are not recurved; it has leaves with long trichomes at the base. Microscopically, the herbs are similar; both having the characteristic Lamiaceous glandular trichomes; the rather subtle differences are described in the Eur. Ph. Both have a characteristic odour of thymol and are used as culinary herbs.

Constituents

The active principle is the volatile oil, which has the major constituent thymol, with lesser amounts of carvacrol, 1,8-cineole, borneol, thymol methyl ether and α-pinene. However, the flavonoids (apigenin, luteolin, thymonin, etc.) and the polyphenolic acids (labiatic, rosmarinic and caffeic) are expected to contribute to the anti-inflammatory and antimicrobial effects.

Therapeutic uses and available evidence

Thyme, and oil of thyme, are carminative, antiseptic, antitussive, expectorant and spasmolytic, and, as such, are used for coughs, bronchitis, sinusitis, whooping cough and similar respiratory complaints. Most of the activity is thought to be due to the thymol, which is expectorant and highly antiseptic. Thymol and carvacrol are spasmolytic and the flavonoid fraction has a potent effect on the smooth muscle of guinea pig trachea and ileum. Thymol (Fig. 24.1) is a popular ingredient of mouthwashes and dentifrices because of its antiseptic and deodorant properties. The oil may be taken internally in small doses of up to 0.3 ml, unless for use in a mouthwash, which is not intended to be swallowed in significant amounts.

Thymol is irritant, and toxic in overdose, and should be used with care.

SAGE, *SALVIA OFFICINALIS* L. (SALVIAE FOLIUM) AND *SALVIA* SPP. EU✲

Salvia officinalis L. (syn. garden or red sage, Lamiaceae) is indigenous to Europe, especially the Mediterranean region, and cultivated extensively. Spanish sage is *S. officinalis* subspp. *lavandulifolia* (Vahl) Gams; Greek sage is *S. triloba* L. fil. The leaves are stalked, 3–5 cm long and 1–2.5 cm broad, oblong or lanceolate and rounded at the base and at the apex. Sage has a strong, characteristic, odour. It is widely used as a culinary herb.

Constituents

Sage contains a volatile oil, with α- and β-thujone as the major components (usually about 50%), and cineole, borneol, camphor, 2-methyl-3-methylene-5-heptene and others. Spanish sage does not contain thujone; Greek sage contains only small amounts. Diterpene bitters picrosalvin (carnosol), carnosolic acid, abietane derivatives called royleanones, and flavonoids such as salvigenin, genkwanin, luteolin and derivatives are present, together with the polyphenolic acids salvianolic, rosmarinic and caffeic acids.

Therapeutic uses and available evidence

An infusion of sage is used as a gargle or mouthwash for pharyngitis, tonsillitis, sore gums, mouth ulcers and other similar disorders. Sage extracts and oil have been reported to be antimicrobial. The flavonoids and phenolic acid derivatives have antiviral and anti-inflammatory activity. Sage has a reputation for enhancing memory, and there is some clinical trial evidence (Scholey et al 2008), and the fact that it has anticholinesterase activity, to support this use.

SENEGA, *POLYGALA SENEGA* L. (POLYGALAE RADIX) EU✲

Senega (snake root, rattlesnake root, *Polygala senega* L., Polygalaceae) is native to the USA. In Chinese medicine, senega may also refer to *P. tenuifolia* Willd.; both species are used for similar purposes. The root is light yellowish-grey with a knotty crown, from which slender stems arise, bearing the remains of rudimentary leaves and buds at the base.

Constituents

The active constituents are triterpenoid saponins, the mixture generally known as 'senegin'. These are based on the aglycones presenegenin, senegenin, hydroxysenegin, polygalacic acid and senegnic acid, including the E- and Z-senegins II, III and IV, E- and Z-senegasaponins a, b and c, and others.

Therapeutic uses and available evidence

Senega is used primarily for chronic bronchitis, catarrh, asthma and croup. The saponins are the active constituents, as with other mucolytic plant drugs, and senega is usually taken orally as an infusion. The saponins also have immunopotentiating activity to protein and viral antigens, and exhibit less toxicity than quillaia saponins. They are anti-inflammatory and antiseptic. Senega extracts, the senegasaponins and the senegins are hypoglycaemic in rodents, the senegasaponins are inhibitors of alcohol absorption, and the senegins also have anticancer and antiangiogenic effects *in vitro* (Arai et al 2011). The dose is usually equivalent to 0.5–1 g of the powdered root.

The saponins are irritant and haemolytic, but taken orally do not appear to pose many problems. Nausea and vomiting are the most common side effects and, in view of the other pharmacological actions, care should be taken with senega when given in high doses or to sensitive individuals.

IVY, *HEDERA HELIX* L. (HEDERAE FOLIUM) EU✲

Ivy is a saponin-containing expectorant. It is a common European plant, found also in northern and eastern Asia and introduced into America. *Hedera helix* (Araliaceae) has dark green leathery leaves, shiny, with 3–4 triangular lobes. The berries are small, purplish-black and globular, with the calyx ring visible at the apex. Both leaves and berries may be used as part of phytothera-peutic preparations. The berries are somewhat toxic if consumed.

Constituents

The actives are saponins based on oleanolic acid, bayogenin and hederagenin, including the hedero-saponins (or hederacosides) B, C and D, and α- and β-hederin, the polyyne falcarinol, and also flavonoids.

Therapeutic uses and available evidence

Ivy extracts are used in preparations for bronchitis and catarrh, as an expectorant. The saponins and sapogenins are the main active ingredients; they are expectorant and antifungal. Few clinical studies have been carried out, and further work is needed (Holzinger and Chenot 2011). One study showed that after 7 days of therapy with dried ivy leaf extract, 95% of patients showed improvement or healing of their symptoms, and it was safe and well-tolerated: the overall incidence of adverse events was 2.1%, mainly gastrointestinal disorders (Fazio et al 2009).

Both the saponin and the flavonoid fractions have spasmolytic effects.

A specific mode of action relevant for respiratory conditions of the saponins has been postulated: hederacoside C (which is converted into α-hederin by esterases) as well as its aglucone hederagenin, acts on G protein-linked β_2-adrenergic receptors of epithelial lung cells, resulting ultimately in an indir-ect β_2-sympathomimetic effect (Hegener 2004). Ivy extracts are often used in cosmetic preparations to treat cellulite, with some success. Ivy saponins are being widely investigated for their antileish-manial, molluscicidal, antimutagenic, antithrombin and anticlastogenic effects. The usual therapeutic dose as an expectorant is 0.3 g of crude drug, or equivalent.

Like all saponin-containing drugs, ivy can be irri-tant and allergenic. These effects are also due at least in part to the falcarinol content.

TOLU BALSAM, *MYROXYLON BALSAMUM* L. (BALSAMUM TOLUTANUM) EU*

The resin, which is collected from incisions in the bark and sapwood of *Myroxylon balsamum* (Fabaceae), is a light brown, fragrant, balsamic resin, softening when warm and becoming brittle when cold. It has a pleasant, sweetish, aromatic, vanilla-like odour.

Constituents

The main constituents of the balsam are cinnamic and benzoic acids, their esters such as benzyl benzo-ate and cinnamyl cinnamate, and esters with resin alcohols, including coniferyl and hydroconiferyl benzoates.

Therapeutic uses and available evidence

Balsam of tolu is expectorant, stimulant and antisep-tic. It is used in cough mixtures and pastilles, and as a lozenge base. Although there is no modern clin-ical evidence, many balsams are used for similar purposes and generally agreed to have a useful ther-apeutic role as expectorants, antiseptics and demul-cents. Balsam of tolu is an ingredient in Friar's balsam, which is used as a steam inhalation and also as a protectant in skin formulations. The antimicro-bial activity is due to the benzyl benzoate and benzyl cinnamate content.

Tolu balsam, like many other balsam resins, can cause allergic reactions.

IPECACUANHA, *CEPHAELIS IPECACUANHA* A. RICH AND *C. ACUMINATA* KARSTEN (IPECACUANHAE RADIX) EU*

'Ipecac' is obtained from the root and rhizome of *Cephaelis ipecacuanha* and C. *acuminata* (Rubiaceae). Rio, Matto Grosso and Brazilian ipecac are used to describe C. *ipecacuanha* (syn. *Psychotria ipecacuanha* Stokes) and Cartagena, Nicaragua or Panama ipe-cac, C. *acuminata*. They are native to tropical central and south America and cultivated in southern Asia. C. *ipecacuanha* root is slender, twisted and reddish brown, up to about 4 mm in diameter, with a char-acteristic ringed appearance. C. *acuminata* is larger, with fewer annulations. The root can be identified microscopically by the characteristic tracheids and bordered pitted xylem vessels, and the needle crys-tals of calcium oxalate (see Eur. Ph.).

Constituents

Both species contain isoquinoline alkaloids as the active principles, usually about 2–3%. The most important are emetine (Fig. 16.6) and cephaeline, with psychotrine and some others.

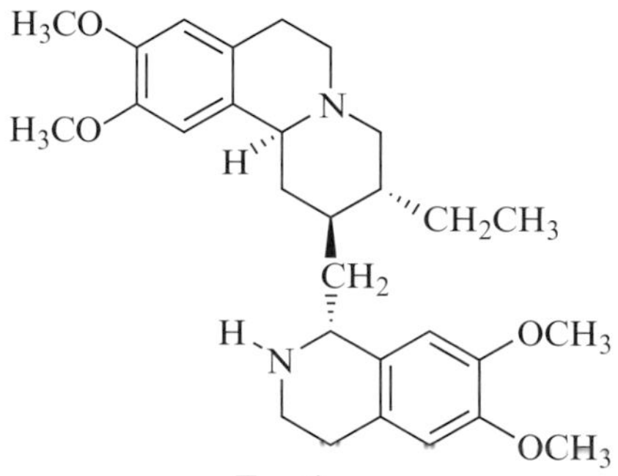

Emetine

Fig. 16.6

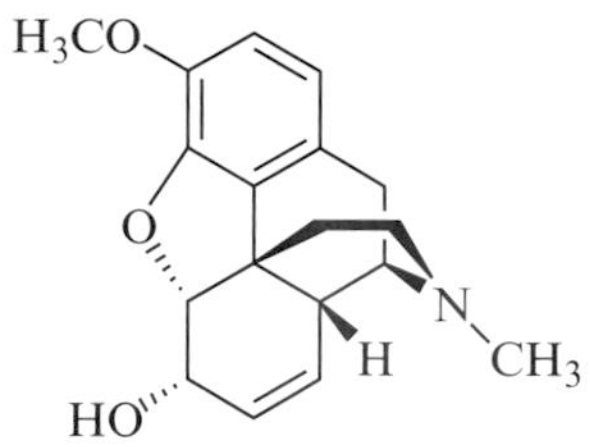

Codeine

Fig. 16.7

Therapeutic uses and available evidence

Ipecac extract is an ingredient of many cough preparations, both elixirs and pastilles, because of its expectorant activity. It is also well known as an emetic and has been employed to induce vomiting in cases of drug overdose, particularly in children. This use is, however, highly controversial (Quang and Woolf 2000). The alkaloids are amoebicidal, but the emetic activity means that they are rarely used for this purpose. There is little clinical evidence for the use of ipecac as an expectorant but it has a long history of traditional use. Ipecacuanha Liquid Extract BP is given at a dose of 0.25–1 ml.

Ipecac causes vomiting in large doses and the alkaloids are cytotoxic.

COUGH SUPPRESSANTS

Cough is a reflex action and a symptom of other diseases such as asthma and colds due to 'nasal drip'. Cough suppressants may be useful in some instances, but efficacy is not fully proven and if expectoration is required, for example to avoid sputum retention, they should not be used. They are not recommended for small children who are highly susceptible to respiratory depression caused by opiates. Codeine and semi-synthetic opiates such as dextromethorphan are the most common antitussives; in severe cases such as in lung cancer, stronger opiates such as methadone may be used.

CODEINE EU✷

Although found in opium (*Papaver somniferum*), codeine (Fig. 16.7) is usually used as the isolated alkaloid, in the form of a salt (usually phosphate)

formulated as a linctus, at a dose of 5–10 mg 4-hourly, to treat cough. The dose for treating diarrhoea and pain is much higher (up to 240 mg daily in divided doses).

Codeine is sedating and constipating. In large doses it may cause respiratory depression and should not be used in hepatic or renal impairment. It is also liable to abuse and is available only on prescription in many countries.

GENERAL PHYTOMEDICINES USED IN COLDS AND INFLUENZA

Some of these herbs have antiviral and anti-inflammatory activity, some are demulcents or stimulate the immune system, and many have several of these properties. They are often used in combination with other ingredients as herbal teas for the supportive or symptomatic therapy of respiratory disease.

DEMULCENTS AND EMOLLIENTS

Many herbal teas, made particularly from flowers and leaves, are used to obtain symptomatic relief from colds and influenza. Some are diaphoretic (induce sweating), some are anti-inflammatory and analgesic, others are mucilagenous and soothing, and many have some antiviral activity due to the polyphenolic constituents. They are used as a general supportive measure and are usually pleasant to take. As well as the plants discussed here, other botanical drugs rich in mucilage are also used for respiratory conditions, for example the lichen 'Icelandic Moss' from *Cetraria islandica* (L.) Ach. (Parmeliaceae).

COLTSFOOT, *TUSSILAGO FARFARA* L. (TUSSILAGO FOLIUM) EU✷

Coltsfoot (Asteraceae) is a common wild plant in Britain and Europe, growing in damp places. The flowers appear in early spring before the leaves. The leaves are hoof-shaped, with angular teeth on the margins, green above and coated with matted, long white hairs on the lower surface. The flowers are bright yellow, with a characteristic scaly pedicel. Both the leaves and flowers are used medicinally.

Constituents

The main constituent is a mucilage composed of acidic polysaccharides, together with flavonoids, triterpenes and sterols. Pyrrolizidine alkaloids, including senkirkine, tussilagine and isotussilagine, may be present in variable amounts, usually very minor (about 0.015%) or absent, depending on source.

Therapeutic uses and available evidence

Coltsfoot is used for pulmonary complaints, irritating or spasmodic coughs, whooping cough, bronchitis, laryngitis and asthma. The polysaccharides are anti-inflammatory and immunostimulating, as well as demulcent, and the flavonoids also have anti-inflammatory and antispasmodic action.

The pyrrolizidine alkaloids are known to cause hepatotoxicity in rats fed daily on high doses, but not on daily low-dose regimens, and appear not to cause damage to human chromosomes *in vitro*. However, samples containing significant quantities of these alkaloids should not be used.

ELDERFLOWER AND ELDERBERRY (FRUIT), *SAMBUCUS NIGRA* L. (SAMBUCI FLOS, SAMBUCI FRUCTUS) EU✷

Sambucus nigra (Adoxaceae or Sambucaceae), the Black or European elder (berry), is a common European hedge tree or shrub. The flowers appear in May as small, creamy-white, flat-topped umbel-like clusters and are followed by small, shiny, purplish-black berries. Most parts of the plant are used, but most commonly the flowers and berries, which are also used to make refreshing drinks and country-style wines. The berries should not be eaten raw as they contain lectins, which can cause gastrointestinal disturbances, but which are destroyed by heat. Related species are toxic (e.g. Danewort, *S. ebulus*).

Constituents

Triterpenes including ursolic and oleanolic acid derivatives, flavonoids (rutin, quercetin, nicotoflorin, hyperoside), and phenolic acids such as chlorogenic acid are the main actives. The flowers contain an essential oil.

Therapeutic uses and available evidence

Elder flowers are used as an infusion or herbal tea, and a mixture with peppermint is a traditional remedy for colds and influenza. They induce perspiration, which is thought to be beneficial in such cases. Recent studies show an *in vitro* activity against several strains of influenza virus, and a clinical study has also demonstrated a reduction in the duration of flu symptoms for the berries (see Vlachojannis et al 2010 for review). The effect was attributed to an increase in inflammatory cytokine production as well as a direct antiviral action. The usual dose is about 3 g of flowers infused with 150 ml of hot water, but is not critical. Elder flowers are non-toxic and no side effects have been reported. Both the berries and the flowers are used to make cordials which are taken medicinally for their reputed antioxidant and antiviral properties.

LINDEN FLOWERS, *TILIA* SPP. (TILIAE FLOS) EU✷

Linden flowers (although called 'lime flowers' they are not related to lime fruit) are from *Tilia platyphylla* Scop., *T. cordata* Mill. and their hybrid (Tiliaceae). They are ornamental trees native to Europe. The pedicel bears 3–6 yellowish-white, five-petalled, fragrant flowers on stalks half-joined to an oblong bract.

Constituents

The flowers contain volatile oil (linalool, germacrene, geraniol, 1,8-cineole, 2-phenyl ethanol and others), flavonoids (hesperidin, quercetin, astralagin, tiliroside), a mucilage of arabinose, galactose and rhamnose polysaccharides, polyphenolics such as chlorogenic and caffeic acids, and GABA (γ-aminobenzoic acid).

Therapeutic uses and available evidence

Linden flowers are used for feverish colds, catarrh, coughs and influenza. They are used as herbal teas to induce diaphoresis (perspiration) like elder and at a similar dose (see above). The polysaccharides are soothing and adhere to epithelial tissue, producing a demulcent effect. The other main use of the flowers is for nervous disorders; the extract is thought to act as an agonist for the peripheral benzodiazepine receptor. There is evidence that components of the aqueous extract of the flowers bind to GABA receptors in rat brain (an effect not due entirely to the GABA content of the extract) and mild sedative effects were confirmed using the elevated maze anxiety test in mice (Anesini 1999). Linden flowers are non-toxic and no side effects have been reported.

MALLOW FLOWER AND LEAVES, *MALVA SYLVESTRIS* L. (MALVAE FLOS AND MALVAE FOLIUM) EU*

The common mallow (*Malva sylvestris* L., Malvaceae) is a wild plant indigenous to southern Europe but naturalized worldwide. The leaves are downy, with 5–7 lobes, and prominent veins on the under surface. The flowers are mauve, with darker veins; both are used for their mucilage content.

Constituents

The main constituents are mucilages, sulphated flavonol glycosides such as gossypin-3-sulphate, hypolaetinglucoside-3'-sulphate and others, and anthocyanins (malvin, the diglucoside of malvidin, and delphinidin).

Therapeutic uses and available evidence

Mallow is a demulcent and pectoral. An infusion is used for colds and coughs, and the mucilage from the leaves is anti-inflammatory with anticomplement activity. Little clinical evidence is available but there is a long tradition of historical use. No adverse effects are known.

MARSHMALLOW LEAF AND ROOT, *ALTHEA OFFICINALIS* L. (ALTHAEAE FOLIUM, ALTHAEAE RADIX) EU*

Both the leaves and the rootstock of the marshmallow (Malvaceae) are used as a demulcent, expectorant and emollient. The plant is a downy perennial reaching up to 2 m in height with leaves broadly ovate or cordate, 10–20 cm long and about 10 cm wide, with 3–7 rounded lobes, palmate veins and a crenate margin. The flowers are pink, five-petalled, up to 3 cm in diameter. The root as it appears in commerce is dried, fibrous, cream-white when peeled, deeply furrowed longitudinally and with some root scars. It is largely tasteless.

Constituents

Both rootstock and leaves are rich in mucilage, consisting of a number of polysaccharides (composed of L-rhamnose, D-galactose, D-galacturonic acid and D-glucuronic acid) and others. It also contains common flavonoids, especially derivatives of kaempferol and quercetin.

Therapeutic uses and available evidence

Both the leaves and root are used internally for coughs and bronchial complaints. Extracts of both are used occasionally for gastric and urinary inflammation in general, and for cystitis. They may be applied externally as a soothing poultice and vulnerary. The mucilages have proven biological activity, including the stimulation of phagocytosis *in vitro*. Antimicrobial and anti-inflammatory activities have also been documented. Several of the polysaccharides isolated from the roots have been found to have antitussive activity. The most common use of extracts of marshmallow root is in the making of confectionery.

PELARGONIUM, *PELARGONIUM SIDOIDES* DC AND *P. RENIFORME* CURT (PELARGONII RADIX) EU*

Pelargonium is obtained from two southern African species, *Pelargonium sidoides* and *P. reniforme* (Geraniaceae) where the tubers, stems and root have been used for centuries to treat a range of infectious conditions.

Constituents

The main active components are hydrolysable tannins, (+)-catechin, gallic acid and methyl gallate, including a unique series of O-galloyl-C-glucosylflavones. Flavonoids including myricetin and quercetin-3-O-beta-d-glucoside, coumarins including scopoletin, umckalin, 5,6,7-trimethoxycoumarin and 6,8-dihy-droxy-5,7-dimethoxycoumarin, are present in both species. A series of benzopyranones has been isolated from *P. sidiodes*, and the pelargoniins (a type of ellagitannin) and a diterpene, reniformin, have been found in *P. reniforme*.

Therapeutic uses and available evidence

In Germany, a standardized extract of *Pelargonium sidioides* (EPs® 7630, also known as Umckaloabo®) is registered by the Federal Institute for Drugs and Medical Devices (BfArM) for the indication 'acute bronchitis' and several randomized, double-blind, placebo-controlled clinical trials support its efficacy in adults and children (Agbabiaka et al 2008). The extract EPs® 7630 has multiple effects which are beneficial in respiratory infections, and include antiviral, antibacterial, immunomodulatory and cyto-protective effects. It also increases the frequency of ciliary beats, thus helping to remove pathogens for the upper respiratory tract, and inhibits the interaction between bacteria and host cells. A recent study has found that EPs® 7630 interferes with the replication of different respiratory viruses including seasonal influenza A virus strains, RSV, human coronavirus, parainfluenza virus and coxsackie virus (Michaelis et al 2011). This extract is also given to athletes to help strengthen the immune system, which can be compromised by extreme exercise, to protect against colds. A study in athletes submitted to intense physical activity found that *Pelargonium sidioides* increased the production of secretory immunoglobulin A in saliva, and decreased levels of both interleukin-15 and interleukin-6 in serum, suggesting a strong modulating influence on the immune response associated with the upper airway mucosa (Luna et al 2011).

IMMUNOSTIMULANTS

Immune stimulation is usually measured using parameters such as an increase in numbers of circulating immune cells, or enhanced phagocytosis after inoculation with a pathogen. It is notoriously difficult to substantiate claims for the prevention of disease, since very large clinical studies are needed for statistical validity, and these are difficult and expensive to perform. However, echinacea is taken widely and the use of an Oriental herb, astragalus, is increasing in the West for the same indications.

ECHINACEA, *ECHINACEA PALLIDA* (NUTT.) BRITT., *E. PURPUREA* MOENCH AND *E. ANGUSTIFOLIA* (DC.) HELL. (ECHINACEAE HERBA, RADIX) EU

Members of the genus *Echinacea* (Asteraceae) are widely distributed in North America and have a long tradition of use, both by the American Indians and the settlers, who developed the first commercial preparations during the 19th century. Both aerial parts and secondary roots are used. The indigenous people used *E. pallida* in particular for a variety of illnesses, such as pain, inflammatory skin conditions and toothache. The three botanical species are used in the preparation of phytomedicines to 'prevent colds and other respiratory infections', as immunostimulants. The complex situation regarding species, quality of products made from them and method of production makes an assessment of the clinical efficacy very difficult. Echinacea is often combined with garlic, for the treatment of colds and allergic rhinitis.

Constituents

Numerous compounds have been identified, but the most pharmacologically relevant ones are not known. All species contain similar types of compounds, although not necessarily the same individual ones. The most important are the caffeic acid derivatives, including echinacoside (Fig. 16.8) (*E. pallida* root), cichoric acid (*E. purpurea* aerial parts) and others, and the alkylamides (found throughout the plant in all three species), which are a complex mixture of unsaturated fatty acid derivatives. Some have a diene or diyne structure (with two unsaturated and two triple unsaturated groups) or a tetraene structure (with four unsaturated groups) linked via an esteramide to a (2)-methylpropane or (2)-methylbutane residue.

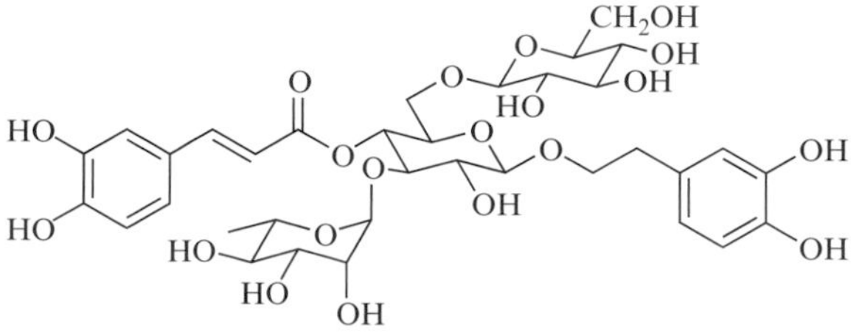

Echinacoside

Fig. 16.8

Therapeutic uses and available evidence

Echinacea preparations are available both as traditional herbal medicinal products used to relieve the symptoms of the common cold and influenza type infections, but also as preparations with a well-established use. There is some evidence in the treatment and prevention of respiratory infections, but more limited evidence for slow healing wounds using topical applications. Clinical evidence for uses as an immunostimulant is available for some of the chemically characterised extracts. Overall a series of meta-analyses showed that Echinacea preparations *seem to be* efficacious both therapeutically (reducing symptoms and duration) and in terms of prophylaxis against the common cold (Shah et al 2007, Woelkart et al 2008). However, *Echinacea* preparations tested in clinical trials differ greatly. There is better evidence that preparations based on the aerial parts of *E. purpurea* might be effective for the early treatment of colds in adults but the results are not fully consistent. A mechanism of action has been postulated by Chicca et al (2009), suggesting that the alkylamides dodeca-2 *E*,4*E*,8*Z*,10*Z*-tetraenoic acid isobutylamide (A1) and dodeca-2*E*, 4*E*-dienoic acid isobutylamide (A2) bind to the cannabinoid-2-(CB2) receptor and are the main anti-inflammatory and immune-modulatory principles, acting in synergy. In addition, alkylamides potently inhibit LPS-induced inflammation in human whole blood and exert modulatory effects on cytokine expression, but these effects are not exclusively related to CB2 binding.

Echinacea appears to be safe, although allergic reactions have been reported. The risk of interactions seems to be very limited (Modarai et al 2007).

ASTRAGALUS, *ASTRAGALUS MEMBRANACEUS* (FISCH.) BGE. (ASTRAGALI RADIX) EU✱

Astragalus membranaceus (Fabaceae) is an herbaceous perennial native to north-eastern China, central Mongolia and Siberia. The drug is known in Chinese medicine as Huang qi. The use of *Astragalus* root as a general tonic dates back to the legendary Chinese emperor Shen-Nong. The root consists of a long cylindrical tap root, which is internally yellowish in colour, but rootlets should be absent.

Constituents

Triterpenoid saponins, the astragalosides I–VIII, and their acetyl derivatives, agroastragalosides I–IV, astramembranins I and II and others; isoflavones including formononetin and kumatakenin, and polysaccharides known as astrogaloglucans.

Therapeutic uses and available evidence

A number of clinical studies, supported by data from over 1000 patients in China, confirm the use of astragalus as an immunostimulant for use in colds and upper respiratory infections. It is also used prophylactically. In China it is also used as an adjunctive in the treatment of cancer, and appears to potentiate the effects of interferon. It also has antioxidant, hepatoprotective and antiviral activity and is used to enhance cardiovascular function (www.thorne.com 2003). Many animal studies have been carried out, but specific data on toxicity are sparse. In general, astragalus is well tolerated but should probably be avoided in autoimmune diseases.

ANDROGRAPHIS, *ANDROGRAPHIS PANICULATA* (BURM.F.) WALL. EX NEES (ANDROGRAPHIS PANICULATAE HERBA)

Andrographis paniculata (Acanthaceae), also known as 'green chiretta', is an erect annual herb found in north-eastern India and many parts of Asia. It is extremely bitter in taste and has been referred to as the 'king of bitters'. It is an important herb in Ayurveda where it is known as kalmegh.

Constituents

The main actives are diterpenes, known as andrographolides, and consist of andrographolide and its many analogues, including neoandrographolide, isoandrographolide, 14-deoxyandrographolide, 14-deoxy-14,15-dehydroandrographolide, 3,19-isopropylideneandrographolide and 14-acetylandrographolide and many others. Flavonoids and polyphenols such as 7-O-methylwogonin, apigenin, onysilin and 3,4-dicaffeoylquinic acid are also present. An alkaloid, andrographine, and a series of sesquiterpene lactones, paniculides A, B, and C, are also present in the root.

Therapeutic uses and available evidence

Andrographis is most commonly used as an immune stimulant, but is also reputed to possess antihepatotoxic, antimicrobial, antithrombogenic, antiinflammatory and anticancer properties (www.thorne.com 2003). Andrographolide has been shown to have immunostimulatory activity, shown by an increase in proliferation of lymphocytes and production of interleukin-2, and the antiinflammatory activity has been demonstrated by an inhibition of NFB,

nitric oxide, PGE2, IL-1β, IL-6, LTB4, TXB2 and histamine (Bao et al 2009, Chandrasekaran et al 2010). In one Chilean study, andrographis herb had a significant drying effect on the nasal secretions of cold sufferers who took 1,200 mg of the extract daily for 5 days (Cáceres et al 1999). A systematic review of the literature has suggested the herb alone (or in combination with Eleutherococcus) may be an appropriate treatment for uncomplicated acute upper respiratory tract infection (Poolsup et al 2004).

References

Agbabiaka, T.B., Guo, R., Ernst, E., 2008. *Pelargonium sidoides* for acute bronchitis: a systematic review and meta-analysis. Phytomedicine 15, 378–385.

Agosti, R., Duke, R.K., Chrubasik, J.E., Chribasik, S., 2006. Effectiveness of *Petasites hybridus* preparations in the prophylaxis of migraine: a systematic review. Phytomedicine 13, 743–746.

Arai, M., Hayashi, A., Sobou, M., et al., 2011. Anti-angiogenic effect of triterpenoidal saponins from *Polygala senega*. J. Nat. Med. 65, 149–156.

Bao, Z., Guan, S., Cheng, C., et al., 2009. A novel antiinflammatory role for andrographolide in asthma via inhibition of the nuclear factor-kappaB pathway. Am. J. Respir. Crit. Care Med. 179, 657–665.

Brattström, A., Schapowal, A., Maillet, I., Schnyder, B., Ryffel, B., Moser, R., 2010. Petasites extract Ze 339 (PET) inhibits allergen-induced Th2 responses, airway inflammation and airway hyperreactivity in mice. Phytother. Res. 24, 680–685.

Cáceres, D.D., Hancke, J.L., Burgos, R.A., Sandberg, F., Wikman, G.K., 1999. Use of visual analogue scale measurements (VAS) to assess the effectiveness of standardized *Andrographis paniculata* extract SHA-10 in reducing the symptoms of common cold. A randomized double blind-placebo study. Phytomedicine 6, 217–223.

Chandrasekaran, C.V., Gupta, A., Agarwal, A., 2010. Effect of an extract of *Andrographis paniculata* leaves on inflammatory and allergic mediators in vitro. J. Ethnopharmacol. 129, 203–207.

Chicca, A., Raduner, S., Pellati, F., Strompen, T., Altmann, K.H., Schoop, R., et al., 2009. Synergistic immunomopharmacological effects of N-alkylamides in *Echinacea purpurea* herbal extracts. Int. Immunopharmacol. 9, 850–858.

Fazio, S., Pouso, J., Dolinsky, D., et al., 2009. Tolerance, safety and efficacy of *Hedera helix* extract in inflammatory bronchial diseases under clinical practice conditions: a prospective, open, multicentre postmarketing study in 9657 patients. Phytomedicine 16, 17–24.

Fleming, R.M., 2008. Safety of ephedra and related anorexic medications. Expert Opin. Drug Saf. 7, 749–759.

Luna Jr., L.A., Bachi, A.L., et al., 2011. Immune responses induced by *Pelargonium sidoides* extract in serum and nasal mucosa of athletes after exhaustive exercise: Modulation of secretory IgA, IL-6 and IL-15. Phytomedicine 18, 303–308.

Michaelis, M., Doerr, H.W., Cinatl Jr., J., 2011. Investigation of the influence of EPs[®] 7630, a herbal drug preparation from *Pelargonium sidoides*, on replication of a broad panel of respiratory viruses. Phytomedicine 18, 384–386.

Modarai, M., Gertsch, J., Suter, A., Heinrich, M., Kortenkamp, A., 2007. Cytochrome P450 inhibitory action of Echinacea preparations differs widely and co-varies with alkylamide content. J. Pharm. Pharmacol. 59, 567–573.

Poolsup, N., Suthisisang, C., Prathanturarug, S., Asawamekin, A., Chanchareon, U., 2004. *Andrographis paniculata* in the symptomatic treatment of uncomplicated upper respiratory tract infection: systematic review of randomized controlled trials. J. Clin. Pharm. Ther. 29, 37–45.

Quang, L., Woolf, A.D., 2000. Past, present, and future role of ipecac syrup. Curr. Opin. Pediatr. 12, 153.

Scholey, A.B., Tildesley, N.T., Ballard, C.G., et al., 2008. An extract of Salvia (sage) with anticholinesterase properties improves memory and attention in healthy older volunteers. Psychopharmacology (Berl) 198, 127–139.

Shah, S.A., Sander, S., White, C.M., Rinaldi, M., Coleman, C.I., 2007. Evaluation of echinacea for the prevention and treatment of the common cold: a meta-analysis. Lancet Infect. Dis. 7, 473–480.

www.thorne.com, 2003. *Astragalus membranaceus*. Monograph. Altern. Med. Rev 8, 72–77.

Vlachojannis, J.E., Cameron, M., Chrubasik, S., 2010. A systematic review on the sambuci fructus effect and efficacy profiles. Phytother. Res. 24 (1), 1–8.

Woelkart, K., Linde, K., Bauer, R., 2008. Echinacea for preventing and treating the common cold. Planta Med. 74, 633–637.

Further reading

Anesini, C., Werner, S., Borda, E., 1999. Effect of *Tilia cordata* Mill. flowers on lymphocyte proliferation. Participation of peripheral type benzodiazepine binding sites. Fitoterapia 70, 361–367.

Hegener, O., Prenner, L., Runkel, F., Baader, S.L., Kappler, J.,

Häberlein, H., 2004. Dynamics of beta2-adrenergic receptor-ligand complexes on living cells. Biochemistry 43, 6190–6199.

Holzinger, F., Chenot, J.F., In press. Systematic review of clinical trials assessing the effectiveness of ivy

leaf (*Hedera helix*) for acute upper respiratory tract infections. Evidence Based Complementary and Alternative Medicine 382789 [Epub 2010 Oct 3].

Chapter 17

The central nervous system

Drugs acting on the central nervous system (CNS) include the centrally acting (mainly opioid) analgesics, anti-epileptics and anti-Parkinson agents, as well as those for psychiatric disorders. Drugs of plant origin are important in all these areas, although not usually for self-medication. They are also of historical interest; for example, the antipsychotic drug reserpine, isolated from *Rauvolfia* species, revolutionized the treatment of schizophrenia and enabled many patients to avoid hospitalization before the introduction of the phenothiazines (such as chlorpromazine) and the newer atypical antipsychotics (olanzapine and risperidone). Unfortunately, reserpine depletes neurotransmitter levels in the brain (it is used as a pharmacological tool in neuroscience for this reason) and so can cause severe depression, and it has recently been implicated in the development of breast cancer. There are no other currently useful antipsychotics obtained from plants and they will not be covered here. Similarly, the useful anti-epileptics are synthetic, with the possible exception of the cannabinoids, from *Cannabis sativa*, which are currently under investigation.

However, for milder psychiatric conditions, phytotherapy can provide useful support. The prevalence of mental health problems, particularly depression and anxiety, in the general population is around one in six people, and around 40% of people with mental health problems will have symptoms of both anxiety and depression. Depression is more common in women than men; around one-half of women and one-quarter of men will be affected by depression at some time. However, other than in mild cases, these disorders are not suitable for self-treatment, and medical supervision is necessary. Sleep disturbances, such as insomnia and early morning awakening, are characteristic of depression and anxiety, although they can also occur independently of mental health problems. Around one-third of adults are thought to experience insomnia, and most do not seek treatment from a physician. Phytotherapy has a role to play in helping to re-establish a regular pattern of sleep. Valerian (Fig. 17.1), for example, has been advocated as a means of alleviating the symptoms of benzodiazepine withdrawal.

Migraine is a common disorder, but can be debilitating. Opioid analgesics are used, and the synthetic 5-HT$_1$ (5-hydroxytryptamine) antagonists (sumatriptan, rizatriptan) are highly effective, although they are not used for the prophylaxis of migraine. Ergotamine is a potent drug used as a last resort in attacks of migraine. Feverfew is sometimes used to prevent attacks, and will be discussed briefly.

In cases of dementia and Alzheimer's disease, natural compounds have played a key role in their symptomatic treatment. Galantamine (from the snowdrop, *Galanthus nivalis*) and derivatives of physostigmine (e.g. rivastigmine) are clinically used as cholinesterase inhibitors. Some plant extracts, such as sage and rosemary, have similar but milder effects and are being investigated for memory improvement. *Ginkgo biloba* has cognition-enhancing properties and can be used for mild forms of dementia.

HYPNOTICS AND SEDATIVES

The difference between a sedative and hypnotic is generally a question of dose. Plant products used in this way are not as potent as synthetic drugs, but neither do they have many of the disadvantages.

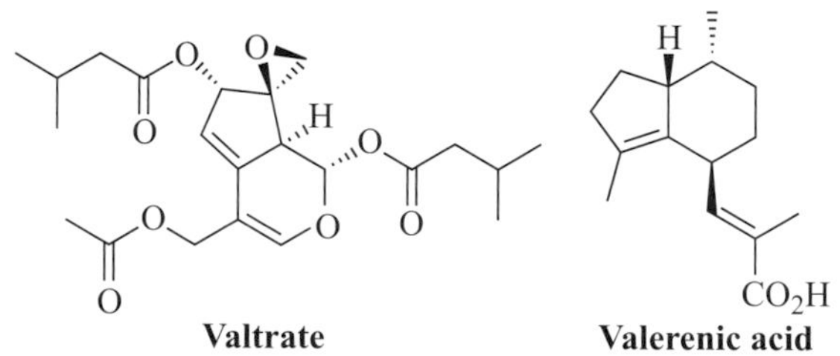

Valtrate   Valerenic acid

Fig. 17.1

However, as with synthetic hypnotics, these medicines are generally intended for short-term use.

HOPS, *HUMULUS LUPULUS* L. (HUMULI LUPULI STROBULI) EU✴

Humulus lupulus (Cannabaceae), often referred to by its common name of hops, has been used traditionally for insomnia, neuralgia and excitability. It is cultivated in several European countries, including England, France and Germany. The part of the plant used pharmaceutically is the female flower heads (known as 'strobiles'). These are composed of overlapping bracts, which enclose the ovary. Hops have a characteristic odour.

Constituents

The main active constituents of hops are the bitter principles found in the oleo-resin. These include the α-acid humulone and the β-acid lupulone, and their degradation products, such as 2-methyl-3-buten-2-ol (Fig. 17.2). Other constituents include flavonoids, chalcones, tannins and volatile oils.

Therapeutic uses and available evidence

Modern pharmaceutical uses of hops include sleep disturbances and restlessness. Sedative and hypnotic activities have been documented *in vivo* (mice) for extract of hops, and for the bitter acid degradation product 2-methyl-3-buten-2-ol. Clinical studies provide some evidence of the hypnotic effects of hops given in combination with the herbal sedative,

2-Methyl-3-buten-2-ol

Fig. 17.2

hypnotic valerian (Zanoli and Zavatti 2008). Antibacterial and antifungal activities have been documented in vitro for certain constituents of hops. Hops are non-toxic, as their use in beer would suggest. Cheers!

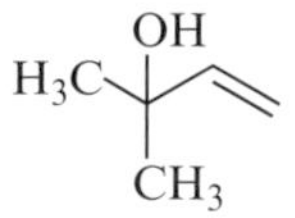

LEMON BALM, *MELISSA OFFICINALIS* L. (MELISSAE FOLIUM) EU✴

Melissa officinalis L. (syn. 'balm' and 'sweet balm', Lamiaceae) has been used traditionally for its sedative effects, as well as for gastrointestinal disorders. The dried leaves are the parts used pharmaceutically. The herb is described in Chapter 17.

Constituents

The volatile oil of melissa contains numerous constituents, mainly monoterpenes, particularly aldehydes (e.g. as citronellal, geranial and neral) and sesquiterpenes (e.g. β-caryophyllene). Flavonoids, including quercetin, apigenin and kaempferol, and polyphenols (e.g. hydroxycinnamic acid derivatives) are also present in the herb. Melissa is listed in the Eur. Ph, which states that the drug contains not less than 4.0% of total hydroxycinnamic derivatives, expressed as rosmarinic acid, calculated with reference to the dried drug.

Therapeutic uses and available evidence

Sedative and antispasmodic effects have been documented for melissa extracts using *in vivo* studies (mice, rats). It is used for nervous or sleeping disorders and functional gastrointestinal complaints. There has been no clinical investigation of the sedative effects of melissa alone in individuals with sleeping disorders. However, clinical trials have explored the effects of melissa in combination with other herbal sedatives (e. g. valerian and hops) and provide some evidence to support the sedative and hypnotic effects of such preparations. Antihormonal effects of balm, mainly antithyroid, have been documented and, recently, cholinergic activity has been found for extracts using human cerebral cortical cell membrane homogenates. Dried lemon balm is usually taken internally in the form of a herbal tea, at a dose of 2–4 g three times a day. Melissa extracts are also applied topically in cases of *Herpes simplex labialis* resulting from HSV-1 infection (see anti-infectives). Lemon balm is regarded as non-toxic, although it should not be used to excess because of the reputed antithyroid activity. For review, see Ulbricht et al 2005.

KAVA, *PIPER METHYSTICUM* FORST. (PIPERIS METHYSTICI RHIZOME)

Piper methysticum (Piperaceae), also known as kava-kava or kawa, has been used in the Pacific Islands, notably Fiji, for hundreds of years. It is a small shrub with heart-shaped leaves and thick, woody roots and rhizomes, which are ground or chewed to release the actives. These are then fermented to make the ceremonial drink Kava, which induces a relaxed sociable state, and is given to visiting dignitaries (including the Pope and the Queen of England). Kava is used medicinally for its tranquillizing properties and numerous other disparate complaints. Recent safety concerns have resulted in Kava products being withdrawn from sale at present (2011), but moves are being made to try to re-introduce it into the EU (Sarris et al 2011).

Constituents

The main components of kava are the kavalactones (also known as kavapyrones), including kavain, dihydrokavain, methysticin, yangonin and desmethoxyyangonin.

Therapeutic uses and available evidence

In vitro studies have previously provided some conflicting data on receptor interactions of kava extract and isolated kavalactones. Current thinking is that kavalactones potentiate $GABA_A$ receptor activity. Other receptor binding studies demonstrate no interaction with benzodiazepine receptors. The efficacy of kava extracts in relieving anxiety is supported by data from several randomized, placebo-controlled, clinical trials, for example an aqueous kava preparation produced significant anxiolytic and antidepressant activity and appeared equally effective in cases where anxiety is accompanied by depression (Sarris et al 2009). Overall, studies indicate reductions in anxiety after 4–12 weeks of treatment with kava extracts at dosages equivalent to 60–240 mg of kavalactones daily.

Kava extracts are generally well tolerated when used at recommended doses for limited periods. However, kava-induced liver injury has been demonstrated in several patients worldwide, and it has been suggested that this is due to inappropriate

quality of the kava raw material (Teschke et al 2011). There may also be a pharmacogenomic component to the toxicity (Sarris et al 2011) and assessment of the causal role of kava is complicated by other factors, including concomitant drugs linked with liver toxicity, and alcohol. There is circumstantial evidence for the roles of toxic metabolites, inhibition of cyclooxygenase (COX) enzymes and depletion of liver glutathione, and pharmacogenomic effects are likely, particularly for cytochrome P450 genes. Experimental and clinical cases of hepatotoxicity show evidence of hepatitis, but the question remains whether this inflammation is caused by components of kava directly, or is due to downstream effects (Zhang et al 2011). A recent study in hepatocytes has shown that kavain has minimal cytotoxicity and methysticin moderate concentration-dependent toxicity, whereas yangonin displayed marked toxicity (Tang et al 2011).

PASSION FLOWER, *PASSIFLORA INCARNATA* L. (PASSIFLORAE HERBA) EU✦

Passion flower (*Passiflora incarnata* L., Passifloraceae) is also known by the common names passion vine, maypop and others. The plant is a climbing vine, native to South America, but now also grown widely including in the USA and India. The dried leafy aerial parts, which normally include the flowers and fruits, are used pharmaceutically. The flower shows a distinctive shape of a cross, and gives the name passion (which refers to Christian connotations rather than romantic). There are numerous curling tendrils and the leaves are three-lobed. The active constituents have not yet been clearly established. The edible passion fruit is from *P. edulis*.

Constituents

The active constituents are not known, but the flavonoids are thought to be important, particularly chrysin and related compounds. These include schaftoside, isoschaftoside, orientin, homoorientin, vitexin, isovitexin, kaempferol, luteolin, quercetin, rutin, saponaretin and saponarin. Alkaloids of the harman type are present in low amounts (the presence of harmine, harmaline, harmol and harmalol has been disputed) as well as β-carbolines. *P. edulis* contains similar types of compounds and cycloartane triterpenoids such as the cyclopassifloic acids and cyclopassiflosides. Passion flower is included in the Eur. Ph. The drug should contain not less than 1.5% of total flavonoids, expressed as vitexin, assayed by a colorimetric method.

Therapeutic uses and available evidence

The historical medicinal uses of passion flower include treatment of insomnia, hysteria, nervous tachycardia and neuralgia. Modern pharmaceutical uses include nervous restlessness and insomnia due to nervous tension, and, specifically based on the THMPD, for the temporary relief of symptoms associated with stress and of mild anxiety.

Animal studies (mice, rats) have documented CNS-sedative effects or reductions in motility for aqueous ethanolic extracts of passion flower and for the constituents maltol and ethylmaltol. Anxiolytic activity has been reported in mice (Sampath et al 2010) and modulation of the GABA system is known to be involved (Appel et al 2010, Elsas et al 2010). Sedative effects are attributed at least in part to the flavonoid, particularly chrysin, content. There are few clinical studies of passiflora; however, a preliminary double-blind randomized trial using 36 patients with generalized anxiety showed the extract to be as effective as oxazepam, but with a lower incidence of impairment of job performance. It has been advocated as an adjunctive therapy for opiate withdrawal symptoms (for review, Miyasaka et al 2007). Generally, passiflora is well tolerated with few side effects; however, isolated reactions involving nausea and tachycardia in one case, and vasculitis in another, have been reported.

VALERIAN, *VALERIANA OFFICINALIS* L. (VALERIANAE RADIX) EU⭐

Valeriana officinalis (Valerianaceae), commonly known as valerian, all-heal, and by many other vernacular (common) names, is among the most well documented of all medicinal plants, particularly in northern Europe. It is an herbaceous plant, reaching about 1 m in height, and is cultivated in many European countries, as well as in Japan and North America. Valerian has a long history of traditional use. Historically, it was used in the treatment of conditions involving nervous excitability, such as hysterical states and hypochondriasis, as well as in insomnia. The parts used pharmaceutically are the root, rhizomes and stolons, which are yellowish grey to pale greyish-brown. The rhizomes may be up to 50 mm long and 30 mm in diameter, whereas the roots may be around 100 mm long and 1–3 mm in diameter.

Valerian root has a characteristic smell, which is usually described as unpleasant.

Constituents

The main components of valerian are the volatile oil and the iridoid valepotriate constituents. The volatile oil contains monoterpenes and sesquiterpenes, such as β-bisabolene, caryophyllene, valeranone, valerianol, valerenol, valerenal, valerenic acid and derivatives (Fig. 17.1). The valepotriate compounds include valtrate, didrovaltrate and isovaltrate. The valepotriates readily decompose on storage and processing to form mainly baldrinal and homobaldrinal, which are also unstable. Valerian also contains alkaloids, including valerianine and valerine, and amino acids such as arginine, γ-aminobutyric acid (GABA), glutamine and tyrosine.

Valerian root is listed in the Eur. Ph., which requires that it contains not less than 5 ml/kg volatile oil for the whole drug, and not less than 3 ml/kg for the cut drug, calculated with reference to the dried drug. It should also contain not less than 0.17% of sesquiterpenic acids, expressed as valerenic acid.

Therapeutic uses and available evidence

In Europe valerian and its various preparations (tablets, tinctures) have been approved for the temporary relief of symptoms of mild anxiety and to aid sleep, and are generally based on traditional use. The sedative effects of valerian root are well documented. *In vivo* studies (in mice) have demonstrated CNS-depressant activity for the volatile oil, the valepotriates and the valepotriate degradation products. The sedative effects of valerian root are thought to be due to the activities of these different components, particularly valerenal and valerenic acid (constituents of the volatile oil), and the valepotriate compounds. Therefore, the profile of these constituents, and their concentrations, in a specific valerian preparation will determine its activity. Biochemical studies have indicated that certain components of valerian, particularly valerenic acid, may lead to increased concentrations of the inhibitory neurotransmitter GABA in the brain by inhibiting its catabolism, inhibiting uptake and/or by inducing GABA release. Increased GABA concentrations are associated with decreased CNS activity, which may, at least partly, explain valerian's sedative activity. It is not clear whether valerian root extracts have effects on the binding of benzodiazepines to receptors. Modern medicinal uses for valerian root preparations are for insomnia, stress and anxiety. Clinical trials have tested the effects of valerian preparations on subjective (e.g. sleep quality) and objective (e.g. sleep structure) sleep parameters, and on measures of stress. Some, but not all, of these studies provide evidence to support the traditional uses of valerian. Several preparations contain valerian root in combination with other herbs reputed to have hypnotic and/ or sedative effects, such as hops (*Humulus lupulus*) and melissa (*Melissa officinalis*) (see Salter and Brownie 2010 for review). It is recommended that valerian preparations should not be taken for up to 2 hours before driving a car or operating machinery; also, the effect of valerian preparations may be enhanced by alcohol consumption. There are isolated reports of hepatotoxicity associated with valerian-containing products, although causality has not been established.

ANTIDEPRESSANTS

ST JOHN'S WORT, *HYPERICUM PERFORATUM* L. (HYPERICI HERBA) EU⁺

St John's wort (Hypericaceae) has a history of medicinal use, particularly as a 'nerve tonic' and in the treatment of nervous disorders. It is commonly used to treat mild and moderate forms of depression and is registered in the UK for the treatment of 'slightly low mood and mild anxiety'.

It is an herbaceous perennial plant native to Europe and Asia. The name St John's wort may have arisen as the flowers bloom in late June around St John's day (24 June). Herbal products containing St John's wort have been among the top-selling herbal preparations in developed countries in recent years. The dried herb (consisting mainly of the flowering tops, including leaves, unopened buds and flowers) is the part used pharmaceutically.

Constituents

St John's wort contains a series of naphthodianthrones, which include hypericin and pseudohypericin, and the prenylated phloroglucinols, such as hyperforin and adhyperforin. Initially, hypericin was considered to be the antidepressant constituent of St John's wort, although evidence has now emerged that hyperforin (Fig. 17.3) is also a major constituent required for antidepressant activity. Further research is necessary to determine which other constituents contribute to the antidepressant effect. The Eur. Ph. states that the drug should contain not less than 0.08% of total hypericins, expressed as hypericin, calculated with reference to the dried drug. Most products containing standardized extracts of St John's wort are still standardized on hypericin content, as hyperforin is fairly unstable. St John's wort also contains other biologically active constituents, such as flavonoids. The leaves and flowers also contain an essential oil, of which the major components are β-caryophyllene, caryophyllene oxide spathulenol, tetradecanol, viridiflorol, α- and β-pinene, and α- and β-selinene.

Therapeutic uses and available evidence

The precise mechanism of action for the antidepressant effect of St John's wort is unclear. Results of biochemical and pharmacological studies have

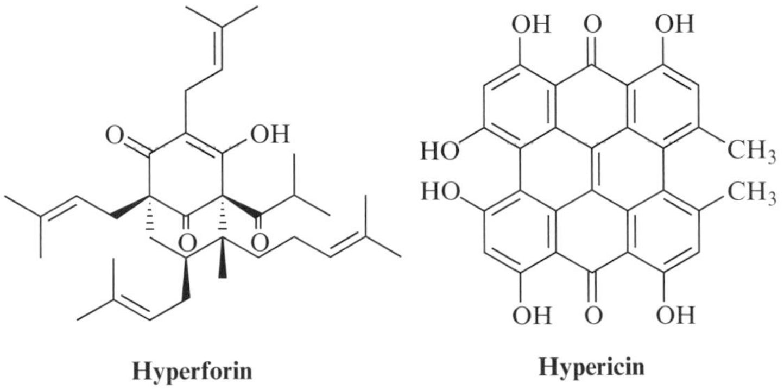

Hyperforin

Hypericin

Fig. 17.3

suggested that St John's wort extracts inhibit synaptosomal uptake of the neurotransmitters, serotonin (5-hydroxytryptamine, 5-HT), dopamine and noradrenaline (norepinephrine) and GABA. Studies involving small numbers of healthy male volunteers have indicated that St John's wort extracts may have dopaminergic activity and effects on cortisol, which may influence concentrations of certain neurotransmitters. Previous *in vitro* studies suggested that St John's wort inhibited monoamine oxidase, although other studies failed to confirm this. Experimental studies involving animal models of depression provide supporting evidence for the antidepressant effects of St John's wort. Evidence from randomized controlled trials indicates that preparations of St John's wort extracts are more effective than placebo, and possibly as effective as conventional antidepressants, in the treatment of mild to moderate depression (for overview, see Linde 2009, Nahrstedt and Butterweck 2010). Generally, a few weeks' treatment is required before marked improvement is seen. St John's wort is not recommended for the treatment of major depression.

Standardized extracts of St John's wort are generally well tolerated when used at recommended doses for up to 12 weeks. Adverse effects reported are usually mild, and include gastrointestinal symptoms, dizziness, confusion and tiredness and, rarely, photosensitivity (due to the hypericin content). However, clinical trials of St John's wort suggest a more favourable short-term safety profile than some conventional antidepressants. Concern has been raised over interactions between St John's wort preparations and certain prescribed medicines, including anticonvulsants, cyclosporin, digoxin, HIV protease inhibitors, oral contraceptives, selective serotonin reuptake inhibitors, theophylline, triptans and warfarin. Patients taking these medicines should stop taking St John's wort and seek medical advice (except in the case of oral contraceptives) as dose adjustment of the prescribed medicines concerned may be necessary. St John's wort should not be used during pregnancy and lactation.

STIMULANTS

CNS stimulants are now rarely employed therapeutically, with the exception of caffeine, although they were important in the treatment of barbiturate poisoning (e.g. picrotoxin) or as a tonic (strychnine). Cola nut extract is used in many herbal tonics and, of course, in the ubiquitous soft drink of the same name. Guarana is an ingredient of some 'energy' drinks and 'healthy' nutritional products. Both cola nut and guarana contain caffeine as the active constituent. Cocaine is more useful medicinally as a local anaesthetic, but its use as a recreational drug is an increasing problem throughout the world.

CAFFEINE EU✷

Caffeine is a methylxanthine derivative found in tea, coffee and cocoa (Fig. 17.4). It is a mild stimulant, and is added to many analgesic preparations to enhance activity, although there is no scientific basis for this practice. High doses may lead to insomnia and a feeling of anxiety, and can induce withdrawal syndrome in severe cases.

COLA NUT, *COLA* SPP. (COLAE SEMEN) EU✷

Cola, or kola nut [*Cola nitida* (Vent.) Schott et Endl., *Cola acuminata* (Beauv.) Schott et Endl., Sterculiaceae], is native to West Africa and extensively cultivated in the tropics, particularly Nigeria, Brazil and Indonesia. The seed is found in commerce as the dried, fleshy cotyledons, without the testa. They are red-brown in colour, convex on one side and flattened on the other, up to 5 cm long and about 2.5 cm in diameter. The cotyledons of C. *acuminata* are generally smaller and divided into 4 or 6 segments.

Cola contains the xanthine derivative caffeine (Fig. 17.4), with traces of theobromine and theophylline. Tannins and phenolics, including catechin, epicatechin, kolatin, kolatein, kolanin, and amines, including dimethylamine, methylamine, ethylamine and isopentylamine, are also present, together with thiamine and other B vitamins.

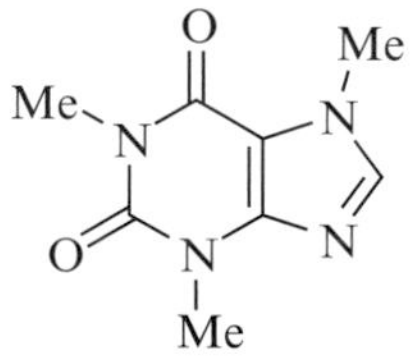

Caffeine

Fig. 17.4

Caffeine is a mild stimulant and has diuretic properties; cola extracts are also astringent and anti-diarrhoeal due to the tannin content. Cola extracts are an ingredient of many tonics for depression and tiredness, and to stimulate the appetite. Cola extract is safe, apart from any effects due to high doses of caffeine (see above).

GUARANA, *PAULLINIA CUPANA* KUNTH. EX H. B. K

Guarana (Sapindaceae) is a vine indigenous to the Amazonian rain forest. The seeds are ground to a paste and used in cereal bars, or extracted and made into a stimulant drink. The effects are similar to those of cola (see above).The main active constituent is caffeine, which was formerly known as guaranine, and other methyl xanthines. It also contains tannins.

COCAINE EU⁂

Cocaine (Fig. 17.5) is a tropane alkaloid extracted from the leaf of coca [*Erythroxylum coca* Lam. and *E. novogranatense* (Morris) Hieron, Erythroxylaceae]. These are shrubs growing at high altitudes in the South-American Andes. The leaf is still chewed by the local people (along with lime to assist buccal absorption), in order to alleviate symptoms of altitude sickness and fatigue. Cocaine is rarely used medicinally, except as a local anaesthetic in eye surgery, but is now a major illicit drug responsible for many health problems and associated crime. The supply and use of cocaine is strictly regulated in most countries.

ANALGESICS

Two types of analgesics are usually recognized: those that act via the CNS (the opioids) and will be discussed briefly here; the non-opiate and

Cocaine

Fig. 17.5

non-steroidal antiinflammatory drugs, which include aspirin, and which will be covered in Chapter 20. It is very common for the two types to be used in combination, for example aspirin with codeine. The opioid analgesics and their derivatives have never been surpassed as painkillers in efficacy or patient acceptability despite their disadvantages. They are obtained from the opium poppy (*Papaver somniferum*) and the most important are still the alkaloids morphine and codeine. Numerous derivatives such as oxycodone, dihydrocodeine, fentanyl, buprenorphine and etorphine have been developed which have different therapeutic and pharmacokinetic profiles, or can be administered via a different route (buccal tablets such as those containing buprenorphine, or transdermal patches, such as with fentanyl). The pharmacology of the opiates is covered in depth in many textbooks and these should be referred to for further information.

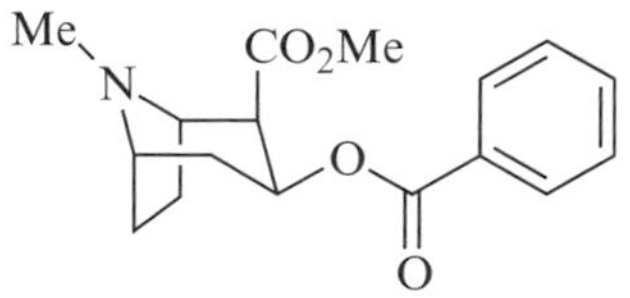

OPIUM, *PAPAVER SOMNIFERUM* L. (OPII CRUDUM; OPII PULVATUS NORMATUS) EU⁂

The opium poppy (*Papaver somniferum*, Papaveraceae) is an annual that is native to Asia, but is cultivated widely for food (the seed and seed oil), for medicinal purposes and as a garden ornamental. It has been used since time immemorial as a painkiller, sedative, cough suppressant and antidiarrhoeal, and features in ancient medical texts, myths and histories. The flowers vary in colour from white to reddish purple, but are usually pale lilac with a purple base spot. The capsules are subspherical, depressed at the top with the radiating stigma in the centre, below which are the valves through which the seeds are dispersed. The seeds are small, greyish and kidney-shaped. The latex, which exudes from the unripe capsule when scored, dries to form a blackish tarry resin, which is known as opium. For pharmaceutical use it can be treated to form 'prepared opium', but opium or the whole dried capsule (known as 'poppy straw') are now used commercially to extract the alkaloids. The supply and use of these products is strictly regulated in most countries. Poppy seeds are used in cooking.

Constituents

Alkaloids represent about 10% of the dried latex. The major alkaloid is morphine (Fig. 17.6), with codeine and thebaine and lesser amounts of very

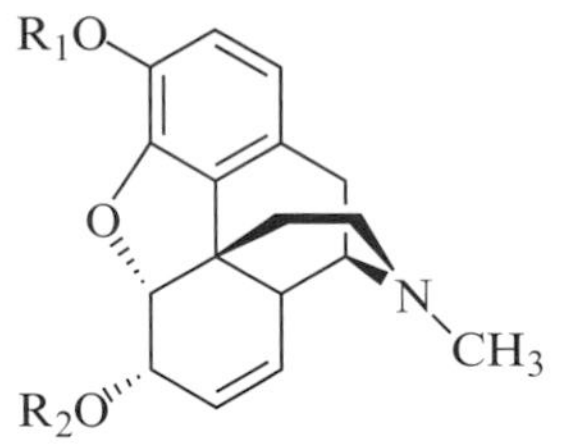

Morphine, $R_1 = R_2 = H$
Codeine, $R_1 = CH_3$, $R_2 = H$

Fig. 17.6

many others including narceine, narcotine, papaverine, salutaridine, oripavine and sanguinarine.

Therapeutic uses and available evidence

Opium has potent narcotic and analgesic properties. The total alkaloidal extract is known as 'papaveretum' and is used for pre-operative analgesia (now with the narcotine removed due to its reported genotoxicity). Morphine is a very potent analgesic, used for severe pain in the short term (e.g. kidney stone), or for terminal illness, and is the starting material for the production of diamorphine (heroin). Codeine is less potent than morphine, although it is a very useful analgesic for moderate to severe pain, in for example for migraine, dental and gynaecological pain. All the opioid analgesics have side effects, which include nausea, constipation and drowsiness; they cause respiratory depression and have a potential for dependence, which varies according to their capacity to induce euphoria. A withdrawal syndrome is common after illicit use (especially with heroin), but less of a problem with medical use.

MIGRAINE

The aetiology of migraine is not fully known and various drugs are used in its treatment. The analgesics mentioned above (particularly codeine) can be used to relieve an attack, although their capacity to induce nausea can cause problems, and aspirin can cause stomach discomfort. The newer synthetic drugs sumatriptan, naratriptan and others are highly effective in acute attacks, and β-blockers and pizotifen taken regularly are used to prevent recurrences. If all else fails, ergotamine can be used in limit doses for acute attacks. There is, however, one herb that has been investigated as a preventative, and this is feverfew.

ERGOTAMINE

Ergotamine is an alkaloid extracted from ergot (*Claviceps purpurea*), a parasitic fungus that grows on cereals, usually rye. It can be used to treat severe migraine that cannot be controlled with other drugs, but it can cause severe adverse reactions and there are restrictions as to the maximum daily and weekly doses. It is not suitable for children.

FEVERFEW, *TANACETUM PARTHENIUM* (L) SCHULTZ BIP. (TANACETI PARTHENII HERBA) EU

Feverfew [syn. *Chrysanthemum parthenium* (L.) Bernh., Asteraceae] is a perennial herb reaching 60 cm, with a downy erect stem. It has been a common garden plant for many centuries and was found in peasants' gardens throughout Europe. It is still a popular medicinal plant in many parts of the world, to treat rheumatism and menstrual problems. The aerial parts are used. The leaves are yellowish-green, alternate, stalked, ovate and pinnately divided with an entire or crenate margin. The flowers, which appear in June to August, are up to about 2 cm in diameter and arranged in corymbs of up to 30 heads, with white ray florets and yellow disc florets and downy involucral bracts.

Constituents

The sesquiterpene lactones are essential for the biological activity, the major one being parthenolide (Fig. 17.7), with numerous others reported from the species (e.g. santamarine). It also contains small amounts of essential oil (0.02–0.07%), with α-pinene and derivatives, camphor and others.

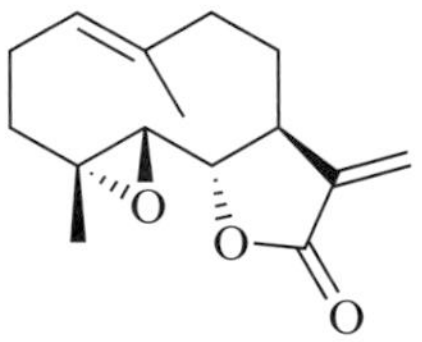

Parthenolide

Fig. 17.7

Therapeutic uses and available evidence

The main use of feverfew today is as a prophylactic and treatment for migraine. The fresh leaves may be eaten, usually with other foods to disguise the nauseous taste, or a standardized extract taken daily to prevent migraine attacks. Although some clinical studies have shown efficacy, others have not, and further work is needed to identify which extracts may be effective (Pittler and Ernst 2004).

Feverfew extracts inhibit secretion of serotonin from platelet granules and proteins from polymorphonuclear leukocytes (PMNs). Since serotonin is implicated in the aetiology of migraine and PMN secretion is increased in rheumatoid arthritis, these findings substantiate the use of feverfew in these conditions. Parthenolide is considered to be the main active constituent. It is a potent inhibitor of NF-kB. The sesquiterpene lactones as a class have an effect on a large number of other targets, including the inhibition of prostaglandin production and arachidonic acid release. This explains the antiplatelet and antifebrile actions to some extent, but in fact feverfew extract with the parthenolide removed also has antiinflammatory activity (Sur et al 2009). Feverfew may produce side effects such as dermatitis, and soreness or ulceration of the mouth. Also, contact dermatitis has been described, especially by workers handling material from this species, caused by the exposure to the allergenic sesquiterpene lactones.

DRUGS USED FOR COGNITIVE ENHANCEMENT AND IN DEMENTIA

There are few effective treatments for improving memory, especially in dementia. Acetylcholinesterase-inhibiting drugs are available to treat Alzheimer's disease with varying degrees of success. Rivastigmine is a reversible, non-competitive inhibitor of acetylcholinesterase. It is a semi-synthetic derivative of physostigmine, an alkaloid found in the Calabar bean (*Physostigma venenosum*), a highly poisonous plant indigenous to West Africa. Galantamine (= galanthamine), an alkaloid extracted from the snowdrop (*Galanthus nivalis*) was introduced around 2001 (Fig. 17.8, Heinrich and Teoh 2004). These drugs appear to slow down progression of the disease for a period of time, but do not cure it, and have side effects making them unacceptable to many patients.

GINKGO, *GINKGO BILOBA* L. (GINKGO FOLIUM) EU*

Ginkgo, the maidenhair tree (Ginkgoaceae), is an ancient 'fossil' tree indigenous to China and Japan and cultivated elsewhere. It is very hardy and is reputed to be the only species to have survived a nuclear explosion. The leaves are glabrous and bilobed, each lobe being triangular with fan-like, prominent, radiate veins. The leaves are used medicinally and the fruits are eaten.

Constituents

Ginkgo contains two major classes of actives, both of which contribute to the activity: ginkgolides A, B and C, and bilobalide, which are diterpene lactones; and the biflavone glycosides such as ginkgetin, isoginkgetin and bilobetin (Fig. 17.9). Ginkgolic acids are present in the fruit but normally only in very minor amounts in the leaf.

Therapeutic uses and available evidence

The most important use of ginkgo is to reduce or prevent memory deterioration, due to ageing and milder forms of dementia, including the early stages of Alzheimer's disease (e.g. Ihl et al 2010). It's enhancement of cognitive processes is thought to be by improving blood circulation to the brain and also due to its antiinflammatory and

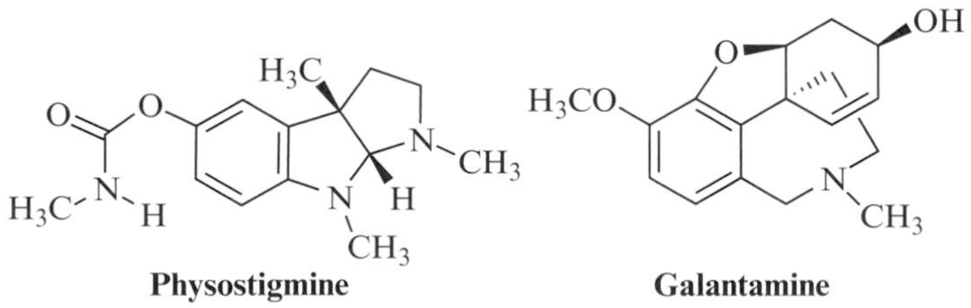

Physostigmine   **Galantamine**

Fig. 17.8

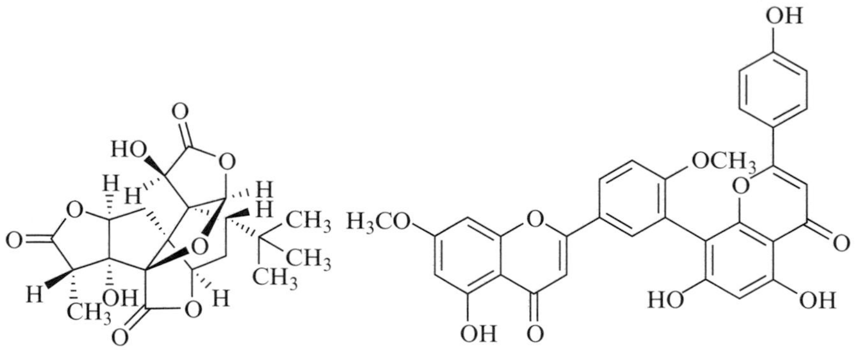

Fig. 17.9

antioxidant effects. Many clinical studies have been carried out (not all of high quality), and the extract has been shown to improve the mental performance in healthy volunteers and geriatric patients where this was impaired (for review, see Weinmann et al 2010). The effects on the CNS are not yet well defined, but include effects on neurotransmitter uptake, neurotransmitter receptor changes during ageing, cerebral ischaemia and neuronal injury.

Inhibition of nitric oxide may play a part. The usual dose of ginkgo (standardized) extracts is 120–240 mg daily. Ginkgo has been reported to cause dermatitis and gastrointestinal disturbances in large doses, although rarely. Allergic reactions in sensitive individuals are more likely to be due to ingestion of the fruits due to the ginkgolic acids, which are usually absent from leaf extracts and ginkgo products, or present only in very small amounts.

References

Appel, K., Rose, T., Fiebich, B., Kammler, T., Hoffmann, C., Weiss, G., 2010. Modulation of the γ-aminobutyric acid (GABA) system by *Passiflora incarnata* L. Phytother. Res. doi:10.1002/ptr.3352. [Epub ahead of print].

Elsas, S.M., Rossi, D.J., Raber, J., et al., 2010. *Passiflora incarnata* L. (Passionflower) extracts elicit GABA currents in hippocampal neurons in vitro, and show anxiogenic and anticonvulsant effects in vivo, varying with extraction method. Phytomedicine 17, 940–949.

Heinrich, M., Lee Teoh, H.L., 2004. Galanthamine from snowdrop – the development of a modern drug against Alzheimer's disease from local Caucasian knowledge. J. Ethnopharmacol. 92, 147–162.

Ihl, R., Bachinskaya, N., Korczyn, A.D., et al., 2010. Efficacy and safety of a once-daily formulation of *Ginkgo biloba* extract EGb 761 in dementia with neuropsychiatric features: a randomized controlled trial. Int. J. Geriatr. Psychiatry [Epub ahead of print 2010 Dec 7].

Linde, K., 2009. St. John's wort – an overview. Forsch. Komplementarmed. 16, 146–155.

Miyasaka, L.S., Atallah, A.N., Soares, B.G., 2007. Passiflora for anxiety disorder. Cochrane Database Syst. Rev. 24:CD004518.

Nahrstedt, A., Butterweck, V., 2010. Lessons learned from herbal medicinal products: the example of St. John's Wort (perpendicular). J. Nat. Prod. 73, 1015–1021.

Pittler, M.H., Ernst, E., 2004. Feverfew for preventing migraine. Cochrane Database Syst. Rev. 1: CD002286.

Salter, S., Brownie, S., 2010. Treating primary insomnia - the efficacy of valerian and hops. Aust. Fam. Physician 39, 433–437.

Sampath, C., Holbik, M., Krenn, L., Butterweck, V., 2010. Anxiolytic effects of fractions obtained from *Passiflora incarnata* L. in the elevated plus maze in mice. Phytother. Res. doi:10.1002/ptr.3332. [Epub ahead of print 2010 Nov 12].

Sarris, J., Kavanagh, D.J., Byrne, G., Bone, K.M., Adams, J., Deed, G., 2009. The Kava Anxiety Depression Spectrum Study (KADSS): a randomized, placebo-controlled crossover trial using an aqueous extract of *Piper methysticum*. Psychopharmacology (Berl) 205, 399–407.

Sarris, J., Teschke, R., Stough, C., Scholey, A., Schweitzer, I., 2011. Re-introduction of Kava *(Piper methysticum)* to the EU: is there a way forward? Planta Med. 77, 107–710.

Sur, R., Martin, K., Liebel, F., Lyte, P., Shapiro, S., Southall, M., 2009.

Anti-inflammatory activity of parthenolide-depleted Feverfew *(Tanacetum parthenium)*. Inflammopharmacol 17, 42–49.

Tang, J., Tang, J., Dunlop, R.A., Rowe, A., Rodgers, K.J., Ramzan, I., 2011. Kavalactones Yangonin and Methysticin induce apoptosis in human hepatocytes (HepG2) in vitro. Phytother. Res. 25, 417–423.

Teschke, R., Sarris, J., Lebot, V., 2011. Kava hepatotoxicity solution: A six-point plan for new kava standardization. Phytomedicine 18, 96–103.

Ulbricht, C., Brendler, T., Gruenwald, J., et al., 2005. Lemon balm *(Melissa officinalis* L.): an evidence-based systematic review by the Natural Standard Research Collaboration. J. Herb. Pharmacotherapy 5, 71–114.

Weinmann, S., Roll, S., Schwarzbach, C., Vauth, C., Willich, S.N., 2010. Effects of *Ginkgo biloba* in dementia: systematic review and meta-analysis. BMC Geriatr. 10, 14.

Zanoli, P., Zavatti, M., 2008. Pharmacognostic and pharmacological profile of *Humulus lupulus* L. J. Ethnopharmacol. 116, 383–396.

Zhang, L.Y., Rowe, A., Ramzan, I., 2011. Does inflammation play a role in kava hepatotoxicity? Phytother. Res. 25, 629–630 doi:10.1002/ptr.3301 [Epub ahead of print 2010 Sep 14].

Chapter 18

Infectious diseases

Plants have been a central part of traditional medicines to cure topical and systemic infections caused by microbes, in particular bacteria. These preparations form the basis of many wound-healing materials in the developing world where the plant is prepared as a crude drug or an extract that is applied topically to improve the healing of a wound. These preparations may have antimicrobial properties and remove the microbes by an antiseptic mechanism and/or they may promote the ability of the wound to repair itself by stimulating cellular growth. Numerous natural products produced by plants also have antiprotozoal and insecticidal activity. Many, especially those containing essential oils, are active against all of these. Intestinal worms can be treated with herbal materials such as wormseed and wormwood (*Artemisia* spp.), but the most effective and least toxic anthelmintic drugs at present are synthetic, so will not be covered here.

There are many reasons why plants are a valuable source of antimicrobial natural products and the most fundamental reason is that they contain intrinsically antimicrobial compounds such as **carvacrol** (Fig. 18.1 and see Chapters 6 and 7) from Thyme (*Thymus vulgaris*, Lamiaceae) which is a monoterpene and is present in the essential oil of this species.

This phenolic monoterpene has a range of antibacterial and antifungal properties (Baser 2008) and may be produced by the plant to protect itself from attack from plant pathogenic microbes and insects that are present in its environment. This is an example of an **intrinsic** or **latent antimicrobial** natural product that the plant produces as a normal part of its chemistry which can be used medicinally. Plants also have the ability to produce antimicrobial

natural products when they are under attack from microbes, herbivores and insects. These compounds are very quickly synthesized by the plant and are called **phytoalexins** which display antimicrobial properties to a wide range of bacteria and fungi. Examples of this phenomenon include the potato, which when inoculated with a fungus synthesizes the antimicrobial coumarin **scopoletin** (Fig. 18.2 and Chapter 6) and the bisbenzyl compound (**3,5-dihydroxy-bisbenzyl**) also depicted in Fig. 18.2, which is produced by a species of yam (*Dioscorea rotundata*, Dioscoreaceae).

This bisbenzyl is very strongly active against a range of Gram-positive and Gram-negative bacteria including *Staphylococcus aureus*, *Bacillus cereus*, *Pseudomonas aeruginosa* and *Escherichia coli* with minimum inhibitory concentrations of 10 mg/L (Fagboun et al 1987). This is astounding activity, particularly against Gram-negative bacteria such as *E. coli* and *P. aeruginosa* which are often impervious to plant antimicrobials.

Plants are also used extensively as topical antimicrobials in many societies and there is an enormous body of primary literature in journals that specialize in ethnomedical research such as the *Journal of Ethnopharmacology*. In the North-Eastern part of Australia the indigenous peoples use the aerial parts of *Eremophila duttonii* (Myoporaceae) as a topical antibacterial preparation (Smith et al 2007) and the active constituent has been isolated and characterized as an unusual serrulatane diterpene (Fig. 18.3).

This compound had activity against *S. aureus* and *S. epidermidis*, both of which are commensal bacteria, common skin organisms and major causative agents in wound infections. It was also active towards the

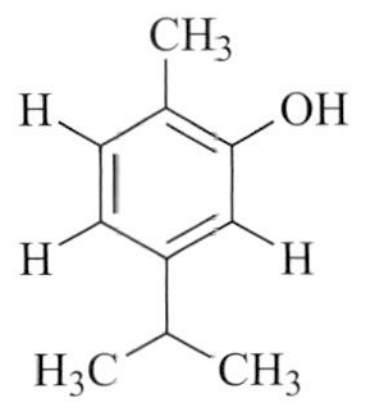

Carvacrol

Fig. 18.1

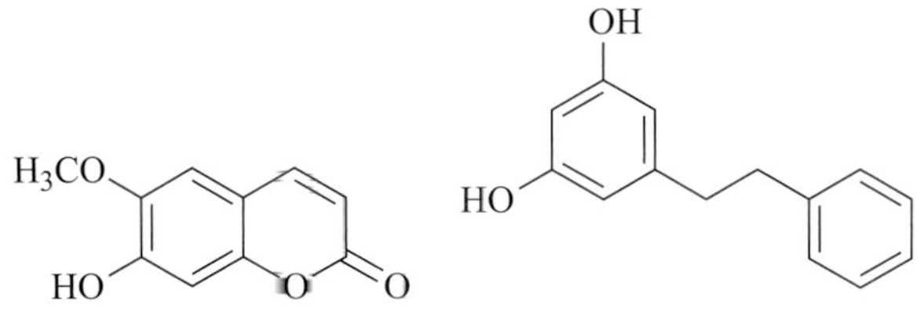

Scopoletin   **3,5-dihydroxy-bisbenzyl from**
                  Dioscorea rotundata

Fig. 18.2

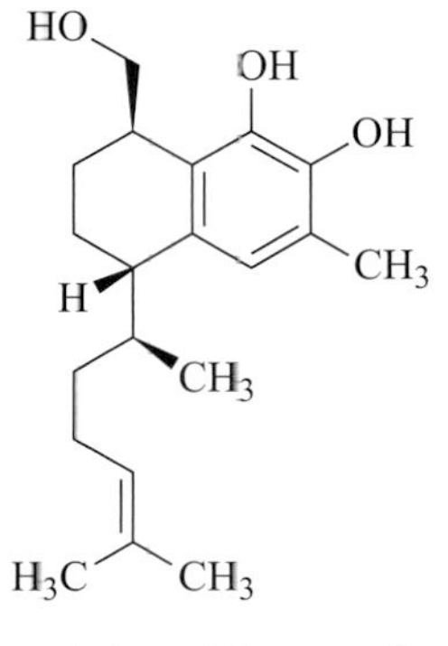

Serrulatane diterpene from
Eremophila duttonii

Fig. 18.3

respiratory pathogen *Streptococcus pneumonia*, one of the main causative agents of pneumonia in adults and children.

Probably the most important reasons that plants produce antibacterial natural products, and why they could be a valuable resource of antimicrobial materials, is that these chemicals are often exceptionally diverse, have stereochemical centres and have extensive functional group chemistry. These factors mean that the compounds will have very distinct shapes, developed by nature over millions of years to bind to protein and DNA targets, and *consequently having*

an inherent biological activity. The readers are urged to consult a new and very important review on natural products highlighting this topic written by Professor Giovanni Appendino and colleagues (Appendino et al 2010). Plant antibacterials are very different in shape and chemistry to existing antibacterial chemotypes (Gibbons 2004, 2008), that are often microbially derived such as erythromycin (Fig. 6.11, Chapter 6) and tetracycline (Fig. 6.8, Chapter 6). This may mean that plant-derived antibacterials could function through a different and as yet undetermined mechanism of action. This would make them valuable where bacterial resistance to conventional antibiotics (beta-lactams, macrolides, tetracyclines) has arisen as these bacteria may be susceptible to these agents by working in a very different way. New agents that function by a different mechanism are currently needed, particularly in bacterial infections such as tuberculosis where the causative organism, *Mycobacterium tuberculosis* may possess multiple resistance to existing antibiotics of choice.

The last reason to look at plants as new antimicrobials is because there are already a number of products and preparations that are on the market. These range in type from food-based materials such as the practically ubiquitous Cranberry products marketed as fruit juices, which may also be used in the management of urinary tract infections, through to high-quality phytomedicines containing bearberry that are used for similar ailments.

We will look at some of the common herbs that are used as antimicrobial products and then cover some of the pure single chemical entities (SCEs) that display promising antimicrobial action.

BROAD-SPECTRUM ANTIMICROBIAL AGENTS

UMCKALOABO (PELARGONIUM), *PELARGONIUM SIDOIDES* DC AND *P. RENIFORME* CURT (PELARGONII RADIX)

Umckaloabo means 'useful for deep cough' in Zulu and this term refers to a medicine used traditionally in South Africa as a treatment for respiratory tract infections. This material is derived from the roots of either *Pelargonium sidoides* or *Pelargonium reniforme* from the Geraniaceae plant family. A decoction of the roots is used to treat chest infections and this material is the subject of a book by Charles Stevens ('Stevens Cure'), a 19th century army officer who contracted pulmonary tuberculosis in

London at the end of the 19th century. He was advised by his physician to move to South Africa where the air quality was much better than in Victorian London which was plagued by 'smog'. Whilst in South Africa he received the Umckaloabo preparation from a traditional healer and this cleared his TB infection. Stevens returned to the United Kingdom and marketed a preparation for TB known as Stevens Consumption Cure.

Constituents

The main active components are hydrolysable tannins, (+)-catechin, gallic acid and methyl gallate, including a unique series of O-galloyl-C-glucosyl-flavones. Flavonoids including myricetin and quercetin-3-O-beta-d-glucoside, coumarins including scopoletin, umckalin, 5,6,7-trimethoxycoumarin and 6,8-dihydroxy-5,7-dimethoxycoumarin, are present in both species. A series of benzopyranones has been isolated from P. sidiodes, and the pelargoniins (a type of ellagitannin) and a diterpene, reniformin, have been found in P. reniforme.

Therapeutic uses and available evidence

Extracts of Pelargonium species have been shown to inhibit the adherence of bacteria to cells of the mucous membrane and there is some published chemistry and biology on methoxylated coumarins (Fig. 18.4) from P. sidoides which have weak antibacterial activity (Kayser and Kolodziej 1997). They have also been shown to interfere with viral replication (Michaelis et al 2011) and to inhibit viral adherence to cells of mucous membrane and to loosen viscous mucus in the respiratory tract. It has also been postulated that these extracts have immuno-modulatory properties. There have been some small

clinical trials on efficacy in reducing the symptoms associated with tonsillitis and bronchitis, particularly amongst children (Matthys et al 2007). These materials are not, however, a replacement for antibiotics, but they may be used as a supplement to ameliorate the symptoms associated with inflammation of the upper respiratory tract (URT).

An ethanolic extract of Pelargonium sidoides is currently marketed by the phytopharmaceutical company Schwabe under the trade name Kaloba. This preparation is marketed to relieve the symptoms of common cold, sore throats and coughs based on long-standing use as a traditional remedy. A number of general practitioners recommend Kaloba as a preparation to reduce the symptoms of soreness associated with URT infections. This extract is also given to athletes to help strengthen the immune system, which can be compromised by extreme exercise, to protect against colds. A study in athletes submitted to intense physical activity found that Pelargonium sidoides increased the production of secretory immunoglobulin A in saliva, and decreased levels of both interleukin-15 and interleukin-6 in serum, suggesting a strong modulating influence on the immune response associated with the upper airway mucosa (Luna et al 2011).

There has also been a study on extracts demonstrating weak antibacterial activity which is due to the presence of the ubiquitous unsaturated fatty acids oleic and linoleic acid against fast-growing species of Mycobacterium; however these compounds are unlikely to be responsible for the 'anti-TB' activity of Steven's cure (Seidel and Taylor 2004).

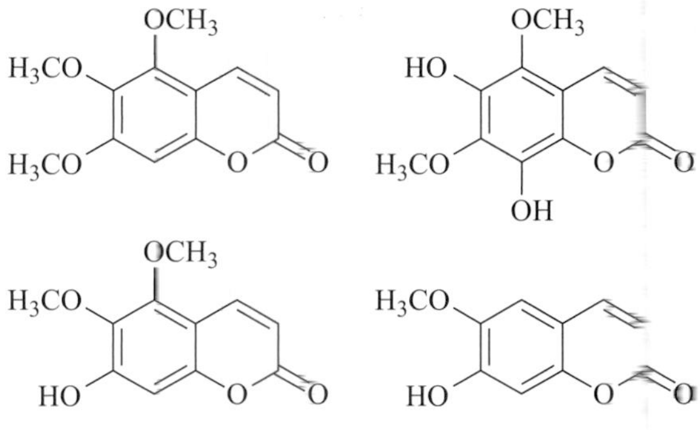

LEMON BALM, MELISSA OFFICINALIS L. (MELISSAE FOLIUM) EU

This plant is a member of the Lamiaceae plant family and has white flowers and the leaves have a highly pungent and aromatic smell being one of the most popular fragrances due to the essential oil of this species. Unfortunately, the plant produces very little essential oil and this accounts for the high cost of genuine lemon balm oil. This species contains phenolic compounds and the oil is rich in mono- and sesquiterpenes and the plant has long use as an antimicrobial and carminative and mild sedative.

There are a number of topical formulations which are marketed for Herpes simplex virus skin lesions and there are clinical data and some in vitro activity has been confirmed with the extracts of Melissa officinalis (Koytchev et al 1999). The herb is generally

Fig. 18.4

well-tolerated, although it has been suggested that long-term use may interfere with thyroid function.

Constituents

Both the polyphenolics and the essential oil are thought to be responsible for the antimicrobial effects. Phenolics include protocatechuic acid, caffeic acid, rosmarinic acid and tannins, in significant amounts, together with flavonoids such as cynaroside, cosmosiin, isoquercitrin and others. The volatile oil consists mainly of α- and β-citral (= neral and geranial), with caryophyllene oxide, linalool, citronellal, nerol, geraniol, germacrene-D, traces of eugenyl acetate, *cis*- and *trans*-β-ocimene, copaene and others.

Therapeutic uses and available evidence

Lemon balm is antimicrobial, carminative and sedative. Hot water extracts have antiviral properties, mainly due to the polyphenolic acids. Topical formulations are used for *Herpes simplex* virus skin lesions, the antiviral activity having been confirmed *in vitro* and also by clinical trial. Aqueous extracts also inhibit division of tumour cells, and tannin-free extracts inhibit protein biosynthesis (for review, see Ulbricht et al 2005). The herb is used as an ingredient of herbal teas, often with other herbs, for nervous disorders and insomnia (see Chapter 17). Lemon balm is well tolerated, although it should not be taken internally in high doses over a long period because of its reputed antithyroid activity.

GARLIC, *ALLIUM SATIVUM* L. (ALLII SATIVI BULBUS) EU

Garlic, and other *Allium* spp. (Alliaceae), have a very long history as both a topical and systemic material to treat various infections. The literature is full of in vitro studies showing efficacy of the extracts and oils of the bulbs of various *Allium* species with activity against various bacteria, fungi and viruses. The family has a long and rich usage as culinary herbs with onions, garlic, shallots and chives all producing antimicrobial sulphur containing natural products, typified by **allicin** and **ajoene** (Fig. 18.5).

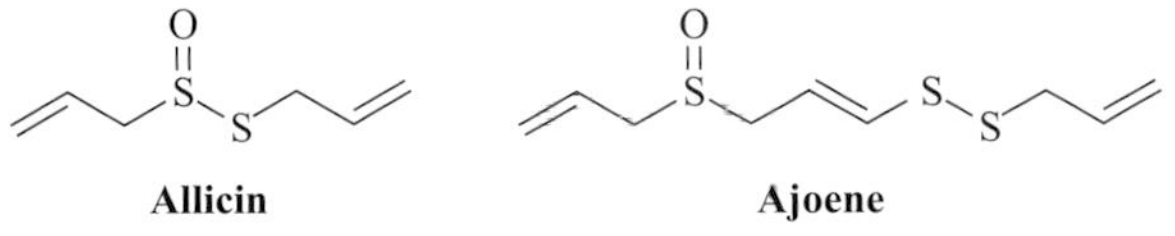

Allicin   **Ajoene**

Fig. 18.5

Garlic has been used clinically for the treatment of tuberculosis with some success in the United States in the 1940s and it has been referred to as Russian penicillin, as a result of its wide use in the former Soviet Union, again with some considerable success as an antibacterial (Bolton et al 1982). The widespread use of garlic has prompted recent investigation of other species which may harbour useful natural products and a number of interesting sulphur-containing antibacterials with very potent antibacterial activity have been isolated, such as the unusual pyridine-*N*-oxide natural products from *Allium stipitatum* (Fig. 18.6, O'Donnell et al 2009). These compounds displayed activity against slow- and fast-growing mycobacteria and a range of *Staphylococcus aureus* species some of which were methicillin-resistant and multidrug-resistant.

Compound 18.6 was also active against *Mycobacterium tuberculosis* with a minimum inhibitory concentration of 0.1 mg/L showing the potential of these natural products and garlic metabolites in general as anti-TB drug-leads.

Constituents

The antimicrobial constituents are the sulphur compounds, which include allicin, allylmethyl trisulphide, diallyl disulphide, diallyl trisulphide, diallyl tetrasulphide, allylpropyl disulphide, and glycosides such as sativoside B1. There are also monoterpenoids present (citral, geraniol, linalool and α- and β-phellandrene) and flavonoids based on kaempferol and quercetin. It is possible that the bulbs of these species, which are the subterranean part of the plant that is the key to reproduction, produce these sulphur natural products as a protection against microbes in their environment.

Therapeutic uses and available evidence

Garlic extracts have been shown to have antibiotic, expectorant and anti-thrombotic properties and many garlic preparations are marketed for their anti-blood clotting properties and to give some protection against atherosclerosis. Preparations from common garlic have also found much use in the treatment for respiratory tract infections, such as common cold, flu and bronchitis. The allyl sulphides, such as allicin and ajoene, are strongly antimicrobial having activity against *Staphylococcus aureus*, *Streptococcus* species and even some Gram-negative bacteria, such as *Helicobacter pylori*, the major bacterial causative agent of stomach ulcers (Harris et al 2001).

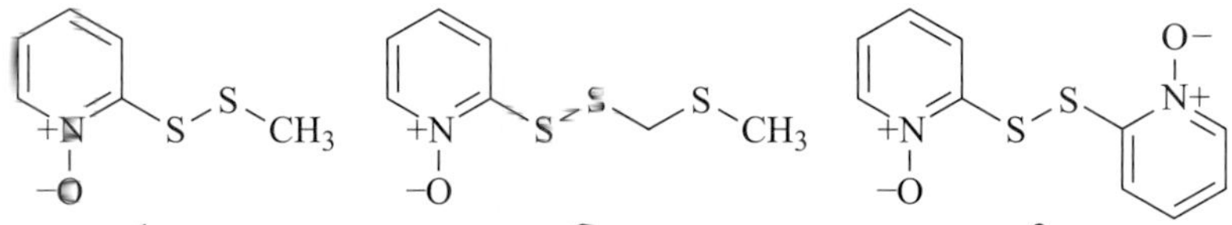

Fig. 18.6

Garlic preparations are generally very well tolerated with low toxicity (other than offensive smell!) although it has been suggested that these materials may have the ability to interfere with anti-platelet drugs.

TEA TREE AND TEA TREE OIL, *MELALEUCA ALTERNIFOLIA* (MAIDEN ET BETCHE.) CHEEL (*MELALEUCAE ATHEROLEUM*) EU

The oil from the leaves and stems of this tree has a long history of traditional usage amongst indigenous peoples of North Australia and New South Wales. This tree grows with other species of Myrtaceae, such as *Eucalyptus*, which are also used topically as an antimicrobial medicine. Over the last 20 years there has been an explosion of usage of tea tree oil products in Europe and the United States and one cannot go into a pharmacy without seeing dozens of preparations including soaps, shampoos, creams, lotions and gels containing this oil, which has a distinctive 'dry' aroma. The leaves and twigs undergo distillation to produce the oil which is pale yellow to colourless. Traditionally the oil is used topically as an antimicrobial for skin infections, to reduce bruising and for insect bites.

Constituents

Tea tree oil is a highly complex mixture of monoterpenes and the major component is terpinen-4-ol (Fig. 18.7), that may be present at concentrations as high as 30%.

Some varieties are rich in 1,8-cineole which is present in *Eucalyptus* oil but the best quality tea tree oils are low in 1,8-cineole and are high in terpinen-4-ol. Other monoterpenes present include γ- and α-terpineol, α- and β-pinene, α-terpineol, limonene and cymene, and the sesquiterpenes cubebol, epicubebol, cubenol, epicubanol and δ-cadinene. The composition of the oil may also depend on the method of distillation.

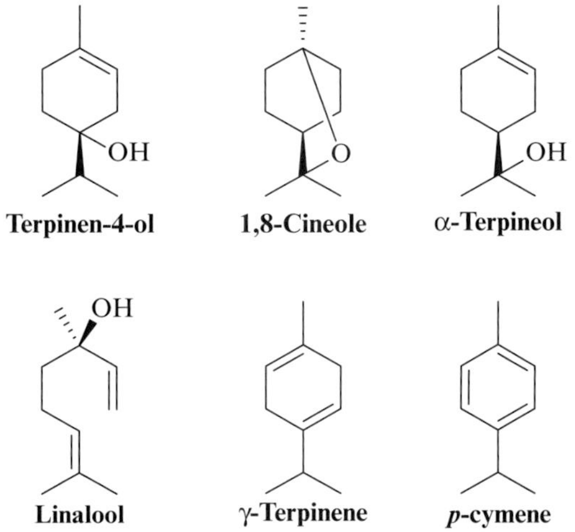

Fig. 18.7

Therapeutic uses and available evidence

Tea tree oil is now used worldwide in the form of skin creams for pimples and acne, pessaries for vaginal thrush, as an inhalation for respiratory disorders and in pastilles for sore throats. It is also popular as a lotion for the treatment of lice and scabies infestations, and for dandruff and other hair and scalp disorders. The oil has broad-spectrum antimicrobial activity against *Staphylococcus aureus*, *Escherichia coli* and various pathogenic fungi and yeasts including *Candida albicans*, and also against the protozoa *Leishmania major* and *Trypanosoma brucei*. There have also been studies conducted at using preparations containing the oil to reduce the spread of MRSA in hospital units (Warnke et al 2009) and there has been much research into the use of this oil as an antiseptic for nursing staff. The most active purified compounds from this oil include terpinen-4-ol, γ-terpinene, α-terpineol and linalool with minimum inhibitory concentrations in the range of 0.125–0.25% v/v (Carson and Riley 1995, Cox et al 2001, Raman et al 1995). These compounds also demonstrated broad-spectrum activity towards Gram-negative bacteria. It was also shown that the non-oxygenated monoterpenes such as γ-terpinene and *p*-cymene (Fig. X.7) reduced the efficacy of terpinen-4-ol by reducing its aqueous solubility (Cox et al 2001). Clinical trials have supported many of the uses of tea tree oil, including for *Herpes labialis*, although most of the studies are rather small (see Carson et al 2006). Undiluted essential oils can cause skin irritation and tea tree oil should be used with care. It should only be taken internally in small doses.

The related manuka tree (*Leptospermum scoparium* J. R. Forst. et G. Forst.) is sometimes referred to as 'New Zealand tea tree', and used for similar purposes.

BEARBERRY, *ARCTOSTAPHYLOS UVA-URSI* L. (UVAE URSI FOLIUM) EU

The leaves of the shrub *Arctostaphylos uva-ursi* (Ericaceae), widely known as Uva Ursi or bearberry, are used to treat cystitis and urethritis, although their use is not supported by evidence from randomized controlled trials.

Constituents

The main constituents are hydroquinone derivatives, notably the glycoside **arbutin**. This compound is hydrolysed in vivo by the enzyme β-glucosidase to give the diphenol, **hydroquinone** (Fig. 18.8). Other constituents include terpenoids such as α- and β-amyrin, flavonoids and tannins.

Therapeutic uses and available evidence

Hydroquinone is the main active component of this material and is a potent phenolic antiseptic. This compound is very active against many bacteria, but in particular those that are liable to cause urinary tract infections such as *Escherichia coli* and *Pseudomonas aeruginosa*. Activity has also been demonstrated against other species such as *Bacillus subtilis* and *Staphylococcus aureus*. Arbutin is hydrolysed by β-glucosidase to yield the active principle hydroquinone, which has antiseptic and astringent properties. Uva-ursi is also mildly diuretic and antilithuric (Beaux et al 1999). Uva ursi preparations

such as Arctuvan require that the urine is alkaline for it to have antiseptic properties and, as such, acidic foods including cranberry juice (see below) should be avoided during treatment. Hydroquinone is a very reactive and biologically active compound and is cytotoxic and mutagenic. High doses and prolonged usage of bearberry products should be avoided and it should not be used during pregnancy or by anyone who has a kidney infection.

CRANBERRY JUICE, *VACCINIUM MACROCARPON* AITON

This is one of the most popular of the plant-derived products with preparations generally being taken in the form of the juice of the berries of *V. macrocarpon* and related species (Ericaceae) or a freeze-dried extract which is then re-suspended in water. Medicinally the berries have been used to treat urinary tract infections and the species is an American plant used traditionally for this purpose. Marketed products include the highly popular Ocean Spray Cranberry Classic and many different fruit juice variants of this product.

Constituents

The chemistry of this plant is still not well understood because it contains many **flavonoid polymers**, in particular the **proanthocyanidins** that are believed to be important for the antibacterial activity of this species (Fig. 18.9).

These proanthocyanidins are exceptionally complex and vary in the number of flavonoid units in the polymer (n may vary considerably in Fig. 18.9), the way in which each of the units is connected and the functional groups present on each unit (R_1 and R_2 groups in the figure may be OH or OMe for example). This can give rise to a highly complex natural product mixture. These compounds are also polar and soluble in water, ethanol and methanol, which can make their analysis by conventional methods such as HPLC and HPLC-MS difficult.

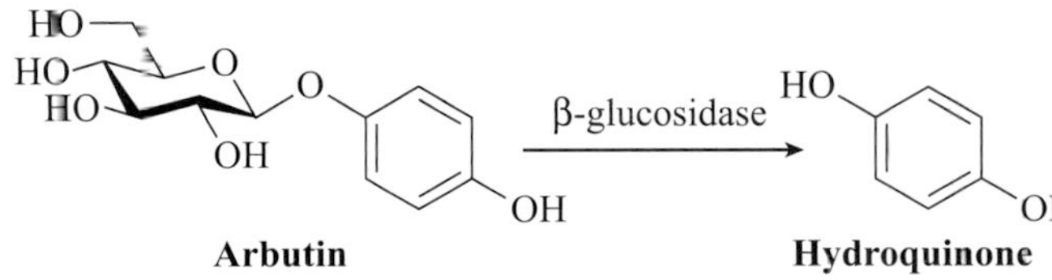

Arbutin   β-glucosidase →   **Hydroquinone**

Fig. 18.8

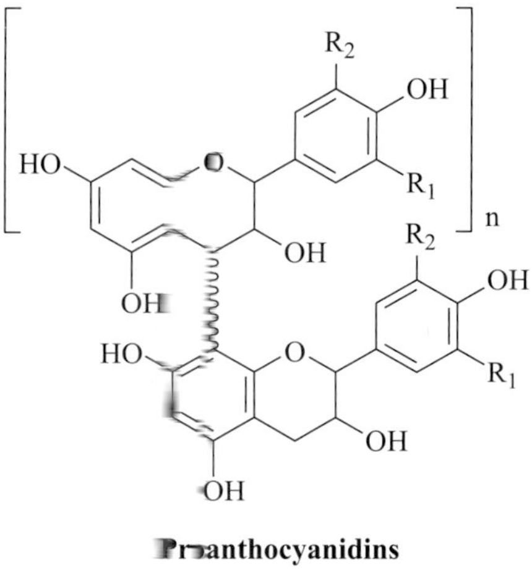

Proanthocyanidins

Fig. 18.9

Tetrahydrocannabinol   Cannabidiol

Fig. 18.10

Therapeutic uses and available evidence

In-vitro experiments with cranberry juice and proanthocyanidins have shown that they have the ability to affect the binding of the bacterium *Escherichia coli*, which is a major causative agent of urinary tract infections, to uroepithelial cells, therefore, inhibition adherence of this bacterium allowing its clearance. Cranberry juice is also thought to act by increasing levels of hippuric acid (a metabolite of benzoic acid) and therefore, acidity of the urine. Clinical studies of cranberry juice have provided equivocal evidence for prevention or treatment of UTIs and the efficacy remains unproven (see Jepson and Craig 2008). Cranberry juice has a high calorific content, and patients with diabetes who wish to use cranberry juice should use sugar-free preparations. Reports that cranberry juice interacts with warfarin are controversial, and are now considered to be unproven (Zikia et al 2010). Cranberries have also been used for unrelated disorders such as kidney stones, and are frequently used in foods.

SINGLE CHEMICAL ENTITY (SCE) AND NOVEL PLANT ANTIBACTERIALS

So far we have looked at herbal products and their extracts as antibacterials, but there is a growing body of literature describing the activities associated with single compounds isolated in bioassay-guided fractionation studies on plants (Gibbons 2004, 2008). These plants may result from random screening,

from a traditional antibacterial use of the plant or the plant material may have been treated prior to the study to elicit phytoalexins.

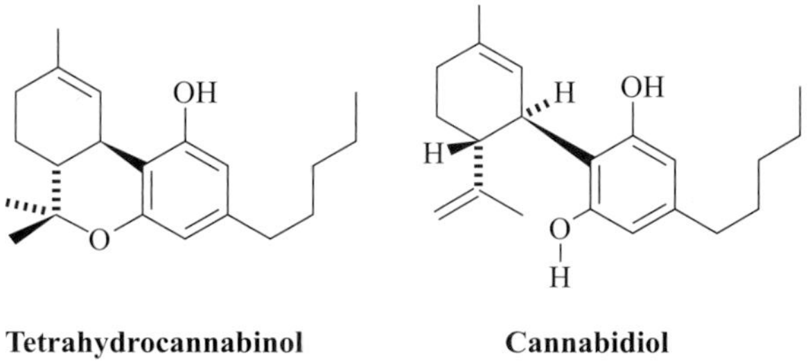

Cannabis sativa has a long history of use as a medicinal material having not only euphoriant, but also antiseptic properties. In Afghanistan there is anecdotal usage of cannabis resin to treat plague and as a topical antimicrobial preparation. There is in vitro evidence to support the antibacterial properties of cannabis as the major components, **tetrahydrocannabinol** and **cannabidiol** (Fig. 18.10) are highly active against Gram-positive bacteria such as *Staphylococcus aureus* and its methicillin-resistant (MRSA) variants (Appendino et al. 2008).

Cannabidiol has the added advantage of also displaying anti-inflammatory activity and this would certainly be advantageous as a wound healing/cleansing preparation. Given the recent marketing authorization in the UK and Canada for Sativex, a licensed cannabis-based medicine used to ameliorate the pain and spasticity associated with multiple sclerosis (MS), there is real opportunity to develop new cannabis-based antibacterials.

There has also been some work on the acylphloroglucinol group of natural products and one of the first members of this class to be elucidated was hyperforin (Fig. 18.11), from St John's wort. This metabolite was studied due to its excellent activity against penicillin- and methicillin-resistant *Staphylococcus aureus* strains with MIC values being 0.1–1 mg/l (Schempp et al 1999).

The acylphloroglucinols are relatively complex natural products based on a cyclic aromatic-derived core with many prenyl groups, which may be either cyclized or oxidized to give a highly functional group rich and chiral class of products such as hyperforin. Other examples from this group include the drummondins (Fig. 18.11) from another species of *Hypericum*, *H. drummondii*, which had potent activity (MIC = 0.39 mg/l, Jayasuriya et al 1991).

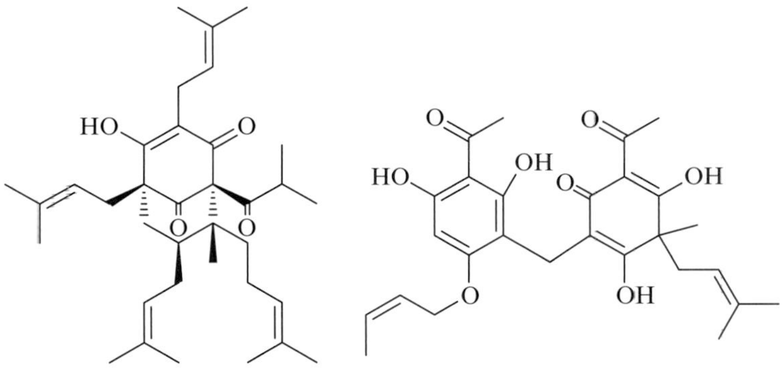

Hyperforin   **Drummondin E**

Fig. 18.11

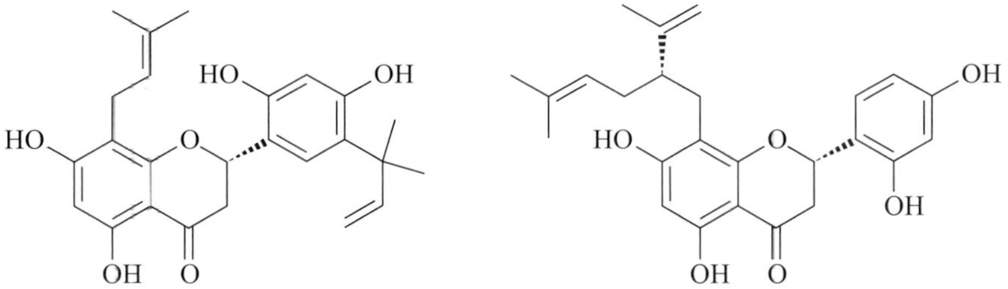

1   **2 Sophoraflavone G**

Fig. 18.12

The flavonoids are probably the most intensively studied natural products in terms of their antimicrobial activity and the flavanones, for example compound **1** (Fig. 18.12), within this class have some very interesting levels of potency and action. Many of these natural products possess prenyl or geranyl groups that presumably contribute to the lipophilicity and membrane solubility of these compounds. This could improve their cellular uptake and enhance their ability to penetrate the bacterial cell.

Compound **1** has excellent potency toward MRSA strains with MIC values of 1.5 mg/l and compound **2** is sophoraflavanone G, which is antibacterial in its own right (MIC = 3.1 mg/l) and also has strong synergism in combination with the glycopeptide antibiotic vancomycin, which is used clinically to treat MRSA infections (Sakagami et al 1998). A combination of sophoraflavanone G with vancomycin could feasibly contribute to better treatment of an MRSA infection and it is conceivable that these lipophilic compounds could be formulated into a topical antiseptic preparation to help with decolonization.

Plants within the Apiaceae family, which includes carrot, coriander, parsnip, caraway and dill, are known to produce polyacetylenic natural products. These compounds have conjugated triple bonds (acetylenes). Some of these metabolites are deadly poisonous, such as **cicutoxin** from Cowbane (*Cicuta virosa*), whereas others such as **falcarindiol** (Fig. 18.13) are present in the roots of these plants and are probably synthesized as a protection against microbes in their environment.

Falcarindiol has a similar shape to **phomallenic acid B**, a fungal-derived antibacterial natural product which has been shown to be an inhibitor of fatty acid synthase-2 (FAS-II) and it is possible that falcarindiol functions in a similar fashion. Falcarindiol is present in many Chinese medicinal plants, and one of these, *Angelica dahurica*, is used to treat acne and this metabolite may in part be responsible for this action as the main bacterial causative agents of acne are the staphylococci and *Propionibacterium acnes*.

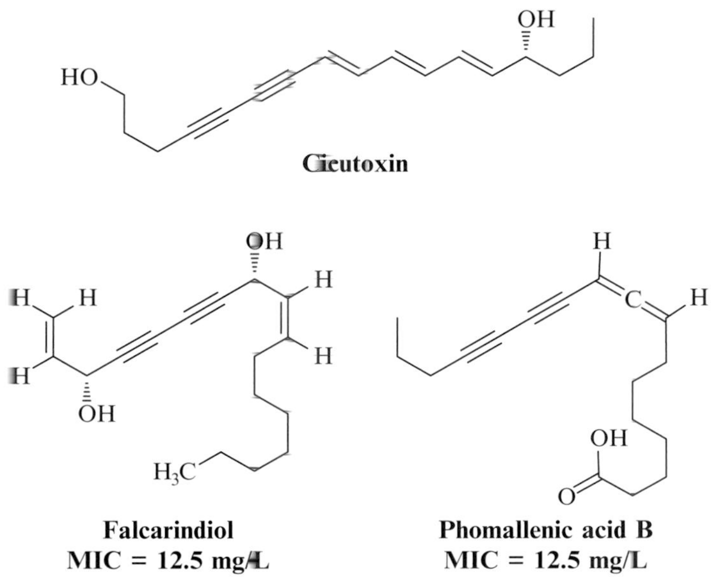

Cicutoxin

Falcarindiol
MIC = 12.5 mg/L

Phomallenic acid B
MIC = 12.5 mg/L

Fig. 18.13

We have already seen that some natural products such as sophoraflavanone G have the ability to potentiate the action of existing antibacterial agents. Bacteria have the ability to remove antibiotics from their cells by a process known as efflux that can make the antibiotic inactive against that strain. Such effluxing strains have proteins on their cell membranes which transport the antibiotics out of the bacterial cell. Some natural products (Fig. 18.14) have been found to inhibit these proteins and stop them from removing the antibiotic and such an action has the potential to restore antibiotic activity.

Plant natural products with the ability to inhibit these processes include tea catechins such as epicatechin gallate, simple diterpenes like totarol, alkaloids such as reserpine and even complex resin oligosaccharides (Fig. 18.14) (Stavri et al 2007).

There is great potential to discover new antimicrobial substances from plants and the chemistry presented by plant sources is very often highly functional and chiral, and these facets are desirable in a drug-lead candidate, assuming supply issues can be overcome. Studies on plant antibacterials require greater depth, particularly with respect to mammalian cytotoxicity (selectivity between microbial and mammalian toxicity) and mechanism of action. Once these issues have been addressed, it is highly likely that plant sources will generate new antimicrobial chemotypes.

ANTIPROTOZOAL AGENTS

The classical antiprotozoal drug, used to treat malaria, is quinine, from *Cinchona* bark. It is still occasionally used to treat the disease, but more importantly it is the template for the production of newer semi-synthetics such as chloroquine and mefloquine, and others now under development. Most of these are also used for malaria prophylaxis. The most recent antimalarial to be introduced clinically is artemisinin (from sweet or annual wormwood, *Artemisia annua*) or the more stable derivative, artemether. Lapacho (taheebo) contains quinones, which are antiprotozoal, although it is often used in South America as an anticancer treatment. Ebony wood (from *Diospyros* spp.) contains naphthoquinones which are used in a similar way by local peoples. Emetine, an alkaloid from *Cephaelis ipecacuanha*, is amoebicidal, but too toxic for clinical use; however, investigations continue into the effect of similar, semi-synthetic compounds for further development. Most of the important protozoal diseases are endemic in the tropics (e.g. bacillary dysentery), and many (e.g. *Leishmania*) involve a non-human vector, which may be an insect, larva or snail. Control of these diseases, therefore, includes the use of pesticides to destroy the vector, improvement in hygiene and water supplies, as well as targeting the parasite. For many developing countries, the

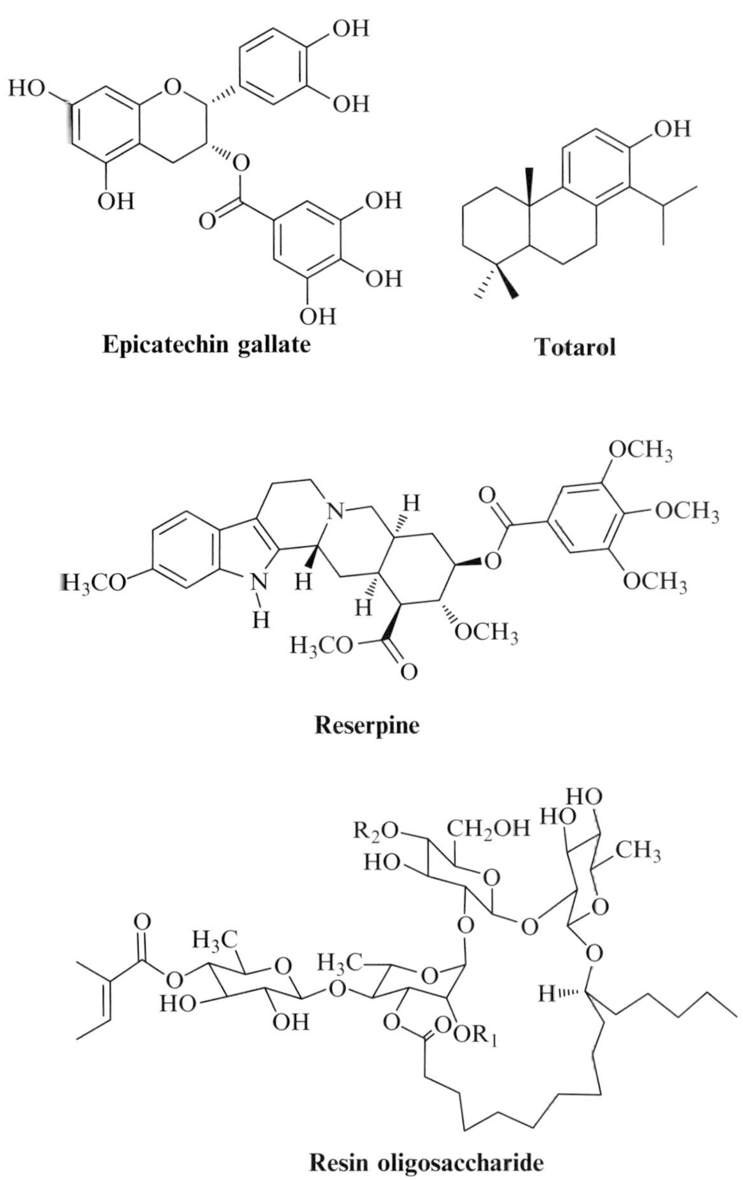

Epicatechin gallate

Totarol

Reserpine

Resin oligosaccharide

Fig. 18.14

use of plant-based anti-protozoals and pesticides represents the best chance of some sort of disease control.

CINCHONA, *CINCHONA* SPP. (CINCHONAE CORTEX) EU*

Trees of the genus *Cinchona* (Rubiaceae) are used as a source of quinine (for structure, see Chapter 1). Red cinchona, 'cinchona rubra', is *C. pubescens*

(= *C. succirubra* Pavon); yellow cinchona, 'cinchona flava', is *C. calisaya Wedd.*, or *C. ledgeriana* Moens. et Trim. Other species and hybrids of the genus *Cinchona* are also used. It has been called Peruvian bark, from the country of origin, and also Jesuit's bark, since it was originally introduced into Europe by Jesuit missionaries. It is native to mountainous regions of tropical America, and cultivated in South-East Asia and parts of Africa. The bark is found in commerce as quills or flat pieces.

The external surface is brownish-grey, usually fissured, and lichens and mosses may be seen as greyish-white or greenish patches.

Constituents

The actives are quinoline alkaloids, the major being quinine (Fig. 18.15), with quinidine, cinchonine, cinchonidine, epi and hydro derivatives of these, quinamine and others. The total alkaloid content of the bark should be not less than 6.5%, with 30–60% being of the quinine type. Identification is by thin-layer chromatography (TLC). The alkaloids are fluorescent.

Therapeutic uses and available evidence

Quinine was primarily used as an antimalarial before the advent of semi-synthetics, which have improved efficacy, especially against resistant strains, different pharmacokinetic profiles and reduced toxicity. The bark was formerly used as a febrifuge, tonic, orexigenic, spasmolytic and astringent, but it is only used now for the extraction of the alkaloids, quinine and its isomer quinidine. Both quinine and quinidine have antimalarial activity, although quinine is more widely used. Both are cardiac anti-arrhythmic agents (see Chapter 15), which limits their usefulness as antimalarials, and quinidine is still used clinically for this purpose. Quinine salts are used for the prevention of night cramps (the dose for this purpose is 200–300 mg of quinine sulphate or bisulphate) and in low doses is an ingredient of some analgesic and cold and flu remedies. Chronic overdosage can result in the condition known as cinchonism, which is characterized by headache, abdominal pain, rashes and visual disturbances. Cinchona and quinine should not be taken in large doses during pregnancy except for treating malaria.

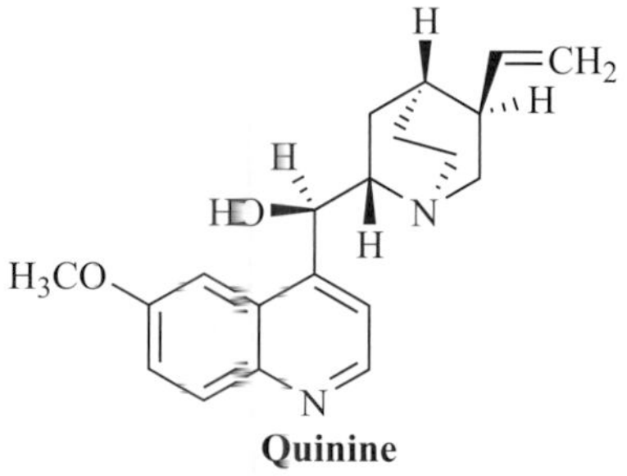

LAPACHO (TAHEEBO, PAU D'ARCO), *TABEBUIA* SPP.

Lapacho is obtained from several species of *Tabebuia* (Bignoniaceae), including T. *avellanedae* Lorentz ex Griseb., T. *rosea* Bertol., T. *serratifolia* (Vahl) Nicholson and others. These are large tropical trees, indigenous to South America. The inner bark is used medicinally. Lapacho is used traditionally for infectious diseases, including protozoal, bacterial, fungal and viral infections, to enhance immune function and for treating various cancers. Lapachol is antiprotozoal against *Leishmania, Trypanosoma* and *Schistosoma* spp., as well as being antiinflammatory.

Constituents

The active constituents are naphthoquinones, the most important being lapachol (Fig. 18.16), with deoxylapachol, α- and β-lapachone and others. It also contains anthraquinones, benzoic acid and benzaldehyde derivatives.

Therapeutic uses and available evidence

Antimicrobial effects are documented against *Candida, Brucella* and *Staphylococcus* spp., and for several viruses. Lapacho is also becoming popular as an anticancer treatment; antitumour activity has been shown in vitro and in vivo and a few uncontrolled trials have been carried out. The evidence available so far is inconclusive and this botanical drug should not be recommended for the treatment of cancer. Semi-synthetic derivatives of lapachol are being prepared in order to increase activity and reduce toxicity. Lapachol is cytotoxic in large doses, and inhibits pregnancy in mice; however, there is little evidence of toxicity for the herb when used in normal doses. For review, see Gómez Castellanos et al 2009.

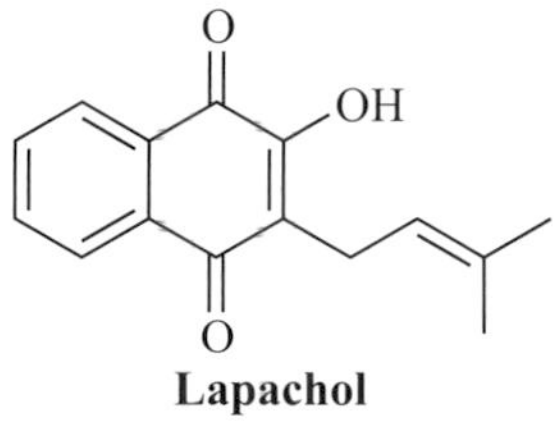

Quinine

Fig. 18.15

Lapachol

Fig. 18.16

SWEET WORMWOOD (SYN. QINGHAOU), *ARTEMISIA ANNUA* L.

Qinghaou (*Artemisia annua* L.), also known as annual wormwood, is a native of temperate parts of Asia, particularly China. It is a prostrate or erect annual with woody stems, pinnately divided leaves and small yellow flowers arranged in panicles. It has a characteristic sweet, aromatic, odour. The herb has been used for thousands of years in China for fevers and disorders of the liver. It is highly effective for the treatment of malaria, especially against resistant strains of *Plasmodium berghei* and *P. falciparum*, and this is now the major use of the plant.

Constituents

The herb contains sesquiterpene lactones, the most important of which is artemisinin (qinghaosu; Fig. 18.17), as well as the arteannuins A–O, artemisitine, artemisinic acid, hydroarteannuin, and others. There is also a volatile oil containing artemisia ketone, cadinene and others, and flavonoids including artemetin.

Therapeutic uses and available evidence

Artemisinin is one of the most rapidly acting antiplasmodial compounds known. Several more stable and effective derivatives, such as artemether, arteether and artesunate have been developed and are being used clinically for both the prophylaxis and treatment of malaria (see Cui and Su 2009). The herb appears to be fairly non-toxic, although cytotoxicity in vitro and teratogenic effects have been observed in mice. There is evidence that the whole herb extract may be superior to isolated artemisinin, since the flavonoids present in the leaves have been linked to suppression of CYP450 enzymes responsible for altering the absorption and metabolism of artemisinin in the body, and also to a beneficial immunomodulatory activity in subjects afflicted with parasitic and chronic diseases (Ferreira et al 2010).

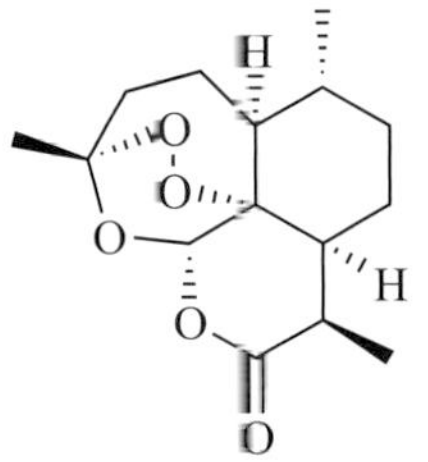

INSECTICIDAL AGENTS

PYRETHRUM (INSECT) FLOWERS, *CHRYSANTHEMUM* SPP.

Chrysanthemum cinerariaefolium (Trev.) Vis., *C. coccineum* Willd. and *C. marshallii* Aschers (Asteraceae) are all known as insect flowers. Dalmation insect flowers are *C. cinerariifolium* [formerly *Pyrethrum cinerarii folium* Trev. or *Tanacetum cinerariifolium* (Trev.) Sch. Bip.]; *C. coccineum* and *C. marshallii* are known as Persian and Causasian insect flowers, respectively. They are indigenous to the Balkans but widely cultivated elsewhere. The unopened flower heads are used; they are about 7 cm in diameter, with creamy-white ligulate florets and yellow tubular florets. There are two or three rows of lanceolate greenish-yellow, hairy bracts and a flat receptacle without paleae.

Constituents

All species contain pyrethrins, which are esters of chrysanthemic and pyrethric acids and are the actives. They are known as pyrethrins I (Fig. 18.18) and II, cinerins I and II and jasmolins I and II.

Therapeutic uses and available evidence

The natural pyrethrins are used to treat lice and scabies infestations and to kill other types of insect (houseflies, etc.) which are not necessarily causes of skin infestation. Pyrethrin I is the most potent of the naturally occurring compounds, although all have a knockdown effect on insects. The natural products have been used to develop semi-synthetic derivatives such as permethrin, phenothrin, tetramethrin, cypermethrin and decamethrin, which can be more potent and offer more chemical stability. All of these have been shown to have clinical efficacy, but the semi-synthetic compounds are more likely to lead to resistance arising

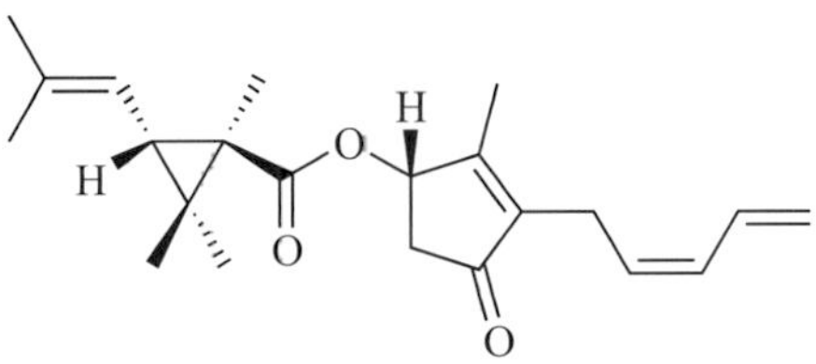

Artemisinin

Fig. 18.17

Pyrethrin I

Fig. 18.18

because of their persistence. Pyrethrum is mostly considered to be harmless to humans and animals, and may be used as a spray, lotion or powder, or fumigant. Pyrethroids are much less toxic to humans than synthetic insecticides, but care should be taken as they can cause irritation or allergic reactions.

QUASSIA WOOD, *PICRASMA EXCELSA* (SW.) PLANCH AND *QUASSIA AMARA* L.

Picrasma excelsa and other species, and *Quassia amara* (Simaroubaceae) are both known as quassia or bitter wood. Jamaica quassia is *P. excelsa*, Surinam quassia is *Q. amara* and Japanese quassia is *P. ailanthoides* Planch. The wood occurs in commerce as logs, chips or shredded; it is whitish, becoming yellow on exposure to the air.

Constituents

Quassia contains quassinoids such as quassin, isoquassin (= picrasmin), neoquassin, 18-hydroxyquassin,

quassinol, quassialactol, quassimarin and similikalactones, nigaki lactones A–N and nigaki hemiacetals A–F, and picrasins B, H, I, J depending on the species. *P. excelsa* and *Q. amara* also contain carboline alkaloids including canthin-6-one and various methoxy and hydroxy derivatives, and *P. ailanthoides* contains a series of picrasidine alkaloids.

Therapeutic uses and available evidence

Quassia is an insecticide, anthelmintic, febrifuge and antimalarial, although efficacy in malaria is unproven. It has been used clinically as a fresh infusion to treat head lice in humans, although little evidence for efficacy is available. The quassinoids are responsible for most of the activity; many of them are insecticidal, cytotoxic and amoebicidal both in vitro and in vivo. Quassia has long been used as flavouring in bitter alcoholic and soft drinks, and has been used to stimulate the appetite. Quassia is non-toxic when applied externally, and relatively safe in small doses when ingested.

References

Appendino, G., Gibbons, S., Giana, A., et al., 2008. Antibacterial phytocannabinoids: a structure-activity study. J. Nat. Prod. 71, 1427–1430.

Appendino, G., Fontana, G., Pollastro, F., 2010. Natural products drug discovery. In: Comprehensive Natural Products II. Elsevier Ltd, London, (Chapter 3.08), pp. 205–236.

Baser, K.H., 2008. Biological and pharmacological activities of carvacrol and carvacrol bearing essential oils. Curr. Pharm. Des. 14, 3106–3119.

Beaux, D., Fleurentin, J., Mortier, F., 1999. Effect of extracts of *Orthosiphon stamineus* Benth, *Hieracium pilosella* L., *Sambucus nigra* L. and *Arctostaphylos uva-ursi* (L.) Spreng. in rats. Phytother. Res. 13, 222–225.

Bolton, S., Null, G., Troetel, W.M., 1982. The medical uses of garlic–fact and fiction. Am. Pharm. 22, 40–43.

Carson, C.F., Riley, T.V., 1995. Antimicrobial activity of the major

components of the essential oil of *Melaleuca alternifolia*. J. Appl. Bacteriol. 78, 264–269.

Carson, C., Hammer, K.A., Riley, T.V., 2006. *Melaleuca alternifolia* (Tea Tree) oil: a review of antimicrobial and other medicinal properties. Clin. Microbiol. Rev. 19, 50–62.

Cox, S.D., Mann, C.M., Markham, J.L., 2001. Interactions between components of the essential oil of *Melaleuca alternifolia*. J. Appl. Microbiol. 91, 492–497.

Cui, L., Su, X.Z., 2009. Discovery, mechanisms of action and combination therapy of artemisinin. Expert Rev. Anti Infect. Ther. 7, 999–1013.

Fagboun, D.E., Ogundana, S.K., Adesanya, S.A., Roberts, M.F., 1987. Dihydrostilbene phytoalexins from *Dioscorea rotundata*. Phytochemistry 26, 3187–3189.

Ferreira, J.F., Luthria, D.L., Sasaki, T., Heyerick, A., 2010. Flavonoids from *Artemisia annua* L. as antioxidants and their potential synergism with artemisinin against

malaria and cancer. Molecules 15, 3135–3170.

Gibbons, S., 2004. Anti-staphylococcal plant natural products. Nat. Prod. Rep. 21, 263–277.

Gibbons, S., 2008. Phytochemicals for bacterial resistance – strengths, weaknesses and opportunities. Planta Med. 74, 594–602.

Gómez Castellanos, J.R., Prieto, J.M., Heinrich, M., 2009. Red Lapacho (*Tabebuia impetiginosa*) – a global ethnopharmacological commodity? J. Ethnopharmacol. 121, 1–13.

Harris, J.C., Cottrell, S.L., Plummer, S., Lloyd, D., 2001. Antimicrobial properties of *Allium sativum* (garlic). Appl. Microbiol. Biotechnol. 57, 282–286.

Jayasuriya, H., Clark, A.M., McChesney, J.D., 1991. New antimicrobial filicinic acid derivatives from *Hypericum drummondii*. J. Nat. Prod. 54, 1314–1320.

Jepson, R.G., Craig, J.C., 2008. Cranberries for preventing urinary tract infections. Cochrane Database Syst. Rev. Jan 23;(1):(CD)001321.

Kayser, O., Kolodziej, H., 1997. Antibacterial activity of extracts and constituents of *Pelargonium sidoides* and *Pelargonium reniforme*. Planta Med. 63, 508–510.

Koytchev, R., Alken, R.G., Dundarov, S., 1999. Balm mint extract (Lo-701) for topical treatment of recurring herpes labialis. Phytomedicine 6, 225–230.

Luna Jr., L.A., Bachi, A.L., 2011. Immune responses induced by *Pelargonium sidoides* extract in serum and nasal mucosa of athletes after exhaustive exercise: Modulation of secretory IgA, IL-6 and IL-15. Phytomedicine 18, 303–308.

Matthys, H., Kamin, W., Funk, P., Heger, M., 2007. *Pelargonium sidoides* preparation (EPs 7630) in the treatment of acute bronchitis in adults and children. Phytomedicine 6, 69–73.

Michaelis, M., Doerr, H.W., Cinatl Jr., J., 2011. Investigation of the influence of EPs® 7630, a herbal drug preparation from *Pelargonium sidoides*, on replication of a broad panel of respiratory viruses. Phytomedicine 18, 384–386.

O'Donnell, G., Poeschl, R., Zimhony, O., et al., 2009. Bioactive pyridine-N-oxide sulphides from *Allium stipitatum*. J. Nat. Prod. 72, 360–365.

Raman, A., Weir, U., Bloomfield, S.F., 1995. Antimicrobial effects of tea-tree oil and its major components on *Staphylococcus aureus, Staph. epidermidis* and *Propionibacterium acnes*. Lett. Appl. Microbiol. 21, 242–245.

Sakagami, Y., Mimura, M., Kajimura, K., et al., 1998. Anti-MRSA activity of sophoraflavanone G and synergism with other antibacterial agents. Lett. Appl. Microbiol. 27, 98–100.

Schempp, C.M., Pelz, K., Wittmer, A., Schöpf, E., Simon, J.C., 1999. Antibacterial activity of hyperforin from St John's wort against multiresistant *Staphylococcus aureus* and Gram-positive bacteria. The Lancet 353, 2129.

Seidel, V., Taylor, P.W., 2004. In vitro activity of extracts and constituents of Pelargonium against rapidly growing mycobacteria. Int. J. Antimicrob. Agents 23, 613–619.

Smith, J.E., Tucker, D., Watson, K., Lloyd Jones, G., 2007. Identification of antibacterial constituents from the indigenous Australian medicinal plant *Eremophila duttonii* F. Muell. (Myoporaceae). J. Ethnopharmacol. 112, 386–393.

Stavri, M., Piddock, L.J.V., Gibbons, S., 2007. Bacterial efflux pump inhibitors from natural sources. J. Antimicrob. Chemother. 59, 1247–1260.

Ulbricht, C., Brendler, T., Gruenwald, J., et al., 2005. Lemon balm (*Melissa officinalis* L.): an evidence-based systematic review by the Natural Standard Research Collaboration. J. Herb. Pharmacother. 5, 71–114.

Warnke, P.H., Becker, S.T., Podschun, R., et al., 2009. The battle against multi-resistant strains: Renaissance of antimicrobial essential oils as a promising force to fight hospital-acquired infections. J. Craniomaxillofac. Surg. 37, 392–397.

Zikria, J., Goldman, R., Ansell, J., 2010. Cranberry juice and warfarin: when bad publicity trumps science. Am. J. Med. 123, 384–392.

Chapter 19

The endocrine system

Phytomedicines are often used in the treatment of hormonal disorders, although they are not a substitute for hormone replacement, whether for insulin in diabetes, or natural female and male sex hormones. They do not have a place in the management of thyroid deficiency either, which should be treated with thyroxine. In diabetic patients, many foods and herbs can help to reduce blood glucose levels and may assist in controlling hyperglycaemia in milder cases of non-insulin dependent diabetes. Phytomedicines are much less potent in effect than the sex hormones, but this can be an advantage, as for example with the phytoestrogens. There are several conditions for which phytomedicines may offer at least some symptomatic relief, for example, premenstrual syndrome, which affects around 20–30% of women for up to 2 weeks before the start of menstruation, and the menopause, which affects all women, usually around the age of 51 years. Certain phytomedicines also have beneficial effects in benign prostatic hyperplasia, which is very common in men over 50 years of age and is characterized by a swollen prostate gland, causing frequent or difficult urination.

HYPOGLYCAEMIC AND ANTIDIABETIC HERBS

Many plants and foods lower blood glucose levels by a variety of mechanisms. Although type 1 diabetes (insulin-dependent diabetes mellitus) must be controlled by injections of insulin, type 2 diabetes (non-insulin-dependent diabetes mellitus) responds well to improvements in diet and hypoglycaemic drugs. Phytomedicines have a part to play and are

very popular in Asia, where a wide range of herbs is used. Complex carbohydrate preparations, such as guar gum, act by inhibiting glucose absorption from the gut and hence preventing the surge in blood glucose that can occur immediately after a meal. This is a feature of high-fibre diets which are also recommended in diabetes, and such diets also have the advantage of regulating blood cholesterol levels.

GUAR GUM, *CYAMOPSIS TETRAGONOLOBUS* (L.) TAUBERT (CYAMOPSIDIS SEMEN) EU✲

Guar gum is obtained from the ground endosperms of the seeds of *Cyamopsis tetragonolobus* (Leguminosae), a plant indigenous to Africa and parts of Asia, producing a yellowish-white flour which can be used to supplement the diet and even made into food items such as pasta. The flour is a source of fibre and used as an adjunct in the treatment of diabetes.

Constituents

These are polysaccharides composed of straight and branched chains of D-galactose and D-mannose polymers.

Therapeutic uses and available evidence

The flour reduces pre- and postprandial glucose levels and is usually given with meals, and may also be of use in lowering blood lipid levels (Butt et al 2007). Like other bulk fibre preparations, it has other clinical effects such as the alleviation of diarrhoea, and it has been advocated as a slimming aid, and this does seem to be justified. It is also used as a thickening and suspending agent in foods, and as a tablet binder. The usual dose of the powdered gum is 5 g given with each meal. Few side effects have been noted, but patients treated with guar sometimes consider it to be rather unpalatable when made into foods.

GYMNEMA, *GYMNEMA SYLVESTRE* R.BR.

Gymnema sylvestre (Asclepidaceae) grows wild in India, Sri Lanka and tropical Africa. It is a large woody climber with small yellow flowers. The leaves, which are ovate and hairy on both surfaces, have a slightly bitter taste, and if chewed this is followed by a remarkable temporary loss of sensitivity to the taste of sugar and other sweeteners. This unusual property has no relation to the hypoglycaemic effects, although may have originally been the rationale for its traditional use.

Constituents

The leaves and root contain saponin glycosides known collectively as 'gymnemic acid', which consists of a mixture of gymnemic acids, gymnemasins, gymnasides, gymnemosides and their aglycones. Gurmarin, a polypeptide is responsible for the desensitization of the palate to sweet tastes.

Therapeutic uses and available evidence

The herb is a traditional treatment for diabetes in India but, although widely used, there is insufficient clinical evidence available to recommend this herb as yet. The antihyperglycaemic properties are due to the gymnemic acids and other saponins. Oral administration of a specific standardized extract OSA(R) (1 g/day, 60 days) induced significant increases in circulating insulin and C-peptide, which were associated with a reduction in fasting and post-prandial blood glucose. In vitro measurements using isolated human islets of Langerhans demonstrated direct stimulatory effects of OSA(R) on insulin secretion from human β-cells, consistent with an in vivo mode of action through enhancing insulin secretion (Al-Romaiyan et al 2010). The leaf extract also has hypolipidaemic activity in human patients and animals fed a high-fat diet (Kanetka et al 2007). The usual dose is up to 4 g of leaf daily. Gymnemic acids are well tolerated, but care should be taken when used in conjunction with other antidiabetic agents.

KARELA, *MOMORDICA CHARANTIA* L.

The bitter gourd or bitter melon, karela (*Momordica charantia*, Cucurbitaceae), is grown throughout India, China, Africa and parts of America. It is a slender, climbing shrub with kidney-shaped, lobed leaves. The fruit resembles a cucumber with numerous ridges or warts and soft spines. It has an intensely bitter taste. Both the leaves and fruit are used medicinally.

The plant is widely used in the treatment of diabetes. The fruit is eaten as a vegetable; the leaf may be made into a type of 'bush tea', called 'cerassie'.

Constituents

The plant contains triterpene (cucurbitane-type) glycosides called momordicosides A–L and the goyaglycosides A–H, as well as momordicin, momordicinin and cucurbitanes I, II and III and goyasaponins I, II and III. Proteins and lectins present include α-, β- and γ-momorcharins and momordins a and b.

Therapeutic uses and available evidence

Both the fruit and the leaf have hypoglycaemic effects. The extract causes hypoglycaemia in animals and human diabetic patients, and several clinical studies have confirmed benefits (see review by Grover and Yadav 2004), but a recent Cochrane review (Ooi et al 2010) states that there is insufficient evidence to recommend it for type 2 diabetes mellitus, and that further studies are required to address issues of standardization and the quality control of preparations. It has also been used to treat asthma, skin infections and hypertension (Grover and Yadav 2004). Contraceptive and teratogenic effects have been described in animals, so care should be taken in pregnant women, although cooking the vegetable may well destroy many of the toxins.

PHYTOESTROGENS

There are many plants that contain oestrogenic substances (phytoestrogens), and pharmacological and epidemiological evidence suggests that they act as mild oestrogens or, in certain circumstances, as anti-oestrogens (by binding to oestrogen receptors and preventing occupation by natural oestrogens). They generally have beneficial effects, including chemopreventive activity. As well as the herbs mentioned below, many pulses (which are legumes) contain phytoestrogens, as do linseed and hops. The main chemical types of phytoestrogen are the isoflavones, coumestans and lignans, and some species of palm even contain similar hormones (e.g. estriol) to those found in the human body. The common occurrence of these substances has implications for men as well as for women, in that the incidence of benign prostatic hyperplasia is lower in men, and menopausal symptoms in women, in societies consuming significant amounts of foods containing these substances in their normal diet. However, a recent case-control study in the UK found no significant associations between phytoestrogen intake and breast cancer risk, although colorectal cancer risk was inversely associated with enterolignan intake in women but not in men (Ward and Kuhnle 2010). Soya phytoestrogen intake may even have a beneficial effect on tumour recurrence (Roberts 2010). As the majority of studies have not involved women with breast cancer and are of short duration, it would be wise for patients with hormone-dependent cancers to avoid taking phytomedicines known to affect hormone levels.

RED CLOVER, *TRIFOLIUM PRATENSE* L.

Red (or pink) clover (Fabaceae) is widely distributed throughout Europe, naturalized in North America and found in many other parts of the world. The flower heads are ovoid, red or pinkish purple, about 2–3 cm in diameter, composed of numerous individual, keeled flowers. The leaflets are trefoil, often with a whitish crescent in the centre. Both the leaves and isolated isoflavones are used medicinally.

Constituents

The major actives are phytoestrogens of two types: the isoflavones genistein (Fig. 19.1), afrormosin, biochanin A, daidzein, formononetin, pratensein, calyconin, pseudobaptigenin, orobol, irilone and

Fig. 19.1

Genistein   Coumestrol

trifoside, and their glycoside conjugates; and the coumestans coumestrol (Fig. 19.1) and medicagol.

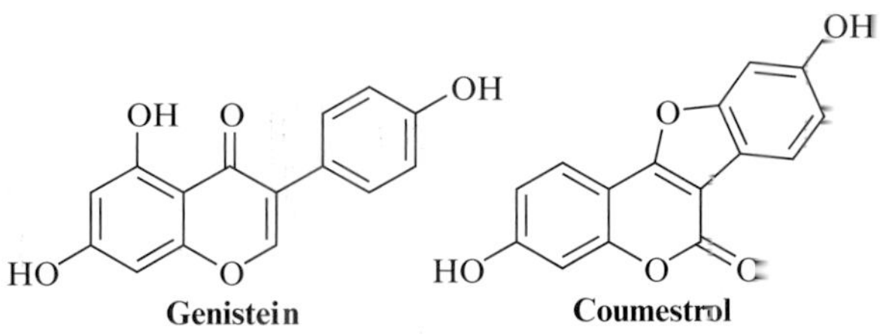

Therapeutic uses and available evidence

Red clover was traditionally used for skin complaints such as psoriasis and eczema, and as an expectorant in coughs and bronchial conditions. However, it has recently been used more as a source of the isoflavones, for a natural method of hormone replacement therapy (for review, see Sabudak and Guler 2009). The isoflavones are oestrogenic in animals but the clinical use for menopausal women has not yet been well supported by clinical studies, except for a marginally significant effect for treating hot flushes in menopausal women (Coon et al 2007). Biochanin A inhibits metabolic activation of the carcinogen benzo(a)pyrene in a mammalian cell culture, suggesting chemopreventive properties. Red clover extracts also inhibit cytochrome P450 3A4 in vitro, which supports such a use. Red clover is considered safe.

SOYA, *GLYCINE* MAX (L.) MERR.

Soya (Fabaceae) is a low-growing, typically leguminous crop plant, producing white or yellow beans. It is an important item of diet in many countries and is used in many ways. For example 'soya milk' is used as a substitute for animal milk in allergic people (especially babies), and can be made into yoghurt. The protein is used as a meat substitute and to make tofu, and is fermented into condiments such as 'soy sauce'. The bean sprouts are eaten raw in salads and used in stir-fry dishes; the flour can be made into bread and cakes.

Constituents

Soya contains phytoestrogens of two chemical types: isoflavones including genistein, daidzein and their derivatives, ononin, isoformononetin and others, and coumestans such as coumestrol (especially in the sprouts). There is a fixed oil composed mainly of linoleic and linolenic acids, and phytosterols including β-sitosterol and stigmasterol.

Therapeutic uses and available evidence

Preparations containing the isolated isoflavones are used medicinally. The available epidemiological evidence suggests that a diet high in soya can reduce menopausal symptoms and prostate enlargement, although clinical trials have not yet proved these benefits.

The isoflavones and coumestans are oestrogenic, and are now being used as a natural form of hormone replacement therapy, although the evidence for this is not conclusive. Dietary inclusion of whole soya foods appears to produce a reduction in some clinical risk factors for osteoporosis, and soy isoflavone supplements moderately decreased the bone resorption marker deoxypyridinoline but did not affect the bone formation markers alkaline phosphatase and serum osteocalcin in menopausal women, although the effects varied between studies (Taku et al 2010).

Cardiovascular disease and lipid profiles in menopausal women have been reported to be improved by consumption of whole soya foods, although results have been conflicting. In an open study of 190 healthy postmenopausal women given 35 mg of soy isoflavones, a reduction in the number of hot flushes was found (Albert et al 2002), but no improvement was seen in women with breast cancer given a beverage containing 90 mg of soy isoflavones. There is still much work to be done on the clinical effects of the isoflavones in soya, but at present it appears that they are beneficial with few adverse effects (for review, see Messina 2010). Opposing advice has been given regarding the safety of dietary phytoestrogen use for women with previous breast cancer. However, as mentioned above, the majority of studies have not been conducted in women with breast cancer and many are of short duration. Soya is considered to be non-toxic.

HORMONAL IMBALANCE IN WOMEN

Although the phytoestrogens can be considered to affect hormone activity, there are other herbal medicines that are considered to have the capacity to regulate hormone levels without necessarily being oestrogenic. Their mechanism of action is generally not known.

BLACK COHOSH, *CIMICIFUGA RACEMOSA* NUTT. (CIMICIFUGAE RACEMOSAE RHIZOME) ⬛✷

Black cohosh (syn. *Actaea racemosa* L., Ranunculaceae) is also known as 'squawroot', because of its traditional use for female complaints. In North America, where the plant originates, it was also used to treat snakebite, hence another synonym, 'black snakeroot'. It has also been used for a variety of disparate disorders, including rheumatism, sciatica, chorea and tinnitus. The parts used medicinally are the rhizomes and roots, which are dark brown in colour.

Constituents

The active components of black cohosh are considered to be the triterpene glycosides, such as actein (Fig. 19.2), 27-deoxyactein and several cimicifugosides; the flavonoids may contribute to the activity.

Therapeutic uses and available evidence

Hormonal and antiinflammatory effects have been described for black cohosh and reductions in serum luteinizing hormone concentrations have been documented for methanolic and lipophilic extracts, but there are conflicting data on the oestrogenic activity of the herb. Although there is some evidence from randomized, placebo-controlled clinical trials, it does not consistently demonstrate an effect of black cohosh on menopausal symptoms, including flushes, and further rigorous trials seem warranted (Borrelli and Ernst 2008). Black cohosh use appears safe in women with previous breast cancer (Roberts 2010), but the majority of studies regarding the efficacy of such herbal treatments have not been conducted in women with breast cancer and many are of short duration. Adverse effects are rare, but may include gastrointestinal disturbance and lowering of blood pressure with high doses. It should be avoided in pregnancy and lactation because of insufficient data.

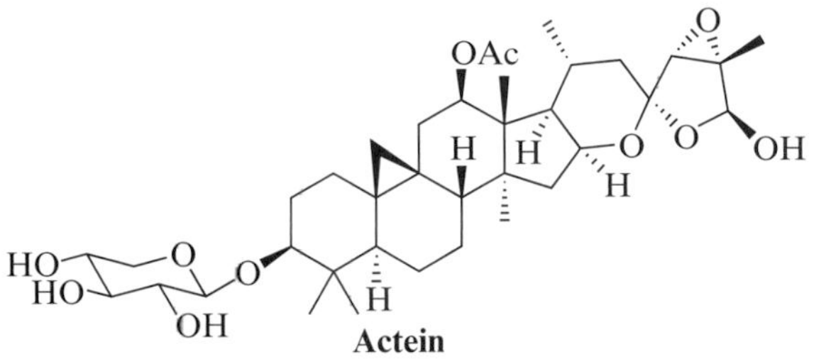

Fig. 19.2

CHASTEBERRY, *VITEX AGNUS-CASTUS* L. (AGNI CASTI FRUCTUS) EU✷

Vitex agnus-castus (Verbenaceae) is also known by the common names 'chasteberry' and 'chaste tree', but is often referred to simply as 'agnus castus'. It has a history of traditional use for menstrual problems, including premenstrual symptoms and dysmenorrhoea, and also for menopausal complaints. It was considered historically to reduce the libido, especially in men, hence the names 'chasteberry', 'agnus castus' (which means 'chaste lamb') and 'monk's pepper'. *Vitex agnus-castus* is native to the Mediterranean. It is a shrub or small tree, which grows to 1–6 m in height. The fruit (berries) is reddish-black and around 2–4 mm in diameter, and is the part used pharmaceutically.

Constituents

The pharmacologically active components of *Agnus castus* have not yet been clearly established, although the diterpene constituents (e.g. rotundifuran) are likely to be important. Flavonoids, mainly vitexin, casticin, and others, such as kaempferol and quercetagetin, iridoids are also present.

Therapeutic uses and available evidence

Extracts of agnus castus and isolated diterpene constituents display dopamine receptor binding activity in vitro. For example, dopaminergic activity and inhibition of prolactin secretion has been demonstrated in vitro for rotundifuran. Dopaminergic activity is associated with inhibition of prolactin synthesis and release. Modern pharmaceutical uses of agnus castus include menstrual cycle disorders, premenstrual syndrome and mastalgia (cyclical breast pain). There is some evidence from randomized controlled trials to support the effects of proprietary preparations of agnus castus in relieving breast pain in women with mastalgia. Alleviation of symptoms of premenstrual syndrome is also supported by results of randomized controlled trials (for example, Ma et al 2010). In addition, clinical studies provide some evidence to support the effects of agnus castus on lowering prolactin concentrations in hyperprolactinaemia. Other studies have reported that agnus castus does not markedly affect prolactin concentrations in women with normal basal prolactin levels. Although evidence from rigorous randomized controlled trials is lacking for agnus castus in

the alleviation of menopausal symptoms, emerging pharmacological evidence supports a role in this context (for review, see Van Die et al 2009).

Agnus castus is generally thought safe, but as with most medicines it is not recommended during pregnancy. It should not be used during lactation as it may suppress milk production; its effects upon neonates are not known.

BENIGN PROSTATIC HYPERPLASIA

Benign prostatic hyperplasia (BPH) is so common in older men that it can almost be considered a normal part of ageing. The symptoms are increased frequency, and difficulty, of micturition (urination). BPH requires a medical diagnosis to eliminate the possibility of prostate cancer, and so self-treatment is only suitable after consultation with a medical practitioner. Severe cases are treated with surgery, which is not always entirely successful, or drug treatment with either specific α-adrenergic-blocking agents or testosterone 5α-reductase inhibitors. α-Blockers relax smooth muscle in BPH and improve urinary flow, but have side effects including drowsiness, syncope and dry mouth. The enzyme 5α-reductase catalyses the conversion of testosterone to the more potent androgen, dihydrotestosterone, and if this is prevented, a reduction in prostate size and consequent improvement in urine flow ensues. Phytotherapy is thought to be as successful (or almost) as synthetic drug treatment, but complete reversal of the enlargement of the prostate is not possible.

NETTLE, *URTICA DIOICA* L. (URTICAE HERBA, RADIX) EU✷

Urtica dioica (Urticaceae) is commonly known as stinging nettle or simply urtica. Traditionally, it has been used to treat a disparate range of conditions, including uterine haemorrhage, epistaxis, cutaneous eruptions, and nervous and infantile eczema, which have little relation to its modern pharmaceutical uses. It has also been used as supportive therapy in rheumatic ailments. The plant grows to around 60–120 cm in height and has serrated leaves with stinging hairs and bristles. The herb and the roots are the parts used pharmaceutically.

Constituents

The phytochemistry of nettle is well documented, although it is not clear precisely which constituents are responsible for the various activities. Lignans present in the root, including pinoresinol, secoisolariciresinol, dehydrodiconiferyl alcohol and neo-olivil, may be important in inhibiting the interaction between sex hormone-binding globulin and 5α-testosterone. Other constituents include lectins, the mixture known as UDA (urtica dioica agglutinin), composed of at least six isolectins, and triterpenes such as olearolic and ursolic acid derivatives. The leaf contains flavonoids, mainly isorhamnetin, kaempferol and quercetin glycosides, and glycoprotein, with indoles such as histamine and serotonin, betaine, acetylcholine, caffeic, chlorogenic and caffeoylmalic acids.

Therapeutic uses and available evidence

Modern uses of nettle extracts are focused mainly on symptom relief in BPH and adjuvant treatment (i.e. in addition to non-steroidal antiinflammatory drugs) in arthritis and rheumatism. Evidence from in vitro and in vivo (mice) studies measuring sex hormone-binding globulin to human prostate membranes, and by inhibition of proliferation of human prostatic epithelial and stromal cells, suggests that nettle root extracts have beneficial effects on BPH tissue. Several compounds from the roots are also known to be aromatase inhibitors, and there is evidence from some clinical trials to support the use of nettle root extracts for relief of symptoms associated with BPH (for review, see Chrubasik et al 2007). Nettle leaf extracts inhibit the pro-inflammatory transcription factor NF-κB, partially inhibit cyclo-oxygenase and lipoxygenase, and inhibit tumour necrosis factor and interleukin-1β secretion stimulated by lipopolysaccharide. Nettle preparations are generally thought of as safe, with few (if any) adverse events being reported.

PYGEUM BARK, *PRUNUS AFRICANA* (HOOK. F.) KALKM. (PRUNI AFRICANI CORTEX)

The African prune (*Pygeum africanum*, Rosaceae) is a tropical evergreen tree indigenous to central and southern Africa. The use of pygeum bark is becoming more widespread throughout Europe and the USA, and is in danger of becoming scarce due to over-harvesting of the bark.

Constituents

The bark contains sterols and pentacyclic triterpenes, including abietic, oleanolic, ursolic and crataegolic acids, N-butylbenzene-sulfonamide, and esters of ferulic acid.

Therapeutic uses and available evidence

Traditionally used for micturition problems and now for BPH, pygeum extract has antiproliferative and apoptotic effects on proliferative prostate fibroblasts and myofibroblasts, but not on smooth muscle cells (Quiles et al 2010). The compound N-butylbenzene-sulfonamide, isolated from *P. africanum*, is a specific androgen receptor antagonist which inhibits both endogenous prostate serum antigen expression and growth of human prostate cancer cells, but does not interact with oestrogen receptors (Papaioannou et al 2010). Clinical studies have shown the extract to be moderately effective, and it may be a useful treatment option for men with lower urinary symptoms consistent with BPH. However, the studies are small, of short duration, use varied doses and preparations, and rarely report outcomes using standardized validated measures of efficacy, so further work is needed (Wilt et al 2002). Acute and chronic toxicity and mutagenicity tests have shown no adverse effects, and the extract appears to be well-tolerated in men when administered over long periods. It is often used in combination with nettle.

SAW PALMETTO, *SERENOA SERRULATA* HOOK. F. (SABALIS SERRULATAE FRUCTUS) EU✤

Serenoa serrulata (Arecaceae) is also known as *Serenoa repens* and *Sabal serrulata*, as well as the common name 'saw palmetto'. Saw palmetto is a small 'fan palm', which produces berries with a diameter of 1–2 cm. The fruit (berries) is the part used pharmaceutically. It has been used traditionally for cystitis and sex hormone disorders, including prostatic enlargement. Most commercial saw palmetto comes from the USA.

Constituents

The phytochemistry of saw palmetto is fairly well known, although precisely which components are responsible for the pharmacological effects have yet to be established. Constituents likely to be important include: the fatty acids capric, caprylic, lauric, oleic, myristoleic, palmitic, linoleic and linolenic acids; the monoacyl glycerides 1-monolaurin and 1-monomyristicin; phytosterols such as β-sitosterol, campesterol, stigmasterol, lupeol and cycloartenol (Fig. 19.3). Long-chain alcohols (farnesol, phytol and polyprenolic alcohols), and flavonoids are present, as well as immunostimulant, high-molecular-weight polysaccharides containing galactose, arabinose, mannose, rhamnose and glucuronic acid.

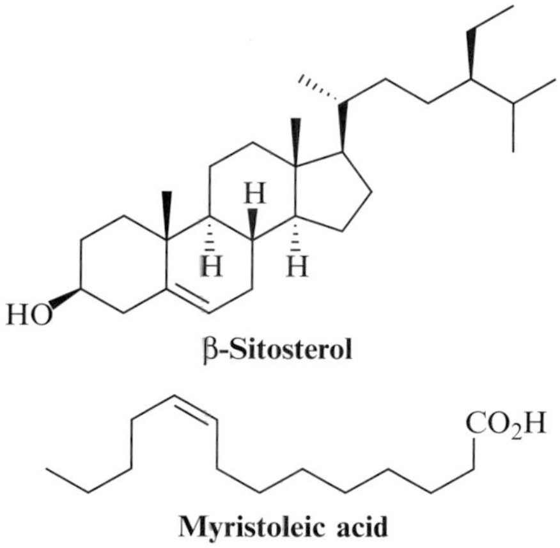

β-Sitosterol

Myristoleic acid

Fig. 19.3

Therapeutic uses and available evidence

Saw palmetto is now mainly used to treat BPH. This is supported by evidence from several randomized controlled trials, which also provided preliminary evidence that extracts (usually liposterolic) achieve improvements similar to those seen with the 5α-reductase inhibitor finasteride (Mantovani et al 2010). However, other studies show no effect and the efficacy is disputed (Barnes 2009; Tacklind et al 2009, Mantovani 2010). Post-marketing surveillance studies suggest that saw palmetto extracts are well tolerated, and comparative clinical studies indicate that they have a more favourable safety profile than finasteride, at least in the short term. Liposterolic

and ethanolic extracts of saw palmetto inhibit 5α-reductase (the enzyme which catalyses the conversion of testosterone to 5α-dihydrotestosterone in the prostate) in vitro; other studies have described beneficial effects in animal models of BPH. Spasmolytic activity, which may also contribute to improvements in BPH, has also been documented in vivo (rats) for an ethanolic extract of saw palmetto. In vitro growth arrest of prostate cancer LNCaP, DU145, and PC3 cells (Yang 2007) and in vivo oestrogenic and antiinflammatory activities have been reported for extracts of saw palmetto, and may be due to the high content of β-sitosterol. The antiinflammatory effects may also be due to the presence of the polysaccharides.

References

Al-Romaiyan, A., Liu, B., Asare-Anane, H., et al., 2010. A novel *Gymnema sylvestre* extract stimulates insulin secretion from human islets in vivo and in vitro. Phytother. Res. 24, 1370–1376.

Albert A, Altabre C, Baró F et al 2002. Efficacy and safety of a phytoestrogen preparation derived from *Glycine max* (L.) Merr in climacteric symptomatology: a multicentric, open, prospective and non-randomized trial. Phytomedicine 9(2):85–92.

Barnes, J., 2009. Saw palmetto. *Serenoa repens*. Also known as Serenoa serrulata, Sabal serrulata and the dwarf palm. J. Prim. Health Care 1, 323.

Borrelli, F., Ernst, E., 2008. Black cohosh (*Cimicifuga racemosa*) for menopausal symptoms: a systematic review of its efficacy. Pharmacol. Res. 58, 8–14.

Butt, M.S., Shahzadi, N., Sharif, M.K., Nasir, M., 2007. Guar gum: a miracle therapy for hypercholesterolemia, hyperglycemia and obesity. CRC Crit. Rev. Food Sci. Nutr. 47, 389–396.

Coon, J.T., Pittler, M.H., Ernst, E., 2007. *Trifolium pratense* isoflavones in the treatment of menopausal hot flushes: a systematic review and meta-analysis. Phytomedicine 14, 153–159.

Chrubasik, J.E., Roufogalis, B.D., Wagner, H., Chrubasik, S., 2007. A comprehensive review on the stinging nettle effect and efficacy profiles. Part II: urticae radix. Phytomedicine 14, 568–579.

Grover, J.K., Yadav, S.P., 2004. Pharmacological actions and potential uses of *Momordica charantia:* a review. J. Ethnopharmacol. 93, 123–132.

Kanetka, P., Singhal, R., Kamat, M., 2007. *Gymnema sylvestre:* a memoir. J. Clin. Biochem. Nutr. 41, 77–81.

Ma, L., Lin, S., Chen, R., Wang, X., 2010. Treatment of moderate to severe premenstrual syndrome with *Vitex agnus castus* (BNO 1095) in Chinese women. Gynecol. Endocrinol. 26, 612–616.

Mantovani, F., 2010. *Serenoa repens* in benign prostatic hypertrophy: analysis of 2 Italian studies. Minerva Urol. Nefrol. 62, 335–340.

Messina, M., 2010. A brief historical overview of the past two decades of soy and isoflavone research. J. Nutr. 140, 1350S–1354S.

Ooi, C.P., Yassin, Z., Hamid, T.A., 2010. *Momordica charantia* for type 2 diabetes mellitus. Cochrane Database Syst. Rev. Feb 17; (2): CD007845.

Papaioannou, M., Schleich, S., Roell, D., et al., 2010. NBBS isolated from *Pygeum africanum* bark exhibits androgen antagonistic

activity, inhibits AR nuclear translocation and prostate cancer cell growth. Invest. New Drugs 28, 729–743.

Quiles, M.T., Arbós, M.A., Fraga, A., de Torres, I.M., Reventós, J., Morote, J., 2010. Antiproliferative and apoptotic effects of the herbal agent *Pygeum africanum* on cultured prostate stromal cells from patients with benign prostatic hyperplasia (BPH). Prostate 70, 1044–1053.

Roberts, H., 2010. Safety of herbal medicinal products in women with breast cancer. Maturitas 66, 363–369.

Sabudak, T., Guler, N., 2009. *Trifolium L.* – a review on its phytochemical and pharmacological profile. Phytother. Res. 23, 439–446.

Tacklind, J., Donald, R., Rutks, I., Wilt, T.J., 2009. *Serenoa repens* for benign prostatic hyperplasia. Cochrane Database Syst. Rev. Apr 15;(2): CD001423.

Taku, K., Melby, M.K., Kurzer, M.S., Mizuno, S., Watanabe, S., Ishimi, Y., 2010. Effects of soy isoflavone supplements on bone turnover

markers in menopausal women: systematic review and meta-analysis of randomized controlled trials. Bone 47, 413–423.

Van Die, M.D., Burger, H.G., Teede, H.J., Bone, K.M., 2009. *Vitex agnus-castus* (Chaste-Tree/Berry) in the treatment of menopause-related complaints. J. Altern. Complement. Med. 15, 853–862.

Ward, H.A., Kuhnle, G.G.C., 2010. Phytoestrogen consumption and association with breast, prostate and colorectal cancer in EPIC Norfolk. Arch. Biochem. Biophys. 501, 170–175.

Wilt, T., Ishani, A., Mac Donald, R., Rutks, I., Stark, G., 2002. *Pygeum africanum* for benign prostatic hyperplasia. Cochrane Database Syst. Rev. (1):CD001044.

Yang, Y., Ikezoe, T., Zheng, Z., Taguchi, H., Koeffler, H.P., Zhu, W.G., 2007. Saw Palmetto induces growth arrest and apoptosis of androgen-dependent prostate cancer LNCaP cells via inactivation of STAT 3 and androgen receptor signaling. Int. J. Oncol. 31, 593–600.

Chapter 20

The reproductive tract

Drugs used in hormonal disorders have been covered in Chapter 19. Other drugs that are used in obstetrics, including substances used in childbirth, and genitourinary disorders and erectile dysfunction in men, will be mentioned briefly here.

PHYTOMEDICINES IN CHILDBIRTH

Taking (any) medicine during pregnancy is generally not advisable as safety of the mother and fetus cannot be guaranteed. Raspberry leaf is included here simply because according to folklore it has a widespread use in facilitating childbirth, and it is often recommended that it be taken during pregnancy for this purpose, but the use cannot be recommended as there is little clinical evidence available to demonstrate either safety or efficacy.

ERGOMETRINE EU✳

Ergometrine (Fig. 20.1) is an alkaloid extracted from ergot (*Claviceps purpurea* Tul.), a parasitic fungus growing on cereals, usually rye. It is used to manage the third stage of labour (in conjunction with oxytocin), and to control postpartum haemorrhage if the placenta has not been completely expelled. It must be used only under the care of a midwife or obstetrician.

RASPBERRY LEAF, *RUBUS IDAEUS* L. (RUBI IDAEI FOLIUM)

Raspberry leaf (*Rubus idaeus*, Rosaceae) 'tea' has been used for centuries to facilitate childbirth, and it is usually recommended that it be drunk freely before and during confinement for maximum benefit. The raspberry shrub is well known and will not be described. It is cultivated in many temperate countries for the fruit.

Constituents

The leaves have not been well investigated, but contain uncharacterized polypeptides and flavonoids, mainly glycosides of kaempferol and quercetin, including rutin.

Therapeutic uses and available evidence

A retrospective observational study on 108 mothers in Australia indicated that a shortening of labour and reduction in medical intervention occurred, with no untoward effects apart from a single case of diarrhoea and anecdotal reports of strong Braxton Hicks contractions. However, a larger, randomized placebo-controlled trial of 192 women by the same authors did not confirm such benefits, although no adverse effects for either mother or baby were noted (Simpson et al 2001). Uterine relaxant effects have been demonstrated in animals (Rojas-Vera et al 2002), and raspberry leaf appears to affect only the pregnant uterus of both rats and humans, with no activity on the non-pregnant uterus. However, no further identification of the active principle(s) has been made and a recent review concludes that in the absence of good clinical data, raspberry leaf cannot be recommended in pregnancy (Holst et al 2009).

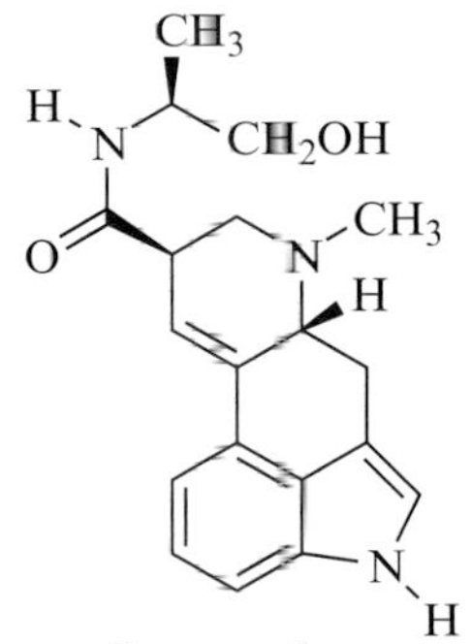

Ergometrine

Fig. 20.1

MALE SEXUAL DYSFUNCTION (IMPOTENCE)

Male impotence (failure to produce a satisfactory or sustainable erection) may result from psychogenic, vascular, neurogenic or endocrine abnormalities (such as diabetes), or drug treatment (e.g. with antihypertensives and antidepressants). It can be treated with either intracavernosal injections of papaverine or alprostadil (prostaglandin E1), intraurethral application (alprostadil) or systemically [sildenafil (Viagra) or apomorphine]. Medical assessment is needed before these drugs are prescribed. Although papaverine is of natural origin, it is only suitable for self-medication after medical diagnosis, but there are several herbal products available, which claim to treat this distressing disorder. The most common are probably epimedium, and yohimbe, a traditional aphrodisiac, and there are others, which are often strange botanical mixtures and usually sold under the description 'Herbal Viagra'. There is no good clinical evidence of efficacy for any of these, although epimedium has some pharmacological actions in common with those of sildenafil (Viagra®), and may have a placebo effect.

EPIMEDIUM BREVICORNUM MAXIM (EPIMEDII HERBA) AND EPIMEDIUM SPP.

Epimedium brevicornum Maxim (Berberidaceae) and related species are also known as 'horny goat weed'. The herb was apparently discovered by the Chinese, who noticed that when goats had eaten it, they were eager to mate, and for this reason they called the herb 'yin yang huo', or 'licentious goat plant'. Epimediums are sprawling, attractive, perennial herbs, with cordate leaves and white, cream, pink, yellow or lavender flowers. Although native to Asia and the Mediterranean region, they are widely cultivated. Epimedium has been used for the treatment of erectile dysfunction in Traditional Chinese Medicine for many years. It is also used to ease menopausal symptoms in women and to treat and prevent osteoporosis.

Constituents

The flavonoids are the active constituents, the most important being icariin and its analogues, with epimedin A, B, and C, and baohuoside I.

Therapeutic uses and available evidence

Icariin has phosphodiesterase type 5 inhibiting effects (the mechanism of action of sildenafil) and may also have neurotrophic effects (Zeng et al 2010, Ma et al 2011). A study of the effects of icariin administered daily to cavernous nerve-injured rats found that the ratio of intracavernous pressure to arterial pressure was significantly higher compared with control (and also single-dose icariin-treated) animals. The penile tissue of rats treated with icariin showed greater positivity for neuronal nitric oxide synthase and calponin, and cultured pelvic ganglia treated with icariin had significantly greater neurite length (Shindel et al 2010). Icariin is also a bone anabolic agent that may exert its osteogenic effects through the induction of bone morphogenetic protein-2 and NO synthesis, subsequently regulating gene expression and contributing to the induction of osteoblast proliferation and differentiation (Hseih et al 2010).

PAPAVERINE EU✦

Papaverine (Fig. 20.2) is an alkaloid extracted from the opium poppy (*Papaver somniferum* L.). It is most often used for the treatment of impotence of

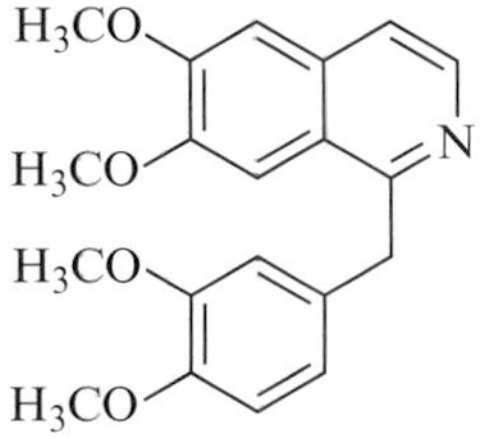

Papaverine

Fig. 20.2

neurological or psychogenic origin. As it must be given by intracavernosal injection, it is normally only used as a last resort when less invasive treatments have failed.

YOHIMBE, *PAUSINYSTALIA JOHIMBE* (K. SCHUM.) PIERRE

Yohimbe bark (Rubiaceae) occurs as flat or slightly quilled pieces, often covered with lichen.

Constituents

The bioactive constituents are indole alkaloids, the major one being yohimbine, together with α- and β-yohimbane, pseudoyohimbine and coryantheine.

Therapeutic uses and available evidence

Yohimbine (Fig. 20.3) is an α-adrenergic blocker and has a wide (but not justified) reputation as a sexual stimulant. It should be used only under the advice of a medical herbalist or physician.

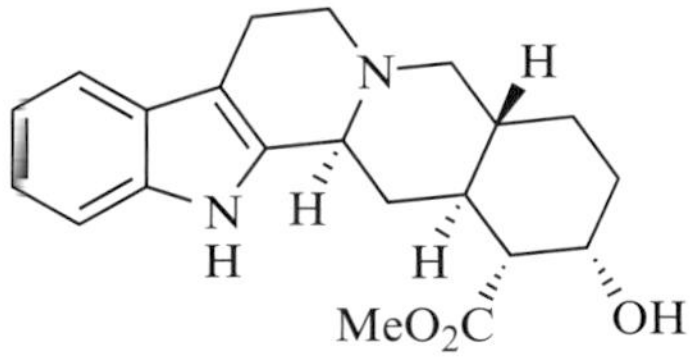

Yohimbine

Fig. 20.3

References

Holst, L., Wright, D., Nordeng, H., Haavik, S., 2009. Raspberry leaf – should it be recommended to pregnant women? Complement. Ther. Clin. Pract. 15, 204–208.

Hseih, T.P., Sheu, S.Y., Sun, J.S., Chen, M.H., Liu, M.H., 2010. Icariin isolated from *Epimedium pubescens* regulates osteoblasts anabolism through BMP-2, SMAD4, and Cbfa1 expression. Phytomedicine 17, 414–423.

Ma, H., He, W., Yang, Y., et al., 2011. The genus Epimedium: An ethnopharmacological and phytochemical review. J. Ethnopharmacol. 134, 519–541.

Rojas-Vera, J., Patel, A.V., Dacke, C.G., 2002. Relaxant activity of raspberry (*Rubus idaeus*) leaf extract in guinea-pig ileum in vitro. Phytother. Res. 16, 665–668.

Shindel, A.W., Xin, Z.C., Lin, G., et al., 2010. Erectogenic and neurotrophic effects of icariin, a purified extract of horny goat weed (*Epimedium* spp.) in vitro and in vivo. J. Sex. Med. (4 Pt 1), 1518–1528.

Simpson, M., Parsons, M., Greenwood, J., Wade, K., 2001. Raspberry leaf in pregnancy: its safety and efficacy in labor. J. Midwifery Womens Health 46, 51.

Zeng, K.W., Ko, H., Yang, H.O., Wang, X.M., 2010. Icariin attenuates β-amyloid-induced neurotoxicity by inhibition of tau protein hyperphosphorylation in PC12 cells. Neuropharmacology 59 (6), 542–550.

Chapter 21

The musculoskeletal system

Short-lived and self-limiting inflammatory disorders are not normally treated with phytomedicines, but recently the use of some botanical preparations for chronic inflammatory conditions has become increasingly widespread. The use of analgesic and antiinflammatory drugs such as paracetamol, aspirin and ibuprofen is common for such conditions, but the side effects of these drugs can limit their acceptability. Non-steroidal antiinflammatory drugs (NSAIDs) act mainly via inhibition of cyclo-oxygenase (COX); enzymes, also known as prostaglandin synthases (PGS). At present three are known, COX-1, COX-2 and COX-3 (a splice variant of COX-1, sometimes referred to as COX-1b). Inhibition of COX-1 (e.g. with aspirin, ibuprofen and diclofenac) reduces levels of the gastroprotective prostaglandins, leading to inflammation of the gastrointestinal lining and even ulceration and bleeding. COX-2, however, is only induced in response to pro-inflammatory cytokines, and is not found in normal tissue (unlike COX-1). It is associated particularly with oedema and the nociceptive and pyretic effects of inflammation. Treatment with inhibitors of COX-2 does not produce such severe gastrointestinal side effects, but there are concerns about their cardiovascular safety. Other targets for treating inflammatory diseases include 5-lipoxygenase (LOX), NF-κB (which is activated in rheumatoid arthritis and other chronic inflammatory conditions), and certain cytokines which inhibit the activity of tumour necrosis factor-α (TNFα). Chronic expression of NO is also associated with various inflammatory conditions, including arthritis.

DRUGS USED IN ARTHRITIS, RHEUMATISM AND MUSCLE PAIN

The classic NSAID, aspirin, was originally developed as a result of studies on salicin, obtained from willow bark (see below and Chapter 15 and – for historical aspects – Chapter 3). Although it was thought at first that the effects of salicin were due only to the hydrolysed product salicylic acid, it is now known that plant antiinflammatory agents tend to have fewer gastrointestinal side effects than salicylates in general. There are also several combination herbal products on the market, for which little clinical data are available, but which are very popular and seem to produce few side effects.

BROMELAIN (ANANASE)

Bromelain is a mixture of proteolytic enzymes extracted from the fruit and stem of the pineapple (*Ananas comosus* L.) and other species of bromeliad (Bromeliaceae). The active constituents are protease-inhibiting enzymes having molecular weights between 5000 and 6000.

Bromelain has been proposed for the treatment of atherosclerosis, dysmenorrhoea, scleroderma, infection and sports injuries. It is antiinflammatory in animal studies and is used clinically to treat bruising, arthritis, joint stiffness and pain, and to improve healing postoperatively, including after dental procedures. It is considered to be an effective alternative to NSAIDs, as shown by a number of clinical trials. A recent study to assess the efficacy of bromelain in controlling the oedema and pain after tooth extraction found it to be effective in treating postoperative oedema after third molar surgery (Inchingolo et al 2010). Bromelain, given once daily in acute tendon injury at a dosage of 7 mg/kg for 14 days, promoted healing by stimulating tenocyte proliferation in rats (Aiyegbusi et al 2011). Bromelain is generally well tolerated, but side effects include minor gastrointestinal upsets.

DEVIL'S CLAW, *HARPAGOPHYTUM PROCUMBENS* DC. EX MEISSNER (HARPAGOPHYTI RADIX) EU*

Devil's claw (Pedaliaceae) has fairly recently been developed into a successful and relatively well-characterized medicine. The name arises from the claw-like appearance of the fruit. The secondary storage roots are collected in the savannahs of southern Africa (mainly the Kalahari Desert) and, while still fresh, they are cut into small pieces and dried. The main exporters are South Africa and Namibia. Devil's claw was used traditionally as a tonic for 'illnesses of the blood', fever, kidney and bladder problems, during pregnancy and as an obstetric remedy for induction or acceleration of labour, as well as for expelling the retained placenta.

Constituents

The most important actives are considered to be the bitter iridoids, harpagide and harpagoside (Fig. 21.1), with 8-*O*-*p*-coumaroylharpagide, procumbide, 6'-*O*-*p*-coumaroylprocumbide, pagide and procumboside; the triterpenoids oleanolic and ursolic acids, β-sitosterol and a glycoside harproside. Other compounds present include phenylethyl glycosides such as verbascoside and isoacteoside, polyphenolic acids (caffeic, cinnamic, and chlorogenic acids), and flavonoids such as luteolin and kaempferol. According to the Eur. Ph. the drug must contain ≥1.2% harpagide and harpagoside, expressed as harpagoside.

Therapeutic uses and available evidence

In Europe, a tea (made from a dose of about 1.5 g/day of the powdered drug) has been used for the treatment of dyspeptic disorders such as indigestion and lack of appetite. This effect is due to the presence of bitter glycosides, the iridoids, which are present in large amounts.

Most pharmacological and clinical research has been conducted using standardized extracts for the treatment of rheumatic conditions and lower back pain. Several clinical studies, including some placebo-controlled double-blind trials, demonstrate the superiority of these extracts to placebo in patients with osteoarthritis, non-radicular back pain and other forms of chronic and acute pain. Other studies show their therapeutic equivalence to conventional forms of treatment. Devil's claw is generally well tolerated and appears to be a suitable alternative to NSAIDs, which often have gastrointestinal side effects (for review, see Barnes 2009, Cameron et al 2009).

The mechanism of action is not fully known: fractions of the extract containing the highest concentration of harpagoside inhibited COX-1 and COX-2 activity and greatly inhibited NO production, whereas in contrast, the fraction containing mainly the other iridoids increased COX-2 and did not alter NO and COX-1 activities. A fraction containing mainly cinnamic acid was able to reduce only NO production (Anauate et al 2010). An extract of *Harpagophytum procumbens* showed a significant antiinflammatory effect in the rat adjuvant-induced chronic arthritis model, and harpagoside dose-dependently suppressed the lipopolysaccharide (LPS)-induced production of inflammatory cytokines (IL-1β, IL-6, and TNF-α) in mouse macrophage cells (Inaba et al 2010). These demonstrate that harpagoside is probably the main active constituent

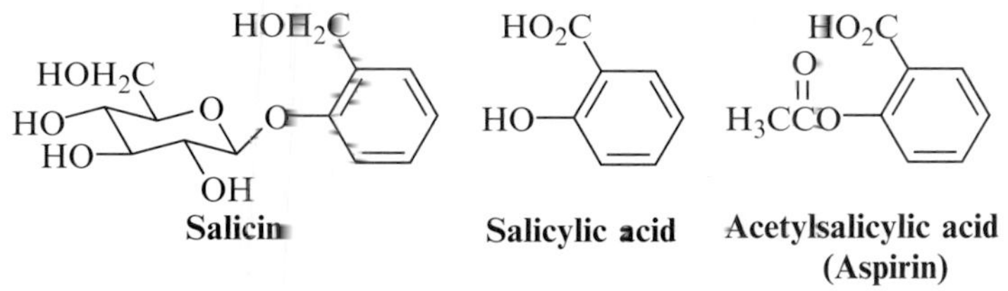

Salicin   Salicylic acid   Acetylsalicylic acid
                                   (Aspirin)

Fig. 21.1

responsible for the effect of devil's claw, but that other components from the crude extract can antagonize or increase the synthesis of inflammatory mediators. In summary, both the pharmacological mechanism and the compounds responsible for this activity have to be investigated further, and by in vivo methods. There are implications for the production methods for preparing devil's claw extracts, and a recent study of the antiinflammatory activity of various commercial products has demonstrated that there is a great difference in their composition, and concludes that the harpagoside content is not a reliable method of predicting the therapeutic efficacy (Ouitas and Heard 2010). Extracts of devil's claw are generally well tolerated but should not be used for patients with gastric or duodenal ulceration. The aqueous extract possesses spasmogenic, uterotonic action on rat uterine muscles (Mahomed and Ojewole 2009), leading credence to the folkloric obstetric uses but suggesting that it should be avoided in pregnant women. Side effects include minor gastrointestinal upsets.

ROSEHIP, *ROSA CANINA* L. (ROSAE PSEUDOFRUCTUS; ALSO KNOWN AS ROSAE FRUCTUS OR ROSAE PSEUDOFRUCTUS CUM FRUCTIBUS)

The fruits of the wild or dog rose, *Rosa canina* (Rosaceae) are known as rosehips, and are botanically 'pseudofruits', composed of achenes enclosed in a fleshy receptacle or hypanthium. The trichomes found inside rose hips are irritant and are often removed before powdering the fruit. There are several types of rosehip preparation available: rosehip and seed (the ripe pseudofruits, including the seed); rosehip (the ripe seed receptacle, freed from seed and attached trichomes), and rosehip seed (the ripe, dried seed). The whole pseudofruit, i.e. rosehip with seed, is most commonly used and widely investigated.

Constituents

Antiinflammatory constituents isolated from rosehip extracts include the triterpene acids, oleanolic, betulinic and ursolic acids; oleic, linoleic and alpha-linolenic acids, and a series of galactolipids which are thought to be a major contributor to the effects (Chrubasik et al 2008b).

Therapeutic uses and available evidence

Traditionally, rose hips were used as a source of vitamin C and were made into syrups for that purpose, but modern use is now focused on their antiinflammatory effects (for review, see Chrubasik et al 2008a). In a pilot surveillance study which included 152 patients with acute exacerbations of chronic pain, mainly of the lower back and knee, patients were recommended rose hip and seed powder at a dose providing up to 3 mg of galactolipid/day for up to 54 weeks. Multivariate analysis suggested an appreciable overall improvement, irrespective of type of pain, and this was reflected for most of the individual measures. There were no serious adverse events (Chrubasik et al 2008b). In a recent double-blind placebo-controlled trial of 89 patients with rheumatoid arthritis, treatment with encapsulated rose-hip powder 5 g daily for 6 months suggested that patients with rheumatoid arthritis may benefit from additional treatment with rose hip (Willich et al 2010). A study comparing powdered rose hip with and without the seeds found that extracts derived from rose hip without fruits were more effective in assays carried out for inhibition of COX-1, COX-2 and 5-LOX-mediated leukotriene B(4) formation, as well as for antioxidant capacity (Wenzig et al 2008). Extracts of rosehips have displayed potent antiinflammatory and antinociceptive activities in several in vivo experimental models (Deliorman Orhan et al 2007, but the mechanism of action and the active constituents are still not fully known. Bioassay-guided fractionation of rosehip powder yielded the triterpene acids, oleanolic acid and ursolic acid, as inhibitors of lipopolysaccharide induced interleukin-6 release (Saaby et al 2011), but these are ubiquitous compounds and may only play a part in the overall activity.

TURMERIC, *CURCUMA DOMESTICA* VAL. (CURCUMAE DOMESTICAE RHIZOMA) 🇪🇺✴

The rhizomes of turmeric (syn. *C. longa* L., Zingiberaceae) are imported as a ready-prepared and ground, dark yellow powder with a characteristic taste and odour. The distinctive colour and presence of starch grains (as both simple and compound grains) and cork make the microscopic identification of the drug relatively straightforward. Turmeric is used in religious ceremonies by Hindus and Buddhists. It is important in the preparation of curry powders and is increasingly being used as a colouring agent because of the increased use of natural ingredients in foods. A related species is Javanese turmeric (*Curcuma xanthorrhiza* Roxb., Curcumae xanthorrhizae rhizoma; Eur. Ph.), which is mostly used for dyspepsia and other gastrointestinal problems.

Constituents

Three classes of compounds are particularly important: the curcuminoids – the mixture known as curcumin (Fig. 21.2) – consisting of several phenolic diarylheptanoids including curcumin, monodemethoxycurcumin and bisdemethoxycurcumin; an essential oil (about 3–5%), containing about 60% sesquiterpene ketones (turmerones), including arturmerone, α-atlantone, zingberene, with borneol, α-phellandrene, eugenol and others; and polysaccharides such as glycans, the ukonans A–D.

Therapeutic uses and available evidence

Turmeric is becoming increasingly popular in the West, as an antiinflammatory and antihepatotoxic agent (see also Chapter 14, Gastrointestinal and biliary system). It is also widely used in Ayurveda and Chinese medicine as an antiinflammatory, digestive, blood purifier, antiseptic and general tonic. It is given internally and also applied externally to wounds and insect bites. Most of the actions are attributable to the curcuminoids, although some of the essential oil components are also antiinflammatory. The efficacy of curcumin and its regulation of multiple targets, as well as its safety for human use, means that turmeric has received considerable interest as a potential therapeutic agent for the prevention and/or treatment of various malignant diseases, arthritis, allergies, Alzheimer's disease and many other inflammatory illnesses (for review, see Zhou et al 2011). Antiinflammatory properties have been documented in numerous pharmacological

models, and the use of turmeric seems promising, despite the limited number of clinical studies and poor bioavailability (for review, see Henrotin et al 2010). Curcumin has been studied as an anticancer drug and inhibits iNOS (inducible nitric oxide synthase) in both in vitro and in vivo mouse models via a mechanism involving the pro-inflammatory transcription factor NF-κB. It has also been shown to inhibit the activation of another transcription factor (AP-1), indicating that curcumin may be a nonspecific inhibitor of NF-κB. Reports also indicate cyclo-oxygenase inhibition and free radical scavenging ability as potential targets (for review, see Epstein et al 2010). Immunostimulant activity, due to the polysaccharide fraction, has been shown, and anti-asthmatic effects have been noted, together with antimutagenic and anticarcinogenic effects. It is the subject of much current research but clinical evidence is urgently needed. Turmeric is well tolerated.

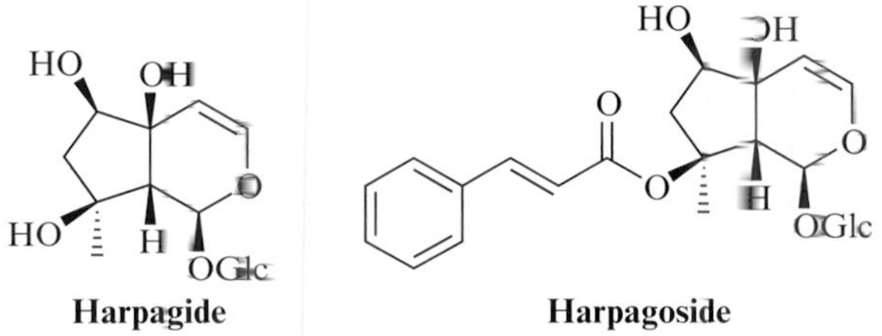

WILLOW BARK, *SALIX* SPP. (SALICIS CORTEX) EU ✷

Salix spp., including *S. purpurea* L., *S. fragilis* L., *S. daphnoides* Vill. and *S. alba* L. (Salicaceae), are the source of the drug 'willow bark'. They are trees and shrubs common in alpine ecosystems, flooded areas and along the margins of streams. Willow bark is a European phytomedicine with a long tradition of use for chronic forms of pain, rheumatoid diseases, fever and headache. As is well known, one of its main compounds, salicin, served as a lead molecule for the development of aspirin (acetylsalicylic acid).

Constituents

Phenolic glycosides, including salicin (Fig. 21.3), phenolic acids, tannins (mainly dimeric and polymeric procyanidins) and flavonoids are the most prominent groups of compounds. The most commonly used willow bark dry extract has a salicin content of 15–18%.

Very few pharmacological studies of individual compounds from willow bark (and their metabolites)

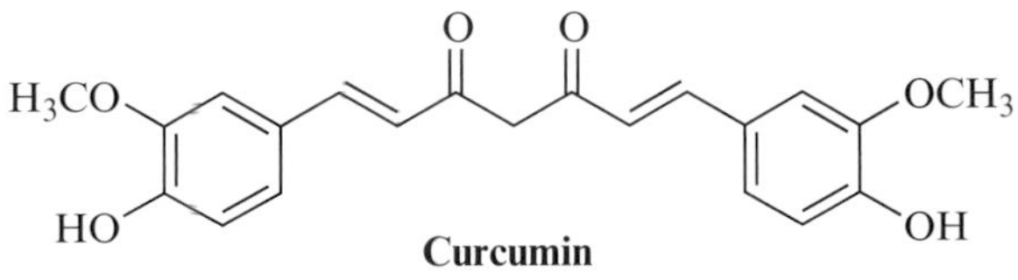

Harpagide

Harpagoside

Fig. 21.2

Curcumin

Fig. 21.3

have been conducted. The extract, however, exerts effects on several pro-inflammatory targets, including both isoforms of cyclo-oxygenase and, recently, willow bark water extract STW 33–1 has been shown to produce a significant inhibition of TNFα and NF-κB in activated monocytes (Bonaterra et al 2010).

Therapeutic uses and available evidence

Willow bark has been studied clinically. The effectiveness of an extract of willow bark (which is licensed as a medicine in Germany) has been shown to be superior to placebo for osteoarthritis and lower back pain, and with fewer side effects than for example aspirin (for review, see Vlachlojannis et al 2009). However, further more stringent clinical and mechanistic studies are needed. In very high doses, the side effects of salicylates may be encountered, although these are rarely seen at therapeutic levels of the extract. In general, the effective dose contains lower amounts of salicylate than would be expected by calculation, and a form of synergy is thought to be operating within the extract.

DRUGS USED IN GOUT

Gout is a very painful, localized inflammation of the joints (particularly those of the thumb and big toe) caused by hyperuricaemia and the consequent formation of needle-like crystals of uric acid in the joint. For prevention, the xanthine oxidase inhibitor allopurinol is the drug of choice, but an alternative is sulfinpyrazone, which increases excretion of uric acid. Prophylactic treatment should never be initiated during an acute attack as it may prolong it. Acute gout is normally treated with indomethacin or other NSAIDs (but not aspirin), but, if inappropriate, colchicine can be used.

COLCHICINE EU✦

Colchine (Fig. 21.4) is a pure alkaloid extracted from the corms and flowers of *Colchicum autumnale* L., the autumn crocus or meadow saffron (Colchicaceae, formerly Liliaceae). The plant grows from bulbs in meadows throughout Europe and North Africa, typically appearing during the autumn, with the fruit developing over winter and being dispersed prior to the first mowing of the meadows. The leaves and the fruit appear during spring. The plant extract

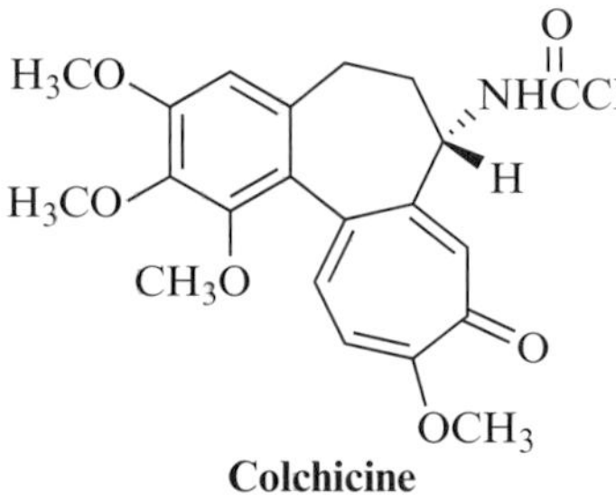

Colchicine

Fig. 21.4

is not used because colchicine is highly toxic and the dose must be rigorously controlled.

Colchicine is used in the acute phase of gout, particularly when NSAIDs are either ineffective or contraindicated (for review, see Schlesinger et al 2009). Colchicine is occasionally also used as prophylaxis for Mediterranean familial fever. It is an important tool for biochemical research, as an inhibitor of the separation of the chromosomes during mitosis (e.g. used in breeding experiments to produce polyploid organisms). Colchicine causes gastrointestinal upsets such as nausea, vomiting, abdominal pain and diarrhoea. The dose is 1 mg initially, followed by increments of 500 µg every 2–3 hours until relief is obtained, to a maximum of 6 mg. The course should not be repeated within 3 days.

TOPICAL ANTI-INFLAMMATORY AGENTS

Most topical antirheumatics are rubifacients, which act by counter-irritation. They are used for localized pain or when systemic drugs are not appropriate. Many contain salicylates, and capsaicin is used for severe pain (e.g. with shingles). They should not be used in children, pregnant or breastfeeding women or with occlusive dressings. Arnica is also widely employed, despite little clinical evidence to support its use.

ARNICA, *ARNICA MONTANA* L. (ARNICAE FLOS) EU✦

Arnica (Asteraceae) is widely used in many European countries, including the UK. The flower heads are the part used, and, as A. *montana* is protected, other species are being investigated as substitutes. Extracts and tinctures are applied topically, for bruising, sprains, swellings and inflammation, usually in the form of a cream or gel.

Constituents

Arnica species are rich in sesquiterpene lactones of the pseudoguianolide type. The most abundant sesquiterpene lactone in *A. montana* is helenalin (Fig. 21.5), with 11α,13-dihydrohelenalin. Flavonoids, including quercetin and kaempferol derivatives, some coumarins and an essential oil are the other groups of natural products found typically in the flower heads of arnica.

Therapeutic uses and available evidence

Extracts of arnica and the pure sesquiterpene lactones with an exocyclic methylene group (e.g. helenalin) have been shown to exert antiinflammatory effects in vivo in animal models, although few clinical studies have been carried out. A randomised, double-blind study in 204 patients with active osteoarthritis of the hands, carried out to compare ibuprofen gel (5%) with arnica gel (50 g tincture/100 g, drug extract ratio 1:20), found that there were no differences in pain relief and hand function after 21 days' treatment between the two groups. Adverse events were reported by five patients (4.8%) on arnica, slightly lower than the ibuprofen group (Widrig et al 2007).

However, a recent trial conducted in 53 subjects who were carrying out eccentric calf exercises found that rather than decreasing leg pain, arnica increased leg pain 24 hours after exercise (Adkison et al 2010). However, this effect did not extend to the 48-hour measurement, and it is not clear how this model relates to most of the clinical situations in which arnica is used. There was no difference in muscle tenderness or ankle range of motion.

Helenalin is well known for its in vitro effects on several transcription factors, including NF-κB and NF-AT. Arnica preparations also suppress matrix metalloproteinase-1 (MMP1) and MMP13 mRNA levels in articular chondrocytes at low concentrations, possibly due to inhibition of DNA binding of the transcription factors AP-1 and NF-kappaB (Jäger et al 2009). The cytotoxicity of the sesquiterpene lactones is well documented, and allergic

Helenalin

Fig. 21.5

reactions may occur. Arnica is used externally, except in homoeopathic preparations, but the sesquiterpene lactones have been shown to be absorbed through the skin (Tekko et al 2006).

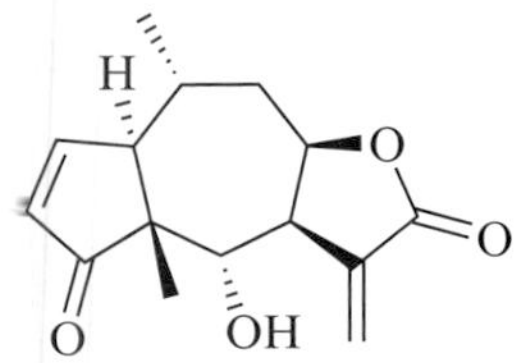

CAPSAICIN

Capsaicin is the pungent oleo-resin of the fruit of the chilli pepper (*Capsicum frutescens* L., and some varieties of *C. annuum* L., Solanaceae), also known as capsicum, cayenne, or hot. Green and red (or bell) peppers and paprika are produced by milder varieties. The plant is indigenous to tropical America and Africa but is widely cultivated.

Constituents

Capsaicin itself is 8-methyl-*N*-vanillyl-non-6-enamide; other capsaicinoids such as dihydrocapsaicin, nordihydrocapsaicin, homodihydrocapsaicin are present in the natural product. These are esters of vanillyl amine with C_8-C_{13} fatty acids.

Therapeutic uses and available evidence

Capsaicin acts on vanilloid receptors, causing inflammation, but it also desensitizes sensory nerve endings to pain stimulation by depleting the neuropeptide Substance P from local C-type nerve fibres. It is used as a local analgesic in the treatment of postherpetic neuralgia, diabetic neuropathy, osteoarthritis and for pruritus (Papoiu and Yosipovitch 2010). In the management of intractable neuropathic pain, it may provide a degree of pain relief to some patients (Derry et al 2009). Capsaicin has long been used in cough and cold remedies, and recent findings that the vanilloid 1 (TRPV1) receptor is a sensor of airway irritation and initiator of the cough reflex (Geppetti et al 2010) may provide a rationale for that usage.

For external use, capsaicin is normally formulated as a cream containing 0.025%, 0.075% or 0.75%. Capsaicin can produce severe irritation. It causes burning on initial application and should not be applied near the eyes, mucous membranes or to broken skin. It should be avoided in children and pregnant or breastfeeding women.

WINTERGREEN OIL, *GAULTHERIA PROCUMBENS* L., *BETULA LENTA* L.

Wintergreen oil is now most often obtained from *Betula lenta* (Betulaceae) rather than *Gaultheria procumbens* (Ericaceae), although both have similar compositions. It has a characteristic odour of methyl salicylate.

Constituents

The oil contains methyl salicylate (about 98%), which is produced by enzymatic hydrolysis of phenolic glycosides during maceration and steam distillation.

Therapeutic uses and available evidence

Methyl salicylate is antiinflammatory and anti-rheumatic. Oil of wintergreen is used mainly in the form of an ointment or liniment for rheumatism, sprains, sciatica, neuralgia and all kinds of muscular pain. Methyl salicylate can cause irritation. It should not be applied near the eyes, mucous membranes or to broken skin, and should be avoided in children and pregnant or breastfeeding women.

NOCTURNAL LEG CRAMPS

Night cramps are common in elderly people, and particularly in patients with liver disease such as cirrhosis.

QUININE EU✦

Quinine is isolated from the bark of *Cinchona* spp. Quinine salts can be effective in reducing their incidence, but should be avoided for routine use in the management of muscle cramps because of their potential for cardiac toxicity. However, in select patients they can be considered once potential side effects are taken into account. It has been recommended that quinine should be used more in patients with cirrhosis, subject to further investigations (Corbani et al 2008). Quinine salts are used in doses of 200–300 mg at bedtime, in ambulatory patients. For further information on quinine, including the structure, see Chapter 18.

References

Adkison, J.D., Bauer, D.W., Chang, T., 2010. The effect of topical arnica on muscle pain. Ann. Pharmacother. 44, 1579–1584.

Aiyegbusi, A.I., Duru, F.I., Anunobi, C.C., Noronha, C.C., Okanlawon, A.O., 2011. Bromelain in the early phase of healing in acute crush Achilles tendon injury. Phytother. Res. 25, 49–52.

Anauate, M.C., Torres, L.M., de Mello, S.B., 2010. Effect of isolated fractions of *Harpagophytum procumbens* D.C. (devil's claw) on COX-1, COX-2 activity and nitric oxide production on whole-blood assay. Phytother Res. 24(9), 1365–1369.

Barnes, J., 2009. Devil's claw (*Harpagophytum procumbens*). Also known as 'grapple plant' or 'wood spider'. J. Prim. Health Care 1, 238–239.

Bonaterra, G.A., Heinrich, E.U., Kelber, O., Weiser, D., Metz, J., Kinscherf, R., 2010. Anti-inflammatory effects of the willow

bark extract STW 33-I (Proaktiv$^{(®)}$) in LPS-activated human monocytes and differentiated macrophages. Phytomedicine 17, 1106–1113.

Cameron, M., Gagnier, J.J., Little, C.V., Parsons, T.J., Blümle, A., Chrubasik, S., 2009. Evidence of effectiveness of herbal medicinal products in the treatment of arthritis. Part I: Osteoarthritis. Phytother. Res. 23, 1497–1515.

Chrubasik, C., Roufogalis, B.D., Müller-Ladner, U., Chrubasik, S., 2008a. A systematic review on the *Rosa canina* effect and efficacy profiles. Phytother. Res. 22, 725–733.

Chrubasik, C., Wiesner, L., Black, A., Müller-Ladner, U., Chrubasik, S., 2008b. A one-year survey on the use of a powder from *Rosa canina* lito in acute exacerbations of chronic pain. Phytother. Res. 22, 1141–1148.

Corbani, A., Manousou, P., Calvaruso, V., Xirouchakis, I., Burroughs, A.K., 2008. Muscle

cramps in cirrhosis: the therapeutic value of quinine. Is it underused. Dig. Liver Dis. 40, 794–799.

Deliorman Orhan, D., Hartevioğlu, A., Küpeli, E., Yesilada, E., 2007. In vivo anti-inflammatory and antinociceptive activity of the crude extract and fractions from *Rosa canina* L. fruits. J. Ethnopharmacol. 112, 394–400.

Derry, S., Lloyd, R., Moore, R.A., McQuay, H.J., 2009. Topical capsaicin for chronic neuropathic pain in adults. Cochrane Database Syst. Rev. 4, CD007393.

Epstein, J., Sanderson, I.R., Macdonald, T.T., 2010. Curcumin as a therapeutic agent: the evidence from in vitro, animal and human studies. Br. J. Nutr. 103, 1545–1557.

Geppetti, P., Patacchini, R., Nassini, R., Materazzi, S., 2010. Cough: the emerging role of the TRPA1 channel. Lung 188, S63–S68.

Henrotin, Y., Clutterbuck, A.L., Allaway, D., et al., 2010. Biological actions of curcumin on articular chondrocytes. Osteoarthritis Cartilage 18, 141–149.

Inaba, K., Murata, K., Naruto, S., Matsuda, H., 2010. Inhibitory effects of devil's claw (secondary root of *Harpagophytum procumbens*) extract and harpagoside on cytokine production in mouse macrophages. J. Nat. Med. 64, 219–222.

Inchingolo, F., Tatullo, M., Marrelli, M., et al., 2010. Clinical trial with bromelain in third molar exodontia. Eur. Rev. Med. Pharmacol. Sci. 14, 771–774.

Jäger, C., Hrenn, A., Zwingmann, J., Suter, A., Merfort, I., 2009. Phytomedicines prepared from Arnica flowers inhibit the transcription factors AP-1 and NF-kappaB and modulate the activity of MMP1 and MMP13 in human and bovine chondrocytes. Planta Med. 75, 1319–1325.

Mahomed, I.M., Ojewole, J.A., 2009. Uterotonic effect of *Harpagophytum procumbens* DC (Pedaliaceae) secondary root aqueous extract on rat isolated uterine horns. J. Smooth Muscle Res. 45, 231–239.

Ouitas, N.A., Heard, C., 2010. Estimation of the relative antiinflammatory efficacies of six commercial preparations of *Harpagophytum procumbens* (Devil's Claw). Phytother. Res. 24, 333–338.

Papoiu, A.D., Yosipovitch, G., 2010. Topical capsaicin. The fire of a 'hot' medicine is reignited. Expert Opin. Pharmacother. 11, 1359–1371.

Saaby, L., Jäger, A.K., Moesby, L., Hansen, E.W., Christensen, S.B., 2011. Isolation of immunomodulatory triterpene acids from a standardized rose hip powder (*Rosa canina* L.). Phytother. Res. 25, 195–201.

Schlesinger, N., Dalbeth, N., Perez-Ruiz, F., 2009. Gout – what are the treatment options? Expert Opin. Pharmacother. 10, 1319–1328.

Tekko, I.A., Bonner, M.C., Bowen, R.D., Williams, A.C., 2006. Permeation of bioactive constituents from *Arnica montana* preparations through human skin in-vitro. J. Pharm. Pharmacol. 58, 1167–1176.

Vlachojannis, J.E., Cameron, M., Chrubasik, S., 2009. A systematic review on the effectiveness of willow bark for musculoskeletal pain. Phytother. Res. 23, 897–900.

Wenzig, E.M., Widowitz, U., Kunert, O., et al., 2008. Phytochemical composition and in vitro pharmacological activity of two rose hip (*Rosa canina* L.) preparations. Phytomedicine 15, 826–835.

Widrig, R., Suter, A., Saller, R., Melzer, J., 2007. Choosing between NSAID and arnica for topical treatment of hand osteoarthritis in a randomised, double-blind study. Rheumatol. Int. 27, 585–591.

Willich, S.N., Rossnagel, K., Roll, S., et al., 2010. Rose hip herbal remedy in patients with rheumatoid arthritis – a randomised controlled trial. Phytomedicine 17, 87–93.

Zhou, H., Beevers, C.S., Huang, S., 2011. The targets of curcumin. Curr. Drug Targets 12, 332–347.

Chapter 22

The skin

Inflammatory and infectious skin diseases have a high prevalence in both developing and developed countries. Anti-infective preparations have been covered separately in Chapter 18. It is in the areas of dry and itchy skin, inflammation and wound healing, that medicinal plants have an important place.

DRY/ITCHY SKIN CONDITIONS AND ECZEMA

Dry and scaly skin conditions are very common and can arise from many causes. Diagnosis should be carried out initially by a medical practitioner in order to exclude infection, infestation or other serious disorders. Emollients, such as oil-based preparations based on arachis oil, or oat extracts, are usually the first line of treatment. Plant extracts are often incorporated into these preparations and can be very useful.

ARACHIS OIL (ARACHIDIS OLEUM RAFFINATUM) EU*

Arachis oil (also known as groundnut or peanut oil) is expressed from *Arachis hypogaea* L. (Fabaceae). It is a fixed oil consisting mainly of glycerides of oleic and linoleic acids. It is an ingredient of emollient creams and bath oils. Peanuts are dangerously allergenic to some individuals, and the oil should be avoided in these patients as a precaution.

OATS, *AVENA SATIVA* L.

Oats (*Avena sativa*, Graminae) are a widely distributed cereal crop. The seeds, with the husks removed, are crushed to form a coarse powder, which is creamy white in colour.

Constituents

Oats contain proteins (prolamines known as avenin, avenalin and gliadin), polyphenols known as avenanthramides, starch and soluble polysaccharides (mainly β-glucans and arabinogalactans), saponin glycosides including avenacosides A and B, and soyasaponin I. The fatty oil is composed of phytosterols including cholesterol, β-sitosterol and Δ^5-avenasterol, avenoleic, oleic, ricinoleic and linoleic acids and vitamin E.

Therapeutic uses and available evidence

Oats are externally emollient, and a colloidal fraction is used in bath preparations for eczema, and itchy or dry skin, often with success, especially if used regularly over a long period. Cells treated with avenanthramides showed a significant inhibition of TNF-alpha-induced NF-kappaB activity and subsequent reduction of interleukin-8 (IL-8) release. Topical application of avenanthramides mitigated inflammation in murine models of contact hypersensitivity and neurogenic inflammation and reduced pruritogen-induced scratching in a murine itch model. Avenanthramides are thus potent anti-inflammatory agents that appear to mediate the anti-irritant effects of oats (Sur et al 2008). The many clinical properties of colloidal oatmeal derive from its variety of chemical constituents: the starches and beta-glucans are responsible for the protective and water-holding functions of oat and the presence of phenolics confers antioxidant and antiinflammatory activity. Some of the oat phenols are also strong ultraviolet absorbers and the cleansing activity of oat is mostly due to saponins (Kurtz and Wild 2007). Together, these make colloidal oatmeal a cleanser, moisturizer, buffer, as well as a soothing and protective antiinflammatory agent (for review, see Cerio et al 2010).

Oat tinctures are also taken internally for their reputed sedative activity, but this has not yet been proven. Ingestion of oats lowers cholesterol levels; an effect attributed to the saponins and polysaccharides.

INFLAMMATORY SKIN CONDITIONS

Allergic reactions, psoriasis, burns, bruising and general inflammation of skin are common. Severe cases are treated with corticosteroids as well as emollient preparations, ideally under medical supervision. However, minor disorders respond well to phytotherapy, with soothing and antiinflammatory herbal products, as outlined below.

ALOE VERA, *ALOE BARBADENSIS* MILL. [SYN. *ALOE VERA* (L.) BURM. F.]

The name 'aloe vera' is usually applied to the gel obtained from the centre of the fleshy leaves of various species of aloe, to differentiate from the anthraquinone-rich exudate or 'aloes', which is used as a purgative. The botanical nomenclature of the genus *Aloe* (Asphodeliaceae) is complex. The succulent, non-fibrous leaves are about 30–40 cm long, up to 5 cm in diameter and occur in a terminal, sessile rosette. It is common practice in the tropics to use the gel and the heated leaves for burns and other inflammatory skin conditions. Aloe vera is added to shampoo, skin creams, 'after sun' preparations (and even washing powder) but normally in concentrations too low to have any therapeutic effect.

Constituents

An ill-defined extract of the fleshy leaves, obtained by cutting open and scraping out the gel, is used in the preparation of externally used products, especially cosmetics. It contains polysaccharides consisting mainly of glucomannans, glycoproteins such as the aloctins, enzymes such as carboxypeptidases and variable amounts of anthraquinone glycosides.

Therapeutic uses and available evidence

Aloe vera gel is used mainly in the form of the pure gel, applied as a lotion. It may be stabilized and a preservative added for this purpose. For dermatological preparations, there is some evidence for antibacterial, antiinflammatory, emollient and moisturizing effects. The polysaccharides are important as soothing and immunostimulating agents. Some of the glycoproteins have similar effects, while the anthraquinone derivatives are antibacterial. Enzymes extracted from aloe vera gel have been shown to be analgesic and inhibit thermal damage and vascular permeability in mice. The fresh leaf pulp is antioxidant and induces carcinogen-metabolizing phase I enzymes. The gel has been reported to be effective in the treatment of stomach and aphthous (mouth) ulcers. Although few good clinical studies are available, aloe vera gel seems to be helpful in the treatment of burns and to aid wound healing (for review, see Maenthaisong et al 2007). Aloe vera cream was found to be at least as effective as 0.1% triamcinolone acetonide in reducing the clinical symptoms of psoriasis in a recent study (Choonhakarn et al 2010), and in UV-induced erythema, aloe vera gel (97.5%) displayed some antiinflammatory effects superior to those of 1% hydrocortisone in placebo gel (Reuter et al 2008), supporting its use as an after-sun treatment and post-radiotherapy emollient.

EVENING PRIMROSE OIL, *OENOTHERA BIENNIS* L. (OENOTHERA BIENNIS OLEUM) AND OTHER SPP.

Oenothera spp. (Onagraceae) are common ornamentals, the use of which, in Western phytomedicine, was inspired by that of the indigenous North American Indians. It is now of the seed oil that is used in the treatment of atopic eczema. The plant is a medium or tall hairy perennial with alternate, lanceolate leaves and relatively large yellow, four-petalled flowers, developing into long elongated capsules containing the seeds from which the oil is extracted.

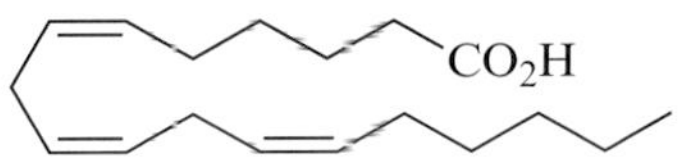

γ-Linoleic acid

Fig. 22.1

Constituents

The seed oil contains about 70% *cis*-linoleic acid and about 9% *cis*-γ-linolenic acid (Fig. 22.1).

Therapeutic uses and available evidence

The fatty oil has been extensively investigated, and its therapeutic benefits ascribed mainly to the γ-linolenic acid content. It is taken internally as well as applied externally. Supplementation with omega-6 essential fatty acids (omega-6 EFAs) is of potential interest in the treatment of atopic dermatitis since patients with atopic dermatitis have been reported to have imbalances in EFA levels. EFAs play a vital role in skin structure and physiology, and deficiency replicates the symptoms of atopic dermatitis. To date, most studies of EFA supplementation in atopic dermatitis have produced conflicting results, although a systematic review has concluded that evening primrose oil has a simultaneous, beneficial effect on itching, crusting, oedema and redness that becomes apparent between 4 and 8 weeks after treatment is initiated. This effect is said to be reduced in association with increasing frequency of potent steroid use (Morse and Clough 2006). The main indications for which clinical evidence exists are: atopic eczema (especially in infants), mastalgia, rheumatoid arthritis and premenstrual syndrome, although the evidence of efficacy is equivocal. Evening primrose oil is usually taken in conjunction with vitamin E to prevent oxidation.

Note: The seed oil of *Borago officinalis* L. (borage, Boraginaceae), also known as Star Flower oil, is used in a similar way to evening primrose oil, but contains 2–3 times more γ-linolenic acid. It seems to provide some benefit to patients with atopic eczema (Foster et al 2010).

MARIGOLD, *CALENDULA OFFICINALIS* L. (CALENDULAE FLOS) ■❋

Calendula officinalis (Scotch or 'pot') marigold is one of the best known medicinal plants of Europe and has a long tradition of pharmaceutical use. Its origin is unclear and it has been cultivated for many centuries. Consequently, many varieties exist and its usage as an ornamental has increased the botanical variance in the species. The flower heads are relatively large, with a diameter of up to 5 cm, and yellow-orange. Some varieties have both ligulate (tongue-shaped) and radiate florets, others have only the ligulate type. The Eur. Ph. (European Pharmacopoeia) requires that only flower heads exclusively containing ligulate florets should be used.

Constituents

Marigold flowerheads contain saponins based on oleanolic acid, including calendasaponins A, B, C and D, and triterpene pentacyclic alcohols such as faradol, arnidiol, erythrodiol, calenduladiol, heliantriols A1, B0, B1 and B2, taraxasterol, lupeol and ursatriol. It also contains flavonoids, including hyperoside and rutin; sesquiterpene and ionone glycosides such as officinosides A, B, C and D, loliolide and arvoside A; a volatile oil and polysaccharides PS-I, -II and -III; and chlorogenic acid.

Therapeutic uses and available evidence

Pharmaceutical uses include inflammatory skin conditions such as topical application for wound healing and after radiotherapy. The flower heads and extracts from them are well known for their antiinflammatory properties, which are mainly due to the lipophilic triterpene alcohols, notably the esters of faradiol. These were demonstrated using in vitro models such as phorbol ester induced mouse ear oedema or croton oil induced irritation. Marigold extract prevented UVB irradiation-induced GSH depletion in the skin of hairless mice after oral administration and increased gelatinase activity, which may be beneficial for skin healing and pro-collagen synthesis (Fonseca et al 2010). Both oral and topical application of *Calendula* flower extract improved healing of excision wounds in rats and reduced the time needed for re-epithelization (Preethi and Kuttan 2009). Extracts stimulated proliferation and migration of fibroblasts at low concentrations (Fronza et al 2009), again supporting its use in wound healing, while the essential oil exerts (in vitro) antibacterial and antifungal effects. Immunostimulant effects have been reported for polysaccharide fractions. Few clinical studies are available to further validate these pharmacological data, although some preliminary studies indicate efficacy.

WITCH HAZEL, *HAMAMELIS VIRGINIANA* L. (HAMAMELIS FOLIUM, AND HAMAMELIS FOLIUM ET CORTEX) EU*

Witch hazel (*Hamamelis virginiana* L., Hamamelidaceae) is indigenous to North America and Canada. The leaves are broadly oval, up to 15 cm long, 7 cm broad, the margin dentate or crenate, the apex acute and the base asymmetrically cordate. The distilled extract, known simply as 'witch hazel', is used as an astringent in skin and eye inflammation.

Constituents

The leaves and bark contain tannins, composed mainly of gallotannins with some condensed catechins and proanthocyanins. These include 'hamamelitannin' which is a mixture of related tannins, including galloylhamameloses and flavonoids.

Therapeutic uses and available evidence

Witch hazel is widely used for the treatment of haemorrhoids, bruises, skin irritation, spots and blemishes and redness of the eye. Hamamelitannin inhibits TNF-mediated endothelial cell death without altering TNF-induced upregulation of endothelial adhesiveness (Habtemariam 2002), which may explain the anti-haemorrhagic use. The proanthocyanidins, gallotannins and gallates are highly active as free radical scavengers. Witch hazel phenolics protected red blood cells from free radical-induced haemolysis and were mildly cytotoxic to 3T3 fibroblasts and HaCat keratinocytes; they also inhibited the proliferation of tumoral SK-Mel 28 melanoma cells at lower concentrations than grape and pine procyanidins (Touriño et al 2008).

Antiviral activity against *Herpes* viruses has been shown, and several clinical studies have demonstrated efficacy of topically applied witch hazel in inflammatory conditions, including UV-irradiated burning and atopic dermatitis (Hughes-Formella et al 2002). An observational study in children (age 27 days to 11 years) with minor skin injuries, diaper dermatitis, or localized inflammation of skin found hamamelis ointment to be as effective as dexpanthenol, and concluded that hamamelis ointment is an effective and safe treatment for certain skin disorders in children up to the age of 11 years (Wolff and Kieser 2007). However, a review of the literature of hamamelis water in women suffering

episiotomy pain following childbirth found it to confer no advantage over ice packs (East et al 2007). Witch hazel is used in after-shave lotions and in cosmetic preparations.

WOUND HEALING

CENTELLA ASIATICA (L.) URBAN (CENTELLAE HERBA) EU*

Centella asiatica (Apiceae), also known as gotu kola, Indian Pennywort, Brahmi and Manduukaparani, is an important medicinal plant throughout the world. The leaves of this small plant are kidney-shaped (reniform), long-stalked with rounded apices. The pinkish to red flowers are borne in small rounded umbels. It is a native of tropical and subtropical Asia and generally grows along streams, ditches and in low wet areas. As a consequence, this makes the species prone to an exposure to sewerage, so there is a risk of high levels of bacterial and other contaminations (including heavy metals). In Sri Lanka and other countries it is an element of the local cuisine, used as a vegetable or in salads.

Constituents

The triterpenes are generally considered to be the major active components. They are mainly pentacyclic triterpenic acids of the ursane- or oleanane-type, and their glycosides, and include asiatic acid, the asiaticosides, madecassic acid, madecassoside, brahmoside, brahmic acid, brahminoside, thankuniside, isothankuniside, centelloside, madasiatic acid, and the centellasaponins. There are some differences depending on the geographical origin of the plant. Flavonoids based on kaempferol and quercetin are present and there is a small amount of essential oil, with α-humulene, β-caryophyllene and bicyclogermacrene as the main constituents.

Therapeutic uses and available evidence

A wide range of pharmacological effects have been reported, including as a general tonic (see also Chapter 25), the most important being its use in skin conditions, including wound healing, inflammation, psoriasis, keloid and the prevention of stretch marks during pregnancy. Creams containing extracts are applied topically, but the herb is also taken internally for mental disorders, to improve memory, for atherosclerosis and to improve venous insufficiency and microangiopathy (for review, see Brinkhaus et al 2000).

Despite the lack of clinical studies, pharmacological studies support the use of Centella in skin conditions. Extracts have been shown to significantly increase the wound breaking strength in a rat incision wound model, improving the rate of epithelization and wound contraction (Shetty et al 2006). Different constituents affect the different phases of wound repair: the triterpenes stimulated extracellular matrix accumulation in rat experimental wounds (Coldren et al 2003), whereas asiatic acid stimulated collagen synthesis, and madecassoside increased collagen secretion (Lee et al 2006). Centella has been suggested as a topical anti-psoriatic agent, and extracts have been shown to inhibit keratinocyte replication. The effect was thought to be due to its two constituent triterpenoid glycosides madecassoside and asiaticoside (Sampson et al 2001).

References

Brinkhaus, B., Lindner, M., Schuppan, D., Hahn, E.G., 2000. Chemical, pharmacological and clinical profile of the East Asian medical plant Centella asiatica. Phytomedicine 7, 427–448.

Cerio, R., Dohil, M., Jeanine, D., Magina, S., Mahé, E., Stratigos, A.J., 2010. Mechanism of action and clinical benefits of colloidal oatmeal for dermatologic practice. J. Drugs Dermatol. 9, 1116–1120.

Choonhakarn, C., Busaracome, P., Sripanidkulchai, B., Sarakarn, P., 2010. A prospective, randomized clinical trial comparing topical aloe vera with 0.1% triamcinolone acetonide in mild to moderate plaque psoriasis. J. Eur. Acad. Dermatol. Venereol. 24, 168–172.

Coldren, C.D., Hashim, P., Ali, J.M., Oh, S.K., Sinskey, A.J., Rha, C., 2003. Gene expression changes in the human fibroblast induced by Centella asiatica triterpenoids. Planta Med. 69, 725–732.

East, C.E., Begg, L., Henshall, N.E., Marchant, P., Wallace, K., 2007. Local cooling for relieving pain from perineal trauma sustained during childbirth. Cochrane Database Syst. Rev (4):CD006304.

Fonseca, Y.M., Catini, C.D., Vicentini, F.T., Nomizo, A., Gerlach, R.F., Fonseca, M.J., 2010. Protective effect of Calendula officinalis extract against UVB-induced oxidative stress in skin: evaluation of reduced glutathione levels and matrix metalloproteinase secretion. J. Ethnopharmacol. 127, 596–601.

Foster, R.H., Hardy, G., Alany, R.G., 2010. Borage oil in the treatment of atopic dermatitis. Nutrition 26, 708–718.

Fronza, M., Heinzmann, B., Hamburger, M., Laufer, S., Merfort, I., 2009. Determination of the wound healing effect of Calendula extracts using the scratch assay with 3T3 fibroblasts. J. Ethnopharmacol. 126, 463–467.

Habtemariam, S., 2002. Hamamelitannin from Hamamelis virginiana inhibits the tumour necrosis factor-alpha (TNF)-induced endothelial cell death in vitro. Toxicon 40, 83–88.

Hughes-Formella, B.J., Filbry, A., Gassmueller, J., Rippke, F., 2002. Anti-inflammatory efficacy of topical preparations with 10% hamamelis distillate in a UV erythema test. Skin Pharmacol. Appl. Skin Physiol. 15, 125–132.

Kurtz, E.S., Wallo, W., 2007. Colloidal oatmeal: history, chemistry and clinical properties. J. Drugs Dermatol. 6, 167–170.

Lee, J., Jung, E., Lim, J., et al., 2006. Asiaticoside induces human collagen I synthesis through TGFbeta receptor I kinase (TbetaRI kinase)-independent Smad signaling. Planta Med. 72, 324–328.

Maenthaisong, R., Chaiyakunapruk, N., Niruntraporn, S., Kongkaew, C., 2007. The efficacy of aloe vera used for burn wound healing: a systematic review. Burns 33, 713–718.

Morse, N.L., Clough, P.M., 2006. A meta-analysis of randomized, placebo-controlled clinical trials of Efamol evening primrose oil in atopic eczema. Where do we go from here in light of more recent discoveries? Curr. Pharm. Biotechnol. 7, 503–524.

Preethi, K.C., Kuttan, R., 2009. Wound healing activity of flower extract of Calendula officinalis. J. Basic Clin. Physiol. Pharmacol. 20, 73–79.

Reuter, J., Jocher, A., Stump, J., Grossjohann, B., Franke, G., Schempp, C.M., 2008. Investigation of the anti-inflammatory potential of Aloe vera gel (97.5%) in the ultraviolet erythema test. Skin Pharmacol. Physiol. 21, 106–110.

Sampson, J.H., Raman, A., Karlsen, G., Navsaria, H., Leigh, I.M., 2001. In vitro keratinocyte antiproliferant effect of Centella asiatica extract and triterpenoid saponins. Phytomedicine 8, 230–235.

Shetty, B.S., Udupa, S.L., Udupa, A.L., Somayaji, S.N., 2006. Effect of Centella asiatica L (Umbelliferae) on normal and dexamethasone-suppressed wound healing in Wistar Albino rats. Int. J. Low. Extrem. Wounds 5, 137–143.

Sur, R., Nigam, A., Grote, D., Liebel, F., Southall, M.D., 2008. Avenanthramides, polyphenols from oats, exhibit anti-inflammatory and anti-itch activity. Arch. Dermatol. Res. 300, 569–574.

Touriño, S., Lizárraga, D., Carreras, A., et al., 2008. Highly galloylated tannin fractions from witch hazel (Hamamelis virginiana) bark: electron transfer capacity, in vitro antioxidant activity, and effects on skin-related cells. Chem. Res. Toxicol. 21, 696–704.

Wolff, H.H., Kieser, M., 2007. Hamamelis in children with skin disorders and skin injuries: results of an observational study. Eur. J. Pediatr. 166, 943–948.

Chapter 23

The eye

Diagnosis of functional disorders of the eye (glaucoma, etc.) should always be carried out by a medical practitioner. The usual precautions when using extracts in the eye (e.g. sterility of eye drops, absence of irritation of solutions etc.) must also be taken. Simple eye lotions containing mildly astringent and soothing plant products are very popular, especially those containing distilled witch hazel and eyebright herb extracts. However, ophthalmology clearly is not an area where phytotherapy is of wider importance.

INFLAMMATION OF THE EYE

Inflammation may be a result of an allergic reaction, infection or irritation due to dust or particles. Simple irritation of the eye can be treated with an eye lotion or drops, usually containing either extract of witch hazel (see Chapter 22), or the herb eyebright.

EYEBRIGHT, *EUPHRASIA OFFICINALIS* L. AND *E. ROSTKOVIANA* HAYNE (EUPHRASIAE HERBA)

Euphrasia spp. (Scrophulariaceae) have a long history of use in eye disorders, as the name would suggest. The herb is found in meadows and grassy places throughout Europe and temperate Asia. The leaves are opposite near the base and alternate above, about 1 cm long, lanceolate, with four or five teeth on each side; the axillary flowers are two-lipped, small and white, often tinged with purple or with a yellow spot.

Constituents

Eyebright contains iridoid glycosides, such as aucubin, geniposide, catalpol, luproside, eurostoside, euphroside, veronicoside, verproside and others; lignans, including coniferyl glucosides and eukovoside; tannins; and polyphenolic acids, including gallic, caffeic and ferulic acids.

Therapeutic uses and available evidence

Extract of *Euphrasia* is a traditional remedy for disorders of the eye such as conjunctivitis. Practically no clinical studies have been carried out, but single-dose eye drops containing extracts of the herb were evaluated in a clinical prospective cohort trial for conjunctivitis, and efficacy and tolerability were deemed 'good to very good' by both patients and physicians (Stoss et al 2000). Overall, the evidence for beneficial effects is very limited.

DISTILLED WITCH HAZEL, AQUA HAMAMELIDIS

Distilled witch hazel is prepared by macerating the dormant and partially dried twigs of *Hamamelis virginiana* L.,(Hamamelidaceae). It is often used in eye drops and eye lotions to soothe the eye and clear redness (for further details, see witch hazel, Chapter 22, Skin).

GLAUCOMA

Glaucoma is always treated under medical supervision. It is associated with increased intraocular pressure and can cause blindness if not treated.

Most of the drugs used are synthetic sympathomimetics, such as dipivefrine and brimonidine, β-blockers such as timolol, or prostaglandin analogues, but there is a useful plant-derived miotic (a substance causing constriction of the pupil), the alkaloid, pilocarpine, which is widely used. It reduces intraocular pressure by opening the drainage channels in the trabecular meshwork, which may be affected by a spasm or contraction of the ciliary muscle.

PILOCARPINE

Pilocarpine (Fig. 23.1) is an alkaloid obtained from Jaborandi leaf (*Pilocarpus microphyllus* Stapf. and other species of *Pilocarpus*, Rutaceae). Pilocarpine is a sympathomimetic agent, causing salivation, tachycardia and other effects if taken systemically. Its main use is in ophthalmic preparations as a miotic, in open-angle glaucoma and to contract

the pupil after the use of atropine (BNF). It is a prescription-only medicine in most countries.

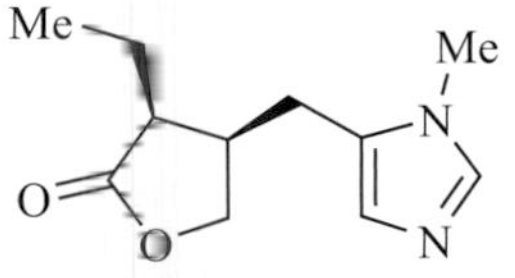

ANTERIOR UVEITIS

Anterior uveitis is an inflammatory disorder of the anterior segment. It is treated (under medical supervision) with atropine or its derivatives, homatropine and tropicamide.

ATROPINE

Atropine (Fig. 23.2) is a tropane alkaloid extracted from deadly nightshade (*Atropa belladonna*, Solanaceae). It is occasionally used as eye drops (0.5%) or ointment (1%) to open the iris for examination or surgical procedures, and to treat anterior uveitis (BNF). See Chapters 4 and 6.

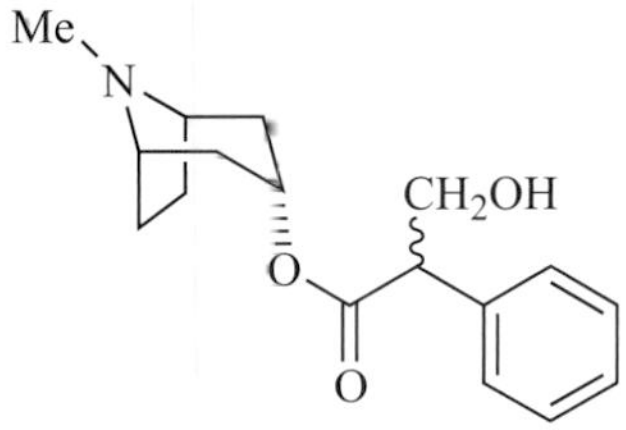

Pilocarpine

Fig. 23.1

Atropine

Fig. 23.2

Reference

Stoss, M., Michels, C., Peter, E., Beutke, R., Gorter, R.W., 2000. Prospective cohort trial of Euphrasia single-dose eye drops in conjunctivitis. J. Altern. Complement. Med. 6, 499.

British National Formulary. Published biannually by the BMJ Group and the Pharmaceutical Press. See also http://bnf.org/bnf/index.htm.

Chapter 24

Ear, nose and orthopharynx

Infections of the ear, nose and throat are treated under medical supervision with antibiotics, but a number of soothing and antiseptic preparations from plant sources are available for use. Decongestants have already been discussed in Chapter 16.

THE EAR

Infections of the ear are treated with either topical or systemic antibiotics. However, the removal of wax from the ear is achieved with the aid of softening agents such as almond, arachis or olive oil (BNF), sometimes followed by ear syringing. For details of arachis oil, see Chapter 22.

ALMOND OIL, *PRUNUS AMYGDALUS* BATSCH (OLEUM AMYGDALI) EU*

Almond oil is obtained from the seed of *Prunus amygdalus* Batsch (Rosaceae). It is a fixed oil, also known as sweet almond oil, and consists of triglycerides, mainly triolein and trioleolinolein, together with fatty acids, including palmitic, lauric, myristic and oleic acids.

OLIVE OIL, *OLEA EUROPEA* L. (OLEUM OLIVAE) EU*

Olive oil is expressed from the fruits of *Olea europea* L. (Oleaceae). Virgin (or cold-expressed) olive oil has a greenish tinge and is used as a food; refined oil is yellowish. Both have a characteristic odour. Olive oil is a fixed oil containing glycerides of oleic acid (about 70–80%), with smaller amounts of linoleic, palmitic and stearic acid glycerides.

THE ORTHOPHARNYX

Simple oral and throat irritation can be treated with an antiinflammatory and antiseptic mouthwash, including the thymol type associated with a visit to the dentist. Many essential oils are used as oral antiseptics, deodorizers and antiinflammatory agents, including mint, clove, eucalyptus and lemon oils, as well as menthol and thymol. These can be incorporated into artificial saliva products, used for relieving dry mouth, which are composed of either animal mucins or hydroxymethoxycellulose derivatives.

THYMOL EU*

Thymol (Fig. 24.1) was originally extracted from thyme (*Thymus* spp.) and is present in many oils, including ajowan, but is now more easily synthesized chemically. It is antiseptic, deodorizing and antiinflammatory and is widely used in dental products (e.g. compound thymol glycerin). Thymol causes irritation in high concentrations when applied externally, and should not be swallowed in significant amounts. Normal doses associated with the herb do not normally cause problems.

PEPPERMINT OIL, *MENTHA* × *PIPERITA* L. (MENTHAE PIPERITAE AETHEROLEUM) EU*

Peppermint oil is antiseptic, deodorizing and antiinflammatory and is widely used in skin and dental products. Other species of mint, such as spearmint, are also used for the same purpose (for botanical and chemical details, see Chapter 14).

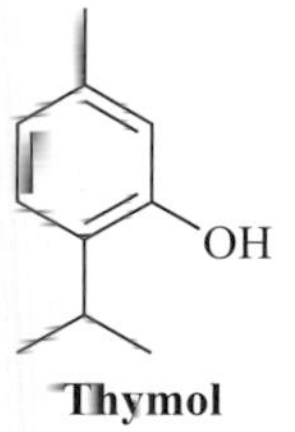

Thymol

Fig. 24.1

Constituents

The major constituents are menthol (30–55%) and menthone (14–32%), with isomenthone (2–10%), menthofuran (1–9%), menthyl acetate (3–5%), 1,8-cineole (6–14%), limonene (1–5%), pulegone (not more than 4.0%) and carvone (not more than 1.0%). Menthol (Fig. 24.2) can cause irritation in high concentrations.

SAGE, *SALVIA OFFICINALIS* L. (SALVIAE FOLIUM) EU✻

The genus *Salvia* is one of the largest of the family Lamiaceae and many of its species, especially those rich in essential oil, have pharmaceutical uses. This common garden plant (garden sage) and culinary shrub has conspicuous blue flowers and relatively large leaves (3–5 cm long, 1–2.5 cm broad), which are oblong or lanceolate, rounded at the base and at the apex, and crenulate at the margin. The young leaves especially are covered with a white layer of fine hairs. The leaves have a characteristic uneven upper surface and prominent lower venation. The taste and odour are characteristic, pungent and aromatic. Sage is a popular culinary herb. *S. triloba* L.f. is also rich in essential oil and has similar topical uses as *S. officinalis* (see also Chapter 16, p. 232).

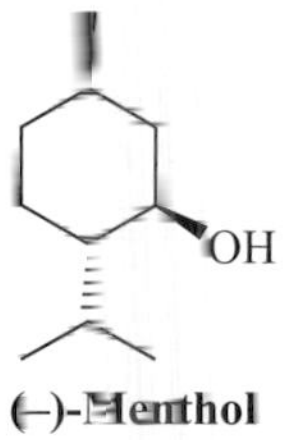

(–)-Menthol

Fig. 24.2

Constituents

The leaves are rich in essential oil with α- and β-thujone as the major components (normally about 50%), with cineole, borneol and others. It also contains rosmarinic acid. Diterpenes and flavonoids are two other important classes of natural products prominent in this species. There are differences in the composition of the essential oil depending on the origin of the plant material.

Therapeutic uses and available evidence

The use of sage leaf, in the form of a tea used as a gargle, is traditional for soothing inflammation of the mucous membranes of mouth and throat. Rosmarinic acid is well known for its antiviral and antiinflammatory effects, sage essential oil is antibacterial and antifungal, and an aqueous extract of sage leaf has been shown to have analgesic and antiinflammatory effects in rats, supporting this use of sage. In the doses used for mouthwashes it is generally considered to be safe. A throat spray containing echinacea and sage was recently compared to a chlorhexidine and lidocaine spray in a multicenter, randomized, double-blind, double-placebo controlled trial involving 154 patients with acute sore throats. They used two puffs every 2 hours, up to 10 times daily until they were symptom-free, for a maximum of 5 days. The main outcome measure was the comparison of response rates during the first 3 days, a response being defined as a decrease of at least 50% of the total symptoms compared to baseline. The echinacea/sage treatment showed similar efficacy to the chlorhexidine/lidocaine spray during the first 3 days, i.e. 63.8% in the echinacea/sage group and 57.8% in the chlorhexidine/lidocaine group. For all assessments of efficacy by the physician and patient, no difference between the two treatments was seen, and both were very well tolerated (Schapowal et al 2009).

CLOVE, *SYZYGIUM AROMATICUM* (L.) MERR. & L.M. PERRY (CARYOPHYLLI FLOS) EU✻

Cloves are obtained from the flower buds of *Syzygium aromaticum* (syn. *Eugenia caryophyllata* Thunb., Myrtaceae) which are collected prior to opening. The buds are brown, about 1–1.5 cm long, with a very characteristic shape, the lower portion consisting of the calyx tube enclosing in its upper half the immature flower. Taste and odour are highly characteristic. On pressing a clove with the fingernail, oil should be exuded. Cloves are used as a culinary spice.

Constituents

The buds are very rich in essential oil (15–20%), consisting mainly of eugenol (Fig. 24.3), usually 85–90%, and numerous minor constituents, including acetyl eugenol, α- and β-caryophyllene, methyl salicylate. Tannins such as eugeniin, casuarictin, tellimagrandin I, and flavonoids, are found in the plant material but not in the oil.

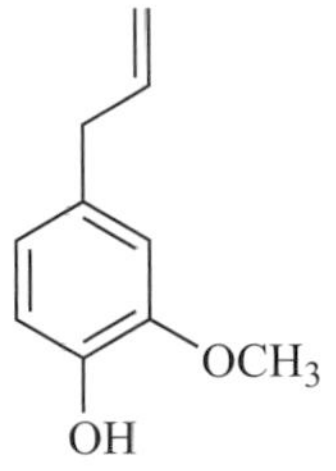

Therapeutic uses and available evidence

Clove oil is used for the symptomatic relief of toothache and is a constituent of many dental preparations. The oil is useful in the treatment of inflammation of the mucous membranes of mouth and throat. It has antiseptic, antispasmodic, anti-

Eugenol

Fig. 24.3

histaminic and anthelmintic properties, many of which are due to the eugenol content. Eugenol inhibits prostaglandin synthesis and the metabolism of arachidonic acid by human polymorphonuclear leukocytes, inhibits smooth muscle activity in vitro and is antiinflammatory (for review, see Chaieb et al 2007). Clove extracts are used in cosmetics and perfumery.

References

British National Formulary. Published biannually by the BMJ Group and the Pharmaceutical Press. See also http://bnf.org/bnf/index.htm.

Chaieb, K., Hajlaoui, H., Zmantar, T., et al., 2007. The chemical composition and biological activity of clove essential oil, Eugenia caryophyllata (*Syzygium aromaticum* L. Myrtaceae): a short review. Phytother. Res. 21, 501–506.

Schapowal, A., Berger, D., Klein, P., Suter, A., 2009. Echinacea/sage or chlorhexidine/lidocaine for treating acute sore throats: a randomized double-blind trial. Eur. J. Med. Res. 14, 406–412.

Chapter 25

Miscellaneous supportive therapies for stress, ageing, cancer and debility

Although their effects are very difficult to evaluate, preventative medicines are extremely popular with patients and are an essential element of most types of Oriental medicine. They have been collected together here as they are generally used for a multitude of disorders, and to prevent degenerative conditions, including ageing and some forms of cancer. Most of the herbs mentioned here originated in Asia and China. In traditional Chinese medicine they are used to treat 'empty' diseases, to restore 'qi' energy and tonify the organs, having a balancing effect on yin and yang rather than affecting only one. They are thought to strengthen the immune system, improve memory and alertness, enhance sexual performance, promote healing and stimulate the appetite. In the West, the most important Chinese herbs are ginseng, ginkgo, astragalus, shizandra, reishi mushroom, baical scullcap and tea. In Ayurveda, some rejuvenating and tonic herbs are called 'rasayanas' and are considered to have a beneficial effect, balancing the tridosha. In Asian medicine, ashwagandha and *Centella asiatica* are very widely used. Many of these herbs contain saponins or steroidal compounds of some kind and it has been suggested that they act in a similar way to corticosteroids or enhance the effect of naturally occurring steroid hormones in the body. This type of drug is known as an adaptogen, and is considered to be a substance helping the body to deal with, or adapt to, stress or other adverse conditions.

While very contentious, this group is a fast growing area of phytotherapy, but use is often based on very limited scientific evidence.

CANCER CHEMOPREVENTION

During the 1960s and 1970s, work done at the University of Minnesota by LW Wattenberg showed that various compounds, especially from fruits and vegetables (indoles and isothiocyanates), could inhibit chemically induced tumours in laboratory animals. Termed 'chemoprophylaxis of carcinogenesis', this was of obvious benefit to maintenance of human health and had enormous dietary significance. After intensive studies using retinoids (vitamin A related natural products), the term 'cancer chemoprevention' was first used.

Cancer chemoprevention can be defined as 'the prevention of cancer in human populations by ingestion of chemical agents that prevent carcinogenesis'. It is also important to differentiate between cancer prevention (e.g. cessation of cigarette smoking) and cancer chemotherapy (the use of cytotoxic drugs after cancer diagnosis). Cancer chemoprevention has now developed into a well-defined discipline. Several recent epidemiological studies have demonstrated that dietary factors may reduce the incidence of cancers. In one study, involving 250,000 people, an inverse correlation was found between the incidence of lung cancer among people who smoke and consume carotene-rich foods. As well as carotenoids, there was a similar finding for vitamin C and oesophageal and stomach cancers; selenium and various cancers; and vitamin E and lung cancer. Epidemiological studies may help to find leads for chemopreventive agents, which can then be tested in laboratory experiments. Almost 600 'chemopreventive' agents are known and they are usually classified as: inhibitors of carcinogen formation (ascorbic acid, tocopherols, phenols), inhibitors of initiation (phenols, flavones) and inhibitors of postinitiation events (β-carotene, retinoids, terpenes). Many are items of food or beverages (e.g. tea) and are sometimes called 'functional foods' or 'nutraceuticals'. Those that are used *purely* as foods are not covered here, but some others can be found in the chapters for which they are most useful (e.g. ginger, Chapter 14; garlic, Chapter 15). Further examples are given in Table 25.1.

Chemopreventive agents may even work in synergy, with several components contributing to the overall effect, which may be the case with plant drugs. This approach has great promise, with both natural products and synthetics being potentially useful. Dietary campaigns by government bodies, the American Cancer Society and others recommend that 5–7 servings of vegetables be consumed daily to function as a source of cancer chemopreventive agents. However, it is not reasonable to assume that chemopreventive agents will safeguard humans from known carcinogenic risks such as smoking. As knowledge of these agents increases they will play an increasing role in cancer prevention. Chemoprevention will not be covered further, apart from tea, as it is a vast subject in its own right. However, there are some useful recent reviews which discuss compounds, mechanisms and future directions available, such as Shu et al (2010), Gullett et al (2010) and Cerella et al (2010). Some data on the chemopreventive effects of garlic, anthocyanins (bilberry) and others can be found in the monographs of these plants.

Table 25.1	Known types of chemopreventive agents	
GROUP	**EXAMPLES**	
Micronutrients	Vitamins A, C and E, selenium, calcium, zinc	
Food additives	Antioxidants	
Non-nutritive molecules	Carotenoids, coumarins, indoles, alkaloids	
Industrial reagents	Photographic developers, herbicides, UV-light protectors	
Pharmaceuticals	Retinoids, antiprostaglandins, antithrombogenic agents, non-steroidal antiinflammatory drugs	
Hormones and antihormones	Dehydroepiandrosterone, tamoxifen	

TONICS, STIMULANTS, ADAPTOGENS AND SUPPORTIVE THERAPIES

AÇAI BERRY, *EUTERPE OLERACEA* MART. (EUTERPE FRUCTUS)

The fruits of the palm *Euterpe oleracea* Martius (açai, Arecaceae) have been acclaimed as having a wide range of health-promoting and therapeutic benefits due to their reportedly high levels of antioxidants. Açai has a history of use as a medicinal plant and as a staple food in many parts of Brazil. Traditionally, it has been used to treat fevers, skin complications, digestive disorders and parasitic infections. In recent years, açai berry has been advertised widely, for example, via the internet.

Constituents

Açai has a relatively high content of polyphenols. Most notable are anthocyanins and flavonoids, as well as fatty acids. Recently, small amounts of lignans have been reported.

Therapeutic uses and available evidence

This botanical drug has become very popular despite a lack of scientific evidence. Clinical data are lacking. The high content of polyphenols has been linked to a range of reported (mostly in vitro) antioxidant, antiinflammatory, antiproliferative and cardioprotective properties. Açai demonstrates promising potential with regard to antiproliferative activity and cardioprotection, but further studies are required (Heinrich et al In press).

ASHWAGANDHA, *WITHANIA SOMNIFERUM* (L.) DUNAL.

Ashwagandha, also known as winter cherry (Solanaceae), is a woody shrub native to the Middle East, Africa and parts of Asia, growing in stony and semi-arid regions; it is cultivated widely. The leaves are elliptical with an acute apex and the flowers campanulate and greenish yellow, developing into red berries enclosed in a papery membrane. The dried root is used medicinally. Ashwagandha has been used in Ayurvedic medicine for over 4000 years, as an adaptogen, sedative and tonic for debility. It is used to enhance fertility in both men and women, and as an aphrodisiac. The name 'ashwagandha' comes from the Sanskrit *ashva* (meaning 'horse') and *gandha* (meaning 'smell'), and refers to the odour of the root. It is also widely used for inflammation, colds, asthma and many other disorders.

Constituents

The root contains steroidal lactones (the withanolides A–Y), withaferin A (Fig. 25.1), withasomniferols A–C and others, phytosterols (such as the sitoindosides) and the alkaloids anahygrine, cuscohygrine, ashwagandhine, ashwagandhinine, withasomnine, withaninine, somniferine and others.

Therapeutic uses and available evidence

Extracts are antioxidant, immunomodulatory and sedative but, despite their wide usage, much of the clinical knowledge is still anecdotal. The few clinical trials which have been carried out are of doubtful quality and cannot be used to confirm efficacy, but they do show that the herb is generally safe. Many of the pharmacological effects have been substantiated in animal studies: for example, the adaptogenic and antistress activity was found to be comparable to that of ginseng, in mice and rats, and immunomodulatory activity has been confirmed. The extract has sedative activity and is reported to be anxiolytic, acting via the GABA-ergic system (Bhattarai et al 2010) and numerous other actions have been documented (for review, see Kulkarni and Dhir 2008). The usual dose of powdered root is 3–6 g daily. Side effects are rare but high doses can cause gastrointestinal irritation.

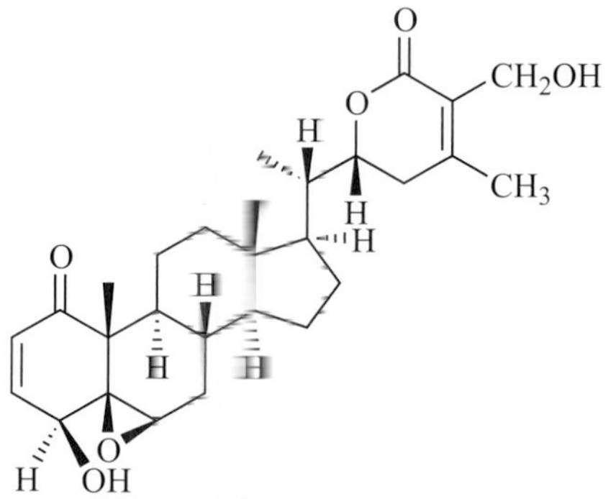

Withaferin A

Fig. 25.1

CENTELLA, *CENTELLA ASIATICA* (L.) URBAN (CENTELLAE HERBA)

The herb has already been described in Chapter 22 (Skin). In addition to the wound healing effects, the plant is considered a 'rasayana' in Ayurvedic medicine; it enhances the immune system and is considered to have a rejuvenating, neurological 'tonic' and mild sedative effect. The immunomodulating effects of the herb have been shown in vitro and in vivo in mice. Studies in rats have shown that asiatic acid has some benefits on memory and learning (Nasir et al 2011), and that the extract can protect against certain types of neurodegeneration (Haleagrahara and Ponnusamy 2010), but in general, evidence for this use is lacking. A small double-blind, placebo-controlled, randomized trial in healthy elderly volunteers in Thailand found that their health-related quality of life was improved and lower extremity strength increased after taking centella extract for 3 months (Mato et al 2009). It may be taken orally, often as an infusion, and applied topically. Other reported effects for the herb include anti-ulcer activity and spasmolytic effects. The powdered leaf is taken at an internal dose of 0.5–1 g daily, or the equivalent in the form of an extract.

GINSENG, *PANAX GINSENG* C.A. MEYER *(PANAX RADIX), ELEUTHEROCOCCUS SENTICOSUS* (RUPR. & MAXIM.) MAXIM. AND RELATED 'GINSENG' SPECIES

Ginseng root in commerce is obtained from *Panax ginseng* C. A. Meyer (Korean or Chinese ginseng, Araliaceae) and other species. American ginseng is from *P. quinquefolius* L., but Siberian ginseng comes from a different but related genus, *Eleutherococcus senticosus* (Rupr. & Maxim.) Maxim. *P. ginseng* is native to China but cultivated widely elsewhere. The root is spindle-shaped, ringed, and divided into two or three equal branches. Red Korean ginseng (from *P. ginseng*) is about 8 years old; it is matured and roasted, and is the most highly regarded form. Ginseng products are liable to adulteration and falsification (often with liquorice), as true ginseng is expensive.

Constituents

All types contain saponin glycosides (the ginsenosides Ra, Rb, Rg_1, Rg_2, Rs, etc.; Fig. 25.2). The ginsenosides are sometimes referred to as the panaxosides, but this nomenclature uses the suffixes A–F, which do not correspond to those of the ginsenosides.

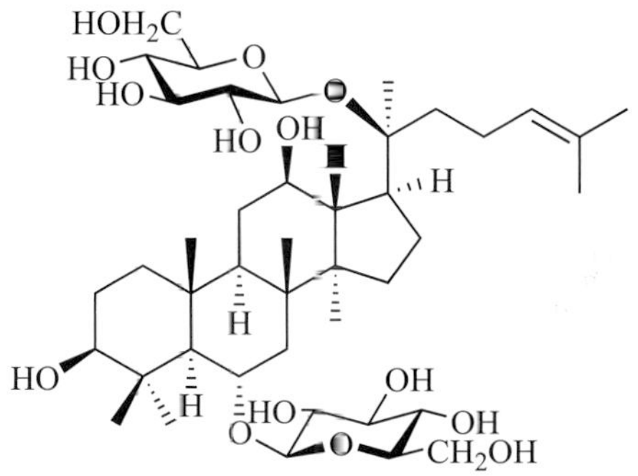

Ginsenoside Rg$_1$

Fig. 25.2

In Siberian ginseng (*Eleutherococcus*), the saponins (eleutherosides A–F) are chemically different, but have similar properties. Glycans (panaxans) also occur in *P. ginseng*. The actual composition of ginseng extracts depends upon the species and method of preparation.

Therapeutic uses and available evidence

Ginseng is taken as a tonic for debility, insomnia, natural and premature ageing, to increase alertness and improve sexual inadequacy, and for diabetes, as well as an adaptogen to relieve stress and improve stamina and concentration. It has been suggested that these effects are due to changes in cholinergic activity and also neuro-protection, as well as antioxidant activity (Wang et al 2007). The adaptogenic effect may be due to the elevation of serum levels of corticosteroids and the reduction of catecholamines, which results in homoeostasis. Ginsenoside Rb$_1$ acts as a central nervous system sedative and Rg$_1$ has antifatigue and stimulant properties. In animals, an extract increases the capacity of skeletal muscle to oxidize free fatty acids in preference to glucose to produce cellular energy, which would support the antifatigue activity seen in conventional exhaustion tests. Ginseng also has a traditional use in diabetes, and the glycans (panaxans A–E) are hypoglycaemic in mice. Other documented effects include immunomodulatory activity, potentiation of analgesia and anticancer effects (by ginsenosides R$_{s3}$ and R$_{s4}$).

Trials of ginseng for improving 'quality of life', including mental health parameters, show beneficial effects for up to 8 weeks of treatment, but as far as cognition is concerned, a recent Cochrane review concludes that further, better quality studies

are needed (Geng et al 2010). Since that review, the results of a placebo-controlled, double-blind, randomized, crossover study assessing the effects of *Panax ginseng* on subjective mood and aspects of 'working' memory processes in healthy young adults, following both single dose and sub-chronic (7 days) ingestion, has been published. Dose-related treatment effects were found: 200 mg slowed a fall in mood, but also slowed responding on a mental arithmetic task across day 1, whereas the 400 mg dose also improved calmness (restricted to day 1) and improved mental arithmetic across days 1 and 8. No evidence of additional benefits, nor attenuation of acute effects, was found with repeated ingestion (Reay et al 2010). The dose is very variable but, in general, for a short course in the young and healthy, 0.5–1 g daily is recommended for up to 20 days; for long-term treatment in the sick or elderly, 0.4–0.8 g daily is more usual. Ginseng is taken widely, and side effects are well documented. They include oestrogenic effects, hypertension and irritability. A 'ginseng abuse' syndrome has been described.

LINGZHI OR REISHI MUSHROOM, *GANODERMA* SPP.

Ganoderma lucidum (Curtis Fr.) P. Karst., *G. japonicum* (Fr. Lloyd) and other species of mushroom (Polyporaceae) grow on tree stumps (mainly conifers) in China, Japan and North America. It is now cultivated for commerce. In China, the fungus is known as lingzhi, and in Japan, as reishi. The fruiting body takes several forms, including a rare, branched or 'antler' type, in addition to the more usual mushroom shape. The colour varies from red, through orange and brown, to black, with the red and antlered varieties being more highly prized. The cap is circular, kidney- or fan-shaped, leathery with a smooth or rippled upper surface, and an under surface that shows the spore tubes. Lingzhi is a very important Chinese medicine; it has been immortalized in Oriental paintings and was used frequently by Taoist monks.

Constituents

The mature fruiting body of the fungus contains a series of triterpenes, mainly lanostanes such as the ganoderic acids A–Z, ganoderals A and B, ganoderiols A and B, epoxyganoderiols A–C, ganolucidic acids A–E, lucidones A–C, lucidenic acids A–M.

Polysaccharides, mainly glucans and arabinoxylo-glucans, and peptidoglycans (known as ganoderans A–C) are also present.

Therapeutic uses and available evidence

Lingzhi is used as an adaptogen and general tonic, in the hope of prolonging life, retarding ageing and generally improving wellbeing and mental faculties. The most common indication is to enhance the immune system, and various animal and clinical studies support such a use. More recently, reishi has been applied as an adjunctive treatment to chemotherapy and radiation in cancer patients, to support immune resistance. The active principles are considered to be the triterpenes and polysaccharides. Extracts inhibit angiotensin-converting enzyme and produce hypotensive effects; cholesterol-lowering effects have been seen in animals. It is also a sedative, liver protectant and cholesterol-lowering agent (for review, see Sanodiya et al 2009). Clinical studies to support the uses are few and some are of doubtful quality.

The dose of the dried fruiting body of the fungus is 6–12 g daily, or the equivalent in extract. Lingzhi is well tolerated, although transient side effects of gastrointestinal disturbance and rashes in sensitive individuals have been reported. Animal studies have shown no toxic effects after long-term high doses, but as with other immune modulators it should probably be avoided in auto-immune disease.

ROSENROOT, *RHODIOLA ROSEA* L. (RHODIOLAE ROSEAE RHIZOMA)

Also known as Golden root, Aaron's rod, *Rhodiola rosea* (Crassulaceae) grows in cold regions of the world, including much of the Arctic, mountainous regions of Central Asia and Europe, and the Rocky Mountains. It is a dioecious perennial reaching 5 to 35 cm in height.

Constituents

The main active constituents of the root and rhizome are monoterpene alcohols and their glycosides, such as salidroside (previously known as rhodioloside or rhodosin), rhodioniside, rhodiolin, rosin, rosavin, rosarin and rosiridin. These compounds are thought to be responsible for the adaptogenic properties of rhodiola. Other phenolic constituents such as p-tyrosol, gallic acid, caffeic acid, chlorogenic acid and flavonoids (catechins and proanthocyanidins)

are present. Geraniol and other essential oil constituents, such as geranyl formate, geranyl acetate, benzyl alcohol and phenylethyl alcohol, give the root its rose-like odour.

Therapeutic uses and available evidence

Rhodiola rhizome preparations exhibit adaptogenic effects, and these include neuroprotective, cardioprotective, anti-fatigue, antidepressive, anxiolytic and CNS stimulating activity. A number of small clinical trials demonstrate that repeated administration of a Rhodiola rosea extract (SHR-5) may exert an anti-fatigue effect and increase mental performance in healthy subjects (measured as an ability to concentrate), and reduce burnout in patients with mild fatigue syndrome. Rhodiola may help in mild to moderate depression and generalized anxiety. Mechanisms of action which may contribute to the clinical effect include interactions with the HPA-system (reducing cortisol levels) and defense mechanism proteins (some heat shock proteins). It does not seem to interact with other drugs and appears to be safe, with only minor adverse effects. For review, see Panossian et al 2010, Panossian and Wikman 2009.

SCHISANDRA, *SCHISANDRA CHINENSIS* (TURCZ.) BAILL. (SCHISANDRAE CHINENSIS FRUCTUS)

The magnolia vine (*Schisandra*, Schisandraceae,) is also known as gomishi in Japan, and Wu-wei-Zi in China. It is a monoecious liana, native to Northern China, Korea, Japan and eastern Russia, usually found climbing round tree trunks. The leaves are elliptical and the flowers cream with a pleasant odour. The fresh berries are scarlet, small and ovoid, hanging in clusters and are the main botanical drug used. When dry they are wrinkled, dark reddish brown, containing a sticky pulp and a yellow kidney-shaped seed. *Schisandra sphenanthera* Rehder & E. H. Wilson is also widely used for similar purposes.

Constituents

The active constituents are lignans, including schizandrin A (=deoxyschisandrin or wuweizu A), schizandrin B (=wuweizu B or γ-schizandrin B; Fig. 25.3), schizandrol A (=schizandrin), schizandrol B (=gomisin A), schisandrin C, schisantherin A (=gomisin C), schisantherin B (=gomisin B), gomisins H, K, L, M, N, schizanhenol, wuweizu C, schisantherin C and others.

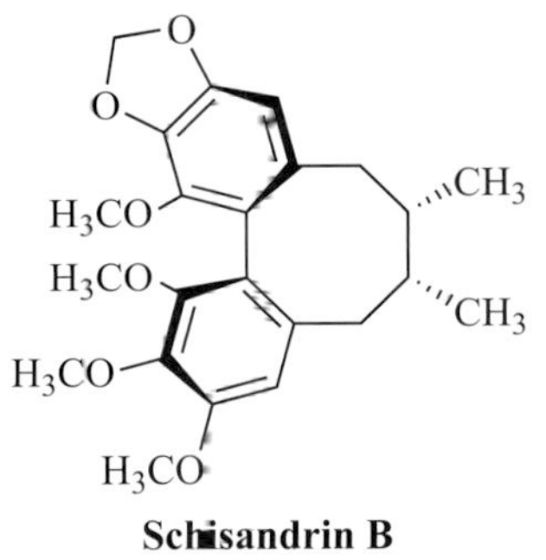

Schisandrin B

Fig. 25.3

Therapeutic uses and available evidence

Schisandra has been used in China since ancient times to prolong life and increase energy ('qi') and act as a general and sexual tonic, especially for men. It is also used to reduce sweating, detoxify the liver, enhance kidney function and suppress cough in lung disease. The adaptogenic and antifatigue properties have been tested in several animal studies; for example, the effect on the physical recovery of racehorses was found to be beneficial, as well as producing a general improvement in performance. Schizanhenol and schizandrin B protect against peroxidative damage associated with ageing and ischaemia in the rat brain, and a human study has suggested that intellectual activity can be enhanced. Many pharmacological studies support the use of schisandra, although few good clinical trials have been performed. Hepatoprotective effects have been documented in animal and cell culture studies. Schizandrin B, schisandrin C and gomisin A reduced liver enzyme levels and prevented histological damage in experimental models of liver injury, inhibited lipid peroxidation and stimulated glycogen synthesis in the liver. Antioxidant and free radical scavenging effects have also been described in vivo and in vitro. Deoxyschisandrin, gomisin A, B and C increase liver cytochrome P450 enzymes, which supports the detoxifying and

anticancer properties attributed to the plant. Antitumour-promoting and antiinflammatory properties have also been shown in skin and the lignans are known to be platelet activating factor antagonists. For review, see Panossian and Wikman (2008, 2009). Daily doses of powdered berry are usually 1.5–6 g or higher if used to treat kidney disease.

Few toxicity studies have been carried out but, although relatively safe, schisandra is reputed to increase gastric acidity and may cause allergy in susceptible individuals. It should be avoided during pregnancy (possible uterine stimulation) and epilepsy.

Skullcap, *Scutellaria baicalensis* Georgi (Scutellaria baicalensis radix)

Scutellaria baicalensis (Huan qin, Lamiaceae) is sometimes known as baical skullcap to differentiate it from American skullcap (*S. laterifolia* L.). It grows in northern China, Siberia and Manchuria. The leaves are opposite, lanceolate and sessile with an acute apex. The flowers are blue, with a helmet-shaped upper lip (hence the name). The root is used medicinally.

Constituents

The root contains flavonoids including baicalin, baicalein, wogonin, chrysin, oroxylin A, skullcapflavones I and II, and others (Fig. 25.4).

Therapeutic uses and available evidence

Skullcap is used for a wide variety of ailments, particularly fevers, infections, jaundice, thirst and nosebleeds, and as an antidote and sedative. Baicalin is antiinflammatory and anti-allergic; it inhibits the formation of lipoxygenase products and, to a lesser extent, cyclo-oxygenase products in leukocytes. It also inhibits the generation of inflammatory cytokines and is synergistic with β-lactam antibiotics against methicillin-resistant *Staphylococcus aureus* in vitro. Extracts of *S. baicalensis* inhibit lipid

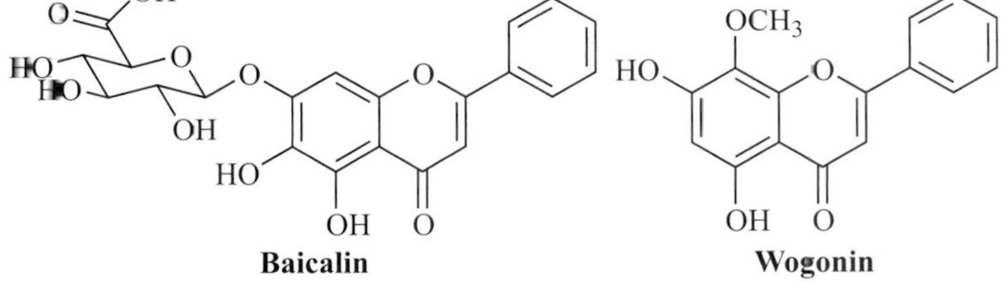

Baicalin   **Wogonin**

Fig. 25.4

peroxidation in rat liver and the herb has been clinically tested in China in patients with chronic hepatitis, where it improved symptoms in over 70% of patients, increasing appetite, relieving abdominal distension and improving the results of liver function tests. Wogonin also suppresses production of hepatitis B virus surface antigen. The flavones interact with the benzodiazepine-binding site of the GABA$_A$ receptor, with wogonin and baicalein being the most potent; this supports the sedative use of the herb. Baicalein is antigenotoxic in vitro and inhibits adhesion molecule expression induced by thrombin and cell proliferation of several types of cells. Wogonin inhibits nitric oxide production in activated C6 rat glial cells, acting via NF-κB inhibition and thus suppressing cell death. It also reduces skin inflammation in mice (induced by phorbol ester expression of COX-2) and inhibits monocyte chemotactic protein-1 gene expression in human endothelial cells. Antioxidant and antibiotic activities have also been reported for extracts. These activities all support the antiinflammatory and other uses of skullcap, although clinical trial evidence is sparse (for review, see Li-Weber 2009, Wang et al 2007). The daily dose of skullcap root is usually 5–8 g. Generally, baical skullcap is well tolerated, but little information as to side effects and contraindications is available.

TEA, *CAMELLIA SINENSIS* (L.) KUNTZE (GREEN TEA LEAVES: THEAE VIRIDIS FOLIUM; BLACK TEA LEAVES: THEAE NIGRAE FOLIUM)

Tea (*Camellia sinensis*, Theaceae) is cultivated in China, India, Sri Lanka, Kenya, Indonesia and elsewhere. Green tea is produced in China and Japan; it is not processed and thus differs from black tea, which is fermented and produced in India, Sri Lanka and Kenya. Oolong tea is partially fermented. The leaf buds and very young leaves are used to prepare the beverage and extracts for medicinal use.

Constituents

Tea contains caffeine, and much smaller amounts of other xanthines such as theophylline and theobromine. The polyphenols are the antioxidant constituents [in green tea these are mainly (−)-epigallocatechin; Fig. 25.5], together with theogallin, trigalloyl glucose. In black tea, they have been oxidized to form the 'tea pigments', the theaflavins, thearubigens and theaflavic acids.

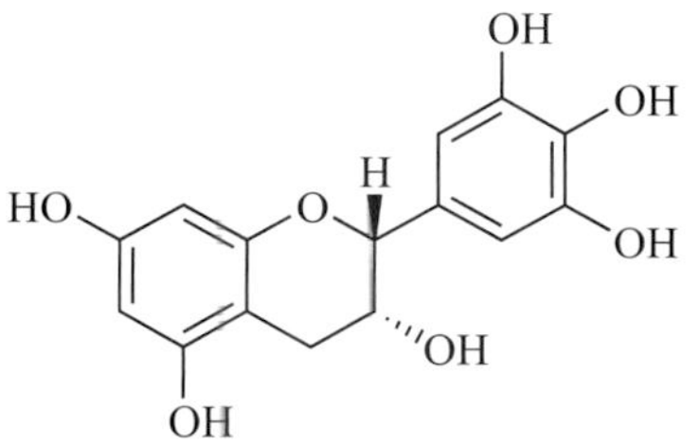

(−)-Epigallocatechin

Fig. 25.5

Therapeutic uses and available evidence

Tea is a stimulant, diuretic, astringent and antioxidant. Green tea is used medicinally more frequently than black tea. The stimulant and diuretic properties are due to the caffeine content, and the astringency and antioxidant effects to the polyphenols (Wang et al 2007).

Tea is useful in diarrhoea, and in China is used for many types of dysentery. The polyphenols in green tea have cancer chemopreventive properties due to their antioxidant capacity. Habitual consumption of green tea is generally associated with a lower incidence of cancer (for review, see Lambert and Elias 2010) and black tea is now known to have similar health benefits, which are ascribed to the tea pigments (for review, see Kumar et al 2010). Anti-inflammatory and antitumour effects have been described, and attributed to inhibition of the transcription factor NF-κB, and the risk of breast and stomach cancers appears to be lower for green tea drinkers. Black tea consumption is associated with a lower risk of death from ischaemic heart disease and has been shown to reverse endothelial dysfunction in coronary heart disease. Tea is also antimicrobial and anticariogenic, and is even reputed to help weight loss. Tea is drunk in nearly every country in the world for its refreshing, mildly stimulating and analgesic effects. There is no recommended dose for tea, and consumption varies widely.

Tea as a beverage is non-toxic in the usual amounts ingested, although it can cause gastrointestinal upsets and nervous irritability, due to the caffeine content. However there is now some concern about the safety of concentrated preparations or excessive consumption of green tea. Cases of hepatotoxicity have been associated with consumption of high doses of green tea-containing dietary supplements (10–29 mg/kg/d p.o.). In most cases, patients presented with elevated serum alanine aminotransferase (ALT) and bilirubin levels and in some cases liver biopsies were performed, and periportal and portal inflammation were observed. All cases resolved following cessation of supplement consumption, and re-injury was observed in some studies when the subject began reusing the same preparations, suggesting a causative effect of the green tea. There is also a case report of a 45-year-old man who developed jaundice and elevated serum ALT following consumption of 6 cups/d green tea infusion for 4 months (reviewed by Mazzanti et al 2009).

References

Bhattarai, J.P., Ah Park, S., Han, S.K., 2010. The methanolic extract of *Withania somnifera* acts on GABAA receptors in gonadotropin releasing hormone (GnRH) neurons in mice. Phytother. Res. 24, 1147–1150.

Cerella, C., Sobolewski, C., Dicato, M., Diederich, M., 2010. Targeting COX-2 expression by natural compounds: a promising alternative strategy to synthetic COX-2 inhibitors for cancer chemoprevention and therapy. Biochem. Pharmacol. 80, 1801–1815.

Geng, J., Dong, J., Ni, H., et al., 2010. Ginseng for cognition. Cochrane Database Syst. Rev. 12: CD007769.

Gullett, N.P., Ruhul Amin, A.R., Bayraktar, S., et al., 2010. Cancer prevention with natural compounds. Semin. Oncol. 37, 258–281.

Haleagrahara, N., Ponnusamy, K., 2010. Neuroprotective effect of *Centella asiatica* extract (CAE) on experimentally induced parkinsonism in aged Sprague-Dawley rats. J. Toxicol. Sci. 35, 41–47.

Heinrich, M., Dhanji, T., Casselman, I., In press. Açai (*Euterpe oleracea* Mart.) – a phytochemical and pharmacological assessment of the species' health claims. *Phytochemistry Letters 4: 10–21*. doi: 10.1016/j.phytol. 2010.11.005.

Kulkarni, S.K., Dhir, A., 2008. *Withania somnifera*: an Indian ginseng. Prog. Neuropsychopharmacol. Biol. Psychiatry 32, 1093–1105.

Kumar, G., Pillare, S.P., Maru, G.B., 2010. Black tea polyphenols-mediated in vivo cellular responses during carcinogenesis. Mini Rev. Med. Chem. 10, 492–505.

Lambert, J.D., Elias, R.J., 2010. The antioxidant and pro-oxidant activities of green tea polyphenols: a role in cancer prevention. Arch. Biochem. Biophys. 501, 65–72.

Li-Weber, M., 2009. New therapeutic aspects of flavones: the anticancer properties of Scutellaria and its main active constituents Wogonin, Baicalein and Baicalin. Cancer Treat. Rev. 35, 57–68.

Mato, L., Wattanathorn, J., Muchimapura, S., et al., 2009. *Centella asiatica* improves physical performance and health-related quality of life in healthy elderly volunteer. Evidence-based Complementary and Alternative Medicine. [Epub ahead of print 2009 Oct 30].

Mazzanti, G., Menniti-Ippolito, F., Moro, P.A., et al., 2009. Hepatotoxicity from green tea: a review of the literature and two unpublished cases. Eur. J. Clin. Pharmacol. 65, 331–341.

Nasir, M.N., Habsah, M., Zamzuri, I., Rammes, G., Hasnan, J., Abdullah, J., 2011. Effects of asiatic acid on passive and active avoidance task in male Sprague-Dawley rats. J. Ethnopharmacol. 134, 203–209.

Panossian, A., Wikman, G., 2008. Pharmacology of *Schisandra chinensis* Bail.: An overview of Russian research and uses in medicine. J. Ethnopharmacol. 118, 183–212.

Panossian, A., Wikman, G., 2009. Evidence-based efficacy of adaptogens in fatigue, and molecular mechanisms related to their stress-protective activity. Current Clinical Pharmacology 4, 198–219.

Panossian, A., Wikman, G., Sarris, J., 2010. Rosenroot (*Rhodiola rosea*): traditional use, chemical composition, pharmacology and clinical efficacy. Phytomedicine 17, 481–493.

Sanodiya, B.S., Thakur, G.S., Baghel, R.K., Prasad, G.B., Bisen, P.S., 2009. *Ganoderma lucidum*: a potent pharmacological macrofungus. Curr. Pharm. Biotechnol. 10, 717–742.

Reay, J.L., Scholey, A.B., Kennedy, D.O., 2010. Panax ginseng (G115) improves aspects of working memory performance and subjective ratings of calmness in healthy young adults. Hum. Psychopharmacol. 25, 462–471.

Shu, L., Cheung, K.L., Khor, T.O., Chen, C., Kong, A.N., 2010. Phytochemicals: cancer chemoprevention and suppression of tumor onset and metastasis. Cancer Metastasis Rev. 29, 483–502.

Wang, C.Z., Mehendale, S.R., Yuan, C.S., 2007. Commonly used antioxidant botanicals: active constituents and their potential role in cardiovascular illness. Am. J. Chin. Med. 35, 543–558.

Epilogue – a personal view

J. David Phillipson

This textbook, *Fundamentals of Pharmacognosy and Phytotherapy*, clearly shows the relevance of plants to pharmacy and to medicine today. In order to understand how plants, either as extracts or as single chemical entities, may continue to play a role in healthcare, it is necessary to consider their past and present uses so that their future potential may be assessed. It is essential that medicinal plant material is carefully characterized and hence it needs to be appreciated which botanical and chemical techniques can be utilized for this purpose.

The clinical utility of plant medicines in developed and developing countries is reviewed within this book, and it is evident that plants are involved in all of the major clinical areas.

CONTINUING CHANGES IN PHARMACEUTICAL EDUCATION

It cannot be denied that pharmacognosy has had a chequered history. Established in 1815, it became an important subject in UK pharmaceutical education from 1842 onwards (Shellard 1981, 1982a, b) and was an essential subject because many of the medical treatments of the day utilized plant-based medicines. The preparation of drugs into medicines was also an important component of the syllabus and in the UK this subject was known as pharmaceutics. Gradually, from the turn of the century, synthetic drugs were introduced into medicine and student courses placed more emphasis on pharmaceutical chemistry, in which physical, organic and inorganic chemistry were taught in relation to pharmaceutical drugs. In the early 1950s, when I was a pharmacy undergraduate, my degree course contained only ten lectures on pharmacology, although the basic sciences of zoology, histology and physiology helped to underpin the emerging pharmacology. At this time, pharmacy undergraduate curricula in the UK were filled to capacity with students facing heavy lecture loads and many hours of laboratory classes.

In the 1950s, medical treatments were undergoing considerable changes. A wave of new synthetic drugs produced new major prescription items, and it was not uncommon for the practising pharmacist to receive on the same prescription form a doctor's request for 500 barbiturate tablets (to put the patient to sleep) and 500 amphetamine tablets (to wake the patient up). With today's knowledge, this seems incredible. At this time, there was a steady decline in the use of herbal drug prescriptions containing tinctures and extracts. The more potent herbal drugs such as opium and digitalis continued to be used, not as tinctures, but as single isolated compounds: the alkaloids morphine and codeine, and the glycoside digoxin. It became far more appropriate to give patients pharmaceutical preparations, mainly in tablets and capsules, with reliable dose control, rather than plant extracts. Also at this time, the sulphonamides and antibiotics had revolutionized the treatment of infectious diseases by providing effective chemotherapy. In this climate of change, it was obvious that pharmaceutical educators asked questions about the future use of medicinal herbs. The active principles of many herbs were not known and it was assumed, by some, that they did not contain any active principles.

Pharmacy is an applied discipline and student courses have to reflect current practice. With a syllabus bursting at the seams, changes were needed and course material had to be re-evaluated. Academics had to face up to the real world. Was it really necessary to include information on herbal drugs that were no longer prescribed by the medical profession? Was botany required in the education of pharmacists, many of whom would spend their future in busy pharmacies dispensing mainly tablets and capsules containing single chemical entities? As course revision followed course revision during the 1960s to 1980s, the inevitable happened and pharmacognosy courses were cut. Some pharmacy degree courses in the UK and USA were developed without any pharmacognosy content. In some UK universities, particularly where pharmacognosy research was active, or where strong-minded academics held positions of power, the subject remained, albeit considerably reduced.

When academic courses go into revision, changes tend to occur in all subject areas. Pharmacology had become a powerful science, was obviously highly relevant in the education of pharmacists, and occupied more time in the curriculum. Pharmaceutical chemistry also came under close scrutiny. Organic chemistry was the bedrock of discovery of synthetic drugs, whereas the analytical techniques for quality assurance of pharmaceuticals relied on physical chemistry. The last 50 years have seen tremendous advances in analytical techniques, particularly in chromatography and spectroscopy. Again, pharmaceutical educators had to balance the time spent in teaching these subjects and their relevance to the practising pharmacist. Academics were asked whether a practising pharmacist would need to synthesize a drug, use a burette, or run an infrared, ultraviolet, nuclear magnetic resonance or mass spectrum.

Pharmaceutics, once majoring in dispensing techniques, was also under scrutiny. Was it really necessary to teach manipulative techniques for the preparation of liquid medicines, tablets, capsules, creams and ointments? Pharmacists would not necessarily have to prepare these in their dispensaries because increasingly they were becoming available from the pharmaceutical industry. As dispensing courses came under consideration, it became increasingly appreciated that, at the point of dispensing a prescription, the pharmacist was the last link between the patient and the doctor. The role of the pharmacist could be seen to be more advisory, and, gradually, the teaching emphasis began to change from product orientation towards patient orientation. Such changes are being made

to pharmacy undergraduate curricula today, when patient care is considered to be of prime importance.

The battles for the major ground of involvement within pharmacy undergraduate curricula continue. As medical and pharmaceutical sciences develop into newer areas such as molecular biology and genomics, then more science is needed within the course – or is it? Today, the contest is not just between the different sciences, but between the science and the practice of pharmacy. The former head of one UK school of pharmacy has publicly expressed his concern to the profession that science is being replaced by too much pharmacy practice within undergraduate courses in the UK (Florence 2002). It is, after all, a balance between competing subjects and, doubtless, as time goes on this balance will ebb and flow. What seems to be of such obvious importance to pharmacy today may well prove to be superseded within the space of a few years.

PHARMACOGNOSY

The evolution of pharmacognosy in the UK from 1842 to 1980 has been thoroughly reviewed in a series of articles (Shellard 1981, 1982a, b). The subject has either declined considerably or become obsolete in pharmacy undergraduate curricula in the UK and USA, but in Continental Europe the rate of change has not been as rapid and it remains a major subject area in many universities. Perhaps the rate of change should not have been so fast in the UK and the USA, and it is difficult to argue that professional courses, such as pharmacy, should not change to meet the current requirements of the profession.

Let us return briefly to the 1950s when it seemed obvious that herbal drugs were outmoded and that their use would decline, perhaps to such an extent that they would no longer be part of the medical armamentarium. In such a climate I chose to do research in pharmacognosy. Why should I go against common sense and the generous advice so freely given by my colleagues? It was because of my fascination with the chemistry of natural substances found in plants. My undergraduate course had opened up a vista of exotic chemicals, including alkaloids and glycosides, which were unlikely targets for commercially viable organic syntheses. In addition, there were many medicinal plants that had not been examined in any great detail for their chemical constituents. At that time, there was a dearth of techniques to aid isolation and structure determination of small quantities of natural products. Paper chromatography was in its infancy, thin-layer chromatography did not seem practicable, and high-performance liquid chromatography had not been invented. Isolation of single chemical entities was mainly achieved by crystallization from plant extracts. Assuming that gram quantities were available, it was then a matter of chemical degradation and identification of fragments of the original molecule in order to fit the pieces together and arrive at a probable chemical structure. Ultraviolet spectroscopy was available in the 1950s, but infrared, nuclear magnetic resonance and mass spectrometry were not. Who could have envisaged that so many chromatographic and spectroscopic techniques would become available within the space of a few decades so that separation of complex mixtures from plants would yield single compounds with relatively easy determination of their chemical structures? Assuming that a new compound had been isolated in the 1950s, it was not easy to assess its biological activity unless gram quantities were available for classical pharmacological investigation. In the 1950s, the time had not yet arrived for detailed investigation of the components and active principles of medicinal plants (Phillipson 1995).

If we fast-forward to the new millennium, it is now possible to work on small quantities of plant material, isolate and determine the chemical structures of single compounds isolated in submicrogram amounts, and test for a range of biological activities in vitro using, for example, radioligand–receptor binding assays, enzyme assays and microbiological tests (Phillipson 1995, 1999a, b, 2007, Verpoorte 2000). There is now a totally different scientific environment in comparison to the 1950s. Natural products are being increasingly recognized as potential sources of new drug leads (Phillipson 1999a, Verpoorte 2000) and some recent examples of biologically active natural product molecules have been highlighted (Kinghorn 2001). Scientific disciplines other than pharmacy now recognize the importance of plants as sources of medicines and have initiated active research programmes.

PUBLIC PERCEPTION OF MEDICINES

The 1950s heralded the age of medicines that acted on the central nervous system, allowing the development of stimulants, hypnotics, anxiolytics and antipsychotics. It became firmly established in the minds of the majority of the people in the developed world that there was a 'pill for every ill'. What is more, in the UK, with the National Health Service, these treatments were not only considered to be our due rights, but they were also free. As time progressed and millions of people received pharmaceutical drugs, it was realized that such therapies were not necessarily without risk. In fact, it became obvious that for all medicines there was invariably a benefit/risk profile. The barbiturates, for example, were replaced by newer drugs which were thought to be safer and without addictive properties. The benzodiazepines had arrived and eventually it was understood that these also could induce dependence in patients. The big bombshell was the withdrawal of thalidomide from clinical use in the early 1960s. This drug was considered to be safe and was used for the treatment of nausea in pregnancy until it was realized that it caused massive birth defects. Governments were forced to respond to public pressure and legislation was enacted worldwide for the stricter control of medicines. In the UK, the Committee on Safety of Drugs (now Commission on Human Medicines) was established, the Medicines Act was passed, and a competent authority for licensing medicines (the Medicines Control Agency, soon to merge with the Medical Devices Agency to become the Medicines and Healthcare Products Regulatory Agency) was set up. In the USA, the Food and Drug Administration was given additional powers.

Many people were alarmed and began to question the role of pharmaceuticals in their lives. It was apparent that there were two major disadvantages in the use of pharmaceuticals: namely, adverse reactions and failure to cure some diseases. Post thalidomide, it was anticipated that such a disaster would never occur again and it was believed that unsafe medicines would no longer be unleashed on the public. Subsequently, as new drugs came on to the market after stringent toxicity studies had been completed, it was discovered that serious adverse effects, some life-threatening, would appear only after a drug had been used in thousands of patients. Even if the adverse effects occurred only in a minority of patients, a drug might have to be withdrawn from use if the adverse effect caused serious health damage or death. Such events produced much public interest and the media was also able to exploit the situation to its advantage.

The general public understood that medicines might cause serious adverse reactions and also realized that many of the chronic diseases were not necessarily being cured As a result, many people began to distrust pharmaceutical medicines and irrationality abounded. Some concluded that all synthetic chemicals were harmful, particularly pharmaceuticals and pesticides, whilst in contrast all natural substances were considered safe. The fact that nature produces many potent toxins, such as strychnine and ricin, was either ignored or forgotten. Hence, an irrational fear of science developed, as well as a failure to appreciate that advances made by the pharmaceutical industry had helped to increase our lifespan and treat many of the diseases that were not alleviated in former generations.

The demand for medicines still exists and for many in the developed world attention has turned to complementary therapies. Millions in recent years have chosen to use herbal medicines and, hence, what was considered to be obsolete in the 1950s is now considered by many to be the saviour of the human race. The pendulum has swung back.

HERBAL MEDICINES

In the 1980s, the pharmacist on the high street in the UK, having seen herbal preparations nearly disappear completely from his shelves, found that health-food shops were opening new premises. This trend occurred during a period of economic depression when many high street shops were closing. Health-food shops sold not only foods and food supplements, but also medicinal herbs and a range of food products linked to health claims (nutraceuticals). Industry responded with packaged products of herbal material in tablet or capsule formulations for the treatment of minor ailments, including coughs, colds, indigestion and sleeping difficulties. The demand for herbal medicines has continued to grow and, in the USA, annual retail sales were estimated to be US$4 billion in 1998 (Barnes et al 2007).

Newspapers, magazines and television programmes continued to extol the virtues of medicinal herbs, often uncritically, and many 'coffee table' books and articles were written. In the UK, pharmacists asked the Royal Pharmaceutical Society of Great Britain to produce more factual information on medicinal herbs, particularly as to their constituents, pharmacology, clinical trials and safety. In response to this request, a book on herbal medicines was published (Newall et al 1996). A much enlarged and illustrated third edition is currently available (Barnes et al 2007). It is evident that several major areas of interest developed in the years between the publications of the first and subsequent editions.

CLINICAL TRIALS

Many of the medicinally used herbs have very little, if any, published clinical data. However, since 1996 there has been a significant increase in the publication of randomized clinical trials on herbs, such as echinacea, garlic, ginkgo and St John's wort. Although some of these clinical trials are flawed by methodological weaknesses, there can be no doubt that clinical interest in medicinal herbs is growing.

USE OF HERB EXTRACTS OR ISOLATED ACTIVE PRINCIPLES

The focus on the isolation of active principles from herbs in the past has led to the view that each individual herb must have an active principle(s). As active principles were isolated, they replaced the use of the herb or its extract for medicinal purposes. It is now increasingly realized that a single active constituent does not necessarily equate medically to the effect of an extract containing the equivalent dose of the active constituent (Williamson 2001).

HERB–DRUG INTERACTIONS

It has been suspected that medicinal herbs, if exerting a clinical effect, may also interact with concurrently used pharmaceutical medicines. One of the most significant series of herb–drug interactions observed in recent years has been that of St John's wort, currently popular for self-treatment of minor depression. Some of these interactions have been so severe as to cause the Committee on Safety of Medicines to issue warnings about the use of this herb with a series of prescription medicines, including the contraceptive pill, digoxin, HIV protease inhibitors, selective serotonin reuptake inhibitors, theophylline and warfarin (Barnes et al 2001).

SAFETY

Every herb used medicinally must be correctly authenticated, assessed for relative freedom from contamination and assayed (when possible) for active principles. Legislation in many countries has aimed to ensure that toxic herbs are regulated and controlled. In recent years, the importation of herbs into Europe from the Indian subcontinent and from the Far East has posed some problems with the safe use of medicinal herbs. This has been highlighted by the inadvertent inclusion of a toxic Aristolochia species in a herbal slimming remedy sold in Belgium. Renal damage has resulted in the need for dialysis and renal transplantation for some patients, and the development of renal carcinomas. What was originally thought to be a Belgian problem has subsequently proved to be a problem for other countries, including the UK. Legislation has been enacted in the UK and in other countries to prohibit the use of Aristolochia species in unlicensed medicines.

LEGISLATION

The quality, safety and efficacy of herbal medicine products (HMPs) have been of concern to many countries worldwide. In 2004, the European Union introduced a new Directive on Traditional Medicinal Products to control HMPs (Directive 2004/24/EC). This Directive comes into force at the end of April 2011, and any traditional herbal medicines not registered in member states will have to be withdrawn from the market. In the UK, the Medicines and Healthcare Products Regulatory Agency (MHRA) established the Herbal Medicines Advisory Committee (HMAC) to provide independent advice on the quality, safety and efficacy of HMPs to the Minister for Health. HMAC has brought together individuals from different disciplines (including clinicians, pharmacognosists, herbalists and toxicologists) who meet regularly with staff of the MRHA.

DEVELOPING COUNTRIES

Despite the strenuous efforts of organizations such as the World Health Organization (WHO) and the Earth Summits on sustainable development held in Rio and 10 years later in Johannesburg (2002), it is evident that the gap between the rich (so-called developed) and poor (so-called developing) countries is as wide as ever. Billions of the world's population live in abject poverty: in 1995 the then Director of WHO defined the world's most deadly disease as poverty (Phillipson 1995, 1999a, 2007). With

insufficient money to purchase medicines, it is not surprising that billions of poor people rely on their own systems of traditional medicine, despite the efforts of national governments and non-governmental organizations to provide access to cheap sources of essential drugs. The majority of traditional medicines are plant-based and there is still a great dearth of knowledge about many of these medicinally used plants. It is feared that deforestation will lead to the extinction of numerous plant species before their medicinal uses have been recorded or validated. Even among those plants that have known medicinal uses, many have not been investigated scientifically in any detail for their chemical constituents or biological effects.

Having spent a career investigating the chemistry of plants and the biological activities of their constituents, it is salutary to be faced with the 'benefit of hindsight'. To some extent, the investigating scientist is trapped in the laboratory with the techniques of the day. For me, the development of chromatographic techniques speeded the isolation of chemicals from plants, the advent of spectroscopic techniques enabled chemical structure determinations to be made, and subsequent development of sensitive biological tests in vitro facilitated the isolation of active compounds (Phillipson 1995, 1999a, b). There was an obvious progression in the research into medicinal plants as each new technique became available. Now, with the benefit of hindsight, it is possible to ask questions about this research. Was it really necessary to isolate all those compounds and determine their chemical structure, despite the fun involved? Should so much effort have been put into programmes of biological testing and fractionation of medicinal plant extracts? Why start investigations from the chemistry and biological action of medicinal plants instead of starting from their clinical use? In part, this last question can be answered because many clinicians were not interested in treating patients with plants when they could utilize the products of the pharmaceutical industry. Today, there has been a change in the attitude of some members of the medical profession who are sufficiently interested to pursue clinical investigations of plants used in traditional medicines. Such investigations, possibly from ethnomedical leads (Heinrich 2000, Heinrich and Gibbons 2001), also require collaboration with scientists authenticating plant material, ensuring batch-to-batch comparability, isolation of biologically active compounds and determination of their chemical structures. Quality assurance of medicinal herbs in developing countries will benefit from such investigations. Recognition of the molecular structures of active principles will enable development of medicines containing single active constituents and facilitate chemical syntheses and production of synthetic molecules of related structure with possible enhanced activity and safety profiles.

CONCLUSIONS

It is estimated that there are some 10–100 million species of organisms living on earth (Verpoorte 2000). Higher plants form a small group of some 250,000 species of which only 6% have been investigated for biological activities and 15% for their chemical constituents. To date, some 139,000 secondary metabolites have been isolated, the major groups being alkaloids (16,833) and terpenes (30,000). Thus, we have only scratched the surface of this wonderful resource of natural chemicals with its vast potential for the development of new drugs for medicinal use. This text, *Fundamentals of Pharmacognosy and Phytotherapy*, gives a fascinating insight into the medicinal use and potential of higher plants, and forms a basis for teaching programmes in the pharmacy undergraduate curriculum. Furthermore, the text shows that there is scope for further research, as ethnobotany, ethnopharmacology and ethnomedicine (sometimes grouped together as 'ethnopharmacy') provide leads for clinicians and scientists to collaborate in producing new medicines for all mankind, whether they are from developing or developed countries.

MAJOR AREAS FOR PHARMACOGNOSY AND PHYTOTHERAPY RESEARCH

Phytomedicines/traditional medicines
Quality assurance
Mode of action
Clinical trials
Safety, including herbal interactions
Herbal pharmacovigilance
Guides for healthcare professionals

New drug development
Ethnobotany
Ethnopharmacology

Ethnomedicine
Phytochemistry
Biological screening
Industrial and clinical collaboration

Biotechnology
Cell cultures for production of pharmaceuticals
Genetic engineering (e.g. production of proteins)

The pharmaceutical industry, always innovative, will continue to investigate promising leads from natural products in their efforts to produce new drug entities. Any putative new drug must meet very strict criteria in comparison with existing clinical drugs. Compounds that do not offer any significant advantages over existing therapy are discarded. The formation of new medicines in developing countries may have quite different priorities. If, for example, a plant is readily available and has the potential to provide inexpensive therapy for the treatment of disease, then a product may well be produced. It is within this particular area of endeavour that scientists, particularly academics, can collaborate with clinicians.

Pharmacognosy, once considered to be moribund, has the potential for a very bright future in this new millennium and it has been forecast that it will provide new lead compounds (Verpoorte 2000). There is already hard evidence to show that plants have relevance to medicine in the 21st century (Kinghorn 2001) and will continue to play an important role in modern medicine (Kinghorn 2002).

The evidence exists, but will it be sufficient to persuade governments and grant-awarding agencies to provide research funding for the investigation of plant-based medicines? Will pharmacognosy and phytotherapy continue to be integral components within the undergraduate and postgraduate curricula of pharmacy schools? One way to provide a resounding 'yes' to both of these questions is to persuade sufficient numbers of young able scientists to become involved in this area of collaborative multidisciplinary scientific endeavour (see Box). Research into natural products has provided many benefits for mankind and there is now a golden opportunity for it to continue making a worthwhile contribution to health care.

References

Barnes, J., Anderson, L.A., Phillipson, J.D., 2001. St John's wort (*Hypericum perforatum* L.): a review of its chemistry, pharmacology and clinical properties. J. Pharm. Pharmacol. 53, 583–600.

Barnes, J., Anderson, L.A., Phillipson, J.D., 2007. Herbal medicines. A guide for healthcare professionals, third ed. Pharmaceutical Press, London.

Florence, A.T., 2002. The profession of pharmacy leaves science behind at its peril. Pharmaceutical Journal 269, 58.

Heinrich, M. 2000. Ethnobotany and its role in drug development. Phytother. Res. 14, 479–488.

Heinrich, M., Gibbons, S., 2001. Ethnopharmacology in drug discovery: an analysis of its role and potential contribution. J. Pharm. Pharmacol. 53, 425–432.

Kinghorn, A.D., 2002. The role of pharmacognosy in modern medicine. Expert Opin. Pharmacother. 3, 77–79.

Kinghorn, A.D., 2001. Pharmacognosy in the 21st century. J. Pharm. Pharmacol. 53, 135–148.

Newall, C.A., Anderson, L.A., Phillipson, J.D., 1996. Herbal medicines. A guide for health-care professionals. Pharmaceutical Press, London.

Phillipson, J.D., 1999a. New drugs from nature – it could be yew. Phytother. Res. 13, 2–8.

Phillipson, J.D., 2007. Phytochemistry and pharmacognosy. Phytochemistry 68, 2960–2972.

Phillipson, J.D., 1999b. Radio-ligand receptor binding assays in the search for bioactive principles from plants. J. Pharm. Pharmacol. 51, 493–503.

Phillipson, J.D., 1995. A matter of some sensitivity. Phytochemistry 38, 1319–1343.

Shellard, E.J., 1981. A history of British pharmacognosy 1842–1980. Pharmaceutical Journal 226, 108, 189, 406.

Shellard, E.J., 1982a. A history of British pharmacognosy 1842–1980. Pharmaceutical Journal 227, 631, 774.

Shellard, E.J., 1982b. A history of British pharmacognosy 1842–1980. Pharmaceutical Journal 228, 78, 371, 536.

Verpoorte, R., 2000. Pharmacognosy in the new millennium: lead finding and biotechnology. J. Pharm. Pharmacol. 52, 253–262.

Williamson, E.M., 2001. Synergistic and other interactions in phytomedicines. Phytomedicine 8, 401–409.

Index

Note: Page numbers followed by *b* indicate boxes, *f* indicate figures and *t* indicate tables.